AF616234

90 0473770 5
TELEPEN

METHODS IN PHARMACOLOGY

Volume 6

Methods Used in Adenosine Research

General Editor: **Arnold Schwartz**
Baylor College of Medicine, Houston, Texas

Volume 1
Edited by **Arnold Schwartz**

Volume 2: PHYSICAL METHODS
Edited by **Colin F. Chignell**

Volume 3: SMOOTH MUSCLE
Edited by **Edwin E. Daniel** and **David M. Paton**

Volume 4A: RENAL PHARMACOLOGY
Edited by **Manuel Martinez-Maldonado**

Volume 4B: RENAL PHARMACOLOGY
Edited by **Manuel Martinez-Maldonado**

Volume 5: MYOCARDIAL BIOLOGY
Edited by **Arnold Schwartz**

Volume 6: METHODS USED IN ADENOSINE RESEARCH
Edited by **David M. Paton**

A Continuation Order Plan is available for this series. A continuation order will bring delivery of each new volume immediately upon publication. Volumes are billed only upon actual shipment. For further information please contact the publisher.

METHODS IN PHARMACOLOGY

Volume 6

Methods Used in Adenosine Research

Edited by

David M. Paton

University of Auckland
Auckland, New Zealand

PLENUM PRESS • NEW YORK AND LONDON

Library of Congress Cataloging in Publication Data

Main entry under title:

Methods used in adenosine research.

(Methods in pharmacology; v. 6)
Includes bibliographies and index.
1. Adenosine. 2. Adenosine—Research—Methodology. I. Paton, David M. (David Murray), 1938- . II. Series. [DNLM: 1. Adenosine. 2. Research—methods. W1 ME9616N v.6 / QU 58 M5928]
QP905.M45 vol. 6 615′.1s [615′.71] 84-26638
[QP625.A27]
ISBN 0-306-41872-X

A Division of Plenum Publishing Corporation
233 Spring Street, New York, N.Y. 10013

Printed in the United States of America

To my wife Beth, our children Heather
and Fiona, and my father Don

Contributors

RAM P. AGARWAL
Section of Medical Oncology
Evans Memorial Department of Clinical Research
Departments of Medicine and Pharmacology and Hubert H. Humphrey Cancer Research Center
Boston University Medical Center
Boston, Massachusetts

ROBERT M. BERNE
Department of Physiology
University of Virginia School of Medicine
Charlottesville, Viriginia

NOEL J. BUCKLEY
Department of Anatomy and Embryology
Center for Neuroscience
University College, London
London, England

GEOFFREY BURNSTOCK
Department of Anatomy and Embryology
Center for Neuroscience
University College, London
London, England

CAROL E. CASS
Cancer Research Group, McEachern Laboratory
University of Alberta
Edmonton, Alberta, Canada

PETER K. CHIANG
Division of Biochemistry
Walter Reed Army Institute of Research
Washington, D.C.

NOEL J. CUSACK
Department of Pharmacology
King's College London
London, England

ADRIAAN DEN HERTOG
Department of Pharmacology
State University
Groningen, The Netherlands

JEFFREY S. FEDAN
Physiology Section
National Institute for Occupational Safety and Health
Department of Pharmacology and Toxicology
West Virginia University Medical Center
Morgantown, West Virginia

BERTIL B. FREDHOLM
Department of Pharmacology
Karolinska Institute
Stockholm, Sweden

ERIC R. HARLEY
Cancer Research Group, McEachern Laboratory
University of Alberta
Edmonton, Alberta, Canada

J. FRANK HENDERSON
Cancer Research Group, McEachern Laboratory
and Department of Biochemistry
University of Alberta
Edmonton, Alberta, Canada

G. KURT HOGABOOM
Department of Pharmacology and Toxicology
West Virginia University Medical Center
Morgantown, West Virginia

LOWIE P. JAGER
Department of Pharmacology
Central Veterinary Institute
Lelystad, The Netherlands

SIMON M. JARVIS
Department of Physiology
University of Alberta
Edmonton, Alberta, Canada

TERRY P. KENAKIN
Department of Pharmacology
The Wellcome Research Laboratories
Burroughs Wellcome Company
Research Triangle Park, North Carolina

S. KUSACHI
Suncoast AHA Chapter Cardiovascular Research Laboratory
Department of Internal Medicine
University of South Florida College of Medicine
Tampa, Florida

H. J. LEIGHTON
Department of Pharmacology
The Wellcome Research Laboratories
Burroughs Wellcome Company
Research Triangle Park, North Carolina

JOHN P. O'DONNELL
School of Pharmacy
West Virginia University Medical Center
Morgantown, West Virginia

R. A. OLSSON
Suncoast AHA Chapter Cardiovascular Research Laboratory
Departments of Internal Medicine and Biochemistry
University of South Florida College of Medicine
Tampa, Florida

ROBERT E. PARKS, JR.
Section of Biochemical Pharmacology
Division of Biology and Medicine
Brown University
Providence, Rhode Island

ALAN R. P. PATERSON
Cancer Research Group, McEachern Laboratory
University of Alberta
Edmonton, Alberta, Canada

DAVID M. PATON
Department of Pharmacology and Clinical Pharmacology
University of Auckland
Auckland, New Zealand

J. D. PEARSON
Section of Vascular Biology
MRC Clinical Research Centre
Harrow, Middlesex, England

ULRICH SCHWABE
Pharmakologisches Institut
der Universität Heidelberg
Heidelberg, Federal Republic of Germany

JOHANNA D. STOECKLER
Section of Biochemical Pharmacology
Division of Biology and Medicine
Brown University
Providence, Rhode Island

T. W. STONE
Department of Physiology
St. George's Hospital Medical School
University of London
London, England

R. D. THOMPSON
Suncoast AHA Chapter Cardiovascular
Research Laboratory
Department of Internal Medicine
University of South Florida College of
Medicine
Tampa, Florida

DIANNE R. WEBSTER
Department of Pharmacology and Clinical
Pharmacology
University of Auckland
School of Medicine
Auckland, New Zealand

DAVID P. WESTFALL
Department of Pharmacology
University of Nevada School of Medicine
Reno, Nevada

THOMAS D. WHITE
Department of Pharmacology
Dalhousie University
Halifax, Nova Scotia, Canada

JAMES D. YOUNG
Department of Biochemistry
Faculty of Medicine
The Chinese University of Hong Kong
Shatin, N.T., Hong Kong

Preface

In their classic paper in 1929, Drury and Szent-Györgyi described a number of the important cardiovascular actions of adenosine. Another thirty years were to pass before the possible physiological role of adenosine in coronary vasodilation was studied by Berne and others. Since then, there has been a tremendous increase in research into the actions of adenosine. Workers from many disciplines have employed a wide variety of techniques, since adenosine is a product of and a substrate for a number of metabolic pathways, is transported into cells, and acts at discrete receptor sites to modulate the activity of adenylate cyclase and to produce important actions on many cells and tissues including platelets, adipocytes, heart, blood vessels, and other smooth muscles.

International symposia on the actions of adenosine were held in 1978, 1981, and 1982, and the proceedings of these symposia have been published (Baer and Drummond, 1979; Daly *et al.*, 1983; Berne *et al.*, 1983). Since it is not the primary purpose of the present volume to review our current understanding of the numerous actions of adenosine, these volumes should be consulted for such details. Rather, the present volume has been planned to provide both graduate students and investigators in pharmacology and related disciplines with a summary of some of the methods now available for the study of the actions of adenosine and, in particular, to highlight their possible uses and limitations.

The volume has been organized into sections dealing with related topics. It is hoped that this format will facilitate use of the volume and that it may introduce readers to techniques they have not used before or provide deeper insights into their use. Space has not allowed coverage to be given to all the methods or topics that might have been included, such as the effects of adenosine on platelet function and on immunological processes. Such omissions are certainly not intended to imply that these actions are unimportant.

As the editor, I am pleased to acknowledge the tremendous support I have received from the contributors to this volume. They come from eight nations and are among the foremost investigators in this research area. Without their expertise and cooperation, this volume would not have been possible. I personally have found the editing of the volume an educational and rewarding experience, and it is hoped that readers will similarly benefit from its use.

The editing of this volume would not have been possible without the careful and thorough assistance I have received from my secretary, Mrs. Brenda Carlson. Her help is gratefully acknowledged, as is that of my colleague, Dr. Dianne R. Webster, and of my other secretarial assistants in Auckland (Mrs. J. Simpson and Mrs. J. Williamson) and Cape Town (Miss F. Clarke).

David M. Paton

Auckland, New Zealand

REFERENCES

Baer, H. P., and Drummond, G. I. 1979. *Physiological and Regulatory Functions of Adenosine and Adenine Nucleotides*. Raven Press, New York.

Berne, R. M., Rall, T. W., and Rubio, R. 1983. *Regulatory Functions of Adenosine*. Martinus Nijhoff, The Hague.

Daly, J. W., Kuroda, Y., Phillis, J. W., Shimizu, H., and Ui, M. 1983. *Physiology and Pharmacology of Adenosine Derivatives*. Raven Press, New York.

Drury, A. N., and Szent-Györgyi, A. 1929. The physiological activity of adenine compounds with especial reference to their action upon the mammalian heart. *J. Physiol.* (*Lond*)., *68*:213–237.

Contents

I

Synthesis and Measurement of Adenosine and Adenine Nucleotide Analogs

Chapter 1

Synthesis of Adenosine and Adenine Nucleotide Analogs

Noel J. Cusack

Department of Pharmacology
King's College London
London, England

I. INTRODUCTION

Analogs of adenosine and adenine nucleotides have proved of considerable value in the elucidation of the pharmacology of naturally occurring purines. Alterations to the purine, ribose, and phosphate moieties have all provided analogs of pharmacological interest, and some of them are considerably more potent receptor agonists and have a more prolonged pharmacological action than the parent nucleosides and nucleotides. This chapter has been written to provide pharmacologists with a general outline of some manipulations peculiar to the chemistry of adenosine and adenine nucleotides and focuses on procedures that are relatively free from unnecessary complexity. The current availability of a large number of key nucleoside intermediates, chemical reagents, and dried purified solvents has eliminated much of the preliminary tedium formerly associated with their preparation. In the descriptions that follow, it is assumed that all solvents are dry and that all reactions are carried out at room temperature unless otherwise stated.

Survival of the molecule during chemical syntheses needs to be considered, and much of the enjoyment to be found in nucleic acid chemistry arises from juggling various protecting groups. The inherent stability of the purine ring means that alterations to substituents can be performed with impunity, and, indeed, it requires special tricks to open it at all. The ribose moiety is more fragile, and sometimes its hydroxyl groups require protection, usually by acetylation. The ribose–purine, and especially the 2′-deoxyribose–purine, linkages are susceptible to cleavage by inorganic acids, and hot acid also hydrolyzes adenosine 5′-triphosphate (ATP) and adenosine 5′-diphosphate (ADP) to adenosine 5′-monophosphate (AMP), and migration of phosphates about the ribose hydroxyls may occur.

The nomenclature of analogs of adenosine and adenine nucleotides is illustrated in Figure 1. For convenience, syntheses of analogs are divided into those that modify the purine base, the ribose sugar, and the phosphate esters.

II. METHODS OF SYNTHESES OF ANALOGS OF ADENOSINE AND ADENINE NUCLEOTIDES

A. Modified Purines

The most accessible and certainly the most secure points for the attachment of various substituents are at the 6, 2, and 8 positions of the purine ring. If leaving groups such as halogens can be generated at these positions, then nucleophilic displacement of halides by amines can place there a whole host of side chains. Of the halogens attached to purines, fluoro is the most reactive and iodo the least reactive, with chloro and bromo of intermediate reactivity. Alternatively, if thio groups can be placed at the 6, 2, or 8 positions, then the sulfur can be derivatized by reactions with alkyl- or aromatic halides.

1. 6-Substituted Purines

6-Chloro nucleosides are obtained by chlorination of 6-oxo nucleosides, such as inosine, with thionyl chloride and dimethylformamide (DMF) in boiling dichloromethane (Žemlicka and Šorm, 1965). Prior protection of the ribose hydroxyls by acetylation with acetic anhydride in pyridine or, in the case of 2′-deoxyribose, trifluoroacetylation with trifluroacetic anhydride is required in this instance, and their deprotection before subsequent reactions is effected without disturbing the 6-chloro group by keeping with ammonia in methanol for several hours (acetyl) or by chromatography on alumina in methanol (trifluoroacetyl) (Robins and Basom, 1973). Displacement of chloride so as to produce adenosine analogs occurs if the ammonia treatment is prolonged to several days, and N^6-substituted adenosine analogs, many of which are pharmacologically active, can be prepared by boiling a solution of the 6-chloro analog in ethanol with five equivalents of the desired amine (Kikugawa *et al.*, 1973a). The reaction can be followed by thin-layer chromatography (TLC) on silica gel developed for 5 cm with 10% methanol in chloroform. Displacement of chloride by hydroxylamine generates N^6-hydroxyadenosine (Giner-Sorolla *et al.*, 1966) and displacement by anhydrous hydrazine generates N^6-aminoadenosine (Johnson *et al.*, 1958). Displacement of chloride from 6-chloro nucleotides by amines may be carried out in aqueous solution buffered to pH 7 if required (Guilford *et al.*, 1972). N^6-substituted analogs can sometimes be prepared from adenosine and adenine nucleotides as starting materials by quarternization of the N^1-ring nitrogen with sufficently reactive alkyl halides

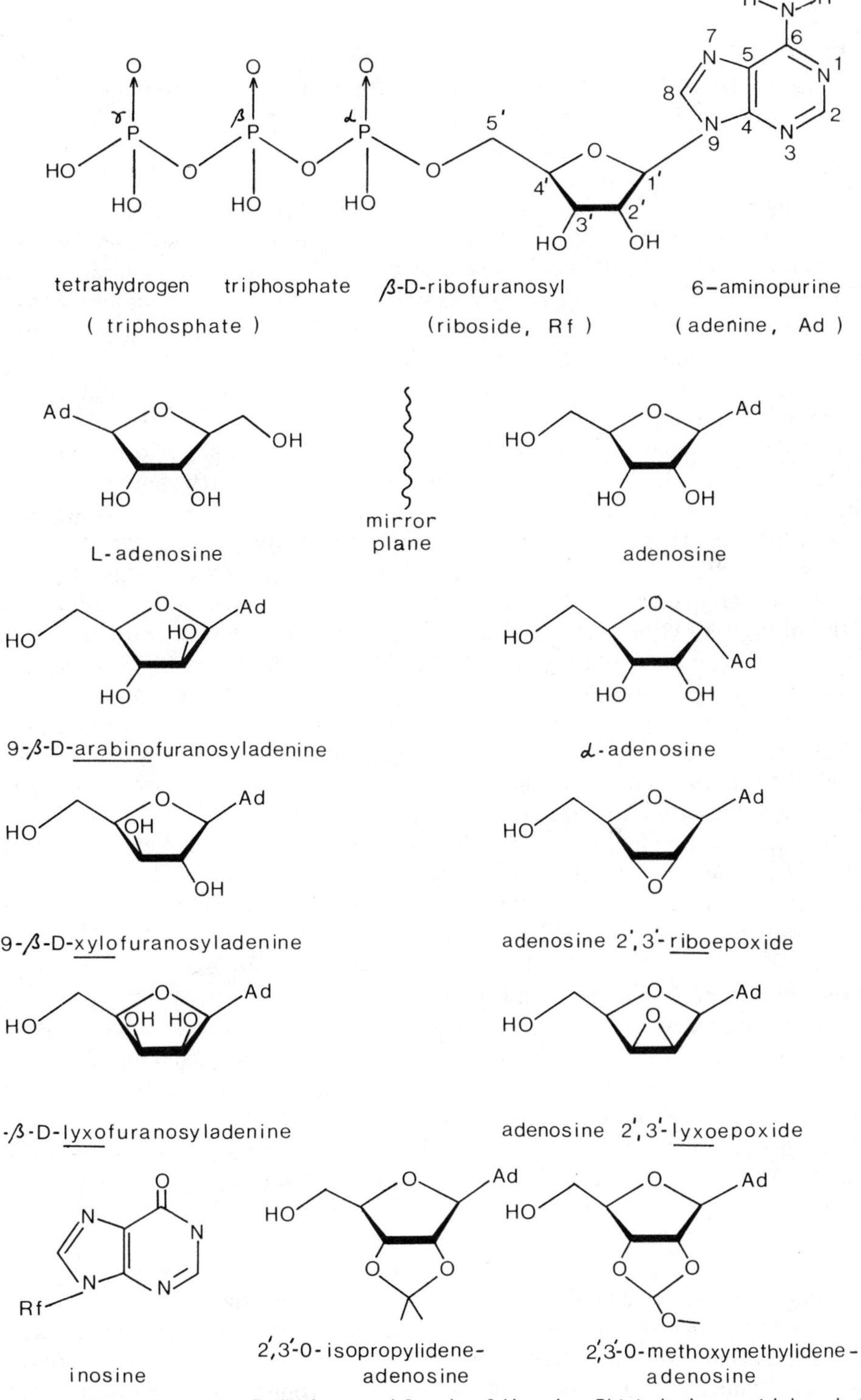

Figure 1. Structure of 9-β-D-ribofuranosyl-6-amino-9-H-purine 5′-tetrahydrogen triphosphate (adenosine 5′-triphosphate, ATP) and of some derivatives of adenosine.

and subsequent rearrangement of the intermediate at alkaline pH (Jones and Robins, 1963). This "Dimroth" rearrangement takes places by scission of the N^1–C^2 bond followed by rotation about the C^5–C^6 bond axis and ring closure (Engel, 1975) and has been used to provide ligands with spacer arms at the N^6 position for affinity chromatography (Lindberg *et al.,* 1973).

6-Chloro nucleosides are converted to 6-iodo derivatives by keeping in concentrated hydroiodic acid at −20°C, to 6-bromo derivatives via 6-thio by treating with thiourea in boiling ethanol followed by bromine in concentrated hydrobromic acid at −15°C (Gerster *et al.,* 1963), and to 6-fluoro derivatives by treatment with dry trimethylamine followed by displacement of the 6-trimethylammonium group with potassium fluoride in DMF at 50°C (Kirburis and Lister, 1971).

6-Chloro nucleosides can be converted to 6-seleno analogs by treatment with selenourea in boiling ethanol (Townsend and Milne, 1970), and 6-thio and 6-seleno nucleotides are obtained from 6-chloro nucleotides by bubbling hydrogen sulfide or hydrogen selenide through their aqueous solution at pH 8 (Broom *et al.,* 1976). Adenosine and adenine nucleotides can be converted directly to 6-thio or 6-seleno analogs by keeping in aqueous pyridine at 65°C with hydrogen sulfide (Meyer *et al.,* 1978) or hydrogen selenide (Shiue and Chu, 1975). S^6-substituted nucleosides and nucleotides are obtained by treating the 6-thio derivatives with a slight excess of the desired alkyl or arylalkyl halide in ammonia and dioxan or in DMF and potassium carbonate (Montgomery *et al.,* 1961). Displacement of chloride from 6-chloro nucleosides by the sodium salts of thiols is an alternative if less convenient procedure for the preparation of S^6-substituted analogs, and similarly the sodium salts of some alcohols give O^6-substituted analogs (Johnson *et al.,* 1958).

6-Methylthio nucleosides and nucleotides in ethanol at 0°C are oxidized by brief treatment with chlorine, and the resulting 6-methylsulfoxide group is very easily displaced by amines to generate S^6-substituted analogs (Wetzel and Eckstein, 1975). Certain S^6-substituted nucleosides, with the ribose hydroxyls protected by acetylation, can have their sulfur atoms plucked out by triphenylphosphine and lithium diisopropylamine in hexamethylphosphoramide (HMPT) at −70°C so as to generate a C^6–C linkage between the purine and the remainder of the side chain (Vorbrüggen and Krolikiewicz, 1976).

6-Oxo groups are best synthesized from adenine nucleosides and nucleotides by a large excess of nitrous acid generated by aqueous acetic acid and 2-methylbutyl nitrite (Holý, 1968). Finally, a 6-position denuded of substituents is obtained by catalytic hydrogenation of 6-chloro derivatives (Brown and Weliky, 1953) or by boiling 6-thio or S^6-substituted derivatives with finely divided ("Raney") nickel in aqueous solution (Fox *et al.,* 1958).

2. 2-Substituted Purines

Many 2-substituted analogs of adenosine and adenine nucleotides exert powerful pharmacological effects and can be derived from 2-chloroadenosine, itself an important adenosine receptor agonist. A key intermediate is 2,6-dichloropurine riboside obtained by diazotization of 2-amino-6-chloropurine riboside with sodium nitrite in concentrated hydrochloric acid at −5°C (Gerster and Robins, 1966). 2-

Chloroadenosine and 2-chloro-N^6-substituted adenosines are obtained by selective displacement of chloride from the much more reactive 6-position of the 2,6-dichloro derivative by ammonia (Schaeffer and Thomas, 1958) or amines (Gough and Maguire, 1967) in methanol for several days, and 2-bromoadenosine analogs are similarly obtained from 2,6-dibromopurine ribosides (Montgomery and Hewson, 1964). The intermediate 2,6-dichloropurine riboside can instead be assembled by melting together the components 2,6-dichloropurine and 2,3,5-tri-*O*-benzoyl-β-D-ribofuranosyl-1-*O*-acetate and heating *in vacuo* at 140°C for 45 min, followed by removal of the benzoyl groups by keeping with ammonia in methanol for several hours (Gough and Maguire, 1967), and the 2,6-dibromopurine riboside can be similarly obtained from 2,6-dibromopurine and a protected ribose derivative in the presence of an acid catalyst (Montgomery and Hewson, 1964). The β configuration of nucleosides arising from these "fusion" reactions is assured by the presence in the ribose component of the 2′-hydroxyl below the plane of the ribose moiety. If it is absent, as in 2′-deoxyribose, then a (separable) mixture of α and β anomers results, while if the 2′-hydroxyl is in the arabinose configuration, above the plane of the sugar, then the resulting nucleoside will have largely the α configuration (Sato *et al.*, 1961). If attempts at assembly by fusion fail, then the silyl method can be tried (Nishimura *et al.*, 1963), which in its simplest application consists of adding trimethylsilyl chloride to a mixture of a protected sugar component, a purine component, and hexamethyldisilazane in boiling acetonitrile (Vorbrüggen and Bennua, 1978), followed by deprotection of the ribose.

2-Thioadenosine can be prepared by heating a solution of 2-chloroadenosine and sodium hydrogen sulfide in DMF at 90°C for 1 day (Kikugawa *et al.*, 1973b), and 2-thio-AMP is obtained in the same way from 2-chloro-AMP (Stone *et al.*, 1976). A very convenient alternative synthesis of 2-thioadenosine consists of treating adenosine N^1-oxide with boiling 5 *M* sodium hydroxide for exactly 15 min to open the pyrimidine ring and heating the crude product with carbon disulfide in aqueous methanol at 120°C for 5 hr in a sealed tube (Kikugawa *et al.*, 1977b). A wide range of S-substituted analogs, some of which are vasodilators (Maguire *et al.*, 1971), are readily prepared by treatment of 2-thioadenosine with the appropriate alkyl- or aryl halides in water or aqueous ethanol containing 1 equivalent of sodium hydroxide (Kikugawa *et al.*, 1973b, 1977a). 2-Thioadenosine is oxidized by iodine solution to the diadenosine disulfide and more aggressively by hydrogen peroxide to the 2-sulfonate (Kikugawa *et al.*, 1973b).

Another procedure involving opening of the pyrimidine ring enables substituents to be joined to the 2 position by carbon–carbon bonds. In this procedure, adenosine N^1-oxide is first benzylated with benzyl bromide in dimethylacetamide for 2 days; the N^1-benzyloxy derivative is kept in water at pH 7 for 8 days and then heated with ammonia in methanol at 80°C for 2 days in a sealed tube; and the N^1-benzyloxy substituent is removed by hydrogenation with Raney nickel for up to 21 days (Montgomery and Thomas, 1972). The resulting 5-amino-4-carboxamidine derivative snaps shut on any alkyl- or aryl aldehydes offered to it and in the presence of oxygen reforms a purine ring bearing a 2-substituent (Meyer *et al.*, 1974).

3. 8-Substituted Purines

These analogs are less interesting than the 6- and 2-substituted analogs since substituents here generally lead to derivatives with greatly reduced pharmacological activity. Direct 8-chlorination of adenosine and adenine nucleotides is effected by tetrabutylammonium iodinetetrachloride in DMF for 1 day (Brentnall and Hutchinson, 1972), and direct 8-bromination is best carried out by addition of a slight excess of bromine to the nucleoside or nucleotide in acetate buffer at pH 4 (Ikehara *et al.*, 1967; Muneyama *et al.*, 1971). 8-Bromo nucleosides and nucleotides are most easily converted to the 8-thio analogs by keeping with sodium hydrogen sulfide in aqueous DMF for several hours (Ikehara *et al.*, 1973) and can be converted to 8-iodo derivatives by iodine in potassium iodide buffered with sodium hydrogen carbonate (Holmes and Robins, 1964). The 8-thio group can be removed with Raney nickel in boiling water for several hours. 8-Fluoroadenosine has only been obtained as an acetylated intermediate, by heating 8-bromo-2′,3′,5′-tri-*O*-acetyladenosine with potassium fluoride in [18]-crown-6-ether in acetonitrile at 120°C for 2 days in a sealed tube, since attempts at deprotection lead to concomitant loss of fluoride (Kobayashi *et al.*, 1976).

Displacement of bromide by amines to generate 8-alkylaminoadenosine is generally achieved by boiling a solution of 8-bromoadenosine in methanol or ethanol containing a large excess of the requisite amine for 16 hr (Long *et al.*, 1976) and 8-bromo-cyclic AMP behaves similarly (Muneyama *et al.*, 1971). Displacement of bromide from 8-bromo-AMP by 1,6-diaminohexane in aqueous solution, by heating in a sealed tube at 140°C for 2 hr, has been used to provide adenine nucleotide ligands having a spacer arm at the 8-position for use in affinity chromatography (Trayer *et al.*, 1974). 8-Hydrazinoadenosine is obtained by boiling 8-bromoadenosine with hydrazine for 2 days (Holmes and Robins, 1965). 8-Azido- adenosine and adenine nucleotides are of interest as photoaffinity analogs, and optimal preparation consists of heating a solution of the 8-bromo derivatives in DMF with a 100-fold excess of triethylammonium azide at 75°C for 10 hr (Holmes and Robins, 1965; Haley and Hoffman, 1974; Czarnecki *et al.*, 1979). 8-Azido derivatives can be rapidly and specifically reduced to 8-amino analogs by 4 equivalents of dithiothreitol in water at pH 8.7 (Cartwright *et al.*, 1976).

S-substituted 8-thio derivatives are prepared by boiling a solution of the 8-bromo analog in methanol containing 5 equivalents of sodium methoxide and a large excess of the desired thiol, while boiling sodium methoxide in methanol alone produces the 8-methoxy derivative (Holmes and Robins, 1965; Muneyama *et al.*, 1971). Conversion of 8-bromo to 8-oxo is achieved by boiling with acetic acid containing sodium acetate. Acetic anhydride is often included, in which case the resulting acetylated 8-oxo derivative is subsequently deprotected with ammonia in methanol (Ikehara *et al.*, 1965; Muneyama *et al.*, 1971).

B. Modified Riboses

Alterations to the ribose moiety will be confined to manipulations involving the three hydroxyl groups, which can be used as points of attachment of substitutents, converted to leaving groups by sulfonation with sulfonyl chloride, or replaced by halogens. The relative ease of displacement of halide from the sugar is the opposite of that of the purine ring, and so iodide is most easily lost while the fluoro group is relatively inert.

1. 5′-Substituted Riboses

Reactions at the 5′-hydroxyl are generally those expected of a primary alcohol and can often be conducted on unprotected adenosine analogs, but if masking the 2′ and 3′ hydroxyls is required, then groups specific for adjacent *cis*-diols are usually employed. The 2′,3′-*O*-isopropylidene group is traditional; it is introduced by stirring the adenosine analog with acetone, 2,2-dimethoxypropane, or both, with sufficient acid catalyst such as toluene-4-sulfonic acid (tosic acid) (Hampton, 1961), and is removed by hydrolysis with formic acid for several hours or with 0.01 M hydrochloric acid overnight. The 2′,3′-*O*-methoxymethylidene group is also common; it is introduced by boiling trimethyl orthoformate containing tosic acid and removed by treatment with 0.01 *M* hydrochloric acid for 2 hr followed by adjustment to pH 9 for 10 min (Griffin *et al.*, 1967).

5′-Chloro-5′-deoxy derivatives are most easily obtained by chlorination of adenosine with a solution of purified thionyl chloride in HMPT overnight, and 5′-bromo-5′-deoxy derivatives are obtained similarly with thionyl bromide (Kikugawa and Ichino, 1971), but 2′-deoxyadenosine is converted to 3′,5′-dideoxy-3′,5′-dihaloadenosine by this procedure (Hogenkamp, 1974). 5′-Deoxy-5′-iodo analogs are obtained by iodination of 2′,3′-*O*-isopropylidene nucleosides with methyltriphenoxyphosphonium iodide in dichloromethane, initially at −70°C (Dimitrijevich *et al.*, 1979). 5′-Alkylthio and 5′-arylthio 5′-deoxyadenosines are obtained from the 5′-chloro derivatives by heating with a solution of the desired thiol in 2 *M* sodium hydroxide for 1 hr (Kikugawa *et al.*, 1972), and delicate 5′-thiols may be synthesized in liquid ammonia containing the sodium salt of the desired thiol (Borchardt *et al.*, 1975). 5′-Deoxyadenosines are obtained by removal of the 5′-chloro group by catalytic hydrogenation (McCarthy *et al.*, 1968), by reduction with tributyltin hydride in tetrahydrofuran (Yang *et al.*, 1977), or by removal of 5′-alkylthio groups with Raney nickel (Robins *et al.*, 1966).

Treatment of 2′,3′-*O*-isopropylideneadenosine with toluene-4-sulfonyl chloride (tosyl chloride) transforms the 5′-hydroxyl to the 5′-*O*-tosyl group, which is readily displaced by nucleophiles as the toluene-4-sulfonate (tosate). Keeping 5′-*O*-tosyladenosine with a large excess of liquid ammonia or of neat amine for several days enables 5′-amino-5′-deoxyadenosine and a variety of its 5′-substituted amino analogs to be prepared (Schmidt *et al.*, 1968). However, displacement of tosate by azide and halides requires that the 6-amino group be first acylated to avoid intramolecular displacement of tosate by N^3 of the purine ring to form a cyclic nucleoside. Heating N^6-acetyl- or N^6-formyl-2′,3′-*O*-isopropylidene-5′-tosyladenosine with sodium iodide, lithium bromide, lithium chloride, or sodium azide provides 5′-deoxy-5′-haloadenosines and 5′-azido-5′-deoxyadenosine, respectively (Jahn, 1965), and selective reduction of the azido group by hydrogen sulfide in aqueous pyridine produces 5′-amino-5′-deoxyadenosine (Adachi *et al.*,

1977). 5′-Cyano-5′-deoxyadenosine can be obtained by displacement of tosate from 2′,3′-*O*-isopropylidene-5′-tosyladenosine with potassium cyanide and [18]-crown-6-ether in methanol, and oxidation of the cyano group by hydrogen peroxide provides a mixture of the 6′-carboxamide and 6′-carboxylic acid (Meyer *et al.*, 1976). 2′,3′-*O*-Isopropylideneadenosine is oxidized to the 5′-aldehyde by dicyclohexylcarbodiimide and dichloroacetic acid in dimethylsulfoxide (DMSO), and, although this aldehyde is extremely reactive, the crude reaction mixture can often be used for subsequent reactions of the aldehyde function (Pfitzner and Moffatt, 1963). Chemical procedures are available for obtaining the pure 5′-aldehyde, which has been used to provide several adenosine analogs with chains extended from the 5′-position (Ranganathan *et al.*, 1974; Hampton and Chawla, 1975). Oxidation of 2′,3′-*O*-isopropylideneadenosine by alkaline permanganate provides, after deprotection, adenosine 5′-carboxylic acid (Harmon *et al.*, 1969), and esterification of this acid by adding thionyl chloride to a suspension of adenosine 5′-carboxylic acid in the appropriate alcohol provides a series of esters, some of which are vasodilators (Prasad *et al.*, 1976). Neat thionyl chloride enables the intermediate 5′-carbonyl chloride to be isolated and addition of this to an excess of the desired amine at −50°C enables a variety of carboxamides to be prepared (Prasad *et al.*, 1980), including adenosine 5′-*N*-ethylcarboxamide (NECA) a potent vasodilator (Stein *et al.*, 1975) and adenosine receptor agonist (Cusack and Hourani, 1981a; Brown *et al.*, 1982; Londos *et al.*, 1980).

2. 2′- and 3′-Substituted Riboses

It is convenient to group alterations to 3′- and 2′-hydroxyls together as they are interrelated to some extent. Because the carbon atoms are chiral, nucleophilic *displacement* inverts the configuration at the 2′ position to arabinofuranosyl, at the 3′ position to xylofuranosyl, and at both the 2′ and 3′ positions to lyxofuranosyl derivatives of adenine (Figure 1). Simple *cleavage* from hydroxyls at these positions leads to retention of configuration of course.

2′- and 3′-*O*-tosyl groups are rather inactive, but inversion of configuration of 2′- or 3′-hydroxyl groups is readily achieved by sulfonation with methanesulfonyl chloride (mesyl chloride) in pyridine, or with trifluoromethanesulfonyl chloride (triflyl chloride) and sodium hydride in tetrahydrofuran at −60°C, displacement of the mesylate or triflate leaving group with sodium benzoate, and alkaline cleavage of the *O*-benzoyl group to reveal the new hydroxyl group. Displacement of triflate from 3′,5′-protected 2′-*O*-triflylarabinofuranosyladenine by the lithium salts of azide, chloride, bromide, or iodide, by tetrabutylammonium fluoride, and by sodium acetate or by potassium thioacetate generates the 2′-azido-2′-deoxy, 2′-deoxy-2′-halo, 2′-*O*-acetyl, and 2′-deoxy-2′-*S*-acetyl analogs of adenosine. Deacetylation of the 2′-thioacetyl group produces the 2′-deoxy-2′-thio analog, while reduction of the 2′-azido group provides 2′-amino-2′-deoxyadenosine after removal of the 3′,5′-protecting groups (Ranganathan, 1977). A similar series of reactions with a 3′,5′-protected 2′-*O*-triflyladenosine produces the corresponding 2′-arabinofuranosyladenines (Ranganathan and Larwood, 1978).

Reactions can be confined to the 2′-hydroxyl by protecting the 3′,5′-hydroxyl groups simultaneously with the 3′,5′-*O*-tetraisopropyldisiloxane-1,3-diyl (TIPS) group, introduced by treating adenosine with the TIPS-dichloride in DMF and imidazole, and cleaved in 10 min by tetrabutylammonium fluoride in tetrahydrofuran (Markiewicz, 1979). The 2′-hydroxyl can be removed altogether by derivatizing 3′,5′-*O*-TIPS-adenosine with phenylchlorothionocarbonate and reducing the product with tributyltin hydride in toluene (Robins and Wilson, 1981). Confining sulfonation to the 2′-hydroxyl can also be achieved by treating adenosine with dibutyltin oxide in DMF to form the 2′,3′-*O*-dibutyltin derivative, which very obligingly dissociates on addition of tosyl chloride and triethylamine to give 2′-*O*-tosyladenosine exculsively (Wagner *et al.*, 1974). After protection of 5′- and 3′-hydroxyl groups, usually with acid labile tetrahydropyranyl or methoxytetrahydropyranyl groups, the 2′-*O*-tosyl can be cleaved with sodium amalgam in aqueous methanol and replaced if desired by the more reactive mesyl or triflyl groups (Ranganathan and Larwood, 1978). However, intramolecular displacement of tosate by, for example, the 8-oxo function of 3′,5′-*O*-diacetyl-2′-*O*-tosyl-8-oxoadenosine generates, after subsequent deacetylation with ammonia in methanol, 8,2′-anhydroarabinosyladenine. This 8,2′-oxygen ring is opened by hydrogen sulfide in methanol to the 8-thio derivative of arabinofuranosyladenine, which can be desulfurized with Raney nickel to 9-β-D-arabinofuranosyladenine (Ara-A), and illustrates one of the many useful reactions of 8,2′-anhydronucleosides (Ikehara and Maruyama, 1975).

Confining the reactions to the 3′-hydroxyl is accomplished in a very pretty way by keeping 2′,3′-*O*-methoxyethylideneadenosine (prepared from trimethyl orthoacetate and adenosine as described in Section B.1 for the methoxymethylidene derivative) in dilute acid to open the 2′,3′-*O*-ketal ring, and allowing the resulting mixture of 2′-and 3′-*O*-acetates to equilibrate when the thermodynamically favored 3′-*O*-acetate crystallizes out. The 2′- and 5′-hydroxyls are then protected by acid-labile methoxytetrahydropyranyl groups, introduced by acid catalyzed addition of 4-methoxydihydropyran, and the 3′-hydroxyl is reexposed by deacetylation with ammonia in methanol (Green *et al.*, 1970).

Opening of 2′,3′-epoxides by nucleophiles occurs from the opposite (least hindered) side of the epoxide ring and with preferential attack at the 3′ position. If the 2′,3′-epoxide ring is below the plane of the sugar, as in ribose epoxides, then sodium azide in DMF opens this from above the ribose ring to generate largely the 3′-azido-3′-deoxy derivative with a xylose configuration (Robins *et al.*, 1974). Similarly, sodium iodide in acetonitrile containing boron trifluoride generates largely 3′-deoxy-3′-iodoxylofuranosyladenine (Mengel and Wiedner, 1976). An easy way to synthesize 2′,3′-ribose epoxides is to boil 2′,3′-*O*-methoxyethylideneadenosine with pivaloyl chloride in pyridine, then simultaneously cyclizing and deprotecting the intermediate by keeping with sodium methoxide in methanol (Robins *et al.*, 1976). Nucleophilic attack on 2′,3′-lyxo epoxides in a similar manner to that described for 2′,3′-ribo epoxides proceeds from below the sugar ring to generate largely the 3′-substituted arabinofuranosyl derivatives (Mengel and Wiedner, 1976).

2′- and 3′-amino-deoxyadenosines are prepared by catalytic hydrogenation of the corresponding azides. Reaction of the 3′-amino-3′-deoxyadenosine with aldehydes followed by reduction of the resulting Schiff bases with sodium borohydride enables a variety of substituents to be placed at the 3′ position (Morr and Ernst, 1979). Another way of placing substituents at the 3′ position makes use of the rather curious behavior of adenosine towards 2-acetoxyisobutyryl halides (Russel *et al.*, 1973). In particular 2-acetoxyisobutyryl iodide generates a 5′-protected-3′-deoxy-3′-iodo-2′-*O*-acetate in the xylose configuration, and the 3′-iodo can be displaced by lithium chloride in DMF with inversion of configuration to give after deprotection 3′-chloro-3′-deoxyadenosine (Jain *et al.*, 1974; Mengel and Wiedner, 1976). Removal of chloride if required to give 3′-deoxyadenosine is best accomplished in this environment with tributyltin hydride, as catalytic hydrogenation can be protracted (Robins *et al.*, 1976).

3. L-*Riboses*

L-Enantiomers of adenosine and adenine nucleotides, in which the naturally occurring β-D-ribofuranosyl moiety is replaced by β-L-ribofuranosyl, are best synthesized by assembly from a purine base and an L-sugar derivative obtained from the commercially available L-xylose or L-arabinose. Fusion of 2,6-dichloropurine with 2,3,5-tri-*O*-benzoyl-β-L-ribofuranosyl-1-*O*-acetate, readily available from L-xylose (Acton *et al.*, 1965), followed by removal of the benzoyl groups and displacement of the 6-chloro group with ammonia in methanol, furnishes the L-enantiomer of 2-chloroadenosine, from which other 2-substituted analogs of L-adenosine can be obtained (Cusack *et al.*, 1979; Cusack and Planker, 1979). L-Adenosine itself is more easily synthesized by stirring the sodium salt of adenine in DMF with 2-*O*-tosyl-5-*O*-trityl-L-arabinose, readily obtained from L-arabinose, and cleaving the 5′-trityl group with hot 80% acetic acid (Holý and Šorm, 1969). L-Adenosine can be utilized as a source of 2-thio-L-adenosine, via L-adenosine N^1-oxide, and provides a route to 2-methylthio-L-adenosine and other S-substituted L-adenosine analogs (Burnstock *et al.*, 1983). The L enantiomer of NECA, L-NECA, can also be synthesized from L-adenosine exactly as described for NECA (Cusack and Hourani, 1981a). These L enantiomers of adenosine and adenine nucleotide analogs have been used to test the stereoselectivity of purine receptors on platelets (Cusack *et al.*, 1979; Cusack and Hourani, 1981a) and smooth muscle (Cusack and Planker, 1979; Brown *et al.*, 1982; Burnstock *et al.*, 1983; Cusack and Hourani, 1984; Hourani, 1984).

C. Modified Phosphates

Most modifications will refer to the 5′-phosphate, -diphosphate, and -triphosphate since these are of most relevance to the pharmacology of adenine nucleotides and are also the easiest to synthesize.

1. *Substituted 5′-Monophosphates*

5′-Monophosphates are most easily synthesized by phosphorylation of unprotected adenosine analogs with phosphoryl chloride (Yoshikawa *et al.*, 1967).

Generally, the adenosine analog is dissolved in trimethyl orthophosphate by heating if necessary, then cooled to 0°C or below, and pure ("doping grade" is ideal) phosphoryl chloride added. The progress of the phosphorylation is monitored by TLC on silica gel developed in 30% methanol in chloroform by the increasing appearance of ultraviolet-absorbing material at the origin. The amount of phosphoryl chloride and length of time required can vary from 3 equivalents and 1 hr (2-methylthioadenosine) to 10 equivalents and 2 days (2-chloroadenosine). The reaction is terminated by pouring onto crushed ice and water and quickly neutralized by addition of triethylamine. 5′-Phosphorothioates can be obtained by using thiophosphoryl chloride in the above procedure (Murray and Atkinson, 1968), and 2-substituted 5′-phosphorothioates and 5′-monophosphates are of interest as specific inhibitors of the actions of ADP on platelets (Gough *et al.*, 1978; Cusack and Hourani, 1982a,b).

Some nucleosides do not survive the acidic conditions of the above phosphorylation procedure. However, nucleoside hydroxyl groups can be phosphorylated under very mild conditions by dianilinidophosphorochloridate in pyridine, and the aniline groups removed from the phosphate under neutral condtions by treatment with 3-methylbutyl nitrite in acetic acid and pyridine for 3 hr (Zielinski and Smrt, 1974). This method of phosphorylation is not specific for the 5′-hydroxyl and may be applied to any chosen hydroxyl provided the other hydroxyls are protected.

AMP can be converted to adenosine 5′-monofluorophosphate by 2,4-dinitro-1-fluorobenzene and tri-*n*-butylamine in DMF for 1 day (Wittman, 1963). An AMP analog having the 5′-oxygen replaced by a carbon atom (homo-AMP) is prepared by mixing 2′,3′-*O*-isopropylideneadenosine 5′-aldehyde (crude reaction mixture, see Section B.1) with the "Wittig" reagent diphenyl triphenylphosphoranylidenemethylphosphonate in DMSO, followed by reduction of the unsaturated linkage and deprotection, to give adenosine 5′-deoxy-5′-methylphosphonate (Jones and Moffat, 1968). The Wittig reagent is prepared from methyltriphenylphosphonium bromide by treatment with 1-butyl lithium in hexane followed by diphenyl phosphorochloridate (Jones *et al.*, 1968). AMP analogs having the 5′-oxygen replaced by sulfur are prepared by displacing bromide from 5′-bromo-5′-deoxyadenosine analogs with aqueous lithium thiophosphate (Morr, 1976). AMP analogs having the 5′-oxygen replaced by nitrogen are easily hydrolyzed, but may be obtained by enzymic cleavage of 5′-amido-5′-deoxy-ATP (Section C.2) (Wilkes *et al.*, 1973).

2. *Substituted 5′-Diphosphates and 5′-Triphosphates*

Analogs of ADP and ATP are usually made in two steps from AMP by first placing a leaving group on to the 5′-monophosphate and then, without isolation of this activated AMP intermediate, displacing the leaving group with the desired orthophosphate or pyrophosphate derivative. Activation of AMP is often best achieved by treatment of a solution of its triethylamine or tri-*n*-butylamine salt in HMPT with a five-fold excess of carbonyldiimidazole (Ott *et al.*, 1967). The reaction can be followed by TLC on cellulose developed by propan-2-ol:*M*

NH_4HCO_3 (7:3) for 6 cm, and on completion the excess carbonyldiimidazole is destroyed by addition of methanol. Addition of the adenosine 5′-phosphorimidazolate to a five-fold excess of the tri-*n*-butylammonium salt of orthophosphate, monofluorophosphate, pyrophosphate, imidodiphosphate, peroxydiphosphate, methylenediphosphonate, or difluoromethylenediphosphonate can provide ADP, adenosine 5′-[β-fluoro]diphosphate, ATP, adenosine 5′-[β,γ-imido]triphosphate, adenosine 5′-[β,γ-peroxy]triphosphate, adenosine 5′-[β,γ-methylene]triphosphate, or adenosine 5′-[β,γ-difluoromethylene]triphosphate, respectively (Ott *et al.*, 1967; Young *et al.*, 1971; Myers *et al.*, 1963; Haley and Yount, 1972; Rosendahl and Leonard, 1982; Blackburn *et al.*, 1981). Many of these AMP and ATP analogs and their 2-substituted congeners are pharmacologically active on platelets (Gough *et al.*, 1972; Cusack and Hourani, 1982a,b) and smooth muscle (Satchell and Maguire, 1975; Burnstock *et al.*, 1983; Cusack and Hourani, 1984; Hourani, 1984). This imidazolate procedure is readily adapted to the syntheses of ^{32}P-radiolabeled analogs, such as 2-methylthioadenosine 5′-[β-^{32}P]diphosphate, suitable for binding studies to some adenine nucleotide receptors (Macfarlane *et al.*, 1983).

Another method of activation, useful if the above procedure fails, is to treat a solution of the tri-*n*-octylammonium salt of AMP in dioxan with excess diphenyl phosphorochloridate followed after 3 hr by displacement of diphenyl phosphate by addition of the desired phosphates in pyridine (Michelson, 1964). All of the di- and triphosphates previously mentioned can be prepared by this method if preferred, and this anion exchange procedure, but not the above imidazolate procedure, can be extended to the synthesis of adenosine 5′-[α-thio]diphosphate and adenosine 5′-[α-thio]triphosphate by addition of phosphate or pyrophosphate to activated adenosine 5′-monophosphorothioate (AMPS) (Eckstein and Goody, 1976). The details set out by Eckstein and Goody (1976) should be adhered to exactly, as for example, changing the first solvent from dioxan to DMF produces ADP or ATP instead (N.J. Cusack, unpublished observations). The α-thio analogs are chiral and therefore exist as pairs of S_p and R_p diastereoisomers which can easily be separated, and have been used to test the stereoselectivity of ectonucleotidases (Cusack *et al.*, 1983), the platelet ADP receptor (Cusack and Hourani, 1981b; 1982b) and P_2-purinoceptors on smooth muscle (Burnstock *et al.*, 1984).

Thiophosphate fails to displace either imidazole or diphenyl phosphate from activated AMP, but displacement by thiophosphate derivatized at sulfur by the base-labile *S*-carbamoylethyl group enables adenosine 5′-[β-thio]diphosphate (ADP-β-*S*) to be synthesized (Goody and Eckstein, 1971). Although adenosine 5′-[β-thio]triphosphate can be obtained as a mixture of S_p and R_p diastereoisomers by addition of ADP-β-*S* to diphenyl phosphorochloridate-activated 2-cyanoethyl phosphate, the yield is low and the isomers cannot be separated. In view of this, it is much more convenient to prepare the S_p and R_p isomers separately by enzymic phosphorylation of ADP-β-*S* by acetate kinase and pyruvate kinase respectively (Eckstein and Goody, 1976; Jaffe and Cohn, 1978). The γ-substituted ATP analog adenosine 5′-[γ-thio]triphosphate is synthesized by addition of ADP to an excess of *S*-carbamoylethyl thiophosphate that has been activated by diphenyl phosphorochloridate followed by removal of the sulfur protecting group (Goody and

Eckstein, 1971). Similarly, adenosine 5′-[γ-fluoro]triphosphate is synthesized by addition of ADP to excess activated monofluorophosphate (Haley and Yount, 1972). The alternative approach, activation of ADP followed by addition of the phosphate analog, is not satisfactory.

Keeping 5′-amino-5′-deoxyadenosine with aqueous sodium metatriphosphate for 2 days provides a 5′-amido analog of ATP, in which the 5′-oxygen is replaced by nitrogen, and enzymic dephosphorylation of this can be used to generate the corresponding 5′-amido analog of ADP (Wilkes *et al.*, 1973). γ-Phenylamido derivatives of ATP are obtained by treating an aqueous solution of ATP at pH 5.6 with a water-soluble carbodiimide, followed by addition of a large excess of the desired aromatic amine (Babkina *et al.*, 1975). Adenosine 5′-[α,β-methylene]diphosphates are synthesized from 2′,3′-*O*-isopropylideneadenosines and methylenediphosphonic acid by keeping with dicyclohexylcarbodiimide in pyridine and tri-*n*-butylamine at 60°C (Myers *et al.*, 1965; Gough *et al.*, 1972).

It should be mentioned that high-performance liquid chromatography can be of great value in studies with analogs of adenosine nucleotides, since even minor alterations on the molecule often have large effects on the retention times. For example, isocratic elution from reverse phase columns enables the R_p and S_p diastereoisomers of the α-thio analogs of ADP and ATP to be easily separated (Cusack and Hourani, 1981b, 1982b), and the retention times of 2-chloro-ATP and 2-methylthio-ATP are nearly three- and sixfold, respectively, that of ATP.

REFERENCES

Acton, E. M., Ryan, K. J., and Goodman, L. 1964. Synthesis of L-ribofuranose and L-adenosine. *J. Am. Chem. Soc., 86:*5352–5354.

Adachi, T., Yamada, Y., Inoue, I., and Saneyoshi, H. 1977. An alternative method of selective reduction of unsaturated nucleoside azides to amines. *Synthesis, 9:*45–46.

Babkina, G. T., Zarytova, V. F., and Knorre, D. G. 1975. Preparation of γ-amides of nucleoside 5′-triphosphates in aqueous solution with water soluble carbodiimide. *Bioorg. Khim. (USSR), 1:*611–615.

Blackburn, G. M., Kent, D. E., and Kolkmann, F. 1981. Three new β,γ-methylene analogues of adenosine triphosphate. *J. Chem. Soc. Chem. Commun., 1981:*1188–1190.

Borchardt, R. T., Huber, J. A., and Wu, Y. S., 1975. A convenient preparation of S-adenosylhomocysteine and related compounds. *J. Org. Chem., 41:*565–567.

Brentnall, H. J., and Hutchinson, D. W. 1972. Preparation of 8-chloroadenosine and its phosphate esters. *Tetrahedron Lett., 1972:*2595–2596.

Broom, A. D., Uchic, M. E., and Uchic, J. T. 1976. Combined enzymatic and chemical approaches to the synthesis of unique polyribonucleotides. *Biochim. Biophys. Acta, 425:*278–286.

Brown, C., Burnstock, G., Cusack, N. J., Meghji, P., and Moody, C. J. 1982. Evidence for stereospecificity of the P_1-purinoceptor. *Br. J. Pharmacol., 75:*101–107.

Brown, G. B., and Weliky, V. S. 1953. The synthesis of 9-β-D-ribofuranosyl-purine and the identity of nebularine. *J. Biol. Chem., 204:*1019–1024.

Burnstock, G., Cusack, N. J., Hills, J. M., MacKenzie, I., and Meghji, P. 1983. Studies on the stereoselectivity of the P_2-purinoceptor. *Br. J. Pharmacol., 79:*907–913.

Burnstock, G., Cusack, N. J., and Meldrum, L. A. 1984. Effects of phosphorothioate analogues of ATP, ADP and AMP on guinea-pig taenia coli and urinary bladder. *Br. J. Pharmacol. 82:*369–374.

Cartwright, I. L., Hutchinson, D. W., and Armstrong, V. W. 1976. The reaction between thiols and 8-azidoadenosine derivatives. *Nucleic Acid Res., 3:*2331–2339.

Cusack, N. J., and Hourani, S. M. O. 1981a. 5′-N-Ethylcarboxamidoadenosine: A potent inhibitor of human platelet aggregation. *Br. J. Pharmacol., 72:*443–447.
Cusack, N. J., and Hourani, S. M. O. 1981b. Effects of R_p and S_p diastereoisomers of adenosine 5′-O-(1-thiodiphosphate) on human platelets. *Br. J. Pharmacol., 73:*409–412.
Cusack, N. J., and Hourani, S. M. O. 1982a. Specific but noncompetitive inhibition by 2-alkylthio analogues of adenosine 5′-monophosphate and adenosine 5′-triphosphate of human platelet aggregation induced by adenosine 5′-diphosphate. *Br. J. Pharmacol., 75:*397–400.
Cusack, N. J., and Hourani, S. M. O. 1982b. Adenosine 5′-diphosphate antagonists and human platelets: No evidence that aggregation and inhibition of stimulated adenylate cyclase are mediated by different receptors. *Br. J. Pharmacol., 76:*221–227.
Cusack, N. J., and Hourani, S. M. O. 1984. Some pharmacological and biochemical interactions of the enantiomers of adenylyl 5′-(β,γ-methylene)-diphosphonate with the guinea-pig urinary bladder. *Br. J. Pharmacol. 82:*155–159.
Cusack, N. J., and Planker, M. 1979. Relaxation of isolated taenia coli of guinea pig by enantiomers of 2-azido analogues of adenosine and adenine nucleotides. *Br. J. Pharmacol., 67:*153–158.
Cusack, N. J., Hickman, M. E., and Born, G. V. R. 1979. Effects of D-and L-enantiomers of adenosine, AMP and ADP and their 2-chloro- and 2-azido-analogues on human platelets. *Proc. Royal Soc. Lond. B, 206:*139–144.
Cusack, N. J., Pearson, J. D., and Gordon, J. L. 1983. Stereoselectivity of ectonucleotidases on vascular endothelial cells. *Biochem. J., 214:*975–981.
Czarnecki, J., Geahlen, R., and Haley, B., 1979, Synthesis and use of azido photoaffinity analogues of adenine and guanine nucleotides. *Methods Enzymol., 56:*642–653.
Dimitrijevich, S. D., Verheyden, J. P. H., and Moffatt, J. G. 1979. Halo sugar nucleosides. 6. Synthesis of some 5′-deoxy-5′-iodo and 4′,5′-unsaturated purine nucleosides. *J. Org. Chem., 44:*400–406.
Eckstein, F., and Goody, R. S., 1976. Synthesis and properties of diastereoisomers of adenosine 5′-(O-1-thiotriphosphate) and adenosine 5′-(O-2-thiotriphosphate). *Biochemistry, 15:*1685–1691.
Engel, J. D. 1975. Mechanism of the Dimroth rearrangement in adenosine. *Biochem. Biophys. Res. Commun., 64:*581–586.
Fox, J. J., Wempen, I., Hampton, A., and Doerr, I. L. 1958. Thiation of nucleosides. I. Synthesis of 2-amino-6-mercapto-9-β-D-ribofuranosylpurine ("Thioguanosine") and related purine nucleosides. *J. Am. Chem. Soc., 80:*1669–1675.
Gerster, J. F., and Robins, R. K. 1966. The synthesis of 2-fluoro- and 2-chloroinosine and certain derived purine nucleosides. *J. Org. Chem., 31:*3258–3262.
Gerster, J. F., Jones, J. W., and Robins, R. K. 1963. Purine nucleosides. IV. The synthesis of 6-halogenated 9-β-D-ribofuranosylpurines from inosine and guanosine. *J. Org. Chem., 28:*945–948.
Giner-Sorolla, A., Medrek, L., and Bendick, A. 1966. Synthesis and biological activity of 9-β-D-ribofuranosyl-6-hydroxylaminopurine. *J. Med. Chem., 9:*143–144.
Goody, R. S., and Eckstein, F. 1971. Thiophosphate analogs of nucleoside di- and triphosphates. *J. Am. Chem. Soc., 93:*6252–6257.
Gough, G., and Maguire, M. H. 1967. Some biologically active N^6-methylated adenosine analogues. *J. Med. Chem., 10:*475–478.
Gough, G., Maguire, M. H., and Penglis, F. 1972. Analogs of adenosine 5′-diphosphate—new platelet aggregators. *Molec. Pharmacol., 8:*170–177.
Gough, G. R., Nobbs, D. M., Middleton, J. C., Penglis-Caredes, F., and Maguire, M. H. 1978. New inhibitors of platelet aggregation. 5′-Phosphate, 5′-phosphorothioate, and 5′-O-sulfamyl derivatives of 2-substituted adenosine analogs. *J. Med. Chem., 21:*520–525.
Green, D. P. L., Ravindranathan, T., Reese, C. B., and Saffhill, R. 1970. The synthesis of oligoribonucleotides. VIII. The preparation of ribonucleoside 2′,5′-bisketals. *Tetrahedron, 26:*1031–1041.
Griffin, B. E., Jarman, M., Reese, C. B., and Sulston, J. E. 1967. The synthesis of oligoribonucleotides. II. Methoxymethylidene derivatives of ribonucleosides and 5′-ribonucleotides. *Tetrahedron, 23:*2301–2313.
Guilford, H., Larsson, P.-O., and Mosbach, K. 1972. On adenine nucleotides for affinity chromatography. *Chemica Scripta, 2:*165–170.

Haley, B. E., and Hoffman, J. F., 1974. Interactions of a photoaffinity ATP analog with cation-stimulated adenosine triphosphatases of human red cell membranes. *Proc. Natl. Acad. Sci. USA, 71:*3367–3371.

Haley, B., and Yount, R. G. 1972. γ-Fluoroadenosine triphosphate. Synthesis, properties, and interaction with myosin and heavy meromyosin. *Biochemistry, 11:*2863–2871.

Hampton, A. 1961. Nucleotides. II. A new procedure for the conversion of ribonucleosides to 2′,3′-O-isopropylidene derivatives. *J. Am. Chem. Soc., 83:*3140–3145.

Hampton, A., and Chawla, R. R. 1975. Syntheses of the epimeric 5′-C-carboxy derivatives of 2′,3′-O-isopropylidene adenosine. *J. Carbohydr. Nucleos. Nucleot., 2:*281–298.

Harmon, R. E., Zenerosa, C. V., and Gupta, S. K. 1969. Permanganate oxidation of purine nucleosides. *Chem. Ind. (Lond.), 1969:*1141.

Hogenkamp, H. P. 1974. Chemical synthesis and properties of analogs of adenosylcobalamin. *Biochemistry, 13:*2736–2740.

Holmes, R. E., and Robins, R. K. 1964. Purine nucleosides. VII. Direct bromination of adenosine, deoxyadenosine, guanosine, and related purine nucleosides. *J. Am. Chem. Soc., 86:*1242–1245.

Holmes, R. E., and Robins, R. K. 1965. Purine nucleosides. IX. The synthesis of 9-β-D-ribofuranosyl uric acid and other 8-substituted purine ribonucleosides. *J. Am. Chem. Soc., 87:*1772–1776.

Holý, A. 1968. Oligonucleotidic compounds. XXIV. Synthesis of 2′,3′-phosphates of inosine, xanthosine, 6-mercapto-9-(β-D-ribofuranosyl)purine, and 2-amino-6-mercapto-9-(β-D-ribofuranosyl)purine. *Collect. Czech. Chem. Commun., 33:*2259–2270.

Holý, A., and Šorm, F. 1969. Oligonucleotidic compounds. XXXIV. Preparation of some β-L-ribonucleosides, their 2′(3′)-phosphates and 2′,3′-cyclic phosphates. *Collect. Czech. Chem. Commun., 34:*3383–3401.

Hourani, S. M. O. 1984. Desensitization of the guinea-pig urinary bladder by the enantiomers of adenylyl 5′-(β,γ-methylene)diphosphonate and by substance P. *Br. J. Pharmacol., 82:*161–164.

Ikehara, M., and Maruyama, T. 1975. Studies of nucleosides and nucleotides. LXV. Purine cyclonucleosides. 26. A versatile method for the synthesis of purine O-cyclo-nucleosides. The first synthesis of 8,2-anhydro-8-oxy-9-β-D-arabinofuranosylguanosine. *Tetrahedron, 31:*1369–1372.

Ikehara, M., Tada, H., and Muneyama, K. 1965. Nucleosides and nucleotides. XXV. Purine cyclonucleosides. 2. Synthesis of 5′-deoxyguanosine via a 5′,8-cyclonucleoside. *Chem. Pharm. Bull. Tokyo, 13:*639–642.

Ikehara, M., Uesugi, S., and Kaneko, M. 1967. Bromination of adenine nucleoside and nucleotide. *J. Chem. Soc. Chem. Commun., 1962:*17–18.

Ikehara, M., Ohtsuka, E., and Uesugi, S. 1973. Nucleosides and nucleotides. LVI. Versatile method for the synthesis of 8-mercaptoadenosine nucleotides. *Chem. Pharm. Bull. Tokyo, 21:*444–445.

Jaffe, E. K., and Cohn, M. 1978. Divalent cation-dependent stereospecificity of adenosine 5′-O-(2-thiotriphosphate) in the hexokinase and pyruvate kinase reactions. The absolute stereochemistry of the diastereoisomers of adenosine 5′-O-(2-thiotriphosphate). *J. Biol. Chem., 253:*4823–4825.

Jahn, W. 1965. Synthese 5′-substituierter adenosinderivate. *Chem. Ber., 98:*1705–1708.

Jain, T. C., Jenkins, I. O., Russel, A. F., Verheyden, J. P. H., and Moffatt, J. G. 1974. Reactions of 2-acyloxyisobutyryl halides with nucleosides. IV. A facile synthesis of 2′,3′-unsaturated nucleosides using chromous acetate. *J. Org. Chem., 39:*30–38.

Johnson, Jr., J. A., Thomas, H. J., and Schaeffer, H. J. 1958. Synthesis of potential anticancer agents. XII. Ribosides of 6-substituted purines. *J. Am. Chem. Soc., 80:*699–702.

Jones, G. H., and Moffatt, J. G. 1968. The synthesis of 6′-deoxyhomonucleoside-6′-phosphonic acids. *J. Am. Chem. Soc., 90:*5337–5338.

Jones, J. W., and Robins, R. W. 1963. Purine nucleosides. III. Methylation studies of certain naturally occurring purine nucleosides. *J. Am. Chem. Soc., 85:*193–201.

Jones, G. H., Hamamura, E. K., and Moffatt, J. G. 1968. A new stable Wittig reagent suitable for the synthesis of α,β-unsaturated phosphonates. *Tetrahedron Lett., 1968:*5731–5734.

Kiburis, J., and Lister, J. H. 1971. Nucleophilic displacement of the trimethylammonio-group as a new route to fluoropurines. *J. Chem. Soc., 1971:*3942–3947.

Kikukawa, K., and Ichino, M. 1971. Direct halogenation of the sugar moiety of nucleosides. *Tetrahedron Lett., 1971:*87–90.

Kikugawa, K., Iizuka, K., Higuchi, Y., Hirayama, H., and Ichino, M. 1972. Platelet aggregation inhibitors. 2. Inhibition of platelet aggregation by 5′-, 2-, 6-, and 8-substituted adenosines. *J. Med. Chem., 15*:387–390.

Kikugawa, K., Iizuka, K., and Ichino, M. 1973a. Platelet aggregation inhibitors. 4. N^6-Substituted adenosines. *J. Med. Chem., 16*:358–364.

Kikugawa, K., Suehiro, H., and Ichino, M. 1973b. Platelet aggregation inhibitors. 6. 2-Thioadenosine derivatives. *J. Med. Chem., 16*:1381–1388.

Kikugawa, K., Suehiro, H., and Aoki, A. 1977a. Platelet aggregation inhibitors. X. S-Substituted 2-thioadenosines and their derivatives. *Chem. Pharm. Bull. Tokyo, 25*:2624–2637.

Kikugawa, K., Suehiro, H., Yanase, R., and Aoki, A. 1977b. Platelet aggregation inhibitors. IX. Chemical transformation of adenosine into 2-thioadenosine derivatives. *Chem. Pharm. Bull. Tokyo, 25*:1959–1969.

Kobayashi, Y., Kumadaki, I., Ohsawa, A., and Murakami, S. 1976. Synthesis of 2′,3′,5′-tris-O-acetyl-8-fluoroadenosine. *J. Chem. Soc. Chem. Commun., 1967*:430–431.

Lindberg, M., Larsson, P.-O., and Mosbach, K. 1973. A new immobilized NAD^+ analogue, its applications in affinity chromatography and as a functioning coenzyme. *Eur. J. Biochem., 40*:187–193.

Londos, C., Cooper, D. M. F., and Wolff, J. 1980. Subclasses of adenosine receptors. *Proc. Natl. Acad. Sci. USA, 77*:2551–2554.

Long, R. A., Robins, R. K., and Townsend, L. B. 1967. Purine nucleosides. XV. The synthesis of 8-amino- and 8-substituted aminopurine nucleosides. *J. Org. Chem., 32*:2751–2756.

Macfarlane, D. E., Srivastava, P., and Mills, D. C. B. 1983. 2-Methylthioadenosine [β-^{32}P]diphosphate. An agonist and radioligand for the receptor that inhibits the accumulation of cyclic AMP in intact blood platelets. *J. Clin. Invest., 71*:420–428.

Maguire, M. H., Nobbs, D. M., Einstein, R., and Middleton, J. C. 1971. 2-Alkylthioadenosines, specific coronary vasodilators. *J. Med. Chem., 14*:415–420.

Markiewicz, W. T. 1979. Tetraisopropyldisiloxane-1,3-diyl, a group for simultaneous protection of 3′- and 5′-hydroxy functions of nucleosides. *J. Chem. Res. (S), 1979*:24–25.

McCarthy, J. R., Robins, R. K., and Robins, M. J. 1968. Purine nucleosides. XXII. The synthesis of angustmycin A (Decoyinine) and related unsaturated nucleosides. *J. Am. Chem. Soc., 90*:4993–4999.

Mengel, R., and Wiedner, H. 1976. Nucleosidtransformationen. 1. Umwandlung von adenosin in 2′- und 3′-azido-, -amino- sowie -chloro-substituierte deoxyadenosine. *Chem. Ber., 109*:433–443.

Meyer, R. B., Shuman, D. A., and Robins, R. K. 1974. A new purine ring closure and the synthesis of 2-substituted derivatives of adenosine cyclic 3′,5′-phosphate. *J. Am. Chem. Soc. 96*:4962–4966.

Meyer, R. B., Stone, T. E., and Heinzel, F. P. 1978. Direct sulfhydrolysis of cyclic AMP: One-step synthesis of the cyclic ribonucleotide of 6-mercaptopurine. *J. Heterocycl. Chem., 15*:1511–1512.

Meyer, W., Böhnke, E., and Follman, H. 1976. Facile preparation of 5′-cyano- and 5-carboxynucleosides. *Angew. Chem. Int. Ed. Engl., 15*:499–500.

Michelson, A. M. 1964. Synthesis of nucleotide anhydrides by anion exchange. *Biochim. Biophys. Acta, 91*:1–13.

Montgomery, J. A., and Hewson, K. 1964. The synthesis of 2-bromoadenosine. *J. Heterocycl. Chem., 1*:213–214.

Montgomery, J. A., and Thomas, H. J. 1972. Nucleosides of 2-azapurines and certain ring analogues. *J. Med. Chem., 15*:182–187.

Montgomery, J. A., Johnston, T. P., Gallagher, A., Stringfellow, Jr., C. R., and Schabel, Jr., F. M. 1961. Comparative studies of the anticancer activity of some S-substituted derivatives of 6-mercaptopurine and their ribonucleosides. *J. Med. Pharm. Chem., 3*:265–288.

Morr, M., 1976, Synthese des 5′-thio-3′-amido-5′,3′-didesoxyadenosine-3′-5′-cyclophosphats, ein cAMP-derivat mit S und N im cyclophosphatring. *Tetrahedron Lett., 1976*:2127–2128.

Morr, M., and Ernst, L. 1979. Aminonucleosidin, VIII. 3′-Amino-3′-desoxyadenosine, 3′,5′-diamino-3′,5′-didesoxyadenosine und N-substituierte derivate. *Chem. Ber., 112*:2815–2828.

Muneyama, K., Bauer, R. J., Shuman, D. A., Robins, R. K., and Simon, L. N. 1971. Chemical synthesis and biological activity of 8-substituted adenosine 3′,5′-cyclic monophosphate derivatives. *Biochemistry, 10*:2390–2395.

Murray, A. M., and Atkinson, M. R. 1968. Adenosine 5′-phosphorothioate. A nucleotide analog that is a substrate, competitive inhibitor, or regulator of some enzymes that interact with adenosine 5′-phosphate. *Biochemistry, 7*:4023–4029.

Myers, T. C., Nakamura, K., and Flesher, J. W. 1963. Phosphonic acid analogs of nucleoside phosphates. I. The synthesis of 5′-adenylyl methylenediphosphonate, a phosphonic acid analog of ATP. *J. Am. Chem. Soc., 85*:3292–3295.

Myers, T. C., Nakamura, K., and Danielzadeh, A. B. 1965. Phosphonic acid analogs of nucleoside phosphates. III. The synthesis of adenosine-5′-methylenediphosphonate, a phosphonic acid analog of adenosine 5′-diphosphate. *J. Org. Chem., 30*:1517–1520.

Nishimura, T., Shimizu, B., and Iwai, I. 1963. A new synthetic method for nucleosides. *Chem. Pharm. Bull. Tokyo, 11*:1470–1477.

Ott, D. G., Kerr, V. N., Hansbury, E., and Hayes, F. N. 1967. Chemical synthesis of nucleoside triphosphates. *Anal. Biochem., 21*:469–472.

Pfitzner, K. E., and Moffatt, J. G. 1963. The synthesis of nucleoside-5′ aldehydes. *J. Am. Chem. Soc., 85*:3027.

Prasad, R. N., Fung, A., Tietje, K., Stein, H. H., and Brondyk, H. B. 1976. Modification of the 5′-position of purine nucleosides. 1. Synthesis and biological properties of alkyl adenosine 5′-carboxylates. *J. Med. Chem., 19*:1180–1186.

Prasad, R. N., Bariana, D. S., Fung, A., Savie, M., Tietje, K., Stein, H. H., Brondyk, H., and Egan, R. S. 1980. Modification of the 5′-position of purine nucleosides. 2. Synthesis and some cardiovascular properties of adenosine-5′-(N-substituted)carboxamides. *J. Med. Chem., 23*:313–319.

Ranganathan, R. 1977. Modification of the 2′-position of purine nucleosides: Syntheses of 2′-α-substituted-2′-deoxyadenosine analogs. *Tetrahedron Lett., 1977*:1291–1294.

Ranganathan, R., and Larwood, D. 1978. Facile conversion of adenosine into new 2′-substituted-2′-deoxy-arabinofuranosyladenine derivatives: Stereospecific syntheses of 2′-azido-2′-deoxy-, 2′-amino-2′-deoxy-, and 2′-mercapto-2′-deoxy-β-D-arabinofuranosyladenines. *Tetrahedron Lett., 1978*:4341–4344.

Ranganathan, R. S., Jones, G. H., and Moffatt, J. G. 1974. Novel analogues of nucleoside 3′,5′-cyclic phosphates. I. 5′-Mono- and dimethyl analogs of adenosine 3′,5′-cyclic phosphate. *J. Org. Chem., 39*:290–298.

Robins, M. J., and Basom, G. L. 1973. Nucleic acid related compounds. 8. Direct conversion of 2′-deoxyinosine to 6-chloropurine 2′-deoxyriboside and selected 6-substituted deoxynucleosides and their evaluation as substrates of adenosine deaminase. *Can. J. Chem., 51*:3161–3169.

Robins, M. J., and Wilson, J. S. 1981. Smooth and efficient deoxygenation of secondary alcohols. A general procedure for the conversion of ribonucleosides to 2′-deoxynucleosides. *J. Am. Chem. Soc. 103*:932–933.

Robins, M. J., McCarthy, J. R., and Robins, R. K. 1966. Purine nucleosides. XII. The preparation of 2′,3′-dideoxyadenosine, 2′,5′-dideoxyadenosine, and 2′,3′,5′-trideoxyadenosine from 2′-deoxyadenosine. *Biochemistry, 5*:224–231.

Robins, M. J., Fouron, Y., and Mengel, R. 1974. Nucleic acid related compounds. 11. Adenosine 2′,3′-*ribo*-epoxide. Synthesis, intramolecular degradation, and transformation into 3′-substituted xylofuranosyl nucleosides and the *lyxo*-epoxides. *J. Org. Chem., 39*:1564–1570.

Robins, M. J., Mengel, R., Jones, R. A., and Fouron, Y. 1976. Nucleic acid related compounds. 22. Transformation of ribonucleoside 2′,3′-O-ortho esters into halo, deoxy, and epoxy sugar nucleosides using acyl halides. Mechanism and structure of products. *J. Am. Chem. Soc., 98*:8204–8213.

Rosendahl, M. S., and Leonard, N. J. 1982. β-γ-Peroxy analogs of adenosine and guanosine triphosphate: Synthesis and biological activity. *Science, 215*:81–82.

Russel, A. F., Greenberg, S., and Moffatt, J. G. 1973. Reactions of 2-acyloxyisobutyryl halides with nucleosides. II. Reactions of adenosine. *J. Am. Chem. Soc., 95*:4025–4030.

Satchell, D. G., and Maguire, M. H. 1975. Inhibitory effects of adenine nucleotide analogs on the isolated guinea-pig taenia coli. *J. Pharmacol. Exp. Ther., 195*:540–548.

Sato, T., Shimadate, T., and Ishido, Y. 1961. Nucleosides and nucleotides. VII. A new method for syntheses of purine ribonucleosides. 1. *Nippon Kagaku Zasshi, 81*:1440–1442.

Schaeffer, H. J., and Thomas, H. J. 1958. Synthesis of potential anticancer agents. XIV. Ribosides of 2,6-disubstituted purines. *J. Am. Chem. Soc., 80*:3788–3742.

Schmidt, R. R., Schloz, U., and Schwille, D. 1968. Synthese 5′-modifizierter Adenosinderivate. *Chem. Ber., 101:*590–594.

Shiue, C.-Y., and Chu, S.-H. 1975. A novel synthesis of 6-seleno-substituted nucleosides, nucleotides and cyclic nucleotides. *J. Chem. Soc. Chem. Commun., 1975:*319–320.

Stein, H. H., Somani, P., and Prasad, R. N. 1975. Cardiovascular effects of nucleoside analogs. *Ann. N. Y. Acad. Sci., 255:*380–389.

Stone, J. V., Singh, R. K., Horák, H., and Barton, P. G. 1976. Sulfhydryl analogues of adenosine diphosphate: Chemical synthesis and activity as platelet-aggregating agents. *Can. J. Biochem., 54:*529–533.

Townsend, L. B., and Milne, G. H. 1970. Synthesis of the selenium congener of the naturally occurring nucleoside guanosine, 6-selenoguanosine. *J. Heterocycl. Chem., 7:*753–754.

Trayer, I. P., Trayer, H. R., Small, D. A. P., and Bottomley, R. C. 1974. Preparation of adenosine nucleotide derivatives suitable for affinity chromatography. *Biochem. J., 139:*609–623.

Vorbrüggen, H., and Bennua, B. 1978. New simplified nucleoside synthesis. *Tetrahedron Lett., 1978:*1339–1342.

Vorbrüggen, H., and Krolikiewicz, K. 1976. C-Substitution of nucleosides with the aid of the Eschenmoser sulphide contraction. *Angew. Chem. Int. Ed. Engl., 15:*689–690.

Wagner, D., Verheyden, J. P. H., and Moffatt, J. G. 1974. Preparation and synthetic utility of some organotin derivatives of nucleosides. *J. Org. Chem., 39:*24–30.

Wetzel, R., and Eckstein, F. 1975. Synthesis and reactions of 6-methylsulfonyl-9-β-D-ribofuranosylpurine. *J. Org. Chem., 40:*658–660.

Wilkes, J. S., Hapke, B., and Letsinger, R. L. 1973. A 5′-amino analog of adenosine diphosphate. *Biochem. Biophys. Res. Commun., 53:*917–922.

Wittman, R. 1963. Die reaktion der phosphosaüren mit 2,4-dinitro-fluobenzol, 1. Eine neue synthese von monofluorophosphorsaüremonoestern. *Chem. Ber., 96:*771–779.

Yang, Y., Hogenkamp, H. P. C., Long, R. A., Revenkar, G. R., and Robins, R. K. 1977. A convenient synthesis of 5′-deoxyribonucleosides. *Carbohydrate Res., 59:*449–457.

Yoshikawa, M., Kata, T., and Takenishi, T. 1967. A novel method for phosphorylation of nucleosides to 5′-nucleotides. *Tetrahedron Lett., 1967:*5065–5068.

Yount, R. G., Babcock, D., Ballantyne, W., and Ojala, D. 1971. Adenylyl imidodiphosphate, an adenosine triphosphate analog containing a PNP linkage. *Biochemistry, 10:*2484–2489.

Zielinski, W. S., and Smrt, J. 1974. Phosphorodianilidates in the synthesis of the deoxyribooligonucleotidic chain. *Collect. Czech. Chem. Commun., 39:*2483–2490.

Žemlicka, J., and Šorm, F. 1965. Nucleic acids components and their analogs. LX. The reaction of chloromethylenedimethylammonium chloride with 2′,3′,5′-tri-O-acetylinosine. A new synthesis of 6-chloro-(9-β-D-ribofuranosyl)purine. *Collect. Czech. Chem. Commun., 30:*1880–1889.

Chapter **2**

The Measurement of Adenosine and Adenine Nucleotides in Tissues and Body Fluids

Dianne R. Webster

Department of Pharmacology and Clinical Pharmacology
University of Auckland School of Medicine
Auckland, New Zealand

I. INTRODUCTION

The measurement of adenosine and adenosine-related compounds is of interest to workers in many different fields. As the purpose of research varies so do the compounds of interest, the sensitivity required of the assay, and the number of possible pitfalls in the difficult task of producing a measurement in an assay that accurately reflects the *in vivo* state. Among the questions to be asked before an assay method is chosen are: what equipment is available? What metabolites are of interest? Are these metabolites different levels of endogenous compounds or do they represent the fate of exogenous compounds? If one is concerned with the fate of exogenous compounds, what concentration is to be used and will direct chemical measurements be suitable or will radiolabel be necessary?

The measurement process may be divided arbitrarily into three parts:

1. Sample collection.
2. Sample preparation for measurement.
3. Measurement by either one of the following:
   a. Specific chemical techniques, e.g., radioimmunoassay, protein binding, or enzymic methods.
   b. General physical properties, e.g., UV absorbance, or radioactivity after a more sophisticated separation process (usually a form of chromatography).

As with all analyses in biological material, the investigator must bear in mind two questions: is the adenosine in the sample a proper reflection of the adenosine *in vivo*? Is all the material measured adenosine and is all the adenosine measured?

II. SAMPLE COLLECTION

As adenosine nucleotides are subject to rapid dephosphorylation and adenosine to either phosphorylation or deamination, care in sample collection is required to obtain samples that are as representative as possible of the *in vivo* concentrations of the adenine-containing compounds.

If recovery experiments are to be done as part of the validation procedure of the assay, the purines of interest should be added as soon as possible after sample collection, preferably before enzyme deactivation procedures are carried out.

A. Tissues

There is general agreement that tissue samples must be frozen as quickly as possible and not be thawed until deproteinized. Liquid nitrogen is the usual cooling agent used for snap-freezing or cooling sampling tongs.

Brain tissue is particularly difficult to sample quickly. It has been reported that lower adenosine levels are obtained in the rat by freezing through the skull rather than through the exposed dura (Nordstrom *et al.*, 1977). A comparison of two freezing methods indicated that an *in situ* technique prevents perturbations in adenosine metabolism caused by hypoxia in the small time delay before the tissue freezes (Winn *et al.*, 1981). The adenosine content of rat brain has been found to be low and uniform in the different regions if the animals are killed and the tissues fixed by microwave radiation (Wojcik and Neff 1982).

B. Blood

Whole blood may be treated as a tissue and snap-frozen, or the whole blood collected directly into acid. If this is done, trichloracetic acid is better than percholoric acid (Jaworek *et al.*, 1974). Plasma levels of adenosine are preferable to serum levels as adenosine is released during the clotting process (Capogrossi *et al.*, 1982), and the anticoagulated sample should be centrifuged immediately after collection as adenosine and other purines are released into the plasma on standing (Tattersall *et al.*, 1983). It has been suggested that 5–10 μM erythro-9-(2-hydroxy-3-nonyl)-adenine (EHNA; Tattersall *et al.*, 1983) or 1 μM deoxycoformycin (dCF; Capogrossi *et al.*, 1982) be added to the blood collection tubes to prevent adenosine deamination in the blood samples. The addition of 2 μM dipyridamole would also inhibit adenosine uptake into blood cells such as human platelets (Dresse *et al.*, 1982). However, the effect of dipyridamole varies with the species and cell type studied. Not only is care needed to preserve the adenosine content of the tissues but also to ensure that the correct sample is being extracted. For example, platelet contamination of peripheral blood mononuclear cell preparations can occur (Goday *et al.,* 1983).

C. Cell Cultures and Incubation Media

It has been shown that washing of cultured cells before extraction leads to a loss of adenine-containing compounds. Fifty percent of cell nucleotides were lost when cultured aortic endothelial cell suspensions were prepared with trypsin-EDTA, even though there was no evidence of cell damage as measured by vital dye exclusion (Pearson and Gordon, 1979). Medium is rapidly removed by pouring off or centrifugation with cooling to 4°C and deproteinization of the monolayer (Pearson and Gordon, 1979; Harmenberg *et al.,* 1983) or pellet (Reinhart and Koroly, 1982). Dilution of the extract by medium remaining around the cells may be corrected for by dilution of [^{14}C]inulin (Plagemann and Wohlheuter, 1981) or [^{14}C]glucose (Brenton *et al.,* 1977). Incubation medium from isolated tissue studies may be collected into tubes containing the deproteinizing agent (Willemot and Paton, 1981a).

D. Urine

Urine for measurement of purines including adenine compounds should be collected with a preservative to prevent bacterial metabolism of the compounds of interest. A suitable preservative is a 50:50 mixture of toluene and light paraffin (Simmonds, 1969). Collection of samples into acid preservative (e.g., HCl) will result in degradation of deoxyadenosine to adenine in patients receiving dCF, for example, or in adenosine deaminase-deficient patients.

III. SAMPLE PREPARATION

Preparation of samples for analysis involves producing an extract suitable for the analysis in which the purines are stable. This involves halting both enzymatic and chemical degradation.

A. Tissue Disintegration

Where this is necessary, it is best done while the tissue is frozen, under liquid nitrogen, or in a mortar and pestle precooled to liquid nitrogen temperature. Cell lysis is achieved by the same agent used as the protein precipitant.

B. Protein Precipitation

The most commonly used agent for deproteinization is perchloric acid (PCA) neutralized by a potassium salt. The range of final perchloric acid concentrations is 0.04–1.0 *M*, but generally about 0.5 *M* neutralized by the stochiometric amount of KOH, $KHCO_3$, K_2CO_3, or KH_2PO_4 or mixtures of two or more of these salts.

Table I. Summary of Some of the Extraction Methods Used for Deproteinization of Tissues before Quantitation of Adenine-Containing Compounds

Tissue	Method	References
Adipose tissue	PCA	Fredholm and Sollevi (1981)
Adrenal gland	PCA	Burke (1982)
Blood, serum, plasma	PCA	Fredholm and Sollevi (1981); Smith and Henderson (1982)
	TCA	Simmonds and Harkness (1981); Simmonds *et al.* (1982)
	Ultrafiltration	Pfadenhauer and Tong (1979); Capogrossi *et al.* (1982)
	EtOH	Holmsen *et al.* (1983)
	$Ba(OH)_2$–$ZnSO_4$	Hutton *et al.* (1981)
	Uranyl acetate	Gardiner (1979)
Bone marrow	Ultrafiltration	Tattersall *et al.* (1983)
Brain	PCA	Gharib *et al.* (1982); Reddington and Pusch (1983)
	EtOH–PCA	Shmukler (1972); Winn *et al.* (1981)
	Microwave–H_2O	Wu and Phillis (1978)
	Microwave–$ZnSO_4$–$Ba(OH)_2$	Wojcik and Neff (1982)
Cell suspensions and cultures	PCA	Brenton *et al.* (1977); Hunting *et al.* (1981); Olsson *et al.* (1982); Reinhart and Koroly (1982)
	TCA	Simmonds *et al.* (1982); Earle and Glazer (1983)
	MeOH–EtOH	Kefford and Fox (1982)
	Boiling EDTA	Plagemann and Wohlheuter (1983)
Heart	PCA	Harmsen *et al.* (1981, 1982)
Kidney	PCA	Fredholm and Hedqvist (1978)
Muscle	PCA	Klabunde (1983)
Nerve	Hot acid	Israel *et al.* (1980)
Perfusate, medium	PCA	Willemot and Paton (1981a)
Skin	PCA	Pruneau *et al.* (1982)
Tissues	PCA–TCA	Wagner *et al.* (1982)
Vas deferens	PCA	Willemot and Paton (1981a,b)

The acid may also be neutralized by an amine and extracted into an organic solvent such as Freon as in the method of Khym (1975).

Trichloracetic acid (TCA) is also used at final concentrations around 0.5 *M*. It is generally removed from the sample by extraction into water-saturated diethylether or amine–Freon mixtures.

Extraction of purines by heat, alcohols, salts, ultrafiltration, and distilled water following microwave fixation of rat brain (Wu and Phillis, 1978) has been described. A summary of some of the published methods is given in Table I.

It is often not stated that precipitants are best added to tissues or plasma with vigorous mixing to prevent the formation of lumps of tissue with protein-denatured exterior and unextracted interior. When acids are used to extract tissues, it is important that the neutralization be carried out as quickly as possible after the acid is added to prevent acid hydrolysis of the nucleotides. This will be minimized if the procedure is done in the cold where possible. Deoxyadenosine is hydrolyzed to adenine in the presence of any acid, making other methods of extraction more suitable if adenine or deoxyadenosine is to be quantitated.

C. Further Purification

When the samples under investigation include many other UV-absorbing compounds other than purines (e.g., urines) or when the purines of interest are a minor component of the total purines (e.g., nucleosides and bases in cellular material), it may be necessary to clean up and concentrate the material. This procedure may sometimes be combined with protein removal.

1. Separation of Nucleotides from Nucleosides and Bases

A number of different adsorption techniques have been used to prepare cleaner nucleoside and base extracts or nucleotide extracts. Nucleotides and other strong anions (e.g., urate) may be selectively adsorbed onto ion exchange resin, e.g., Dowex AG1-X2 (Kuttesch *et al.*, 1978; Klabunde, 1983), Aminex A6 (Olsson *et al.*, 1982), or Zerolit 225 (Harkness *et al.*, 1983). Other workers have used alumina (Harmsen *et al.*, 1981) or charcoal (Watkinson *et al.*, 1979). DEAE-cellulose has been used to absorb nucleotides for subsequent fractionation into nucleotide classes (Reinhart and Koroly, 1982).

Small plastic columns filled with packings similar to thosed used in high-performance liquid chromatography (HPLC) columns (Sep-Pak®, Waters Associates) have been used to separate nucleosides (Harmenberg *et al.*, 1983) and *S*-adenosylmethionine and *S*-adenosylhomocysteine (Gharib *et al.*, 1982). These studies utilized the C-18 Sep-Pak. Silica Sep-Paks have been used for nucleotide separations (Lothrop and Uziel, 1980).

An elegant method for the separation of adenosine and other ribose sugars (molecules that include a planar *cis*-diol in their configuration) by affinity chromatography was described by Gerhke and colleagues (1978). It has been used by a number of other groups to facilitate measurement of adenosine in low concentrations (Pfadenhauer and Tong, 1979; Fredholm and Sollevi, 1981). A commercial form of the gel is available (Biorad Affi-Gel 601).

D. Concentration

All the commonly used methods of concentrating aqueous solutions have been applied to extracts containing purines. Rotary evaporation both with (Hirschhorn *et al.*, 1981) and without (Simmonds, 1969) N_2 protection has been used. Freeze-drying of column extracts is another way to concentrate the purine for measurement and has been widely used (Earle and Glazer, 1983; Harkness *et al.*, 1983). The protein-free extract after ultrafiltration was concentrated by blowing with an air stream (Capogrossi *et al.*, 1982). The ideal solvent for reconstitution of the dried extract, if the sample is to be analyzed by HPLC and if it is suitable with regard to such things as pH (for sample stability), is the initial mobile phase of the chromatography.

IV. SPECIFIC METHODS OF MEASUREMENT

A. Enzymatic Methods

The enzymatic methods for measuring adenosine-based compounds depend on the conversion of one compound to another with different UV or visible absorbance or fluorescence characteristics. The classic source for enzymic methods is *Methods of Enzymatic Analysis* (Bergmeyer, 1974). Some of the relevant references are listed in Table II.

Some samples are suitable for direct enzymic determinations of adenosine-based compounds; some need to be deproteinated, whereas some require further purification or concentration (Bockman *et al.*, 1976). Hypoxanthine, inosine, and adenosine can be analyzed in the same sample by sequential addition of enzymes (Olsson, 1970).

Fluorimetric measurement of β-nicotinamide adenine dinucleotide phosphate, reduced form (NADPH) has been used to measure AMP, ADP, and ATP in brain extracts (Lowry *et al.*, 1964). The hydrogen peroxide produced when hypoxanthine and xanthine are oxidized to uric acid can be coupled to dichlorofluorescein, thus allowing the fluorimetric determination of small amounts of hypoxanthine, adenosine, and inosine if adenosine deaminase (ADA) and purine nucleoside phosphorylase (PNP) are also used (Gardiner, 1979; Tattersall *et al.*, 1983).

B. Bioluminescence

The firefly luciferin–luciferase bioluminescence assay is the most sensitive method available for the measurement of ATP. It is specific for ATP although substances that alter the amount of ATP present will interfere with the assay, e.g., ADP if myokinase is present or creatine phosphate if creatine kinase is present (Strehler, 1974). A variety of nucleotide triphosphates at a range of concentrations has been shown not to interfere with the assay (Moyer and Henderson, 1983).

The light produced may be measured by a fluorimeter (Strehler, 1974), scintillation counter (Stanley and Williams, 1969; Strehler, 1974), or chemiluminometer (White and Leslie, 1982). Because of the specificity of the method if the ATP-containing solution is not turbid, ATP may be measured directly without deproteinization. This fact has led to the method being modified to give continuous levels of ATP so that production or consumption of ATP can be studied without serial sampling or replicate experiments (Lundin *et al.*, 1976; White and Leslie, 1982).

If myokinase and pyruvate kinase are added, AMP and ADP may be converted to ATP, and thus each of these adenine nucleotides can be measured by

Table II. Summary of Enzymic Methods for Adenosine-Related Compounds from Bergmeyer

Compound	Enzymes	Measure	Author(s)
A	Guanase, xanthine oxidase	Uric acid, 293 nm	Naher (1974)
H, X	Xanthine oxidase	Uric acid, 280, 293 nm	Jorgensen (1974)
H, X	Xanthine oxidase	Formazan, 540 nm	Fried and Fried (1974)
UA	Uricase	Uric acid, 293 nm	Schiebe *et al.* (1974)
AR	ADA	AR, 265 nm	Mollering and Bergmeyer (1974)
HR	PNP, xanthine oxidase	Uric acid, 293 nm	Coddington (1974)
ATP	Phosphoglycerate kinase	NADH, 340 nm	Jaworek *et al.* (1974)
ATP	Hexokinase, glucose-6-phosphate dehydrogenase	NADPH, 340 nm	Lamprecht and Trautschold (1974)
ATP	Tetrahydrofolate synthetase	5,10-methenyl-tetrahydrofolic acid, 350 nm	Rabinowitz (1974)
AMP, ADP	Myokinase, pyruvate kinase, lactate dehydrogenase	NADH, 340 nm	Jaworek *et al.* (1974)
ATP and ADP	Phosphoglycerate kinase, myokinase glyceraldehyde, phosphate dehydrogenase	NADH, 340 nm	Gruber *et al.* (1974)
Adenosine phosphates	Phosphatase, ADA	AR, 265 nm	Mollering and Bergmeyer (1974)
ATP	Luciferase	Light	Strehler *et al.* (1974)
cAMP	Protein binding	Radioactivity	Michal and Wunderwald (1974)

the luciferase reaction (Kimmich *et al.*, 1975). Alternatively, adenylate kinase and pyruvate kinase may be used for the conversion (Spielmann *et al.*, 1981).

It has been shown that the luciferin–luciferase preparation may contain an ATP contamination, in which case a correction can be made for the resting luminescence prior to the addition of sample (Silinsky, 1975). The enzyme preparations used for conversion of AMP and ADP to ATP may also contain variable amounts of contaminating adenine nucleotides (Spielmann *et al.*, 1981).

C. DNA Polymerase Assay

It is difficult to measure deoxyATP (dATP) in the presence of ATP unless it is present in large amounts as in dCF inhibition or ADA-deficient erythrocytes. Measurement of normal physiological concentrations of dATP is possible with the DNA polymerase assay (Kefford and Fox, 1982). Several modifications to the method have been suggested (Hutton *et al.*, 1981). A good recent review of the method has been published (Hunting and Henderson, 1981).

D. Radioligand Binding

A sensitive method for measuring adenosine is the radioligand binding method (Olsson *et al.*, 1978). It is not widely used because of the difficulty of preparing suitable antisera.

V. NONSPECIFIC METHODS OF MEASUREMENT

A. Ion-Exchange Chromatography

Ion-exchange chromatography is used in several different ways in the analysis of adenine-containing compounds. The use of ion exchange in HPLC and sample preparation are discussed elsewhere in this chapter. Ion exchange as an analytical method has two uses: first, the separation of purines for subsequent counting when a radiotracer has been used; second, the separation of purines for subsequent determination by UV absorption.

1. Anion Exchange

Anion exchange chromatography is used more often than cation exchange. Neutralized tissue extracts chromatographed on anion exchange columns with gradient elution have provided good nucleotide separations for radioactivity measurements. Nucleotides from blood were separated on Bio Rad AG 1-X8 chloride with HCl gradient (Fredholm, 1975). A step gradient of HCl was used to separate adenosine and the adenine nucleotides on a Dowex AG1-X4 column (Israël *et al.*, 1980). Bio-Rad AG 1-X8 and a $KHCO_3$ gradient have also been used (Zimmerman, 1978).

The direct measurement of adenine-containing compounds in urine from patients with ADA deficiency or adenine phosphoribosyltransferase (APRT) deficiency is possible by ion exchange, since there are increased amounts of the metabolites present and usually at least a moderate volume of urine available. A column of Bio Rad AG 1-X8 and elution with an HCl gradient followed by concentration of the column eluate fractions, electrophoresis, and UV spectroscopy to quantitate and identify each compound has been used to measure dAR and other urinary purines in ADA deficiency (Simmonds *et al.,* 1979) and adenine, 8-hydroxyadenine, 2,8-dihydroxyadenine and other urinary purines in APRT deficiency (Van Acker *et al.,* 1977).

2. *Cation Exchange*

Cation exchange has been used to quantitate purines in urine of ADA-deficient patients. The purines were eluted from a Bio Rad AG 50-X4 column with a gradient of HCl. The compounds were identified and quantitated directly by the absorbances and absorbance ratios at 250, 260, 275,and 290 nm (Mills *et al.,* 1978). Adenosine and deoxyadenosine metabolites after red cell incubations were also separated this way (Mills *et al.,* 1981).

B. Paper and Thin-Layer Chromatography

Paper and thin-layer chromatography (TLC) have been mainly used to separate the metabolic products of a radiolabeled precursor. The purines are generally chromatographed with unlabeled carriers, visualized by absorbance or fluorescnece of UV light and quantitated by scintillation counting. The products after ^{32}P-orthophosphate labeling were visualized by autoradiography (Reinhart and Koroly, 1982). In may cases a single system does not separate all the compounds of interest, and a second development is necessary in either the same or the second dimension, or the use of two complementary systems.

Chromatographic systems for the separation of metabolites after incubations with labeled adenine have been described (Crabtree and Henderson, 1971; Jhamandas and Dumbrille, 1980; Van Den Berghe *et al.,* 1980; Brosh *et al.,* 1982). Suitable systems for separation of metabolites after incubations with adenosine are given by a number of authors (Baer and Vriend, 1981; Willemot and Paton, 1981a; Brosh *et al.,* 1982; Bakhle and Chelliah, 1983; Reddington and Pusch, 1983). After incubation with adenine nucleotides, the products have been separated by TLC (Pearson *et al.,* 1980; Willemot and Paton, 1981b), as have the metabolites of dAR (Plagemann and Wohlheuter, 1983) and orthophosphate (Reinhart and Koroly, 1982).

A possible metabolite of adenine, adenosine, or adenine nucleotides in nonhuman, nondalmatian dog systems that is often ignored in analyses is allantoin, possibly because it has negligible UV absorption at the wavelengths used for the detection of purine with intact purine-ring nuclei. It has, however, been included in some systems (Van Den Berghe *et al.,* 1980; Brosh *et al.,* 1982).

Another possible route of adenosine metabolism is through the synthesis of *S*-adenosylhomocysteine (SAH). The system of Reddington and Pusch (1983) includes SAH and *S*-adenosylmethionine (SAM) as does that of Schrader *et al.* (1981).

The acid-soluble nucleosides and bases in myocardium have been separated by TLC and quantitated directly on the plate by scanning the fluorescence quenching of the plates with a spectrodensitometer (Parker *et al.*, 1973).

C. High-Performance Liquid Chromatography

High-performance liquid chromatography has evolved from open column chromatography in the last 15 years. The improved column-packing materials have made possible faster (30 min for separation of purine nucleotides) and more sensitive (down to a few picomoles per injection without concentration of the sample) analyses of adenine-containing compounds and other purines and pyrimidines.

The range of adenosine-related compounds and the range of their concentrations is so wide that it is impossible to measure them all simultaneously. Furthermore, the range of possible interfering compounds varies so much with the tissue, the preparation method, and the compounds of interest to the investigator that it is impossible to give a single HPLC method as the method of choice for each particular class of compound.

1. Separation of Nucleosides and Bases

The most widely used method for the separation of nucleosides and bases is reversed-phase chromatography. The selection of which C_{18} column to use (with regard to percent loading of the silanol groups with $-C_{18}$ chains and the capping of the remainder with $-CH_3$ residues) will affect the subtleties of the separation. The most commonly used reversed-phase column is the μBondapak C-18 (Waters Associates) but many others are used successfully.

The selection of mobile phase to elute the compounds of interest is important, particularly with regard to pH, since the purines bind best to the stationary phase when they have no overall charge. The most frequently used eluant is an ammonium or potassium phosphate buffer of about 10 m*M* at a pH approximately 5.5, although 4–100 m*M* and pHs from 3.05 to 6.10 have been used successfully. It is generally necessary to have a proportion of an organic solvent in the mobile phase to increase the speed of elution of nucleosides. If an isocratic (single solvent) separation is suitable, 1–20% methanol has been used in the mobile phase or up to 40% methanol has been used in gradient elutions. A combination of acetate buffer and acetonitrile has also been used to separate nucleosides (Harmenberg *et al.*, 1983).

A single report has been made of the separation of adenosine using high-performance affinity chromatography on a boronate-modified silica column (Glad *et al.*, 1980).

The separation of adenosine with *S*-adenosylmethionine and *S*-adenosylhomocysteine has been achieved with the use of reversed-phase chromatography of ion-paired purines. Use has been made of heptane sulphonic acid as the ion pair reagent (Gharib *et al.*, 1982) and octanesulphonic acid (Wagner *et al.*, 1982).

A more specific and sensitive method for adenosine measurement involves conversion to the etheno derivative with subsequent chromatographic separation with fluorescent detection (Kuttesch *et al.*, 1978; Wojcik and Neff, 1982).

2. *Separation of Nucleotides*

High-performance liquid chromatography separation of nucleotides has been achieved mostly with modifications of the open-column strong ion exchange methods. Most methods use Partisil 10 SAX column-packing (Whatman) and elute the nucleotides with a gradient from about 10 m*M* potassium or ammonium phosphate to about 0.8 *M* potassium phosphate, or, for reasons of economy, make the high-concentration eluant of 0.3 *M* potassium phosphate and 0.5 *M* potassium chloride. The separation may be optimized by manipulation of the buffer pHs. Some use the same pH (4.1: Klabunde and Mayer, 1979; 3.7: Earle and Glazer, 1983); some use pH increases (2.85–4.40: Harmsen *et al.*, 1982; 4.0–4.5: Hunting *et al.*, 1982; 3.4–4.3: Webster and Whaun, 1981), whereas some favor pH gradient decreases (5.0–3.1: Pon and Ogilvie, 1981).

Ion exchange nucleotide separations have also been reported using citrate concentration gradient (Khym, 1975; Cohen *et al.*, 1980). An important consideration in the choice of high-concentration buffer in separations at moderate to high sensitivity is the availability of a salt containing a low enough contamination with UV-absorbing impurities that the baseline does not show an unacceptable rise through the chromatogram. Ion-pair chromatographic separation of nucleotides is increasingly being used. Tetrabutylammonium phosphate has been used as the ion pair reagent by some workers (Juengling and Kammermeir, 1980; Harkness *et al.*, 1983), and the use of 11-aminoundecanoic acid has been described (Knox and Jurand, 1981).

Extensive developmental work has been required to produce chromatographic separations of bases, nucleosides, and nucleotides in a single run. This has been achieved using a tetraborate–ammonium chloride system (Bakay *et al.*, 1978) and by adding magnesium ions and Tris to a reversed-phase system (Armiger *et al.*, 1983).

It is much easier to separate standard compounds where they exist in approximately equal quantities than from biological media where other interfering compounds are present and the compounds of interest may differ in concentration 1000 times or more. It is therefore suggested that biological samples be included at an early stage of the method development. A summary of some methods which have been successfully used in biological material is given in Table III.

3. *Detection Methods*

The most widely used detection method in purine HPLC is UV absorbance, usually at 254 nm. This is nonspecific and detects pyrimidines, creatinine, and aromatic amino acids. Dual wavelength detection and good sample preparation and chromatography improve the specificity.

The sensitivity and specificity of HPLC measurements are increased with the use of fluorescence detection, as this allows variability of both the excitation and emission wavelengths. When this is combined with prechromatographic derivatization to the etheno-adenine compounds, small amounts of adenine-containing compounds may be determined in body cells and fluids (Kuttesch *et al.*, 1978) and tissues (Wojcik and Neff, 1982).

Table III. Some HPLC Separations That Have Been Used to Analyze Biological Samples[a]

Purine separated	Type of chromatography	Sample	References
P, PR	RP g phosphate/MeOH	Serum	Hartwick *et al.* (1979a,b); Agarwal *et al.* (1982)
P, PR, cAMP	RG g phosphate/MeOH	Urine, culture medium	De Abreu *et al.* (1982)
P, PR	RP g phosphate/MeOH	Erythrocytes, lymphocytes, plasma	Simmonds *et al.* (1982)
P, PR	RP i phosphate/MeOH	Plasma, CSF	Simmonds and Harkness (1981)
P, PR	RP i phosphate/MeOH	Blood, plasma after nucleotides removed with alumina	Harmsen *et al.* (1981)
PR	RP g phosphate/MeOH	Muscle: or nucleotides removed on Bio-red AG 1 × 8 formate columns	Klabunde (1983)
PR	RP i acetate/MeCN	GMK cells after SepPak cleanup	Harmenberg *et al.* (1983)
PR	RP i phosphate/MeOH	Rat brain	Nordstrom *et al.* (1977)
PR, SAM	RP i phosphate/MeOH	Plasma, urine	Hutton *et al.* (1981)
P, PR, PXP	SAX g tetraborate/NH_4Cl	Fibroblasts	Bakay *et al.* (1978)
P, PR, PXP	RP g phosphate/Mg^{2+}/Tris	Myocardium	Armiger *et al.* (1983)
PXP	WAX i phosphate	Tetrahymena cells	Reinhart and Koroly (1982)
PXP	WAX g citrate	S-49 cells	Cohen *et al.* (1980)
PXP	SAX g phosphate	Erythrocytes	Webster and Whaun (1981)

PXP	SAX g phosphate/KCl	Lymphocytes	Brenton *et al.* (1977)
PXP	SAX g phosphate/KCl	Muscle	Klabunde and Mayer (1979)
PXP	RP i t-butylammonium phosphate/MeOH	Plasma, urine, leukocytes, erythrocytes	Harkness *et al.* (1983)
PXP	RP i t-butylammonium phophate/MeCN	Cardiac tissue	Juengling and Kammermeir (1980)
PXP	SAX g phosphate/KCl	Skin	Pruneau *et al.* (1982)
PXP	SAX g phosphate	Heart	Harmsen *et al.* (1982)
PXP	SAX g phosphate/KCl	Lymphocytes	Earle and Glazer (1983)
PXP	SAX g phosphate/KCl	Brain	Shmukler (1972)
PXP, dPXP	SAX g phosphate/KCl	Erythrocytes, lymphocytes	Simmonds *et al.* (1982)
PTP, dPTP	SAX i phosphate/KCl	Erythrocytes	Smith and Henderson (1982)
PTP, PXP	SAX i,g phosphate/KCl	CHO cells	Hunting *et al.* (1981)
SAM, PR	RP i phosphate/MeOH	Plasma, urine	Hutton *et al.* (1981)
SAM, SAH, PR	RP i heptanesulphonic acid/MeOH	Rat brain after SepPak separation	Gharib *et al.* (1982)
SAM, SAH	RP g octanesulphonic acid, EDTA, phosphate/McCN	Prostate, hepatoma cells	Wagner *et al.* (1982)
SAM	RP i heptane sulphonic acid, EDTA acetate/EtOH	Adrenals	Burke (1982)
cPMP	RP i,g phosphate/MeOH	Urine	Krstulovic *et al.* (1979)

[a] Abbreviations: P, purine base (H, X, A, UA); PR, purine nucleoside (mostly AR, HR, dAR); PXP, purine nucleotides (mostly ATP, ADP, AMP); dPXP, deoxyadenosine nucleotides; RP, reversed-phase; SAX, strong anion exchange; WAX, weak anion exchange; g, gradient; i, isocratic separation.

The use of on-line radiochemical detection has been limited. Bakay and colleagues (1978) used a detector of their own design to quantitate the specific activities of purine nucleotides, nucleosides and bases present in cells after incubation with [^{14}C]hypoxanthine, whereas Webster and Whaun (1981) used a commercially available detector (Flo-one, Radiomatic Instruments, USA) in series with a UV detector. Using either solid or liquid scintillation systems and state-of-the-art electonics, high counting efficiencies are now possible for ^{3}H as well as ^{14}C (e.g. Radiodetector, Reeve Analytical Ltd., Glasgow, UK). This method will give increased information and speed of analysis in many radiotracer studies.

4. *Quantitation*

Both peak height and peak area have been shown to be linear with injected amounts of purine over a wide concentration range for both ion exchange and reversed-phase chromatography with UV detection, so that either of these methods is suitable for quantitation.

5. *Peak Identification*

A peak appearing at the retention time of adenosine may be adenosine, adenosine and another compound, or something else altogether. Thus, peak identity should be confirmed by a method other than retention times. The methods available include the following.

Standard addition. Co-chromatography with authentic compounds will often produce alterations of peak shape if the peak is not of the added compound, even if they have identical retention times.

Peak shift. The use of enzymic peak shift is well described and conditions included by Hartwick and co-workers (1979b). The use of ADA for adenosine and modified adenine nucleoside identification is most often used (Argarwal *et al.*, 1982; Wojcik and Neff, 1982). Nucleotides have been hydrolyzed with alkaline phosphatase and the nucleosides rechromatographed (Cohen *et al.*, 1980) or with the serial degradation of the glucose–hexokinase system (Pruneau *et al.*, 1982). The reaction conditions of periodate with the *cis*-diol configuration of ribose has also been used (Hartwick *et al.*, 1979a,b). A method of peak-shift identification has been reported (Gharib *et al.*, 1982) for *S*-adenosylmethionine and *S*-adenosylhomocysteine.

Another method of peak shift utilizes the changes in retention times that occur when changes in the pH of the mobile phase change the ionic state of purine compounds (Simmonds and Harkness, 1981).

Spectra and absorbance ratios. The purine and pyrimidine bases have characteristic absorption maxima and shape of absorption spectrum. Stopped flow scanning of the absorption spectrum of peaks of interest has been reported (Hartwick *et al.*, 1979a,b). An easier parameter to measure routinely is the ratio of UV absorbance of the peaks at two different wavelengths. This can be done simultaneously with two detectors in series or using a commercially available dual wavelength detector (e.g., the Waters Associates Model 440). The wavelengths generally used are 254 and 280 nm. The advantage of this method of peak identity confirmation is that it can be done on each run routinely, and it checks all peaks on every run. Sometimes two compounds that appear as one peak at one wavelength show as a shouldered peak at the second wavelength as well as an altered wavelength absorption ratio.

Peak shape. Alteration of peak shape, e.g., shouldering, is indicative of coelution of two or more compounds. In reversed-phase systems, adenine chromatographs with a characteristic tailing (Simmonds and Harkness, 1981). More detail may be found in two excellent reviews (Brown *et al.,* 1980; Zakaria and Brown, 1981).

Internal standard. Since the recovery of added purines from biological samples is generally good, little use is made of internal standards in quantitation. Because of the distinctive peak it produces especially when absorbance measurements are made simultaneously at 280 and 254 nm, uric acid in human samples has been used as a reference for the retention times of other compounds (Simmonds and Harkness, 1981). Allopurinol is a possible internal standard for nucleoside and base measurements and xanthosine diphosphate for nucleotide measurements.

An example of the use of an HPLC method is that in use in our laboratory for the study of 5′AMP metabolism by the guinea-pig ileum. This tissue primarily degrades exogenous purines. Consequently the method measures 5′AMP, adenosine, inosine, hypoxanthine, xanthine, and uric acid. The tissue is suspended in an organ bath containing 3.0 ml balanced salt solution and the purine and enzyme inhibitors when these are used. Aliquots (100 μl) of medium are removed at various time intervals and further degradation stopped by the addition of TCA (10 μl, 50%) with mixing. The TCA is extracted into water-saturated diethylether until the pH is about 4.0. Recovery of the above purines is quantitative. Fifty-microliter samples are injected onto a μBondapak C-18 column (Waters Associates) protected by a precolumn filled with pellicular octadecylsilane (ODS) packing and eluted with a linear gradient from 0–20% methanol in potassium dihydrogen phosphate, 67 m*M*, natural pH. The gradient is complete in 12 min. Purines and other compounds are detected by UV absorbance at 254 and 280 nm and 0.01 absorbance units full scale (AUFS) (M440 dual channel detector, Waters Associates) and identified by retention time and absorbance ratio. Occasional samples also are cochromatographed with a mixture of authentic compounds and adenosine verified by peak shifts to inosine (incubation with a calculated amount of calf intestinal ADA, Type III, Sigma Chemical Company pH 7.4, 37°C, 30 min). Quantitation is by comparison of peak height with external standard solutions and the limit of easy detection is about 2 pmoles per injection.

D. Electrophoresis

A method developed for separating urinary purines (Simmonds, 1969) by electrophoresis on silica–cellulose plates in borate buffer has been used to separate adenine-containing compounds after incubation of erythrocytes with adenosine and deoxyadenosine (Sahota *et al.*, 1980). Electrophoresis and HPLC have been used together to separate adenosine incubation products (Perret and Dean, 1977).

Substrates and reaction products found in studies of adenosine and inosine–guanosine phosphorylase assays were separated by electrophoresis on paper in ammonium diborate (Divekar, 1976).

Adenine-containing compounds present after the incubation of platelets with adenine or adenosine have been separated on paper by electrophoresis in citrate buffer (Sixma *et al.*, 1976; Doni, 1981).

E. Isotachophoresis

Isotachophoresis has been used to separate purines in serum (Oerlemans *et al.*, 1980) and urine in children with inborn errors of metabolism including APRT and ADA deficiencies (Simmonds *et al.*, 1980). Adenine nucleotides and other metabolites (lactate, phosphocreatine, inorganic phosphate) have also been quantitated using this technique (Brolsma *et al.*, 1982).

F. Pulse-Labeling

Nucleotides and other phosphate-containing compounds in platelets have been pulse-labeled with ^{32}P-phosphate and the radiolabeled compounds separated by various chromatographic methods. Since ^{32}P is uniformly distributed among the various phosphate-containing compounds the amount of radioactivity is proportional to the amount of the compound present. This method has the advantage of measuring only the metabolizing pools and not, for example, the ADP storage pool of platelets (Holmsen *et al.*, 1983).

G. Nuclear Magnetic Resonance

[^{31}P]-NMR has been used to measure ATP and creatine phosphate in whole rat heart (Ingwall *et al.*, 1982).

VI. CONCLUSION

The sensitivity of each method is difficult to describe, as it is dependent on the degree of prior purification of concentration of the sample and often on the instrumentation used. The most sensitive methods are luciferin–luciferase for ATP, which can detect 0.1 pmole (Spielman *et al.*, 1981), DNA polymerase for dATP, which can easily detect 0.5 pmole (Lindberg and Skoog, 1970) and the radioligand-binding method for adenosine, which can detect 1.0 pmole (Olsson *et al.*, 1978). HPLC methods depend for their sensitivity on instrumentation but 1–10pmoles per injection depending on the peak shape and wavelength used for measurement should be possible. A possible source of error when small quantities of nucleotides are being measured is adsorption of the nucleotides onto syringes being used for their measurement (Goswami and Pande, 1981).

ACKNOWLEDGMENTS

D.R.W. was supported by a grant from the Medical Research Council of New Zealand. The expert secretarial assistance of Mrs. Brenda Carlson and Mrs. Joanne Williamson and the literature supplied by Alphatech Systems (NZ) Ltd. are gratefully acknowledged.

REFERENCES

Agarwal, R. P., Major, P. P., and Kufe, D. W. 1982. Simple and rapid high performance liquid chromatographic method for analysis of nucleosides in biological fluids. *J. Chromatogr., 231*:418–424.

Armiger, L. C., Seelye, R. N., Morrison, M. A., and Hollis, D. G. 1984. Comparative biochemistry and fine structure of atrial and ventricular myocardium during autolysis *in vitro*. *Basic Res. Cardiol., 79*:218–229.

Baer, H. P., and Vriend, R. 1981. Effects of adenosine transport inhibitors in smooth muscle. *Proc. West. Pharmacol. Soc., 24*:131–133.

Bakay, B., Nissenen, E. A., Sweetman, L., and Nyhan, W. L. 1978. Analysis of radioactive and nonradioactive purine bases, purine nucleosides and purine nucleotides by high speed chromatography on a single column. *Monogr. Hum. Genet., 10*:127–137.

Bakhle, Y. S., and Chelliah, R. 1983. Metabolism and uptake of adenosine in rat isolated lung and its inhibition. *Br. J. Pharmacol., 79*:509–515.

Bergmeyer, H. U. (Ed.). 1974. *Methods of Enzymatic Analysis,* Vol. 4, 2nd English ed. Academic Press, New York.

Bockman, E. L., Berne, R. M., and Rubio, R. 1976. Adenosine and active hyperemia in dog skeletal muscle. *Am. J. Physiol., 230*:1531–1537.

Brenton, D. P., Astrin, H. K., Cruikshank, M. K., and Seegmiller, J. E. 1977. Measurement of free nucleotides in cultured human lymphoid cells using high-pressure liquid chromatography. *Biochem. Med., 17*:231–247.

Brolsma, M. F. J., Oerlemans, F. T. J., Verberg, M. P., and de Bruyn, C. H. M. M. 1982. Isotachophoretic analysis of some compounds involved in energy metabolism in normal and pathological human muscle extracts. *J. Clin. Chem. Clin. Biochem., 20*:352.

Brosh, S., Boer, P., and Sperling, O. 1982. Effects of fructose on synthesis and degradation of purine nucleotides in isolated rat hepatocytes. *Biochem. Biophys. Acta, 717*:459–464.

Brown, P. R., Krstulovic, A. M., and Hartwick, R. A. 1980. Current state of the art in the HPLC analyses of free nucleotides, nucleosides and bases in biological fluids. In: *Advances in Chromatography,* Volume 18, pp. 101–138. Ed. by Giddings, J. C., Grushka, E., Cazes, J., and Brown, P. R.) Marcel Dekker, New York.

Burke, W. J. 1982. A highly sensitive assay for S-adenosylmethionine by high performance chromatography. *Anal. Biochem., 122*:258–261.

Capogrossi, M. C., Holdiness, M. R., and Israili, Z. H. 1982. Determination of adenosine in normal human plasma and serum by high performance chromatography. *J. Chromatogr., 227*:168–173.

Coddington, A. 1974. Inosine. In: *Methods of Enzymatic Analysis,* Volume 4, pp. 1932–1934. Ed. by Bergmeyer, H. U. Academic Press, New York.

Cohen, M. B., Maybaum, J., and Sadee, W. 1980. Analysis of purine ribonucleotides and deoxyribonucleotides in cell extracts by high-performance liquid chromatography. *J. Chromatogr. 198*:435–441.

Crabtree, G. W., and Henderson, J. F. 1971. Rate-limiting steps in the interconversion of purine ribonucleotides in Ehrlich ascites tumor cells *in vitro*. *Cancer Res., 31*:985–991.

De Abreu, R. A., van Baal, J. M., De Bruyn, C. H. M. M., Bakkeren, J. A. J. M., and Schretlen, E. D. A. M. 1982. High-performance liquid chromatographic determination of purine and pyrimidine bases, ribonucleosides, deoxyribonucleosides and cyclic ribonucleotides in biological fluids. *J. Chromatogr., 229*:67–75.

Divekar, A. Y. 1976. Adenosine phosphorylase activity as distinct from inosine-guanosine phosphorylase activity in sarcoma 180 cells and rat liver. *Biochem. Biophys. Acta, 422:*15–28.

Doni, M. G. 1981. Adenosine uptake and deamination by blood platelets in different mammalian species. *Haemostasis, 10:*79–88.

Dresse, A., Chevolet, C., Delapierre, D., Masset, H., Weisenberger, H., Bolzer, G., and Heinzel, H. 1982. Pharmacokinetics of dipyridamole (Persantine) and its effect on platelet adenosine uptake in man. *Eur. J. Clin. Pharmacol., 23:*229–234.

Earle, M. F., and Glazer, R. I. 1983. 2′deoxycoformycin toxicity in murine spleen lymphocytes. *Mol. Pharmacol., 23:*165–170.

Fredholm, B. B. 1975. Release of adenosine-like material from isolated perfused dog adipose tissue following sympathetic nerve stimulation and its inhibition by adrenergic α-receptor blockade. *Acta. Physiol. Scand, 96:*422–430.

Fredholm, B. B., and Hedqvist, P. 1978. Release of ^{3}H-purines from [^{3}H]-adenine labelled rabbit kidney following sympathetic nerve stimulation and its inhibition by α-adrenoceptor blockade. *Br. J. Pharmacol., 64:*239–245.

Fredholm, B. B., and Sollevi, A. 1981. The release of adenosine and inosine from canine subcutaneous adipose tissue by nerve stimulation and noradrenaline. *J. Physiol., 313:*351–367.

Fried, R., and Fried, L. W. 1974. Hypoxanthine and xanthine. Colorimetric measurement. In: *Methods of Enzymatic Analysis,* Volume 4, pp. 1945–1950. Ed. by Bergmeyer, H. V. Academic Press, New York.

Gardiner, D. G. 1979. A rapid and sensitive fluorimetric assay for adenosine, inosine, and hypoxanthine. *Anal. Biochem., 95:*377–382.

Gehrke, C. W., Kuo, K. C., Davis, G. E., Suits, R. D., Waalkes, T. P., and Borek, E. 1978. Quantitative high-performance liquid chromatography of nucleosides in biological materials. *J. Chromatogr. 150:*455–476.

Gharib, A., Sarda, N., Chabannes, B., Cronenberger, L., and Pacheco, H. 1982. The regional concentrations of S-adenosyl-L-methionine, S-adenosyl-L-homocysteine, and adenosine in rat brain. *J. Neurochem., 38:*810–815.

Glad, M., Ohlson, S., Mansson, L., Mansson, M.-O., and Mosbach, K. 1980. High-performance liquid affinity chromatography of nucleosides, nucleotides and carbohydrates with boronic acid-substituted microparticulate silica. *J. Chromatogr., 200:*254–260.

Goday, A., Simmonds, H. A., Webster, D. R., Levinsky, R. J., Watson, A. T., and Hoffbrand, A. V. 1983. Importance of platelet-free preparations for evaluating lymphocyte nucleotide levels in inherited or acquired immunodeficiency syndromes. *Clin. Sci., 65:*635–643.

Goswami, T., and Pande, S. V. 1981. Syringes are unsuitable for pipetting submicromolar solutions of nucleoside triphosphates because of adsorbtion. *Anal. Biochem., 117:*336–338.

Gruber, W., Möllering, H., and Bergmeyer, H. V. 1974. Analytical differentiation of purine and pyrimidine nucleotides. Determination of ADP, ATP and sum of GTP and ITP in biological material. In: *Methods of Enzymatic Analysis,* Volume 4, pp. 2078–2087. Ed. by Bergmeyer, H. U. Academic Press, New York.

Harkness, R. A., Simmonds, R. J., and Coade, S. B. 1983. Purine transport and metabolism in man: The effect of exercise on concentrations of purine bases, nucleosides and nucleotides in plasma, urine, leucocytes and erthrocytes. *Clin. Sci., 64:*333–340.

Harmenberg, J., Larsson, A., and Hagberg, C. E. 1983. Reversed-phase high-performance liquid chromatography (HPLC) of nucleosides with special reference to deoxythymidine. *J. Liq. Chromatogr., 6:*655–666.

Harmsen, E., de Jong, J. W., and Serruys, P. W. 1981. Hypoxanthine production by ischemic heart demonstrated by high-pressure liquid chromatography of blood purine nucleosides and oxypurines. *Clin. Chim. Acta, 115:*73–84.

Harmsen, E., de Tombe, P. P., and de Jong, J. W. 1982. Simultaneous determination of myocardial adenine nucleotides and creatine phosphate by high-performance liquid chromatography. *J. Chromatogr., 230:*131–136.

Hartwick, R. A., Assenza, S. P., and Brown, P. R. 1979a. Identification and quantitation of nucleosides, bases and other uv-absorbing compounds in serum, using reversed-phase high performance liquid chromatography, I. Chromatographic methodology. *J. Chromatogr., 186:*647–658.

Hartwick, R. A., Krstulovic, A. M., and Brown, P. R. 1979b. Identification and quantitation of nucleosides, bases and other uv-absorbing compounds in serum, using reversed phase high performation liquid chromatography II. Evaluation of human sera. *J. Chromatogr., 186:*659–676.

Hirschhorn, R., Roegner-Maniscako, V., Kuritsky, L., and Rosen, F. S. 1981. Bone marrow transplantation only partially restores purine metabolites to normal in adenosine deaminase-deficient patients. *J. Clin. Invest., 68:*1387–1393.

Holmsen, H., Dangelmaier, C. A., and Akkerman, J. -W. N. 1983. Determination of level of glycolytic intermediates and nucleotides in platelets by pulse-labelling with [^{32}P] orthosphosphate. *Anal. Biochem., 131:*266–272.

Hunting, D., and Henderson, J. F. 1981. Determination of deoxynucleoside triphosphates using DNA polyerase: A critical evaluation. *Can. J. Biochem., 59:*723–727.

Hunting, D., Hordern, J., and Henderson, J. F. 1981. Quantitative analysis of purine and pyrimidine metabolism in Chinese hamster ovary cells. *Can. J. Biochem., 59:*838–847.

Hutton, J. J., Wigninton, D. A., Coleman, M. S., Fuller, S. A., Limouze, S., and Lamplin, B. C. 1981. Biochemical and functional abnormalities in lymphocytes from an adenosine deaminase-deficient patient during enzyme replacement therapy. *J. Clin. Invest., 68:*413–421.

Ingwall, J. S., Fossel, E. T., Kloner, R. F., and Goldhaber, S. Z. 1982. A supplement of inosine aids the salvage of rodent myocardium injured by hypoxia. *J. Clin. Chem. Clin. Biochem., 20:*378.

Israël, M., Lesbats, B., Manaranche, R., Meunioe, F. M., and Frachon, P. 1980. Retrograde inhibition of transmitter release by ATP. *J. Neurochem., 34:*923–932.

Jaworek, D., Gruber, W., and Bergmeyer, H. V. 1974. Adenosine-5-triphosphate. Determination with 3-phosphoglycerate kinase. In: *Methods of Enzymatic Analysis,* Volume 4, pp. 2097–2101. Ed. by Bergmeyer, H. V. Academic Press, New York.

Jhamandas, K., and Dumbrille, A. 1980. Regional release of [^{3}H]adenosine derivatives from rat brain *in vivo:* Effect of excitory amino acids, opiate agonists and benzodiazepines. *Can. J. Physiol. Pharmacol., 58:*1262–1278.

Jørgensen, S. 1974. Hypoxanthine and xanthine. UV assay. In: *Methods of Enzymatic Analysis,* Volume 4, pp. 1941–1945. Ed. by Bergmeyer, H. U. Academic Press, New York.

Juengling, E., and Kammermeir, H. 1980. Rapid assay of adenine nucleotides or creatine compounds in extracts of cardiac tissue by paired-ion reverse-phase high-performance liquid chromatography. *Anal. Biochem., 102:*358–361.

Kefford, R. F., and Fox, R. M. 1982. Purine deoxynucleoside toxicity in non-dividing human lymphoid cells. *Cancer. Res., 42:*324–330.

Khym, J. X. 1975. An analytical system for rapid separation of tissue nucleotides at low pressures on conventional ion exchanger. *Clin. Chem., 21:*1245–1253.

Kimmich, G. A., Randles, J., and Brand, J. S. 1975. Assay of picomole amounts of ATP, ADP and AMP using the luciferase enzyme system. *Anal. Biochem., 69:*187–206.

Klabunde, R. E. 1983. Effect of dipyridamole on post ischemic vasodilation and extracellular adenosine. *Am. J. Physiol., 244:*H273–H280.

Klabunde, R. E., and Mayer, S. E. 1979. Effects of ischemia on tissue metabolites in red (slow) and white (fast) skeletal muscle of the chicken. *Circ. Res., 45:*366–373.

Knox, J. H., and Jurand, J. 1981. Zwitterion-pair chromatography of nucleotides and related species. *J. Chromatogr., 203:*85–92.

Krstulovic, A. M., Hartwick, R. A., and Brown, P. R. 1979. Reversed-phase liquid chromatographic separation of 3′,5′-cyclic ribonucleotides. *Clin. Chem., 25:*235–241.

Kuttesch, J. F., Schmalstieg, F. C., Nelson, J. A. 1978. Analysis of adenosine and other adenine compounds in patients with immunodeficiency diseases. *J. Liq. Chromatogr., 1:*97–109.

Lamprecht, W., and Trautschold, I. 1974. Adenosine-5′-triphosphate. Determination with hexokinase and glucose-6-phosphate dehydrogenase. In: *Methods of Enzymatic Analysis,* Volume 4, pp. 2101–2110. Ed. by Bergmeyer, H. U. Academic Press, New York.

Lindberg, U., and Skoog, L. 1970. A method for the determination of dATP and dTTP in picomole amounts. *Anal. Biochem., 34:*152–160.

Lothrop, C. D., and Uziel, M. 1980. Rapid preparation of nucleotides from acid-soluble pools by chromatography on silica, as exemplified with acid extracts of cultured cells. *Clin. Chem., 26:*1430–1434.

Lowry, O. H., Passonneau, J. V., Hasselberger, F. X., and Schulz, D. W. 1964. Effect of ischemia on known substrates and cofactors of the glycolytic pathway in brain. *J. Biol. Chem., 239:*18–30.

Lundin, A., Rickardsson, A., and Thore, A. 1976. Continuous monitoring of ATP-converting reactions by purified firefly luciferase. *Anal. Biochem., 75:*611–620.

Michal, G., and Wunderwald, P. 1974. Adenosine-3′:5′-monophosphate, cyclic. In: *Methods of Enzymatic Analysis,* Volume 4, pp. 2136–2143. Ed. by Bergmeyer, H. U. Academic Press, New York.

Mills, G. C., Goldblum, R. M., Newkirk, K. E., and Schmalsteig, F. C. 1978. Urinary excretion of purines, purine nucleosides and pseudouridine in adenosine deaminase deficiency. *Biochem. Med., 20:*180–199.

Mills, G. C., Goldblum, R. M., and Schmalstieg, F. C. 1981. Catabolism of adenine nucleotides in adenosine deaminase deficient erythrocytes. *Life Sci., 29:*1811–1820.

Möllering, H., and Bergmeyer, H. U. 1974. Adenosine. In: *Methods of Enzymatic Analysis,* Volume 4, pp. 1917–1922. Ed. by Bergmeyer, H. U. Academic Press, New York.

Moyer, J. D., and Henderson, J. F. 1983. Nucleoside triphosphate specificity of firefly luciferase. *Anal. Biochem., 131:*187–189.

Näher, G. 1974. Adenine and Guanine. In: *Methods of Enzymatic Analysis,* Volume 4, pp. 1909–1915. Ed. by Bergmeyer, H. U. Academic Press, New York.

Nordstom, C. -H., Rehncrona, S., Siesjö, B. K., and Westerberg, E. 1977. Adenosine in rat cerebral cortex: Its determination, normal values, and correlation to AMP and cyclic AMP during short-lasting ischemia. *Acta. Physiol. Scand, 101:*63–71.

Oerlemans, F., Verheggen, T., Mikkers, F., Everaerts, F., and De Bruyn, C. H. M. M. 1980. Analysis of serum purines and pyrimidines by isotachophoresis. In: *Purine Metabolism in Man III,* 122B, pp. 429–433. Ed. by Rapado, A., Watts, R. W. E., and De Bruyn, C. H. M. M. Plenum Press, New York.

Olsson, R. A. 1970. Changes in content of purine nucleoside in canine myocardium during coronary occlusion. *Circ. Res. 26:*301–306.

Olsson, R. A., Davis, C. J., Gentry, M. K., and Vomacka, R. B. 1978. A radioligand-binding assay for adenosine in tissue extracts. *Anal. Biochem., 85:*132–138.

Olsson, R. A., Saito, D., and Steinhart, C. R. 1982. Compartmentalization of the adenosine pool of dog and rat hearts. *Circ. Res., 50:*617–626.

Parker, J. C., Jones, C. E., and Smith, E. E. 1973. Determination of acid-soluble nucleosides and bases in myocardium by thin-layer methods. *J. Chromatogr., 79:*360–363.

Pearson, J. D., and Gordon, J. L. 1979. Vascular endothelial and smooth muscle cells in culture selectively release adenine nucleotides. *Nature,* 281:384–386.

Pearson, J. D., Carleton, J. S., and Gordon, J. L. 1980. Metabolism of adenine nucleotides by ectoenzymes of vascular endothelial and smooth-muscle cells in culture. *Biochem. J., 190:*421–429.

Perrett, D., and Dean, B. 1977. The function of adenosine deaminase in human erythrocyte. *Biochem. Biophys. Res. Comm., 77:*374–378.

Pfadenhauer, E. H., and Tong, S. -D. 1979. Determination of inosine and adenosine in human plasma using high-performance liquid chromatography and a boronate affinity gel. *J. Chromatogr., 162:*585–590.

Plagemann, P. G. W., and Wohlheuter, R. M. 1981. 2-Deoxycorformycin inhibition of intracellular phosphorylation of adenosine in Novikoff rat hepatoma cells. *Biochem. Pharmacol., 30:*417–426.

Plagemann, P. G. W., and Wohlheuter, R. M. 1983. 5′-Deoxyadenosine metabolism in various mammalian cell lines *Biochem. Pharmacol., 32:*1433–1440.

Pon, R. T., and Ogilvie, K. K. 1981. Simultaneous analysis of nucleosides and nucleotides by high performance liquid chromatography. *J. Chromatogr., 205:*202–205.

Pruneau, D., Wülfert, E., Pascal, H., and Baron, C. 1982. High-performance liquid chromatographic procedure for measuring ATP and ADP levels in tissue microbiopsy: Application to rat wound healing proliferative tissue. *Anal. Biochem., 119:*274–280.

Rabinowitz, J. C. 1974. Adenosine-5-triphosphate. Determination with formyltetrahydrofolate synthetase. In: *Methods of Enzymatic Analysis,* Volume 4, pp. 2110–2111. Ed. by Bergmeyer, H. U. Academic Press, New York.

Reddington, M., and Pusch, R. 1983. Adenosine metabolism in a rat hippocampal slice preparation: incorporation into S-adenosylhomocysteine. *J. Neurochem., 40:*285–290.

Reinhart, M. P., and Koroly, M. J. 1982. Analysis of nucleotides from Tetrahymena by high-performance liquid chromatography. *Anal. Biochem., 119:*392–396.

Sahota, A., Simmonds, H. A., Potter, C. F., Watson, J. G., Hugh-Jones, K., and Perrett, D. 1980. Adenosine and deoxyadenosine metabolism in the erythrocytes of a patient with adenosine-deaminase deficiency. In: *Purine Metabolism in Man III,* 122A, pp. 397–401. Ed. by Rapado, A., Watts, R. W. E., and De Bruyn, C. H. M. M. Plenum Press, New York.

Schiebe, P. E., Bernt, E., ànd Bergmeyer, H. U. 1974. Uric Acid. In: *Methods of Enzymatic Analysis,* Volume 4, pp. 1951–1958. Ed. by Bergmeyer, H. U. Academic Press, New York.

Schrader, J., Schütz, W., and Bardenheuer, H. 1981. Role of S-adenosylhomocysteine hydrolase in adenosine metabolism in mammalian heart. *Biochem. J., 196:*65–70.

Shmukler, H. W. 1972. The rapid chromatographic analysis of free nucleotides from rat brain. *J. Chromatogr. Sci., 10:*38–40.

Silinsky, E. M. 1975. On the association between transmitter secretion and the release of adenine nucleotides from mammalian motor nerve terminals. *J. Physiol., 247:*145–162.

Simmonds, H. A. 1969. Two-dimensional thin-layer high-voltage electrophoresis and chromatography for the separation of urinary purines, pyrimidines and pyrazolo pyrimidines. *Clin. Chim. Acta, 23:*319–330.

Simmonds, H. A., Sahota, A., Potter, C. F., Perrett, D., Hugh-Jones, K., and Watson, J. G. 1979. Purine metabolism in adenosine deaminase deficiency. In: *Enzyme Defects and Immune Dysfunction.* Ciba Foundation Symposium 68 (new series), pp. 255–262. Excerpta Medica, Amsterdam.

Simmonds, H. A., Sahota, A., and Payne, R. 1980. A rapid screening method for inborn errors of purine and pyrimidine metabolism using isotachophoresis in *Purine Metabolism in Man III,* 122B, pp. 421–427. Ed. by Rapado, A., Watts, R. W. E., and De Bruyn, C. H. M. M. Plenum Press, New York.

Simmonds, H. A., Webster, D. R., Perrett, D., Reiter, S., and Levinsky, R. J. 1982. Formation and degradation of deoxyadenosine nucleotides in inherited adenosine deaminase deficiency. *Bioscience Rep., 2:*303–314.

Simmonds, R. J., and Harkness, R. A. 1981. High-performance liquid chromatographic methods for base and nucleoside analysis in extracellular fluids and in cells. *J. Chromatogr., 226:*369–381.

Sixma, J. A., Lips, J. P. M., Trieschnigg, A. M. C., and Holmsen, H. 1976. Transport and metabolism of adenosine in human blood platelets. *Biochim. Biophys. Acta, 443:*33–48.

Smith, C. M. and Henderson, J. F. 1982. Deoxyadenosine triphosphate accumulation in erythrocytes of deoxycoformycin-treated mice. *Biochem. Pharmacol., 31:*1545–1551.

Spielmann, H., Jacob-Müller, U., and Schulz, P. 1981. Simple assay of 0.1-1.0 pmol of ATP, ADP and AMP in single somatic cells using purified luciferin-luciferase. *Anal. Biochem., 113:*172–178.

Stanley, P. E., and Williams, S. G. 1969. Use of the liquid scintillation spectrometer for determining adenosine triphosphate by the luciferase enzyme. *Anal. Biochem., 29:*381–392.

Strehler, B. 1974. Adenosine triphosphate and creatine phosphate. Determination with luciferase. In: *Methods of Enzymatic Analysis,* Volume 4, pp. 2112–2126. Ed. by Bergmeyer, H. V. Academic Press, New York.

Tattersall, M. H. N., Slowiaczek, P., and DeFazio, A. 1983. Regional variation in human extracellular purine levels. *J. Lab. Clin. Med., 102:*411–420.

Van Acker, K. J., Simmonds, H. A., Potter, C. F., and Cameron, J. S. 1977. Complete deficiency of adenine phosphoribosyltransferase. Report of a family. *N. Engl. J. Med., 297:*127–132.

Van Den Berghe, G., Bontemps, F., and Hers, H. -G. 1980. Purine catabolism in isolated rat hepatocytes. Influence of coformycin. *Biochem. J., 188:*913–920.

Wagner, J., Danzin, C., and Mamont, P. 1982. Reversed-phase ion pair liquid chromatographic procedure for the simultaneous analysis of S-adenosylmethionine, its metabolites and the natural polyamines. *J. Chromatogr., 227:*349–368.

Watkinson, W. P., Foley, D. H., Rubio, R., and Berne, R. M. 1979. Myocardial adenosine formation with increased cardiac performance in the dog. *Am. J. Physiol., 236:*H13–H21.

Webster, H. K., and Whaun, J. M. 1981. Application of simultaneous uv-radioactivity high performance liquid chromatography to the study of intermediary metabolism. I. Purine nucleotides, nucleosides and bases. *J. Chromatogr., 209:*283–292.

White, T. D., and Leslie, R. A. 1982. Depolarization-induced release of adenosine 5′-triphosphate from isolated varicosities derived from the myenteric plexus of the guinea pig small intestine. *J. Neuroscience, 2:*206–215.

Willemot, J., and Paton, D. M. 1981a. Metabolism and presynaptic inhibitory effects of adenosine in rat vas deferens. *J. Auton. Pharmacol., 1:*217–224.

Willemot, J., and Paton, D. M. 1981b. Metabolism and presynaptic inhibitory effects of 2′, 3′ and 5′adenine nucleotides in rat vas deferens. *Arch. Pharmacol., 317:*110–114.

Winn, H. R., Rubio, R., and Berne, R. M. 1981. Brain adenosine concentration during hypoxia in rats. *Am. J. Physiol., 241:*H235–H242.

Wojcik, W. J., and Neff, N. H. 1982. Adenosine measurement by a rapid HPLC-Fluorometric method: Induced changes of adenosine content in regions of rat brain. *J. Neurochem., 39:*280–282.

Wu, P. H., and Phillis, J. W. 1978. Distribution and release of adenosine triphosphate in rat brain. *Neurochem. Res., 3:*563–571.

Zakaria, M., and Brown, P. R. 1981. High performance liquid column chromatography of nucleotides, nucleosides and bases. *J. Chromatogr., 226:*267–290.

Zimmerman, H. 1978. Turnover of adenine nucleotides in cholinergic synaptic vesicles of the torpedo electric organ. *Neuroscience, 3:*827–836.

Chapter **3**

The Demonstration and Measurement of Adenosine Triphosphate Release from Nerves

Thomas D. White

Department of Pharmacology
Dalhousie University
Halifax, Nova Scotia, Canada

I. INTRODUCTION

A. Brief History of ATP Release from Nerves

In 1953, Holton and Holton observed that antidromic stimulation of the great auricular nerve of the rabbit ear perfused with Locke's solution resulted in a specific increase in the optical density at 260 nm in samples of venous effluent. The differences in absorption spectra of samples of venous effluent were "typical of those produced by substances containing purine and pyrimidine rings, including ATP and its break-down products." Later, Holton and Holton (1954) showed similar time courses for vasodilation caused by antidromic stimulation of the sensory nerve and that caused by injections of ATP. In a subsequent study, Holton (1959) demonstrated, using firefly luciferin–luciferase, that ATP was liberated when the great auricular nerve was stimulated. All these results led the Holtons to propose that ATP might be released from sensory nerve endings and have a possible role in chemical transmission. Notwithstanding the recent evidence that substance P may also be a likely candidate for the transmitter involved in the vasodilation responses following antidromic stimulation of sensory nerves (Gazelius *et al.*, 1981), the studies of the Holtons stand out as the first to suggest a possible transmitter function for ATP or its derivatives.

In 1962, Abood *et al.* demonstrated a release of ^{32}P-labeled orthophosphate and ATP when frog nerve or muscle was stimulated electrically. They related the release of ATP to the depolarization of these excitable tissues and speculated whether outflux of ATP was secondary to excitation or served some primary function in the excitatory event.

In the early 1970s, Burnstock and his colleagues proposed that a purine nucleotide, possibly ATP, might be the nonadrenergic, noncholinergic inhibitory neurotransmitter in vertebrate gastrointestinal smooth muscle (see Burnstock, 1979, for a review). Unfortunately, the results of some recent studies do not support this hypothesis (Westfall *et al.*, 1982; Bauer and Kuriyama, 1982). Nevertheless, tetrodotoxin-sensitive release of radiolabeled adenosine derivatives has been demonstrated during field stimulation of intestinal preparations following incubation with [^{3}H]adenosine (Su *et al.*, 1971; Rutherford and Burnstock, 1978) and a small tetrodotoxin-sensitive release of endogenous ATP has been reported into superfusates from electrically stimulated guinea pig taenia coli (Burnstock *et al.*, 1978). However, a recent study with taenia coli bathed or superfused with medium containing firefly luciferin–luciferase failed to demonstrate tetrodotoxin-sensitive release of ATP (White *et al.*, 1981).

Finally, there is evidence that ATP may be co-released from cholinergic (Silinsky, 1975; Morel and Meunier, 1981) and noradrenergic (Katsuragi and Su, 1980) nerve terminals in a variety of neuromuscular preparations, where it or its major metabolite, adenosine, might have functional significance. Release of ATP or adenosine, or both, from preparations of brains has also been described by numerous groups (see Phillis and Wu, 1981; Stone, 1981, for reviews) and possible functions for adenosine and, to a lesser extent, ATP in the CNS have been postulated.

The functional significance of released ATP has not, in many cases, been determined. However, it seems unlikely that an energetically valuable molecule such as ATP would be released from nerves merely as an accident of exocytosis with no physiological consequences. In the periphery, ATP apparently acts at specific P_2 receptors distinguishable from P_1 adenosine receptors in a variety of smooth muscle preparations (Burnstock, 1983). Adenosine triphosphate facilitates the interaction of acetycholine with its receptor at the neuromuscular junction (Ewald, 1976). Extracellular ATP is, as the Holtons showed, a potent vasodilator, and the recent work of Jahr and Jessell (1983) suggests that ATP excites a subpopulation of rat dorsal horn neurones, raising once again the possibility that ATP might be a neurotransmitter in nociceptive pathways. Following release, ATP is rapidly hydrolyzed extracellularly by a Mg^{2+}- or Ca^{2+}-dependent ATPase whose function has yet to be determined (Nagy *et al.*, 1983). Following further degradation by ecto-ATPases and nucleotidases, ATP is ultimately converted to adenosine, which appears to act at P_1 receptors to inhibit the release of certain transmitters (Fredholm *et al.*, 1982; Su, 1983), relax some smooth muscle preparations (Burnstock 1983), and inhibit nueronal activity in the CNS (Phillis *et al.*, 1974, 1975; Phillis and Wu, 1981).

B. Why Study ATP Release from Nerves?

Most neurotransmitters or modulators are not evenly distributed in the brain or peripheral tissues. Where a relatively high concentration of a particular substance occurs, one might suspect a possible physiological role in that tissue. Unfortunately, because of the ubiquitous occurrence of ATP in all cells, total tissue contents of ATP are unlikely to reveal a possible function for ATP as a transmitter or modulator. Only a relatively small proportion of total cellular ATP probably is released during neuronal activity, and ATP content could reflect the intracellular rather than the extracellular requirements for ATP. The problem is compounded in heterogeneous preparations when one realizes that non-neuronal cells also contain and require ATP for normal cellular functions.

Release of ATP, rather than ATP content, is obviously a much more important criterion to be satisfied if one wishes to investigate a possible transmitter or modulator function for ATP in a system. A variety of techniques have been developed over the years to detect the release of ATP. All have certain shortcomings. One of the major problems in studying ATP release is that extracellular ATP is very rapidly metabolized to ADP, AMP, and adenosine in many tissues, so that the levels of extracellular ATP detected are very low. Increases in extracellular adenosine levels could reflect increases in the release of ATP but may also indicate that adenosine itself might be released either presynaptically or postsynaptically in certain tissues.

In this chapter, I outline several methods currently used to detect ATP or adenosine release, give some examples where they have been employed, and discuss the strengths and weaknesses of the various techniques. No attempt is made to provide a complete bibliography of all instances where a particular technique has been employed. Finally, some conclusions are reached regarding the suitability, or lack of suitability, of certain methods for studying the release of ATP.

II. TECHNIQUES FOR EVOKING ATP RELEASE FROM NERVES

A. Criteria for Transmitterlike Release

1. Ca^{2+}-Dependency

Numerous studies have demonstrated that the depolarization-induced release of putative neurotransmitters is dependent on extracellular Ca^{2+}; the corollary to this is that lack of requirement for extracellular Ca^{2+} would be strong evidence against a particular release process being neurosecretory. Therefore, it is important to demonstrate that depolarization-evoked release of ATP from neuronal preparations shows dependency on extracellular Ca^{2+}. Normally, this can be determined by simply omitting Ca^{2+} from the incubation medium, but sometimes the addition of low concentrations of EGTA (e.g., 1 m*M*) to chelate residual Ca^{2+} is necessary to completely abolish release.

2. *Tetrodotoxin Sensitivity*

Under normal physiological conditions *in vivo,* the release of neurotransmitters is thought to result from the propagation of action potentials that invade the terminal, depolarize it, and elicit the influx of Ca^{2+}, which triggers the release process. The propagation of the action potential in nerve results from a rapid increase in Na^+ conductance consequent to the opening of "fast" Na^+ channels in the axonal membrane. Prevention of these increases in Na^+ conductances should block the generation of action potentials and hence the release of transmitters from nerve terminals.

Tetrodotoxin (TTX), a neurotoxin isolated from the puffer fish, specifically blocks Na^+ channels in excitable tissues (Narahashi *et al.*, 1964; Kao, 1966) and can be used to determine if the release process is triggered by the opening of Na^+ channels in the neuronal membrane. Normally, less than 2×10^{-6} *M* TTX should be more than adequate to block propagated action potentials in nerve, and higher concentrations should be avoided since most preparations of TTX available commercially contain large amounts of citrate that could complex extracellular Ca^{2+} and interfere with release by this means. It should be noted that TTX will not prevent the release of transmitters triggered by direct depolarization of nerve endings, such as occurs when the extracellular K^+ concentration is elevated or the nerve terminals are stimulated electrically at parameters sufficient to directly depolarize their membranes.

B. Releasing Techniques

1. *Electrical Stimulation*

Electrical stimulation of nerves to generate propagated action potentials that invade the axon terminals and elicit Ca^{2+}-dependent release of transmitters should be the closest to "physiological" of all the techniques used to evoke ATP release. Unfortunately, electrical stimulation is often not convenient, especially with suspensions of synaptosomes where extremely large currents must be applied to to evoke release, presumably because the current density per synaptosome in the suspension is very low. This limitation can be circumvented to some extent by depositing the synaptosomes as beds onto nylon gauze and then stimulating with electrodes placed on either side of the gauze. Kuroda and McIlwain (1974) used this technique to study the uptake and release of [^{14}C]adenine derivatives from cortical synaptosomes, but found that 5×10^{-7} *M* TTX only reduced evoked release of radiolabel by 50%, suggesting that some direct electrical depolarization of the synaptosomes might have occurred.

Even with intact tissues such as guinea pig taenia coli and vas deferens, TTX-resistant release of ATP has been observed during transmural stimulation at parameters normally thought to evoke "physiological" release of transmitters (White *et al.*, 1981). Failure of TTX to block release is evidence against it resulting from propagated action potentials in nerve and raises the possibility that the stimulating conditions directly depolarized nerve and muscle in the preparations. Studies of this type demonstrate the importance of experiments with TTX in defining the nature of the electrically evoked release process.

Numerous studies of the electrically evoked release of purines have been reported from peripheral and central nerve preparations. The techniques for electrical stimulation of nerve range from field stimulation (Kuroda and McIlwain, 1974), to transmural stimulation (Burnstock *et al.*, 1978; Daval and Barberis, 1981; White *et al.*, 1981; Fredholm *et al.*, 1982), to *in situ* stimulation by electrodes within cortical cups (Sulakhe and Phillis, 1975), to stimulation of discrete nerve pathways both peripherally (Silinsky, 1975) and centrally (Schubert *et al.*, 1976). Stimulation of discrete pathways offers two major advantages over less specific stimulation techniques. The first of these is that discrete pathways are much easier to define in terms of the presence of known transmitters and the synaptic connections present. The second advantage is that the released material (ATP or nucleosides) can be collected at a site remote from the site of electrical stimulation. This method ensures that the release observed originates as a result of propagated impulses along neurons and is not due to local artefacts of electrical stimulation in the immediate vicinity of the electrodes.

2. *Depolarization with Veratridine*

The veratrum alkaloid, veratridine, depolarizes excitable tissues by activating the Na^+ channels present in the cell membranes. Therefore, one would expect veratridine to produce a depolarization of nerve that is quite similar to physiological depolarization insofar as it is mediated by changes in Na^+ conductances. A number of other neurotoxins also activate Na^+ channels (see Catterall, 1980, for a review). Veratridine has been used to release ATP or radiolabeled adenosine derivatives from a variety of neuronal preparations (White, 1978; Fredholm and Vernet, 1979; Jhamandas and Dumbrille, 1980; Bender *et al.*, 1981). It has the advantage over electrical depolarization that it can be applied to suspensions of nerve endings as well as to intact tissues.

The major drawback to the use of veratridine is that it does not mimic exactly physiological depolarizations. Firstly, veratridine at the concentrations normally used (10–50 μM) not only triggers the opening of Na^+ channels but maintains them open for unphysiologically long periods of time (Ulbricht, 1969). Secondly, veratridine may activate Na^+ channels in tissues where the Na^+ channels do not usually function. For example, Villegas *et al.* (1976) have demonstrated the presence of Na^+ channels sensitive to veratrine alkaloids in the membranes of Schwann cells surrounding squid giant axons. Thirdly, the veratridine-induced release of endogenous ATP from brain synaptosomes is actually increased, rather than decreased, in a Ca^{2+}-free medium (White, 1978). A similar enhancement of veratridine-induced release of GABA from brain preparations in the absence of Ca^{2+} has been reported (see Minchin, 1980, for a review). It should be noted, however, that the veratridine-induced release of ATP from varicosities isolated from the myenteric plexus of the ileum, in contrast to brain synaptosomes, is dependent on extracellular Ca^{2+} (White and Leslie, 1982). Finally, recent studies suggest that while veratridine activates Na^+ channels in cultured neuroblastoma cells, it also blocks Ca^{2+} channels in these cells (Romey and Ladzunski, 1982). For all the above reasons, it would seem that veratridine may not be the pharmacological equivalent of electrical stimulation and that one must be cautious in interpreting the results of experiments where veratridine has been used to depolarize cells.

3. Depolarization with Elevated Extracellular K^+

Elevating the extracellular K^+ concentration depolarizes all cells (not just excitable cells) by diminishing the magnitude of the outward-directed K^+ chemical gradient across the cell membrane (Goldman, 1943). Elevating the extracellular K^+ concentration has been the most popular means of evoking the release of neurotransmitters and numerous studies have described the K^+-evoked release of ATP or radiolabeled adenosine derivatives from central and peripheral neuronal preparations (see Stone, 1981; Phillis and Wu, 1981; Su, 1983, for reviews). In most cases, release by K^+ exhibits Ca^{2+}-dependency, although Fredholm and Vernet (1979) have reported a Ca^{2+}-independent release of purines from hypothalamic synaptosomes depolarized by elevated extracellular K^+.

The major advantage of K^+ depolarization is its simplicity; one merely elevates extracellular KCl by 20–50 m*M* to elicit a measurable release of ATP. Moreover, K^+ depolarization can be applied to all neuronal preparations, including suspensions of synaptosomes. The disadvantages of K^+ depolarization are twofold. Firstly, it does not resemble physiological depolarization of nerves since it is not mediated through Na^+ channels. Secondly, elevating the extracellular K^+ concentration of the incubation medium depolarizes all cells, whether neuronal or non-neuronal, so that K^+ depolarization lacks specificity. Nevertheless, the technique has been so widely used in studies of transmitter release that it remains a very useful and convenient means of releasing ATP or other purines from nerves.

4. A23187

A23187 is a Ca^{2+} ionophore that promotes the entrance of Ca^{2+} into cells and triggers neurosecretion in a wide variety of preparations. It is a useful drug for demonstrating that Ca^{2+} entry rather than depolarization *per se* is responsible for stimulating secretion. Katsuragi and Su (1980) have described a Ca^{2+}-dependent efflux of [^{3}H]purines when ^{3}H-adenosine-labeled rabbit pulmonary arteries were exposed to 5 μM A23187.

III. DETECTION OF RELEASE OF ATP OR ITS DERIVATIVES FROM NERVES

A. Radiolabel Techniques

1. Method

The use of radiolabel techniques has been the most widely used method for studying ATP or adenosine release. The reader is referred to the reviews by Phillis and Wu (1981), Stone (1981), and Su (1983) for specific examples. It is simple and convenient, but it suffers from some rather serious shortcomings that are discussed below.

Typically, the tissue is preincubated with 0.1 μM [^{3}H]adenosine (specific activity 10–40 Ci/mmole) or, in some cases, [^{3}H]adenine or [^{14}C]adenosine for 1–120 min to allow the accumulation of radiolabeled adenosine, inosine, AMP, and ATP in the tissue. [^{3}H]-ATP makes up by far the greatest proportion of radiolabeled purine in most tissues (as much as 90%), indicating that the [^{3}H]adenosine is rapidly incorporated into the nucleotide intracellularly. Following loading, the tissue is washed or superfused for variable periods of time to establish a stable rate of resting release of ^{3}H into the medium. Superfusion systems are ideally suited for such purposes. Samples are collected and radioactivity determined by liquid scintillation spectrometry. Once a stable resting release is established, the preparation is stimulated electrically or depolarized with veratridine or KCl as discussed above, and samples of superfusate or supernatant are collected and assayed for radioactivity. Poststimulus samples should also be collected to determine the recovery of [^{3}H]purine release to resting levels.

2. *Advantages*

The method is simple, sensitive and does not require specialized equipment other than a liquid scintillation spectrometer and perhaps a superfusion apparatus of some sort.

3. *Disadvantages*

There are two major disadvantages to experiments with radiolabeled adenosine-loaded cells. The first of these also applies to the other methods, with the exception of the direct-detection method utilizing firefly luciferin–luciferase; namely, that very little ATP (or in this case [^{3}H]-ATP) is detected in superfusates or bathing media following depolarization. The assumption is usually made that [^{3}H]-ATP is released and then rapidly metabolized primarily to [^{3}H]adenosine extracellularly. However, a number of studies have suggested that adenosine may also be released in its own right (Fredholm and Vernet, 1979; Fredholm and Hedqvist, 1980; Pons *et al.*, 1980). This possibility has been reviewed by Phillis and Wu (1981). For instance, Pons *et al.* (1980) reported that the veratridine-induced stimulation of cAMP formation in brain slices, which is thought to be mediated by extracellular adenosine insofar as it is blocked by the adenosine receptor antagonist 8-phenyltheophylline, was unaffected when ectonucleotidase activity was inhibited. They concluded that the adenosine released by veratridine must have been released as adenosine rather than as a nucleotide such as ATP. Maire *et al.* (1982) have also described a release of nucleosides during electrical stimulation of rabbit nonmyelinated nerve axons (without terminals) preincubated with [^{3}H]adenosine; these nucleosides were apparently not derived from the extracellular breakdown of ATP. Finally, Fredholm *et al.* (1982) have presented evidence that [^{3}H]adenosine released from rat vas deferens by nerve stimulation may originate as adenosine postsynaptically from the muscle rather than presynaptically from the nerve. Clearly, one must be cautious in assuming that radiolabeled purines collected extracellularly are necessarily derived from radiolabeled ATP that was released and then degraded extracellularly.

The second and perhaps more serious limitation of the radiolabel method is that the actual amounts of purines released cannot be determined. Even estimates of the relative amounts of nucleotides or nucleosides collected in superfusates are probably not justified, since one has no knowledge of the intracellular specific activities of the radiolabeled compounds during release. Estimates of the specific activities of purines released into the medium are usually out of the question; if one could assay the unlabeled compounds released into the medium, there would be no need for radiosotopic methods in the first place.

Calculation of the amounts of purine released based on the specific activity of the radiolabeled adenosine used to load the tissue is totally unfounded since it will not reflect the true specific activity of the purine intracellularly. It should be pointed out that this erroneous tactic is not unique to studies of purine release but has been applied in numerous studies of transmitter release processes from nerves preloaded with radiolabeled neurotransmitters or precursors. It is quite incorrect.

B. High-Performance Liquid Chromatography (HPLC) with Ultraviolet (UV) Detection

1. Method

Fredholm and Vernet (1979) have described a technique for determining the release of endogenous, unlabeled purines from synaptosomes into superfusates using HPLC with UV detection. Synaptosomes are layered on top of 200 μl of Sephadex G-15 in a plastic 1 ml syringe plugged on the bottom with cotton. A moveable plunger, pierced by plastic tubing is placed 2 cm above the synaptosomal layer and the chamber immersed in a water bath at 37°C. The synaptosomes are superfused with medium at a rate of 0.3 ml/min with a peristaltic pump and 2-min fractions collected in plastic tubes. The synaptosomes are depolarized either (1) by elevating the KCl in the medium to 30 m*M* and decreasing the NaCl by an equivalent amount to maintain isotonicity, (2) by including 10 μ*M* veratridine, or (3) by electrical stimulation with square wave pulses of 2-msec duration at 50 Hz and 10–20 mA current between silver coil electrodes located at a distance of 2 cm. Supernatant (100 μl) is chromatographed isocratically on a 10 μm-bondapack C18 reversed-phase column with 5 m*M* ammonium phosphate (pH 6.0) containing 15% methanol, and the purines are detected by absorbance at 254 nm with a UV absorbance detector. Fredholm and Vernet (1979) reported a slight release of endogenous adenosine, inosine, and hypoxanthine from synaptosomes exposed to veratridine using this technique.

2. Advantages

This method detects endogenous purines. High-performance liquid chromatography with UV detection is widely available in many laboratories.

3. *Disadvantages*

This HPLC procedure gives a relatively poor (flattened) peak shape and a long retention time for adenosine and does not separate ATP from ADP. Use of a gradient (Chapman *et al.*, 1981) may improve separation. The limits of detection with UV detection, although not stated, appear quite poor. Finally, the origin of these nucleosides are unknown, so that they may or may not give a measure of ATP release.

C. High-Performance Liquid Chromatography with Fluorescence Detection

1. *Method*

Wojcik *et al.* (1981) and Wojcik and Neff (1982, 1983) have described a method for derivatizing purine-containing compounds to fluorescent ethenoderivatives by reaction with chloroacetaldehyde. The derivatives can then be separated by HPLC and detected with a fluorescence detector.

Chloracetaldehyde is added to standards and samples in 1.5-ml conical plastic tubes to obtain a final concentration of 220 μM chloracetaldehyde to produce the etheno derivatives. The tubes are capped, mixed, and placed in a boiling water bath for 20 min. The product is chromatographed at 2 ml/min on a reverse-phase column (C18) with 50 mM acetate buffer (pH 4.5) containing 6.5% (vol/vol) acetonitrile and 2 mM 1-octane sulfonic acid (Na-salt, Sigma Chemical Co.). Fluorescence is detected with an excitation at 270 nm and a band pass emission filter to cut off light below 418 nm.

This method provides excellent separation of adenosine from the nucleotides (Figure 1). Wojcik and Neff (1982) point out that the 1-N^6-ethenoadenosine peak can be identified either by altering its retention time by varying the ionic strength and pH of the buffer or by changing the concentrations of the octane sulfonic acid or acetonitrile. Moreover, incubation with adenosine deaminase (A-6648 type V, Sigma; pH 7.5 at room temperature for 10 min) before derivatization will selectively destroy adenosine.

In practice, Wojcik and Neff usually deproteinate their samples with 10 volumes of 0.25 M $ZnSO_4$ and 10 volumes of 0.25 M $Ba(OH)_2$. This also serves to precipate out most of the ATP and 5′AMP (Wojcik *et al.*, 1981), leaving cyclic 3′,5′AMP, adenosine, and ADP. Wojcik and Neff (1983) have used this assay to detect the release of adenosine from rat striatal slices. We have established this assay in our laboratory and can detect as little as 100 fmole adenosine in 20 μl samples. We have also detected the release of endogenous adenosine from rat brain synaptosomes using this technique (W. MacDonald and T. D. White, unpublished observations).

2. *Advantages*

The method is simple and sensitive and detects endogenous purines. The separation of purine compounds and the peak shapes are good. High-pressure

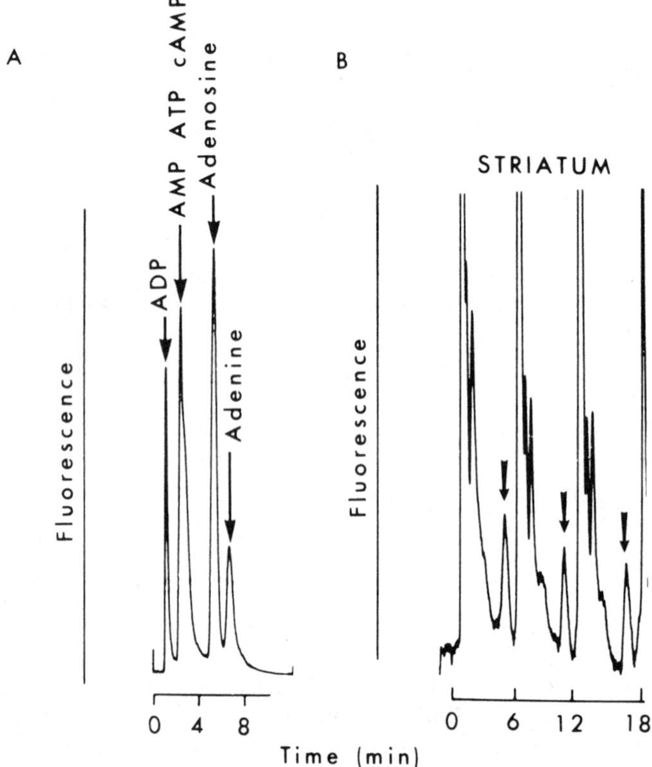

Figure 1. (A) Chromatogram of derivatized adenine-containing standards using HPLC with fluorescence detection. (B) Typical chromatogram of adenine-containing compounds in microwaved rat striatal samples. Arrow indicates adenosine. From Wojcik and Neff (1982), with permission.

liquid chromatography is widely available and fluorescence detectors are relatively inexpensive.

3. Disadvantages

This method is not useful for ATP release, since the nucleotide is rapidly metabolized extracellularly. In any event, deproteinization with $ZnSO_4$–$Ba(OH)_2$ removes ATP from the sample.

D. Two Alternative Methods for Detection of Adenosine

Two new methods for detecting adenosine in biological tissues have been described. To date, these methods have not been applied to studies of adenosine release.

In the first method (Slowiaczek and Tattersall, 1982), adenosine is detected by reaction with a series of enzymes (adenosine deaminase, guanase, peroxidase) to form H_2O_2, which reacts with dichlorofluorescein reagent. The fluoresence is monitored in a fluorescence spectrophotometer; 10 pmoles adenosine can be detected.

In the second method (Newby and Sala, 1982), adenosine is detected by a specific radioimmunoassay. This method can be used to assay large numbers of samples. The major disadvantage of all radioimmunoassays is that they are only as good as the antisera produced, and, in this case, the antibodies do no have affinities as high as one would wish.

Neither of the above methods offer significant advantages over the HPLC–fluorescent method for adenosine, but they might be of some value to laboratories where HPLC is unavailable.

E. Firefly Luciferin–Luciferase Assay for ATP

Certain organisms, notably the firefly, possess the unique ability to produce light by a chemical reaction that requires ATP. In the case of the firefly, the reaction is as follows (Karl and Holm-Hansen, 1976):

$$\text{E (luciferase)} + \text{LH}_2 \text{ (luciferin)} + \text{MgATP} \rightarrow \text{E-LH}_2\text{-AMP} + \text{PP}$$

$$\text{E-LH}_2\text{-AMP} + \text{O}_2 \rightarrow \text{oxyluciferin} + \text{E} + \text{CO}_2 + \text{AMP} + h\nu$$

This provides a very sensitive and specific means of assaying ATP, since the detection of chemiluminescence is inherently much more sensitive than either absorbance or fluorescence spectrophotometry. Several excellent reviews on the use of the luciferin–luciferase assay for ATP have been published and the reader is referred to these for details (Lundin and Thore, 1975; McElroy and Deluca, 1981).

The detection system involves the placing of a cuvette adjacent to a photomultiplier tube in a light-tight chamber. Reagents can be injected into the cuvette by a Hamilton syringe inserted through a rubber septum. In most cases, the rapid injection provides adequate mixing of the reagents. The ATP then reacts with luciferin–luciferase to produce light that is detected by the photomultiplier and recorded. The maximum peak of chemiluminescence obtained bears a linear relationship to the amount of ATP present through a wide range of ATP concentrations (Lundin and Thore, 1975).

In some early studies, liquid scintillation counters were employed to monitor ATP chemiluminescence. However, anyone who anticipates assaying large numbers of samples should obtain some form of chemiluminometer. These cost much less than a scintillation counter, do a better job, and are much more convenient to use. There are a number of chemiluminometers available commercially. I am most familiar with the Chem Glow chemiluminometer (American Instrument Co., Silver Springs, MD), which is a relatively simple apparatus. Some newer instruments offer more sophisticated electronics and data analysis. It is essential that the chemiluminometer have a good mixing system for injected reagents. Be wary of instruments in which only a few microliters of reagent are mixed with a few microliters of sample by microliter syringe; reproducibility of peak height obtained following injection will be compromised with too small volumes.

1. Assay of ATP Released into Medium

a. Method. Numerous studies of the release of ATP have utilized the firefly luciferin–luciferase chemiluminescence assay. The original work of Holton and Holton (1953) used the firefly luminescence method to measure ATP in perfusates of rabbit ears. Silinsky (1975) described a release of ATP or ADP into the bathing medium when the phrenic nerve serving the rat hemidiaphragm was stimulated, and Boyne (1976) detected ATP release from cholinergic vesicles isolated from *Torpedo* electric organ. Finally, as was mentioned above, Burnstock *et al.* (1978) reported a release of ATP into superfusion medium when guinea pig taenia coli or bladder strips were electrically stimulated transmurally.

We have used a simple method to assay the ATP contents of superfusates (Chaudhry *et al.*, 1984), which I describe below. This particular method is only slightly modified from that described by Li and White (1977).

The contents of a vial containing crude luciferin–luciferase equivalent to 50 mg of dried firefly lanterns (Sigma, FLE 50) are reconstituted with 10 ml H_2O to give 5 mg/ml crude extract in 0.01 *M* $MgSO_4$ and 0.25 *M* potassium arsenate buffer. This solution can be stored for 1–2 days at 0–4°C without appreciable loss of activity. Storage serves to reduce the background chemiluminescence of the crude extract (Lundin and Thore, 1975). Before use, 1 mg/ml of crystalline D-luciferin (Sigma) is added to the firefly extract. Addition of D-luciferin greatly increases the net light emitted per unit of ATP in solution (Karl and Holm-Hansen, 1976). Five milliliters of fortified luciferin–luciferase are placed in a gas-tight Hamilton syringe held in a repeating dispenser (American Instruments Co., Silver Spring, MD) situated on top of the reaction chamber of a Chem Glow photometer (American Instruments Co., Silver Spring, MD). The repeating dispenser permits at least one sample to be assayed per minute. A 6 × 50 mm glass cuvette containing 0.5 ml of superfusion medium is placed in the reaction chamber and 0.1 ml of luciferin–luciferase reagent rapidly injected into the cuvette. The maximum peak height of chemiluminescence, which occurs within 1–2 sec at 25°C, is detected on an Aminco photomultiplier and recorded. Standard solutions of ATP in incubation medium are assayed in a similar manner. This method detects as little as 10^{-12} *M* ATP in 0.5 ml of superfusion medium (Chaudhry *et al.*, 1984).

Some argument can be made for using purified luciferase rather than crude firefly lantern extracts such as FLE-50. Purified preparations are less likely to be contaminated with L-luciferin or AMP, both of which may interfere with the assay (Lundin and Thore, 1975). Consequently, these purified enzymes produce a relatively constant light signal without substantial decay. However, if one measures the maximum peak height of chemiluminescence, this is probably not a problem. We have not encountered any difficulties with the crude preparations, which are much less expensive than purified luciferase.

b. Advantages. The firefly luciferin–luciferase assay is a simple and specific method for measuring endogenous ATP in incubation medium, with sensitivities in the order of 10^{-12} *M* ATP in 0.5 ml of sample. One should be able to assay 60 samples per hour with an appropriate repeating dispenser system.

c. Disadvantages. Once again, the major disadvantage of this assay is that much of the released ATP is rapidly hydrolyzed following release, so that very little residual ATP may be detected in media or superfusates. The assay requires the purchase or manufacture of specialized equipment (e.g., a chemiluminometer). D-Luciferin used in the assay is expensive.

2. "On-Line" Direct Detection of ATP Release

All of the aforementioned methods for studying ATP release from nerves suffer from the limitation that very little ATP is detected in perfusates, presumably because the released ATP is rapidly degraded extracellularly by ecto-ATPases or nucleotidases. In 1976, Israel *et al.* described an ingenious method for directly and continuously detecting the release of ATP from the electric organ of *Torpedo marmorata* during electrical stimulation of its motor nerve. They superfused the organ with incubation medium containing crude luciferin–luciferase and directly detected the release of ATP by monitoring the light produced from the ATP–luciferin–luciferase reaction with a photomultiplier. Presumably, the luciferase, which has a high affinity for ATP, reacts with released ATP before the latter can be degraded by ecto-ATPases or nucleotidases. In the case of the *Torpedo* electric organ, most of the ATP appeared to be released postsynaptically from the muscle rather than from the nerve (Israel *et al.,* 1976).

In fact, Israel *et al.* (1976) were not the first to detect directly the release of ATP from cells incubated in medium containing luciferin–luciferase. In 1973, Detwiler and Feinman directly detected the thrombin-induced release of ATP from human blood platelets incubated in medium containing crude firefly extract.

The study of Israel *et al.* (1976) prompted us to see if this method could be applied to synaptosomal preparations, where a postsynaptic source for release of ATP would be eliminated. Synaptosomes prepared from rat brains were incubated in medium containing luciferin–luciferase fortified with added D-luciferin and the release of ATP detected in response to elevated K^+ and veratridine (White 1977, 1978). K^+-evoked release was Ca^{2+} dependent, but veratridine-evoked release was actually augmented rather than reduced in the absence of extracellular Ca^{2+} (White, 1978). We have since employed this method to studies of the regional distribution of ATP in brain (Potter and White, 1980), the possibility of co-release with a variety of transmitters in brain (White *et al.,* 1980; Potter and White, 1982), and, more recently, the release of ATP from varicosities isolated from the myenteric plexus of guinea pig ileum (White and Leslie, 1982). In the latter preparation, the veratridine-evoked release of ATP, unlike that with brain synaptosomes, requires extracellular Ca^{2+}. Subsequent studies have demonstrated that acetylcholine can also initiate the release of ATP from isolated myenteric varicosities (White, 1982; White and Al-Humayyd, 1983) and that much of the evoked release, including that caused by K^+ and veratridine, may originate from noradrenergic terminals present in the preparation (Al-Humayyd and White, 1983).

In other studies, K^+-evoked release of ATP from cholinergic synaptosomes isolated from the *Torpedo* electric organ has been described (Morel and Meunier, 1981). Tetrodotoxin-resistant release of ATP has been detected when guinea-pig taenia coli and vas deferens (White *et al.*, 1981) and rabbit bladder detrusor strips (Chaudhry *et al.*, 1984) were superfused with medium containing luciferin–luciferase and stimulated transmurally using platinum ring electrodes.

a. Method. The method for detecting ATP release described here is taken from White (1978). We usually suspend synaptosomes in a Krebs–Henseleit bicarbonate medium but have also used Tris-buffered media. The synaptosomal suspension should not be too concentrated (less than 4 mg protein/ml) or quenching of the light emitted from the ATP–luciferin–luciferase reaction can occur. Into a 6 × 50 mm cylindrical cuvette are placed 0.5 ml of synaptosomal suspension and 0.02 ml of fortified luciferin–luciferase enzyme preparation. The latter should be prepared daily by adding 0.2 ml synthetic D-luciferin (5 mg/ml H_2O, stored at −20°) to 0.2 ml of crude firefly lantern extract (50 mg Sigma FLE 50 in 2 ml H_2O). The crude firefly extract can be stored at 4°C for several days. Fortification of the luciferin in the crude extract by purified D-luciferin is essential for the detection of ATP release, presumably because the crude firefly extract is deficient in D-luciferin (Karl and Holm-Hansen, 1976).

The cuvette is placed into the reaction chamber of a Chem Glow chemiluminometer (American Instruments Co., Silver Spring, MD) and let stand until a fairly constant level of background light emission is attained, usually 1–2 min. Release studies are usually performed at temperatures at or below 30°C, since we have found that higher temperatures inactivate the enzyme. The synaptosomes are depolarized by rapidly injecting 0.01 ml of appropriate drugs (e.g., KCl, veratridine, neurotransmitters, and others). It is essential that the drugs be injected rapidly to ensure adequate mixing or the results obtained may be inconsistent. We have also found that the drugs must be dissolved in incubation medium rather than water, or light artifacts occur, presumably because of tonicity changes.

The release of ATP into the incubation medium is detected by monitoring the light emitted from the ATP–luciferin–luciferase reaction with an Aminco photomultiplier and recorded on a pen-recorder (Figures 2 and 3). Standard solutions of ATP are also injected into each synaptosomal suspension to determine the sensitivity of detection of the system. This must be done for each determination, not only to detect day-to-day variations but to ensure that the drugs being studied do not affect the production of light from the ATP–luciferin–luciferase reaction.

Unfortunately, difficulties are encountered in quantitating the actual amounts of ATP that are released, especially in the case of the veratridine-induced release of ATP from brain synaptosomes, which has a prolonged duration of light response compared with injections of ATP standards (Figures 2 and 3). However, semiquantitative comparisons can be made of the amounts of ATP released based on the maximum peak heights of chemiluminescence produced (Potter and White, 1980). The maximum peak height of light response to injected ATP is directly proportional to the concentration of ATP injected into the medium (White, 1978), indicating that the amount of chemiluminescence above background observed at a given moment probably gives an accurate measure of the concentration of ATP

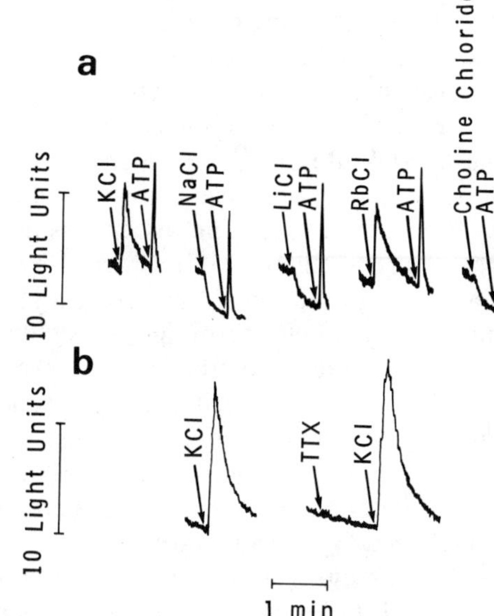

Figure 2. Direct detection of KCl-induced release of ATP from rat brain synaptosomes incubated with luciferin–luciferase. (a) KCl, NaCl, LiCl, RbCl, or choline chloride increased by 23 m*M*. ATP injected as an internal standard to give 9.4×10^{-10} *M*. (b) TTX (4×10^{-7} *M*) did not prevent release of ATP by KCl. From White (1978).

present in the medium at that time. Moreover, the maximum peak heights of chemiluminescence produced by increasing extracellular KCl concentrations are proportional to the log [K^+] and consequently to the degree of depolarization produced (Goldman, 1943). A similar relationship exists for veratridine-induced responses (Potter and White, 1980). From these observations, it follows that the maximum peak height of the light response to KCl or veratridine can be compared with the maximum peak heights in response to known concentrations of ATP and the release of ATP expressed as maximum concentration of ATP achieved in the cuvettes following depolarizations. These values can be standardized against the synaptosomal protein contents or, alternatively, against the occluded lactate dehydrogenase content of the preparation, the latter presumably providing a measure of the yield of synaptosomes (Potter and White, 1980).

Quantitation of the actual amount of ATP released should be possible by integrating the area under the curve and comparing this to responses to ATP

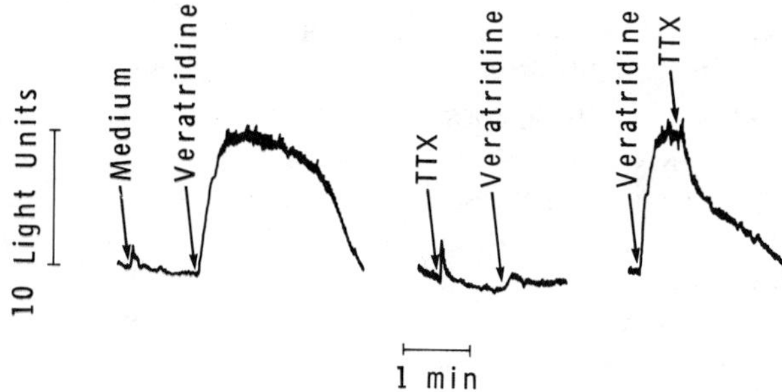

Figure 3. Direct detection of veratridine-induced release of ATP from rat brain synaptosomes incubated with luciferin–luciferase. Veratridine (5×10^{-5} *M*) released ATP by a TTX (4×10^{-7} *M*)-sensitive mechanism. From White (1978).

standards (M. Warenycia and T. D. White, unpublished observations). This is difficult for the long duration responses of brain synaptosomes to veratridine but should be applicable to shorter duration release evoked by KCl.

Release of ATP has been directly detected from smooth muscle preparations superfused with medium containing luciferin–luciferase and stimulated transmurally (White *et al.*, 1984; Chaudhry *et al.*, 1984). The tissue is suspended between two platinum ring electrodes of 2 mm diameter and 1 cm apart and attached by thread to an isometric force transducer within 12 × 15 mm cylindrical cuvettes placed in the chamber of a Chem Glow chemiluminometer with the top removed. The tissue is superperfused, using a Harvard infusion pump, with incubation medium containing luciferin–luciferase (0.67 mg/ml crude firefly extract, Sigma FLE-50, and 0.2 mg/ml synthetic D-luciferin). Medium is withdrawn from the bottom of the cuvette by a peristaltic pump. The entire system, including force transducer and chemiluminometer, is covered with a box and shrouded with black cloth to render the system light-tight. Simultaneous recordings of light produced by the ATP–luciferin–luciferase reaction and mechanical responses of the tissue are recorded on a Grass polygraph.

This technique detected a release of ATP that preceded the mechanical response of the tissue, suggesting it was not the result of muscle movement. However, the release of ATP was not prevented by TTX, indicating that it was not the result of propagated action potentials in nerve (White *et al.*, 1981; Chaudhry *et al.*, 1984).

b. Advantages. This direct method for detecting ATP release offers a number of advantages over other techniques. It very sensitively and specifically detects endogenous ATP release; it is "on-line" and therefore provides short-term temporal indications of release; it avoids collecting and assaying; and it should detect the ATP before the nucleotide can be rapidly degraded by ecto-ATPases.

c. Disadvantages. Although the relative release of ATP can be determined, quantitation of the actual amounts of ATP released is difficult, especially in the case of the superfusion systems. Specialized equipment (a chemiluminometer) is required, and the D-luciferin is costly.

IV. CONCLUSIONS

The advantages and disadvantages of the various methods for detecting the release of ATP or its metabolites from nerve are summarized in Table I. Although radiolabel techniques are simple and sensitive and have been widely used, they are not quantitative and may not accurately reflect the release of endogenous purines. High-performance liquid chromatography with fluorescence detection (Wojcik and Neff, 1982) appears, on balance, to be the method of choice for measuring the release of endogenous adenosine into incubation medium. The firefly luciferin–luciferase assay is highly sensitive and specific for ATP. However, only the "on-line" direct-detection method using luciferin and luciferase in the incubation medium appears capable of detecting the release of ATP before the ATP is rapidly degraded extracellularly by ecto-ATPases and nucleotidases. The

Table I. Methods for Studying the Release of ATP or Adenosine from Nerve

Method	Advantages	Disadvantages	References
Radiolabel technique	Simple, sensitive, inexpensive	Detects little [^{3}H]ATP release, assumes [^{3}H] nucleosides derived from released ATP, does not detect endogenous purines, non-quantitative	Numerous, see reviews by Phillis and Wu (1981), Stone (1981), Su (1983)
HPLC with ultraviolet detection	Simple, detects endogenous purines, quantitative, inexpensive	Poor peak shape for adenosine, poor sensitivity, detects little ATP release, assumes nucleosides derived from released ATP	Fredholm and Vernet (1979), Chapman *et al.* (1981)
HPLC with fluorescence detection	Simple, sensitive, detects endogenous purines, especially useful for adenosine, quantitative, inexpensive	Detects little ATP release, assumes nucleosides derived from released ATP	Wojcik *et al.* (1981), Wojcik and Neff (1982, 1983)
Enzymic-fluorometric method for adenosine	Fair sensitivity, detects endogenous adenosine, quantitative	Expensive, does not detect ATP, assumes adenosine derived from released ATP	Slowiaczek and Tattersall (1982)
RIA for adenosine	Assays large numbers of samples, quantitative	Difficult to prepare antisera, fair sensitivity, does not detect ATP, assumes adenosine derived from released ATP	Newby and Sala (1982)
Luciferin–luciferase assay of ATP in medium	Simple, specific for ATP, very sensitive, assays large numbers of samples, quantitative	Detects little ATP release because ATP degraded extracellularly, requires specialized equipment, D-luciferin is expensive	Silinsky (1975), Boyne (1976), Burnstock *et al.* (1978), Chaudhry *et al.* (1984)
"On-line," direct detection of ATP release with luciferin–luciferase	Simple, very sensitive, specific for ATP, provides temporal indications of release, detects ATP before it can be degraded extracellularly, semiquantitative	Difficult to quantitate, requires specialized equipment, D-luciferin is expensive	Israel *et al.* (1976), White (1977, 1978), Potter and White (1980), Morel and Meunier (1981), White *et al.* (1981)

"on-line" assay offers other advantages, in that it is simple, avoids sampling, and permits continuous monitoring of the release event.

The choice of the tissue preparation in which to study ATP release depends on the questions one wishes answered. Intact tissues, such as nerve–muscle preparations, are more physiological. Accordingly, they are also more complex and the results obtained are difficult to interpret. One must determine if release is presynaptic in origin or occurs postsynaptically from the end organ. Brain slices contain numerous synaptic interconnections that make interpretation of results difficult. Synaptosomal preparations avoid problems of postsynaptic ATP release and synaptic interactions. However, with the exception of electroplax preparations, synaptosomes are heterogeneous, consisting of terminals from a wide variety of nerves; they are also difficult to stimulate electrically.

Electrical stimulation is the method of choice for evoking transmitter release from neural preparations, although clear-cut TTX-sensitivity must be established if one is to conclude that the ATP release is mediated by the propagation of action potentials in nerve. Depolarization with elevated K^+ is convenient and has been widely used. Recent studies suggest that one must be cautious in using veratridine to evoke the release of ATP and other transmitters from nerves. In all cases, a requirement for extracellular Ca^{2+} should be established before one can conclude that the evoked release of ATP or other purines resembles neurosecretion.

REFERENCES

Abood, L. G., Koketsu, K., and Miyamoto, S. 1962. Outflux of various phosphates during membrane depolarization of excitable tissues. *Am. J. Physiol., 202:*469–474.

Al-Humayyd, M., and White, T. D. 1983. Release of ATP from noradrenergic varicosities isolated from guinea-pig myenteric plexus (Abstr.). *J. Neurochem. 41*(Suppl.):S79.

Bauer, V., and Kuriyama, H. 1982. The nature of non-cholinergic, non-adrenergic transmission in longitudinal and circular muscles of the guinea-pig ileum. *J. Physiol., 332:*375–391.

Bender, A. S., Wu, P. H., and Phillis, J. W. 1981. The rapid uptake and release of [^{3}H]adenosine by rat cerebral cortical synaptosomes. *J. Neurochem., 36:*651–660.

Boyne, A. F. 1976. Isolation of synaptic vesicles from *Narcine brasiliensis* electric organ: Some influences on release of vesicular acetylcholine and ATP. *Brain Res., 114:*481–491.

Burnstock, G. 1979. Past and current evidence for the purinergic nerve hypothesis. In: *Physiological and Regulatory Functions of Adenosine and Adenine Nucleotides,* pp. 3–32. Ed. by Baer, H. P., and Drummond, G. I. Raven Press, New York.

Burnstock, G. 1983. A comparison of receptors for adenosine and adenine nucleotides. In: *Regulatory Function of Adenosine,* pp. 49–62. Ed. by. Berne, R. M., Rall, T. W., and Rubio, R. Martinus Nijhoff, Boston.

Burnstock, G., Cocks, T., Kasakov, L., and Wong, H. K. 1978. Direct evidence for ATP release from non-adrenergic, non-cholinergic ("purinergic") nerves in the guinea-pig taenia coli and bladder. *Eur. J. Pharmacol., 49:*145–149.

Catterall, W. A. 1980. Neurotoxins that act on voltage-sensitive sodium channels in excitable membranes. *Ann. Rev. Pharmacol. Toxicol., 20:*15–43.

Chapman, A. G., Westerberg, E., and Siesjo, B. K. 1981. The metabolism of purine and pyrimidine nucleotides in rat cortex during insulin-induced hypoglycemia and recovery. *J. Neurochem., 36:*179–189.

Chaudhry, A., Downie, J. W., and White, T. D. 1984. Tetrodotoxin-resistant release of ATP from superfused rabbit detrusor muscle during electrical field stimulation in the presence of luciferin–luciferase. *Can. J. Physiol. Pharmacol., 62:*153–156.

Daval, J. L., and Barberis, C. 1981. Release of radiolabeled adenosine derivatives from superfused synaptosome beds. *Biochem. Pharmacol., 30:*2559–2567.
Detwiler, T. C., and Feinman, R. D. 1973. Kinetics of the thrombin-induced release of adenosine triphosphate by platelets. Comparison with release of calcium. *Biochemistry, 12:*2462–2468.
Ewald, D. A. 1976. Potentiation of postjunctional cholinergic sensitivity of rat diaphragm muscle by high-energy-phosphate adenine nucleotides. *J. Membrane Biol., 29:*47–65.
Fredholm, B. B., and Hedqvist, P. 1980. Modulation of neurotransmission by purine nucleotides and nucleosides. *Biochem. Pharmacol., 29:*1635–1643.
Fredholm, B. B., and Vernet, L. 1979. Release of ^{3}H-nucleosides from ^{3}H-adenine labeled hypothalamic synaptosomes. *Acta. Physiol. Scand., 106:*97–107.
Fredholm, B. B., Fried, G., and Hedqvist, P. 1982. Origin of adenosine released from rat vas deferens by nerve stimulation. *Eur. J. Pharmacol., 79:*233–243.
Gazelius, B., Brodin, E., Olgart, L., and Panopoulos, P. 1981. Evidence that substance P is a mediator of antidromic vasodilatation using somatostatin as a release inhibitor. *Acta. Physiol. Scand., 113:*155–159.
Goldman, D. E. 1943. Potential impedance and rectification in membrane. *J. Gen. Physiol., 27:*37–60.
Holton, P. 1959. The liberation of adenosine triphosphate on antidromic stimulation of sensory nerves. *J. Physiol., 145:*494–504.
Holton, F. A., and Holton, P. 1953. The possibility that ATP is a transmitter at sensory nerve endings. *J. Physiol., 119:*50–51P.
Holton, F. A., and Holton, P. 1954. The capillary dilator substances in dry powders of spinal roots: A possible role of adenosine triphosphate in chemical transmission from nerve endings. *J. Physiol., 126:*124–140.
Israel, M., Lesbats, B., Meunier, F. M., and Stinnakre, J. 1976. Postsynaptic release of adenosine triphosphate induced by single impulse transmitter action. *Proc. R. Soc. Lond. B., 193:*461–468.
Jahr, C., and Jessel, T. M. 1983. ATP excites a subpopulation of rat dorsal horn neurones. *Nature, 304:*730–733.
Jhamandas, K., and Dumbrille, A. 1980. Regional release of [^{3}H]adenosine derivatives from rat brain *in vivo:* Effect of excitatory amino acids, opiate agonists, and benzodiazepines. *Can. J. Physiol. Pharmacol., 58:*1262–1278.
Kao, C. Y. 1966. Tetrodotoxin, saxitoxin and their significance in the study of excitation phenomena. *Pharmacol. Rev., 8:*997–1049.
Karl, D. M., and Holm-Hansen, O. 1976. Effects of luciferin concentration on the quantitative assay of ATP using crude luciferase preparations. *Anal. Biochem., 75:*100–112.
Katsuragi, T., and Su, C. 1980. Purine release from vascular adrenergic nerves by high potassium and a calcium ionophore, A-23187. *J. Pharmacol. Exp. Ther., 215:*685–690.
Kuroda, Y., and McIlwain, H. 1974. Uptake and release of [^{14}C]adenine derivatives at beds of mammalian cortical synaptosomes in a superfusion system. *J. Neurochem., 22:*691–699.
Li, P. P., and White, T. D. 1977. Rapid effects of veratridine, tetrodotoxin, gramicidin D, valinomycin and NaCN on the Na^+, K^+ and ATP contents of synaptosomes. *J. Neurochem., 28:*967–975.
Lundin, A., and Thore, A. 1975. Analytical information obtainable by evaluation of the time course of firefly bioluminescence in the assay of ATP. *Anal. Biochem., 66:*47–63.
Maire, J. C., Medilanski, J., and Straub, R. W. 1982. Uptake of adenosine and release of adenine derivatives in mammalian non-myelinated nerve fibres at rest and during activity. *J. Physiol., 323:*589–602.
McElroy, W. D., and DeLuca, M. 1981. The chemistry and applications of firefly luminescence. In: *Bioluminescence and Chemiluminescence: Basic Chemistry and Analytical Applications,* pp. 179–186. Ed. by DeLuca, M. E., and McElroy, W. D. Academic Press, New York.
Minchin, M. C. W. 1980. Veratrum alkaloids as transmitter-releasing agents. *J. Neurosci., 2:*111–121.
Morel, N., and Meunier, F. M. 1981. Simultaneous release of acetylcholine and ATP from stimulated cholinergic synaptosomes. *J. Neurochem., 36:*1766–1773.
Nagy, A., Shuster, T. A., and Rosenberg, M. D. 1983. Adenosine triphosphatase activity at the external surface of chicken brain synaptosomes. *J. Neurochem., 40:*226–234.

Narahashi, T., Moore, J. W., and Scott, W. 1964. Tetrodotoxin blockage of sodium conductance on lobster giant axons. *J. Gen. Physiol., 47:*965–974.

Newby, A. C., and Sala, G. B. 1982. A new procedure for haptenizing adenosine leading to a more specific radioimmunoassay method. *Biochem. J., 208:*603–610.

Phillis, J. W., and Wu, P. H. 1981. The role of adenosine and its nucleotides in central synaptic transmission. *Progr. Neurobiol., 16:*187–239.

Phillis, J. W., Kostopoulos, G. K., and Limacher, J. J. 1974. Depression of corticospinal cells by various purines and pyrimidines. *Can. J. Physiol. Pharmacol., 52:*1226–1229.

Phillis, J. W., Kostopoulos, G. K., and Limacher, J. J. 1975. A potent depressant action of adenine derivatives on cerebral cortical neurones. *Eur. J. Pharmacol., 30:*125–129.

Pons, F., Bruns, R. F., and Daly, J. W. 1980. Depolarization-evoked accumulation of cyclic AMP in brain sites: The requisite intermediate adenosine is not derived from hydrolysis of released ATP. *J. Neurochem., 34:*1319–1323.

Potter, P., and White, T. D. 1980. Release of adenosine 5′-triphosphate from synaptosomes from different regions of rat brain. *Neuroscience, 5:*1351–1356.

Potter, P., and White, T. D. 1982. Lack of effect of 6-hydroxydopamine pretreatment on depolarization-induced release of ATP from rat brain synaptosomes. *Eur. J. Pharmacol., 80:*143–147.

Romey, G., and Lazdunski, M. 1982. Lipid-soluble toxins thought to be specific for Na^+ channels block Ca^2 channels in neuronal cells. *Nature, 297:*79–80.

Rutherford, A., and Burnstock, G. 1978. Neuronal and non-neuronal components in the overflow of labelled adenyl compounds from guinea-pig taenia coli. *Eur. J. Pharmacol., 48:*195–202.

Schubert, P., Lee, K., West, M., Deadwyler, S., and Lynch, G. 1976. Stimulation-dependent release of ^{3}H-adenosine derivatives from central axon terminals to target neurones. *Nature, 260:*541–542.

Silinsky, E. M. 1975. On the association between transmitter secretion and the release of adenine dinucleotides from mammalian motor nerve terminals. *J. Physiol., 247:*145–162.

Slowiaczek, P., and Tattersall, M. H. N. 1982. The determination of purine levels in human and mouse plasma. *Anal. Biochem., 125:*6–12.

Stone, T. W. 1981. Physiological roles for adenosine and adenosine triphosphate in the nervous system. *Neuroscience, 6:*523–555.

Su, C. 1983. Purinergic neurotransmission and neuromodulation. *Ann. Rev. Pharmacol., Toxicol., 23:*397–411.

Su, C., Bevan, J. A., and Burnstock, G. 1971. ^{3}H-adenosine triphosphate: Release during stimulation of enteric nerves. *Science, 173:*337–339.

Sulakhe, P. V., and Phillis, J. W. 1975. The release of [^{3}H]adenosine and its derivatives from cat sensorimotor cortex. *Life Sci., 17:*551–556.

Ulbricht, W. 1969. The effect of veratridine on excitable membranes of nerve and muscle. *Ergebn. Physiol., 61:*19–61.

Villegas, J., Sevcik, C., Barnola, F. V., and Villegas, R. 1976. Grayanotoxin, veratrine, and tetrodotoxin-sensitive sodium pathways in the Schwann cell membrane of squid nerve fibres. *J. Gen. Physiol., 67:*369–380.

Westfall, D. P., Hogaboom, G. K., Colby, J., O'Donnell, J. P., and Fedan, J. S. 1982. Direct evidence against a role of ATP as the nonadrenergic noncholinergic inhibitory neurotransmitter in guinea pig tenia coli. *Proc. Natl. Acad. Sci., 79:*7041–7045.

White, T. D. 1977. Direct detection of depolarization-induced release of ATP from a synaptosomal preparation. *Nature, 267:*67–68.

White, T. D. 1978. Release of ATP from a synaptosomal preparation by elevated extracellular K^+ and by veratridine. *J. Neurochem., 30:*329–336.

White, T. D. 1982. Release of ATP from isolated myenteric varicosities by nicotinic agonists. *Eur.J. Pharmacol., 79:*333–334.

White, T. D., and Al-Humayyd, M. 1983. Acetylcholine releases ATP from varicosities isolated from guinea pig myenteric plexus. *J. Neurochem., 40:*1069–1075.

White, T. D., and Leslie, R. A. 1982. Depolarization-induced release of adenosine 5′-triphosphate from isolated varicosities derived from the myenteric plexus of the guinea pig small intestine. *J. Neurosci., 2:*206–215.

White, T., Potter, P., and Wonnacott, S. 1980. Depolarization-induced release of ATP from cortical synaptosomes is not associated with acetylcholine release. *J. Neurochem., 34:*1109–1112.

White, T., Potter, P., Moody, C., and Burnstock, G. 1981. Tetrodotoxin-resistant release of ATP from guinea-pig taenia coli and vas deferens during electrical field stimulation in the presence of luciferin–luciferase. *Can. J. Physiol. Pharmacol., 59:*1094–1100.

Wojcik, W., Olianas, M., Paranti, M., Gentleman, S., and Neff, N. H. 1981. A simple fluorometric method for cAMP: Application to studies of brain adenylate cyclase activity. *J. Cyclic Nucleotide Res., 7:*27–35.

Wojcik, W. J., and Neff, N. H. 1982. Adenosine measurement by a rapid HPLC-fluorometric method: Induced changes of adenosine content in regions of rat brain. *J. Neurochem., 39:*280–282.

Wojcik, W. J., and Neff, N. H. 1983. Location of adenosine release and adenosine A2 receptors to rat striatal neurons. *Life Sci., 33:*755–763.

II

Adenosine Metabolism

Chapter **4**

The Study of Adenosine Metabolism in Isolated Cells and Tissues

J. Frank Henderson

Cancer Research Group
McEachern Laboratory
and Department of Biochemistry
University of Alberta
Edmonton, Alberta, Canada

I. INTRODUCTION

Meaningful studies of adenosine metabolism in isolated animal cells and tissues rely on a thorough understanding of the pathways of adenosine metabolism, on an appreciation of the complications involved in measuring the rates of these pathways, and on a knowledge of the criteria that must be met by methods for the preparation of biological systems and for incubation and extraction. These points are considered herein, together with the several experimental approaches to the study of adenosine metabolism that are commonly used; in addition, a number of methods for the separation of adenosine and its metabolites are given.

A. Primary Pathways of Adenosine Metabolism

The major pathways of adenosine metabolism are relatively simple. Thus, there are two main routes of adenosine utilization, phosphorylation to adenylate by adenosine kinase and deamination to inosine by adenosine deaminase. There are also two main routes of adenosine formation, dephosphorylation of adenylate by 5′-nucleotidases or phosphatases and cleavage of adenosylhomocysteine by adenosylhomocysteine hydrolase. These four routes may be depicted as follows:

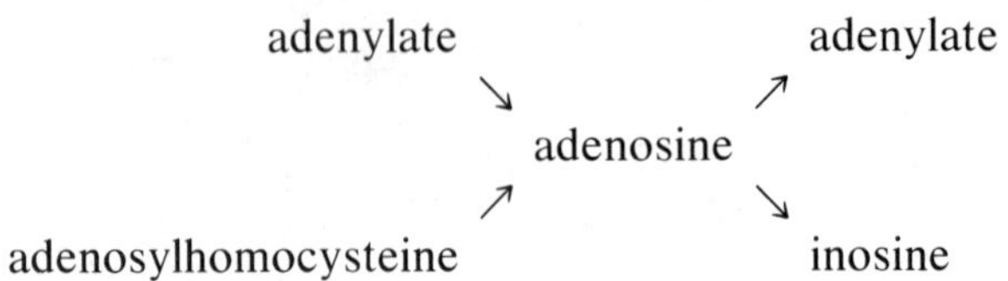

B. Minor and Secondary Pathways

The quantitative measurements of the primary pathways of adenosine metabolism in intact cells and tissues is complicated by a number of factors, particularly the existence of minor pathways of adenosine metabolism and of secondary routes of metabolism that affect the precursors and products of adenosine metabolism.

The interconversion of adenosylhomocysteine and adenosine is reversible, although this reaction in cells usually proceeds predominantly in the direction of adenosine formation. Adenosylhomocysteine formation from adenosine is not promoted (or only slightly increased) by raising the adenosine concentration, but it can be accelerated by the addition of homocysteine.

Another reaction that must be noted is the reversible conversion of adenosine and adenine, apparently by a nucleoside phosphorylase (adenosine + phosphate $\rightleftharpoons$ adenine + ribose-1-phosphate). In most systems this appears to be a quantitatively minor reaction, but its rate is considerably increased as a result of mycoplasma infection.

Other pathways, which probably are of minor importance in most experimental systems, include the formation of adenosine from 3′-adenylate and from adenosine end-groups in RNA.

The study of adenosine metabolism in intact cells and tissues is also complicated by the further metabolism of the adenylate and inosine that are the immediate products of adenosine utilization. Adenylate is readily converted to the corresponding di- and triphosphates, and ATP usually is the quantitatively most important product of adenosine phosphorylation. In some systems an appreciable amount of ATP derived from adenosine may also be incorporated into RNA, converted to coenzymes such as adenosylmethionine or NAD, or both. Adenylate itself may also be deaminated to inosinate and this nucleotide may be further transformed to guanine nucleotides and dephosphorylated to inosine; in most systems this pathway is considerably less important than phosphorylation of adenylate. These reactions are outlined as follows:

ATP ⟶ RNA, coenzymes
↑
ADP
↑
adenylate ⟶ inosinate ⟶ ⟶ guanine nucleotides
↓
inosine

The inosine formed by the deamination of adenosine is also readily metabolized by cells. The primary reaction is phosphorolysis to hypoxanthine; there is little or no phosphorylation of inosine in mammalian tissues. The hypoxanthine so formed may be further metabolized to xanthine and uric acid if xanthine oxidase is present, and the uric acid converted to allantoin if urate oxidase is present. Alternatively, the hypoxanthine may react with phosporibosyl pyrophosphate to form inosinate, and this nucleotide may be converted to both adenine and guanine nucleotides. These reactions are outlined as follows:

inosine ⟶ hypoxanthine ⟶ inosinate
↓
xanthine ⟶ uric acid ⟶ allantoin

The metabolism of the precursors of adenosine formation in intact cells and tissues also needs to be considered. Both adenylate and adenosylhomocysteine normally are present in low concentrations, and both are produced from the same major metabolite, ATP (ATP → ADP → adenylate; ATP → adenosylmethionine → adenosylhomocysteine). In addition, adenylate is also produced by the metabolism of various adenine nucleotide coenzymes and is a product of RNA degradation by certain nucleases.

Examination of these several sets of reactions also makes it apparent that adenosine participates in several *cycles* of metabolism. One such cycle is simply: adenosine ⇆ adenylate. Two others involve the phosphorylation of adenosine to ATP and the subsequent conversion of ATP back to adenosine via both adenylate and adenosylhomocysteine:

adenosine → ATP → adenylate → adenosine
adenosine → ATP → adenosylhomocysteine → adenosine

C. Experimental Approaches

Because adenosine metabolism in intact cells and tissues is in fact so much more complicated than its primary reactions would suggest, and because the immediate precursors of adenosine (adenylate and adenosylhomocysteine) do not enter cells at appreciable rates, experimental studies of this subject usually take two quite distinct approaches. The more common experimental design is to measure the metabolism of exogenously supplied adenosine. The other approach is to study the metabolism of endogenous adenosine and the cycles of adenosine metabolism. These two topics will be considered separately here.

Studies of the metabolism of both exogenous and endogenous adenosine often are aided by the use of inhibitors of one or the other major route of adenosine utilization, deamination and phosphorylation, and this matter will be considered briefly. (A more extensive discussion of adenosine deaminase inhibitors is found elsewhere in this volume, as is a consideration of adenosine uptake into cells and inhibitors of this process.)

II. BIOLOGICAL SYSTEMS

Isolated cells and tissues that have been used in studies of adenosine metabolism include the following: erythrocytes, platelets, and leukocytes derived from blood;

cultured cells in suspension and monolayer cultures; tissue slices; disaggregated cells from tissues, e.g., hepatocytes; and isolated perfused organs, particularly heart. The methods used to prepare these cells and tissues for biochemical studies will not be considered here; however, some general comments will be made regarding matters that specifically effect adenosine metabolism.

ATP concentrations must be maintained at satisfactory levels and rates of adenosine formation must not be appreciably accelerated during the process of preparing the biological system for study. In some cases, this will mean that glucose, oxygen, and phosphate should be present, that the preparation should be done rapidly, or that the system should be chilled; systems vary in their characteristics. Another requirement is that minimal damage be done to cells so that enzymes of adenosine metabolism do not leak into the medium. Finally, it should be noted that incubations have been carried out at a wide range of cell densities; for example, erythrocytes have been studied at concentrations of between 2 and 40%. The cell density used will affect the incubation times and adenosine concentrations that are appropriate and will also affect the incubation conditions needed to maintain satisfactory ATP concentrations.

III. EXOGENOUS ADENOSINE

Adenosine metabolism often is thought of simply in terms of exogenous adenosine, the adenosine supplied to an experimental system by the investigator. In this case, the only major pathways of metabolism to be considered are deamination of adenosine to inosine and its phosphorylation to adenylate. A variety of factors affect the measurement of these pathways, and a number of analytical methods have been applied to this problem.

A. Incubation Conditions

The conditions used for the incubation of isolated cells and tissues, or those used for the perfusion of isolated organs, can affect studies of adenosine metabolism in the following ways: by altering the concentration of adenosine originally present in the cells or its rate of synthesis, or both; by altering the availability of ATP for adenosine phosphorylation; or by altering the relative rates of metabolism of the products of adenosine phosphorylation and deamination. Factors that are particularly important are, first, glucose, oxygen, and anything else that might affect the concentration and generation of ATP, and, second, the concentration of phosphate that is present.

If the concentration of ATP and its rate of generation in the biological system under study are not satisfactory, adenine nucleotides will break down, and this occurrence may, depending on the system, lead to some accumulation of adenosine, which could lead to an unexpected dilution of specific activity of added radioactive adenosine. A second potential consequence of decreased availability of ATP is lowered rates of phosphorylation of adenosine, adenylate, and ADP.

Finally, lowered ATP concentrations might be associated with increased metabolism of adenylate by deamination to inosinate.

The status of an experimental system with respect to its energy requirements is most easily assessed by measuring the ratio of the concentrations of ATP and ADP; this ratio should be 5 or greater for satisfactory results.

Inorganic phosphate can have several effects on studies of adenosine metabolism. First, very low phosphate may reduce the rate of ATP generation. Second, the phosphorolysis of inosine is phosphate dependent; hence, the balance between inosine and hypoxanthine can be affected by phosphate concentration. Phosphate is also a required allosteric activator of phosphoribosyl pyrophosphate synthetase and is, therefore, an important determinant of the availability of phosphoribosyl pyrophosphate; this property affects the relative amount of conversion of hypoxanthine to inosinate. Finally, in at least some systems, high phosphate concentrations inhibit the dephosphorylation of purine nucleotides (Whelan and Bagnara, 1979), whereas moderate phosphate concentrations may stimulate adenosine phosphorylation (Hawkins *et al.,* 1980). The uptake of phosphate by cells is not a rapid process, and intracellular phosphate concentrations often are lower than those in the medium.

B. Extracellular Adenosine Metabolism

If the object of the experiments under consideration is to measure the metabolism of adenosine in a particular cell or tissue, then it is important to exclude or minimize its metabolism in the medium. Though the phosphorylation of adenosine is not likely to occur, extracellular deamination can be a quantitatively very important process. One cause of such undesired metabolism is the use of incubation media that contain sera that have adenosine deaminase activity; bovine sera, for example, whether fetal, newborn, or adult, are high in adenosine deaminase. This problem can be alleviated by using horse serum, which has very low or no adenosine deaminase activity (though each lot should be checked), by inactivating this enzyme activity by heating at 56°C for some hours (Schwartz *et al.*, 1974), or by treating the serum or medium with an inhibitor of adenosine deaminase (see below).

A second problem that sometimes occurs is that adenosine deaminase may be released into the medium from the cells that are being used. This usually occurs when tissue slices or tissues disaggregated by enzyme or mechanical treatment are being used, as the preparations inevitably contain damaged or ruptured cells. In such cases it is helpful to incubate the cell preparation once or twice for 15 to 30 min, after which the medium is discarded and replaced with fresh medium. The experiment is then begun when leakage of adenosine deaminase has reached a minimum level.

Some types of cells, e.g., lymphocytes and lymphoblasts, also tend to become leaky or to lyze entirely when incubated in the absence of protein or when washed by resuspension in protein-free solutions. This outcome may be prevented or minimized by the addition of 1–5% bovine serum albumin to these solutions. (Some preparatives of bovine serum albumin contain adenosine deaminase activity, however, so it is necessary to assay each lot.) The same cells may even release adenosine deaminase when incubated in complete cell culture media.

C. Commercial Preparations of Adenosine

All commercial preparations of adenosine should be checked for purity and if necessary repurified before used; reverse-phase high-performance liquid chromotography (HPLC) is a particularly convenient purification method. Radioactive preparations that have been stored for some time should be rechecked before use.

Radioactive preparations that have been used or that are available include [8-^{4}C]adenosine, [U-^{14}C]adenosine, [8-^{3}H]adenosine, [2-^{3}H]adenosine, [2,8-^{3}H]adenosine, and [2,8,5′-^{3}H]adenosine. [U-^{14}C]Adenosine and adenosine containing tritium in the 5′ position are satisfactory for the measurement of adenosine phosphorylation. However, upon phosphorolysis of the inosine formed by deamination of adenosine, the label in the ribose moiety will be separated from that in the base; the radioactive sugar phosphates and other metabolites formed from the ribose moiety will therefore have to be separated from other metabolites.

Tritiated compounds need to be lyophilized periodically to remove tritiated water formed by tritium–hydrogen exchange; such exchange also diminishes the specific activity of the radioactive adenosine. The rate of this exchange is said to be different for 2-labeled adenosine than for that labeled at the 8 position. Tritium in the 2 position of adenosine will be lost upon the oxidation of inosinate to xanthylate and of hypoxanthine to xanthine; this loss may be an advantage or disadvantage, depending on the design of the experiment.

D. Adenosine Concentration

An extremely important factor to be considered in studies of adenosine metabolism in intact cells is the concentration of adenosine that is used. Among the factors to be considered is the requirement in most types of experiments that the added adenosine not be used up prior to the end of the incubation; thus, the relationships among incubation time, mass of tissue used, and adenosine concentration need to be determined. In addition, it has been found that high concentrations of adenosine inhibit adenosine phosphorylation in some biological systems (Hawkins *et al.*, 1980) and, in some cases, that the addition of high concentrations of adenosine leads to accelerated rates of ATP breakdown (Henderson *et al.*, 1979). Furthermore, in some tissues the activity of adenosine deaminase is much greater than that of adenosine kinase; thus, a prolonged incubation time may be required to produce measurable amounts of adenine nucleotides. During a long incubation, however, high deaminase activity may lead to a substantial reduction in adenosine concentration.

The most important fact, however, is the complex relationships that are now known to exist between adenosine concentration and the rates of the two principal reactions of its utilization, namely, deamination and phosphorylation. The most recent study of this subject has shown three patterns of adenosine metabolism (Snyder and Lukey, 1982). Thus, one group of tissues predominantly phosphorylates adenosine over a wide range of concentrations; mouse liver, brain, and heart are in this group. In a second group (mouse lung, kidney, skeletal muscle, and erythrocytes), phosphorylation is more rapid than deamination at low adenosine concentrations, whereas deamination is greater than phosphorylation at high substrate concentrations. Finally, in still other tissues (mouse spleen leukocytes and thymocytes), deamination is quantitatively the more important reaction at all adenosine concentrations. Inasmuch as relative activities and properties of adenosine deaminase and adenosine kinase are known to vary among tissues and among species, these relationships need to be established in each biological system.

E. Extraction Conditions

Before the final extraction of metabolites, cells sometimes are concentrated and separated from the incubation medium; they may or may not also be washed by resuspension in fresh medium or other solutions. These steps may be taken to produce a concentrated extract, to restrict the final extract to intracellular metabolites, or to remove unused extracellular adenosine, for example, so that it does not interfere with the subsequent separation and measurement of metabolites. Care must be taken to see that such procedures do not lead to cell leakage or lysis and do not lead to any breakdown of nucleotides; as previously stated, this requirement can be verified by measuring ATP:ADP ratios.

The immediate product of adenosine deamination, namely, inosine, and several of its potential metabolites (hypoxanthine, xanthine, uric acid, and allantoin) readily diffuse out of cells; hence, at the end of an incubation, most of these products will be found in the medium, rather than inside the cells. Failure to measure these metabolites in the medium will result in inaccurate estimates of adenosine deamination; therefore, if cells are separated from medium and washed at the end of the incubation, it is necessary to measure metabolites in cells, medium, and wash solutions. (This problem however, does not apply to the measurement of adenosine phosphorylation, as the products of this reaction do not diffuse out of the cells.)

Metabolites finally are extracted under conditions that also stop enzyme activity; usually 0.4 *M* perchloric acid is used, though trichloracetic acid or methanol or boiling aqueous buffer have also been employed. Homogenization of the biological preparation in the extractant may or may not be necessary. Isolated perfused tissues often are quickly frozen to liquid nitrogen temperature and ground to a power before extraction. The extraction should be allowed to proceed for 15–30 min at 4–10°C for maximum recovery of metabolites. If perchloric acid has been used, it is then necessary to bring the extract to neutral pH (pH 5–8) in order to prevent the breakdown of nucleotides. This traditionally has been done using KOH, K_2CO_3 or KOH in $KHCO_3$; precipitated $KClO_4$ is then removed after brief storage at between −20 and 4°C. More recently, however, the perchlorate anion has been extracted into a solution of Alamine in Freon*; this procedure is rapid,

* Alamine 336: The McKerson Corp., 3776 North Dunlop St., Arden Hills, Minnesota 55112; Freon-TF: E.I. du Pont de Nemours and Co., Inc.

simple, produces extracts of more uniform pH (ca. pH 5), and makes a more salt-free extract (Khym, 1975). Some systems (e.g., monolayer cultures) require considerably larger volumes of extractant, such as perchloric acid, than others; if the volume should have to be reduced for subsequent analysis, care needs to be taken that breakdown of nucleotides does not take place.

When monolayer cultures are used, cells may be extracted either *in situ* or following removal from the substratum and centrifugation. In the latter case, the method of harvesting is important: Delhotal *et al.* (1983) have recently shown that ATP concentrations are higher when trypsinization is used instead of scraping. Alternatively, the medium may be removed rapidly and cells chilled quickly both by placing the plate on ice water and by addition of ice-cold saline; after removal of the saline, cold perchloric acid is then added.

It is useful to evaluate the extraction procedure used by measuring the ATP:ADP ratio.

F. Separation and Detection of Metabolites

It is evident that adenosine phosphorylation in intact cells and tissues cannot be assessed simply by measuring adenylate, nor its deamination merely by measuring inosine; the metabolism of both products is sufficiently complex that a number of metabolites have to be measured. The usefulness as well as the sensitivity of different analytical methods will depend on whether radioactive or nonradioactive adenosine is used as substrate, as well as on other requirements of the biological system and experimental design. The most important consideration, of course, is whether it is necessary to measure both phosphorylation and deamination together or only one of these reactions.

1. Radioactive Adenosine

Measurements of adenosine deamination using radioactive adenosine are very sensitive and, with recent developments in methodology, relatively simple. Deamination of adenosine is followed by measuring radioactivity in inosine and hypoxanthine, and, if necessary in particular systems, that in xanthine, uric acid, allantoin, and inosinate as well. Phosphorylation is followed by measuring radioactivity in adenylate, ADP, and ATP; in some systems it may also be necessary to measure radioactivity in other ribonucleotides, in adenine-containing coenzymes, and in RNA. When both reactions are being measured, it obviously is necessary to separate all of the appropriate metabolites and measure their radioactivity.

Separation methods that have been used in recent studies of adenosine metabolism include paper chromatography, thin-layer chromatography (TLC), HPLC, and electrophoresis. A selection of these methods, as reported in recent publications, is given in Tables I to V; the original papers should be consulted for details, and these methods need to be evaluated in each laboratory.

Methods of measuring the conversion of the ribose moiety of [U-^{14}C]adenosine to $^{14}CO_2$ are given by Nordeen and Young (1976).

Table I. Paper Chromatography Systems

Conditions	Compounds separated	References
Isobutyric acid, 1.0 *M* ammonia, 0.1 *M* EDTA[a] (100:160:1.6)	Adenine nucleotides, adenosine, adenine	Lerner and Rubinstein (1970)
1 *M* ammonium acetate, pH 5.0, 95% ethanol (3:7)	Adenine nucleotides, adenosine	Plagemann (1971)
Saturated ammonium sulfate, 0.05 *M* phosphate buffer, pH 6.0, isopropanol (79:19:2)	Adenosine, inosine, adenine, hypoxanthine	Plagemann (1971)
85% saturated aqueous ammonium bicarbonate	Adenosine, inosine, adenine, hypoxanthine	Plagemann (1971)
1-Butanol, water, ammonia (86:14:1)	Adenosine, inosine, adenine, hypoxanthine	Rowe *et al.* (1978)

[a] EDTA, ethylenediaminetetraacetate.

In presenting results of studies of the metabolism of radioactive adenosine, phosphorylation may be equated to the sum of radioactivity (per unit time and unit cell mass) in adenylate + ADP + ATP (plus other metabolites when necessary); deamination may be equated to the sum of radioactivity in inosine + hypoxanthine (plus other metabolites if necessary).

2. *Nonradioactive Adenosine*

Adenosine phosphorylation is usually followed by measuring the increase in ATP concentrations; standard HPLC or enzymatic methods may be used. Deamination may be assessed by measuring ammonia formation (Agarwal *et al.*, 1976), or by the enzymatic assay of inosine or hypoxanthine, or both, or by obtaining some measure of the ribose-1-phosphate formed upon phosphorolysis of inosine (e.g., lactate accumulation or carbon dioxide formation). Because relatively standard methods can be used, and because this approach is less sensitive than when radioactive adenosine is used, it will not be considered further.

IV. INHIBITORS OF ADENOSINE METABOLISM

The experimental study of adenosine metabolism is greatly aided by the ability to inhibit either or both of the major pathways of adenosine metabolism, namely, phosphorylation and deamination. Unfortunately, few of the most useful inhibitors are as yet commercially available.

A. Inhibition of Adenosine Deaminase

The most commonly used inhibitors of adenosine deaminase activity in intact cells and tissues are coformycin, deoxycoformycin (covidarabine) and erythro-9-(2-hydroxy-3-nonyl) adenine (EHNA); these compounds are considered in greater

Table II. One-Dimensional Thin Layer Chromatography (TLC) Systems

Conditions	Compound separated	References
Cellulose		
0.05 aqueous ammonia	Adenine nucleotides, adenosine, inosine, hypoxanthine	Burridge *et al.* (1977a)
1-Butanol, methanol, water, ammonia (60:20:20:1)	Adenine nucleotides, adenosine, inosine plus hypoxanthine	Lomax and Henderson (1972)
1.8 *M* ammonium formate, 2% boric acid, pH 7.0	Adenosine, inosine, adenine, hypoxanthine	Rappaport and Zamecnik (1978)
1-Butanol, propionic acid, water (100:50:70)	Adenosine, inosine, adenine, hypoxanthine	Rappaport and Zamecnik (1978)
Water-saturated 1-butanol, 15 *N* ammonia (100:1)	Adenosine, inosine, hypoxanthine	Bessler *et al.* (1981–1982)
1-Butanol, propionic acid, 4% boric acid (40:25:35)	Adenine nucleotides, adenosine, inosine, adenine, hypoxanthine	Snyder and Lukey (1982)
Silica gel		
1-Butanol, ethyl acetate, methanol, 25% ammonia (7:4:3:3)	Adenosine, adenine, hypoxanthine, inosine, cAMP, adenylate plus ADP plus ATP, adenosylhomocysteine	Schrader and Gerlach (1976), Schrader *et al.* (1981)
1-Butanol, water, ammonia (86:14:1)	Adenosine, adenine, inosine, hypoxanthine	Rowe *et al.* (1978)
1-Butanol, acetone, 33% ammonia, water (50:40:3:15)	Nucleosides, bases	Kolassa *et al.* (1977)
1-Propanol, methanol, 33% ammonia, water (45:15:30:10)	Adenine nucleotides	Kolassa *et al.* (1977)
PEI-cellulose[a]		
0.1 *M* sodium chloride	Adenosine, inosine, hypoxanthine	Namm (1973)
70% 1-propanol	Adenine nucleotides, inosine, hypoxanthine, xanthine	Wong and Henderson (1972)
0.5, 2.0, and 4.0 *M* sodium formate pH 3.4	Adenylate, inosinate, ADP, ATP, GDP, GTP, guanylate, xanthylate	Crabtree and Henderson (1971)
1.25 *M* sodium chloride	Adenylate, ADP, ATP	Jones *et al.* (1972)
0.2 *M* lithium chloride	Adenylate, ADP, ATP, adenosine, inosine, adenine	Willers *et al.* (1982)
0.2 *M* ammonium bicarbonate; then water	Adenylate, ADP, ATP, adenosylmethionine, adenosylhomocysteine, adenosine	Reddington and Pusch (1983)
Isobutanol, ethanol, water (2:1:1)	Adenosylhomocysteine, adenosine, inosine, adenine, hypoxanthine	Reddington and Pusch (1983)

[a] PEI, polyethyleneimine.

Table III. Two-Dimensional Thin-Layer Chromatography (TLC) Systems

Conditions	Compounds separated	References
Cellulose		
1st: acetonitrile, 0.1 *M* ammonium acetate, pH 7.0, ammonia (60:30:10) 2nd: 1-butanol, methanol, water, ammonia (60:20:20:1)	Ribonucleosides, bases	Crabtree and Henderson (1971), Henderson *et al.* (1974)[a]
1st: (a) methanol, (b) methanol, 1-propanol, 25% ammonia, 1% EDTA[b] (3:5:2:6) 2nd: isobutyric acid, 25% ammonia, 1% EDTA (200:9:114)	Ribonucleotides, ribonucleosides, bases	Seipel and Reichert (1977)
PEI-cellulose		
1st: 0.1 *M* sodium chloride 2nd: 1.0 *M* sodium chloride	Ribonucleotides, ribonucleosides, bases	Namm (1973)
1st: 90% formic acid, methanol, water (30:90:15) 2nd: 70% 1-propanol	Ribonucleotides, ribonucleosides, bases	Burridge *et al.* (1977b).

[a] This system has also been used by Smith *et al.* (1977) for the measurement of radioactivity in allantoin.
[b] EDTA, ethylenediamine tetraacetate.

Table IV. Paper Electrophoresis

Conditions	Compounds separated	References
0.045 *M* citrate buffer, pH 4.8; 300 V, 4 hr	Adenylate, AMP, ATP, inosinate, hypoxanthine	Manohar *et al.* (1967)
Pyridine, acetic acid, water, pH 3.5 (1:5:94); 100 V/cm, 40 min	Adenylate, cAMP, ADP, ATP, inosinate, adenine, adenosine, inosine plus hypoxanthine	Shimizu *et al.* (1972)
0.05 *M* sodium citrate, pH 4.6, containing 5 m*M* magnesium sulfate; 25 V/cm	Ribonucleotides, adenine	Dean and Perrett (1976)
0.05 *M* sodium borate, pH 9.0; 3000 V, 90 min	Adenine nucleotides, adenosine, adenine, inosine, hypoxanthine	Meyskens and Williams (1971)
0.05 *M* sodium borate, pH 9.0; 2250 V, 2 hr	Ribonucleosides, bases	Benke and Dittmar (1976)

Table V. High-Performance Liquid Chromatography (HPLC)

Conditions	Compounds separated	References
Reverse-phase		
10 SCX column; 50 m*M* ammonium phosphate, pH 3.0	Ribonucleosides, bases	Whelan and Bagnara (1979)
0.05 column; linear gradient of 10 to 30% B in A: A = 10 m*M* KH_2PO_4; B = 10 m*M* KH_2PO_4, pH 4.9, in 30% methanol	Ribonucleosides	Agarwal *et al.* (1982)
μBondapak C-18 column; 50 m*M* potassium phosphate, pH 6.0, containing 14% methanol	Adenosine, inosine, hypoxanthine	Fredholm and Lerner (1982)
μBondapak C-18 column; 0.05 *M* ammonium phosphate, pH 6.0	Ribonucleotides, ribonucleosides, bases	Ronca-Testoni and Borghini (1982)
Ammonium phosphate: 1st, 0.01 *M*, pH 3.3; 2nd, 0.013 *M*, pH 3.85; 3rd, 0.3 *M*, pH 4.5	Ribonucleotides	Ronca-Testoni and Borghini (1982)
Ion-exchange[a]		
0.002 *M* KH_2PO_4, pH 5.6, to 0.18 *M* KH_2PO_4, plus 0.13 *M* KCl, pH 4.5		Dean and Perrett (1976)
5 m*M* KH_2PO_4, pH 4.0, to 0.3 *M* KH_2PO_4, plus 0.6 *M* KCl, pH 4.5		Kaufman *et al.* (1977)
10 to 500 m*M* NH_4HPO_4, pH 4.0		Whelan and Bagnara (1979)

[a] All procedures listed below are linear gradient systems for the separation of nucleotides.

detail elsewhere in this volume. Although the binding constands for coformycin and deoxycoformycin are ca. 10^{-11} *M*, and that for EHNA ca. 1–6 × 10^{-9} *M* (reviews: Glazer, 1980; Agarwal, 1982), the concentrations that have to be used in experiments using intact cells are in the range 1–10 μ*M;* the entry of these inhibitors into cells is relatively slow.

When used at the minimum concentration required for inhibition of adenosine deaminase activity, the three compounds considered here are relatively specific for this enzyme. At higher concentrations, however, they may inhibit several other aspects of purine metabolism (Henderson *et al.*, 1977).

In studies using exogenous adenosine, it usually is necessary or preferable to carry out a pre-incubation of cells with adenosine deaminase inhibitor, and then to remove unused inhibitor by replacement of the medium prior to addition of the adenosine. This allows the inhibitor to enter the cells and inhibit adenosine deaminase; as adenosine, coformycin and deoxycoformycin compete for entry into cells, it is undesirable for the inhibitors to be present in the medium when the adenosine is added.

The inhibition of adenosine deaminase activity may or may not lead to increased phosphorylation of the added adenosine; this depends on the biological system, adenosine concentration and other factors. However this possibility should always be considered.

B. Inhibition of Adenosine Kinase

Two compounds have been useful for the inhibition of adenosine phosphorylation in intact cells, namely, 4-amino-5-iodo 7-β-D-ribofuranosyl 7H-pyrrolo(2,3-d)pyrimidine (iodotubercidin) (Lomax and Henderson, 1973; Bontemps *et al.*, 1983) and 6-*N*-phenyladenosine (Divekar and Hakala, 1971; J. F. Henderson and K. Boldt, unpublished observations). Relatively high concentrations of these inhibitors are required, ca. 100–400 μM for iodotubercidin and ca. 400 μM for *N*-phenyladenosine. *N*-Phenyladenosine is not a substrate for adenosine kinase; the question whether it is for iodotubercidinis has not been studied. At the concentrations stated above, these compounds have not accelerated ATP breakdown in Ehrlich ascites tumor cells *in vivo,* however, both compounds produced some inhibition of purine biosynthesis *de novo* (Smith, 1975).

V. ENDOGENOUS ADENOSINE

Studies of the metabolism of endogenous adenine may in the first place be carried out simply by measuring the concentration of adenosine under different experimental conditions and, perhaps, in the presence and absence of inhibitors of the major pathways of adenosine utilization. Methods for such studies are considered elsewhere in this volume.

Of concern here, however, are methods by which radioactive adenosine is produced in intact cells and its metabolism studied, without the addition of exogenous radioactive adenosine. Most commonly, cells are incubated with radioactive adenine in order to label intracellular ATP; the adenine is then removed by replacement of the medium in order that radioactive ATP synthesis not continue during the course of the experiments (Lomax and Henderson, 1973). During subsequent incubation the amount of radioactivity in adenosine and its metabolites can then be determined. If desired, the rate of adenosine formation from ATP can be accelerated by interfering with ATP generation, e.g., by addition of 2-deoxyglucose or fructose, or, in the absence of glucose, by anaerobiosis or by addition of inhibitors of oxidative phosphorylation. Again, such experiments may be carried out in the presence and absence of inhibitors of adenosine metabolism.

Technical requirements for such experiments include the ability to label ATP to such an extent that there subsequently will be measurable radioactivity in adenosine and its metabolites and good "energy status" in control cells so that the rate of adenosine formation from ATP will be "normal."

VI. CONCLUSIONS

Good methods now exist for the study of the metabolism of exogenous adenosine in isolated cells and tissues, and the criteria that have to be met to obtain meaningful results are reasonably clear. Considerable species and tissue differences are to be expected, and these need to be explored further. The relevance of studies of exogenous adenosine metabolism in isolated preparations to endogenous adenosine metabolism *in vitro* and *in vivo* and to exogenous adenosine metabolism *in vivo* has yet to be determined. It is important to note, however, that normal plasma and tissue levels of adenosine *in vivo* are ca. 0.5–5 μM.

Some aspects of the metabolism of endogenous adenosine can be studied fairly well. However, further developmental work needs to be done in this area, and in particular the study of the several cycles of adenosine metabolism remains a challenge.

ACKNOWLEDGMENT

The preparation of this review was supported by the National Cancer Institute of Canada.

REFERENCES

Agarwal, R. P. 1982. Inhibitors of adenosine deaminase. *Pharmacol. Ther., 17:*399–429.

Agarwal, R. P., Crabtree, G. W., Parks, R. E. Jr., Nelson, J. A., Keightley, R., Parkman, R., Rosen, F. S., Stern, R. C., and Polmar, S. H. 1976. Purine nucleoside metabolism in the erythrocytes of patients with adenosine deaminase deficiency and severe combined immunodeficiency. *J. Clin. Invest., 57:*1025–1035.

Agarwal, R. P., Major, P., and Kufe, D. W. 1982. Simple and rapid high-performance liquid chromatographic method for analysis of nucleosides in biological fluids. *J. Chromatogr., 231:*418–424.

Benke, P. J., and Dittmar, D. 1976. Purine dysfunction in cells from patients with adenosine deaminase deficiency. *Pediat. Res., 10:*642–646.

Bessler, H., Brosh, S., Sperling, O., Djaldetti, M., and Moroz, C. 1981–1982. The metabolism of adenosine and distribution of adenosine receptor lymphocytes in two human circulating T cell subsets. *J. Immunopharmacol., 3:*265–275.

Bontemps, F., Van den Berghe, G., and Hers, H. -G. 1983. Evidence for a substrate cycle between AMP and adenosine in isolated hepatocytes. *Proc. Natl. Acad. Sci. USA, 80:*2829–2833.

Burridge, P. W., Paetkau, V., and Henderson, J. F. 1977a. Studies of the relationship between adenosine deaminase and immune function. *J. Immunol., 119:*675–678.

Burridge, P. W., Woods, R. A., and Henderson, J. F. 1977b. Purine metabolism in *Saccharomyces cerevisiae*. *Can. J. Biochem., 55:*935–941.

Crabtree, G. W., and Henderson, J. F. 1971. Rate-limiting steps in the interconversion of purine ribonucleotides in Ehrlich ascites tumor cells *in vitro*. *Cancer Res., 31:*985–991.

Dean, B. M., and Perrett, D. 1976. Studies on adenine and adenosine metabolism by intact human erythrocytes using high performance liquid chromatography. *Biochim. Biophys. Acta, 437:*1–15.

Delhotal, B., Lemonnier, F., Couturier, M., and Lemonnier, A. 1983. Influence of two cell harvesting methods on intracellular ATP and amino acid concentrations in human fibroblast cultures. *Biochimie, 65:*121–125.

Divekar, A. Y., and Hakala, M. T. 1971. Adenosine kinase of sarcoma 180 cells. N^6-Substituted adenosines as substrates and inhibitors. *Mol. Pharmacol., 7:*663–673.

Fredholm, B. B., and Lerner, U. 1982. Metabolism of adenosine and 2′-deoxy-adenosine by fetal mouse calvaria in culture. *Med. Biol., 60:*267–271.

Glazer, R. I. 1980. Adenosine deaminase inhibitors: Their role in chemotherapy and immunosuppression. *Cancer Chemother. Pharmacol., 4:*227–235.

Hawkins, C. F., Kyd, J. M., and Bagnara, A. S. 1980. Adenosine metabolism in human erythrocytes: A study of some factors which affect the metabolic fate of adenosine in intact red cells *in vitro. Arch. Biochem. Biophys., 202:*380–387.

Henderson, J. F., Fraser, J. H., and McCoy, E. E. 1974. Methods for the study of purine metabolism in human cells *in vitro. Clin. Biochem., 7:*339–358.

Henderson, J. F., Brox, L., Zombor, G., Hunting, D., and Lomax, C. A. 1977. Specificity of adenosine deaminase inhibitors. *Biochem. Pharmacol., 26:*1967–1972.

Henderson, J. F., Zombor, G., Burridge, P. W., Barankiewicz, G., and Smith, C. M. 1979. Relationships among purine nucleoside metabolism, adenosine triphosphate catabolism, and glycolysis in human erythrocytes. *Can. J. Biochem., 57:*873–878.

Jones, C. E., Parker, J. C., and Smith, E. E. 1972. Determination of myocardial acid-soluble nucleotides on anion-exchange thin layers. *J. Chromatr., 64:*378–382.

Kaufman, I. A., Hall, N. F., DeLuca, M. A., Ingwall, J. S., and Mayer, S. E. 1977. Metabolism of adenine nucleotides in the cultured fetal mouse heart. *Am. J. Physiol., 233:*H282–H288.

Khym, J. X., 1975. An analytical system for rapid separation of tissue nucleotides at low pressures on conventional anion exchangers. *Clin. Chem., 21:*1245–1252.

Kolassa, N., Stengg, R., and Turnheim, K. 1977. Salvage of adenosine, inosine, hypoxanthine, and adenine by the isolated epithelium of guinea pig jejunum. *Can. J. Physiol. Pharmacol., 55:*1039–1044.

Lerner, M. H., and Rubinstein, D. 1970. The role of adenine and adenosine as precursors for adenine nucleotide synthesis by fresh and preserved human erythrocytes. *Biochim. Biophys. Acta, 224:*301–310.

Lomax, C. A., and Henderson, J. F. 1972. Phosphorylation of adenosine and deoxyadenosine in Ehrlich ascites carcinoma cells resistant to 6-(methylmercapto)purine ribonucleoside. *Can. J. Biochem., 50:*423–427.

Lomax, C. A., and Henderson, J. F. 1973. Adenosine formation and metabolism during adenosine triphosphate catabolism in Ehrlich ascites tumor cells. *Cancer Res., 33:*2825–2829.

Manohar, J. V., Denstedt, O. F., and Rubinstein, D. 1967. The metabolism of the erythrocyte. XVII. Mechanism of incorporation of adenine into and resultant elevation of ATP and ADP in human erythrocytes. *Can. J. Biochem., 45:*1153–1161.

Meyskens, F. L., and Williams, H. E. 1971. Adenosine metabolism in human erythrocytes. *Biochim. Biophys. Acta, 240:*170–179.

Namm, D. H. 1973. Myocardial nucleotide synthesis from purine bases and nucleosides. Comparison of the rates of formation of purine nucleotides from various precursors and identification of the enzymatic routes for nucleotide formation in the isolated rat heart. *Circ. Res., 33:*686–695.

Nordeen, S. K., and Young, D. A. 1976. Glucocorticoid action on rat thymic lymphocytes. Experiments utilizing adenosine to support cellular metabolism lead to a reassessment of catabolic hormone actions. *J. Biol. Chem., 251:*7295–7303.

Plagemann, P. G. W. 1971. Nucleotide pools of Novikoff rat hepatoma cells growing in suspension culture. I. Kinetics of incorporation of nucleosides into nucleotide pools and pool sizes during growth cycle. *J. Cell. Physiol., 77:*213–240.

Rappaport, E., and Zamecnik, P. C. 1978. Increased incorporation of adenosine into adenine nucleotide pools in serum-deprived mammalian cells. *Proc. Natl. Acad. Sci. USA, 75:*1145–1147.

Reddington, M., and Pusch, R. 1983. Adenosine metabolism in a rat hippocampal slice preparation: incorporation into S-adenosylhomocysteine. *J. Neurochem., 40:*285–290.

Ronca-Testoni, S., and Borghini, F. 1982. Degradation of perfused adenine compounds up to uric acid in isolated rat heart. *J. Mol. Cell. Cardiol., 14:*177–180.

Rowe, J. N., Van Dyke, K., and Stitzel, R. W. 1978. Purine salvage pathways for the biosynthesis *in vitro* of adenine nucleotides in the guinea pig vas deferens. *Biochem. Pharmacol., 27:*45–51.

Schrader, J., and Gerlach, E. 1976. Compartmentation of cardiac adenine nucleotides and formation of adenosine. *Pflügers Arch., 367:*129–135.

Schrader, J., Schutz, W., and Bardenheuer, H. 1981. Role of S-adenosylhomocysteine hydrolase in adenosine metabolism in mammalian heart. *Biochem. J., 196:*65–70.

Schwartz, P. M., Shipman, C. Jr., and Drach, J. C. 1974. Extensively heat-inactivated calf serum: A tissue culture media supplement devoid of adenosine deaminase activity. *In Vitro, 9:*385.

Seipel, S., and Reichert, U. 1977. Two-dimensional thin-layer chromatography-autoradiography of intracellular purine interconversion products. *J. Chromatogr., 135:*485–488.

Shimizu, H., Tanaka, S., and Kodama, T. 1972. Adenosine kinase of mammalian brain: Partial purification and its role for the uptake of adenosine. *J. Neurochem., 19:*687–698.

Smith, C. M. 1975. Relative importance of alternative pathways of purine nucleotide biosynthesis in Ehrlich ascites tumor cells *in vivo*. M. Sc. Thesis, University of Alberta, p. 39.

Smith, C. M., Rovamo, L. M., Kekomaki, M. P., and Raivio, K. O. 1977. Purine metabolism in isolated rat hepatocytes. *Can. J. Biochem., 55:*1134–1139.

Snyder, F. F., and Lukey, T. 1982. Kinetic considerations for the regulation of adenosine and deoxyadenosine metabolism in mouse and human tissues based on a thymocyte model. *Biochim. Biophys. Acta, 696:*299–307.

Whelan, J. M., and Bagnara, A. S. 1979. Factors affecting the rate of purine ribonucleotide dephosphorylation in human erythrocytes. *Biochim. Biophys. Acta, 563:*466–478.

Willers, I., Singh, S., and Goldde, H. W. 1982. Purine metabolism in fibroblasts of patients with Duchenne's muscular dystrophy. *Human Heredity, 32:*233–239.

Wong, P. C. L., and Henderson, J. F. 1972. Purine ribonucleotide biosynthesis, interconversion and catabolism in mouse brain *in vitro*. *Biochem. J., 129:*1085–1094.

Chapter **5**

Ectonucleotidases

Measurement of Activities and Use of Inhibitors

J. D. Pearson

Section of Vascular Biology
MRC Clinical Research Centre
Harrow, Middlesex, United Kingdom

I. INTRODUCTION

The concept that nucleotidases are present at the cell surface with their active sites accessible to extracellular substrates is nearly 40 years old. Rothstein and Meier (1948) showed that yeast cells possess ectoenzymes capable of catabolizing ATP and ADP, and the demonstration of an ecto-ATPase activity in mammalian nerve cells and red blood cells followed shortly thereafter (Abood and Gerard, 1954; Herbert, 1956). Esner *et al.* (1958) were among the first to use the electron microscope in combination with histochemical techniques to localize ATPase and 5′-nucleotidase (AMPase) activities at the plasma membrane. The cellular specificity of ectonucleotidases was also under investigation; for example, Cummins and Hydén (1962) noted the presence of ecto-ATPase in glial cells but its absence in neurons.

The last decade has seen a great increase in publications concerning ectonucleotidases, particularly 5′-nucleotidase. The known cellular distribution of ectonucleotidase activities has been greatly expanded; the detailed biochemistry of some of the these enzymes has been elucidated; and 5′-nucleotidase has been extensively purified. In the following sections of this chapter, I outline the methods that have been used to study ectonucleotidases, with their advantages and drawbacks, and then summarize what is known of the properties of the enzymes.

Although this book is concerned primarily with methods, I have included a discussion of the possible physiological (and pathological) roles of the ectonucleotidases (Section VIII). This topic is particularly significant because the presence of these enzymes immediately raises as yet unresolved questions concerning the occurrence and function of extracellular nucleotides.

II. EXPERIMENTAL CRITERIA FOR THE IDENTIFICATION OF ECTONUCLEOTIDASES

A. Presence of Ectonucleotidase

Before any detailed characterization of an ectonucleotidase can be performed, it is essential to establish that the activity under investigation is indeed due to an ectoenzyme. The list of appropriate criteria given below is based on those enumerated by De Pierre and Karnovsky (1974a,b) and Newby *et al.* (1975), who were studying ectonucleotidases on granulocytes and fat cells, respectively. It may not be feasible to carry out all of the types of experiments noted in the list, but the conclusion that the activity is due to an ectonucleotidase will be strengthened as more of the following criteria are satisfied.

1. Enzyme Acts on Extracellular Substrate

Demonstrating that a substrate is metabolized at the cell surface is simpler if the substrate is known to be confined to extracellular space: compounds metabolized by ectoenzymes may, if they cross the plasma membrane, also be substrates for intracellular enzymes. Nucleotides do not normally cross intact cell membranes, but can do so under certain conditions (see below).

2. Cellular Integrity Is Maintained

This criterion can be verified in several ways; the most common has been to determine that no measureable release of a cytoplasmic enzyme (such as lactate dehydrogenase) occurs, although it is also desirable (see above) to monitor the permeability of the cell membrane to molecules of a comparable size to the nucleotide substrate. Several biological stimuli (particularly proteases, but also ATP itself at high concentrations) can render the plasma membrane permeable to nucleotides (Rozengurt and Heppel, 1979; Pearson and Gordon, 1979).

3. Enzyme Releases Products Extracellularly

Although ectoenzymes usually release their products into the extracellular medium, it might be postulated that an ectonucleotidase directly transports one or more products of the reaction across the plasma membrane or donates a product to a membrane component. For example, it has been noted that adenosine produced from AMP by the action of ecto-5′-nucleotidase can be taken up more efficiently by cells than exogenously supplied adenosine. There is, however, no evidence that the enzyme is also an adenosine carrier (see Section VIII). Similarly, although some cells possess protein kinases as ectoenzymes, which are capable of transferring the terminal phosphate from extracellular ATP to membrane protein (see Section VII), ectonucleotidases release phosphate to the extracellular medium (De Pierre and Karnovsky, 1974b).

4. Cells Do Not Release Nucleotidase Activity to the Extracellular Medium

Continuous release of enzyme implies that the cell synthesizes and secretes the enzyme to the extracellular space (i.e., it does not physiologically function at the cell surface). Release of declining amounts of activity on repeated washing suggests either that cell integrity has been compromised (i.e., an intracellular nucleotidase is leaking out) or, if cells are demonstrably not permeable, that the measured activity may be attributable to a soluble enzyme bound loosely to the outside of the plasma membrane but originating elsewhere (e.g., in plasma, as may well be the case for ecto-(adenosine deaminase) activity on vascular endothelium (Andy and Kornfeld, 1982; Hellewell and Pearson, 1983). It has also been found that certain cells *in vitro* can release ectoenzymes to the extracellular medium as a consequence of the loss of microvesicles of plasma membrane (Trams *et al.* 1981).

5. Enzyme Structure or Activity Can Be Modified by Nonpenetrating Reagents

At least six types of reagent, usually inhibitors, have been used to affect ectoenzymes.

1. Anti-5′-nucleotidase antibodies have been shown to inhibit selectively and completely 5′-nucleotidase in membrane vesicles and intact cells (Gurd and Evans, 1974; Newby *et al.*, 1975).
2. Suramin, a nonpenetrating trypanocidal drug (Wilson and Wormall, 1949), inhibits ectonucleotidases in intact cells (Smolen and Weissmann, 1978).
3. Diazotized sulphanilic acid, another nonpenetrating reagent (Berg, 1969) inhibits ectonucleotidases in various cell types (e.g., see De Pierre and Karnovsky, 1974a,b; Smolen and Weissmann, 1978; Carraway *et al.*, 1980; Smith *et al.*, 1981).
4. Nucleotide analogs, which are not permeant in intact cells, are powerful and selective inhibitors of ectonucleotidases; e.g., adenosine-α,β-methylene-diphosphonate (APCP) blocks 5′-nucleotidase (Burger and Lowenstein, 1970).
5. Certain lectins stimulate or inhibit ectonucleotidase; e.g., concanavalin A potently inhibits 5′-nucleotidase when the enzyme is purified or in intact cells (Riordan and Slavik, 1974; Stefanovic *et al.*, 1975).
6. Lactoperoxidase-catalyzed radioiodination of the external face of the plasma membrane, followed by copurification of enzyme activity and ^{125}I, is a technique of general applicability to ectoenzymes. It has been used to locate nucleotide pyrophosphatase in the hepatocyte (Evans, 1974).

It should be noted, with the exception of nucleotide analogs, where competitive inhibition has been established, that none of these approaches in itself proves that the active site of the enzyme faces outwards—merely that modification of the enzyme molecule (or possibly alteration of its activity by effects on neighbouring molecules) can be achieved by agents acting outside the cell.

6. *No Additional Enzyme Activity Is Found When Cells Are Broken*

This criterion will be met only if the enzyme concerned is localized exclusively as an ectoenzyme. It should also be pointed out that under certain conditions intracellular activity may represent a pool of newly synthesized or recycled ectoenzyme that is in the process of transport to its functional site at the plasma membrane (Stanley *et al.*, 1980; Widnell *et al.*, 1982).

B. Specificity of Ectonucleotidase

Experiments should be performed to determine whether ectonucleotidase activity is due in part to nonspecific ectophosphatase activity and to eliminate any such activity from contributing to specific ectonucleotidase assays. These experiments are particularly necessary in cytochemical studies of the cellular localization of nucleotidases (see Section IIIF). The proportion of measured activity that may be due to nonspecific phosphatase varies considerably; for example, cultured vascular endothelial cells exhibit little or no nonspecific phosphatase at neutral pH, whereas in isolated granulocytes a substantial minority of measured nucleotidase activity can be due to nonspecific phosphatase (Pearson *et al.*, 1980; De Pierre and Karnovsky, 1974b). The general approach used to improve the specificity of the nucleotidase assay, where necessary, is either to inhibit nonspecific phosphatase or to supply it with a saturating level of a substrate that it cleaves with higher affinity than the nucleotide substrate. Thus, 1–10 m*M* *p*-nitrophenylphosphate or β-glycerophosphate has been added (De Pierre and Karnovsky, 1974b; Pearson *et al.*, 1980), each of which is a good substate for phosphatases (Van Belle, 1972), or levamisole, a specific inhibitor of alkaline phosphatase (Van Belle, 1972) has been used (De Pierre and Karnovsky, 1974a; Smith and Peters, 1981).

In addition, it is clearly important to attempt to delineate the nucleotide substrate specificity of the ectonucleotidase being studied, as well as to investigate the nature of products formed. For example, the designation of an enzyme as a ecto-ADPase, when all that is known is that ADP is converted to AMP, could be misleading (see, e.g., Smith *et al.*, 1980a; Montague *et al.*, 1984). Unless it is also known that phosphate is liberated and that ATP is not being formed, the activity could be due to ecto-adenylate kinase, i.e., ADP + ADP $\rightleftharpoons$ ATP + AMP. More importantly, unless it can be shown that the same enzyme does not catabolize ATP with a similar (or greater) affinity or that it can be characterized more fully in other ways, it might be more appropriately named an ecto-ATPase.

III. EXPERIMENTAL METHODS FOR THE MEASUREMENT OF ECTONUCLEOTIDASE ACTIVITIES

A. Enzyme Sources

Isolated or cultured cells have been used most commonly to detect ectonucleotidases. These systems have the advantage that the criteria required to demonstrate ectoenzyme activity can most easily be met and the intact cells can be used to characterize the substrate and inhibitor profiles of the ectonucleotidases. They can also often be used as the starting material for further purification of the enzyme concerned: homogeneous populations of cells can be isolated in sufficient quantity from several sites (e.g., blood cells, myocardial cells, adipocytes, hepatocytes); alternatively, cultured cell populations can be propagated in large numbers (e.g., fibroblasts, smooth muscle cells, vascular endothelial cells, tumor cells), although it must be borne in mind that the phenotypic expression of ectonucleotidases in cultured cells may not quantitatively reflect the level in the same level cell type *in vivo*; indeed, substantial changes in the levels of 5′-nucleotidase have been reported both as cells are isolated and as cells age in culture (Sun *et al.*, 1975, 1979; Hayes *et al.*, 1979; Lieberman *et al.*, 1982; Chesterman *et al.*, 1983).

Once sufficient characteristics of an ectonucleotidase are known to distinguish it from any similar intracellular enzymic activity, then large scale purification can be performed starting with whole tissues, as has been done for 5′-nucleotidase (see Section IV). Two potential problems exist in this approach. Firstly, the tissue of origin is not a homogeneous cell population; thus, the purified enzyme is likely to be that from the cell type in which it is most prevalent, and neither the relative cellular distribution of activity nor its possible regulatory or other differences between cell types can be determined. Secondly, ectoenzymes are membrane proteins, and, if purified completely, their activity may not reflect that *in vivo*; e.g., the lipid environment of 5′-nucleotidase can regulate its activity (see Section IV).

Although the catabolism of exogenous nucleotides can be readily studied in isolated pieces or slices of tissue (e.g., muscle strips), the attribution of breakdown to ectonucleotidases is more difficult to assess than with isolated cells, primarily because of the uncertain contribution from intracellular enzymes released by damaged or dying cells. As with whole organ enzyme preparation, biochemical studies will not reveal which cell type within the tissue is responsible for the measured activity. This question can best be addressed by light or, preferably, electron microscopic cytochemical techniques (see subsection F below).

It was noted over 30 years ago that circulating nucleotides were degraded efficiently on a single passage through a capillary bed (Binet and Burstein, 1950). Since then, the use of organ perfusion and tracer dilution studies has demonstrated that nucleotides circulating in the bloodstream are metabolized by enzymes at the surface of the vascular endothelium (Hoffman and Okita, 1965; Williamson and Di Pietro, 1965; Baer and Drummond, 1968; Ryan and Smith, 1971; Crutchley *et al.*, 1978). These studies, which have been confirmed by the cytochemical localization of nucleotidases to the endothelial plasmalemma (Marchesi and Barrnett, 1963; Hoff and Graf, 1966; Smith and Ryan, 1970; Borgers *et al.*, 1971; Nakatsu and Drummond, 1972; Wilson *et al.*, 1982), in conjunction with the emerging importance of circulating adenosine as a local vasodilator hormone (see Berne, Chapter 18, this volume), have led to an increasing interest in the physiological role of these endothelial ectoenzymes. Various perfused organ preparations have therefore been used to characterize ectonucleotidases (Frick and Lowenstin, 1976; Cooper *et al.*, 1979; Ronca-Testoni and Borghini, 1982; Chelliah and Bakhle, 1983).

B. Thin-Layer Chromatography

Separation of nucleotides and nucleosides by thin-layer chromatography (TLC) has proved to be one of the most convenient and versatile methods for screening the catabolism of nucleotides. It is equally applicable to radiolabeled or unlabeled substrates; plates containing a UV fluorescent dye are usually used, after the addition of appropriate unlabeled markers if necessary, and the separated compounds are visualized and then extracted for measurement by scintillation spectrometry or by chemical assay. If isolated cells or tissues, rather than purified ectonucleotidases, are being studied, TLC has the advantage that the complete spectrum of possible reactions involving the substrate (e.g., the sequential degradation of ATP → ADP → AMP → adenosine) can be investigated at once as each compound can be separated. For routine assay of a single enzyme, the measurement of released phosphate by one of the techniques outlined in subsection D below may be more convenient. Three TLC systems in common use are described here.

1. Separation of Nucleotides and Nucleosides on Silica Gel by the System of Norman et al. (1974)

This solvent system separates ATP, ADP, IMP, AMP, inosine, and adenosine. Adenosine and hypoxanthine are not well separated. The method is highly reproducible; with 20-cm plates it has a running time of a minimum of about 5 hr but works as well or better if left overnight. It has been used successfully by several research groups (e.g., Crutchley *et al.*, 1978; Cooper *et al.*, 1979; Pearson *et al.*, 1978, 1980; Schütz *et al.*, 1981; Cusack *et al.*, 1983).

2. Separation of Nucleotides from Nucleosides on Silica Gel by the System of Pull and McIlwain (1972)

In this solvent system nucleotides remain at the origin, while inosine, hypoxanthine and adenosine are well separated: it is therefore useful for 5′-nucleotidase assays. With 20-cm plates the running time is 3–4 hr. Elution of nucleotides and nucleosides from silica gel, in this method or the previous one, is easily achieved with a small volume of dilute (0.1 *M*) HCl (Cusack *et al.*, 1983).

3. *Separation of Nucleotides on Polyethyleneimine (PEI)-Cellulose by the Methods of Randerath and Randerath (1964)*

By adjusting the solvent system used, pairs of nucleotides differing only in their bases can be separated. For example, GTP, ATP, GDP, ADP, GMP, and AMP can all be separated on a single 20-cm run in less than 3 hr, by using 1*M* LiCl with 1*M* HCOOH as solvent. Alternatively, good separation of ATP, ADP, and AMP can be achieved in about 45 min on a 10-cm run by using 0.5*M* LiCl with 1.5*M* HCOOH as solvent. In practice, the disadvantages of PEI–cellulose in comparison with silica gel TLC are threefold: the reproducibility is not as good without very strict attention to details such as the use of fresh solvents for each run; AMP and adenosine are not easily well separated; and quantitative elution of the nucleotides requires concentrated LiCl, which then has to be diluted (to prevent subsequent phase separation) before addition to scintillation fluid, thus necessitating the use of larger volumes of scintillation fluid per sample (see Cusack *et al.*, 1983). An additional problem in our laboratory was the inability to separate nucleotides on PEI-cellulose from samples containing neutralized trichloracetic acid, although this is not a problem with silica gel plates (Pearson *et al.*, 1978). Several workers have, however, successfully used PEI-cellulose in nucleotidase studies, including samples extracted with perchloric acid (Dieterle *et al.*, 1978; Dosne *et al.*, 1978; Fox *et al.*, 1981).

C. High-Performance Liquid Chromatography

Over the last decade, highly sensitive techniques for the separation of nucleotides, nucleosides, and bases by high-performance liquid chromatography (HPLC) have been developed (for a review, see Brown *et al.*, 1980). Although the major advantage of HPLC is its great resolving power when applied to complex mixtures, it can also provide a valuable tool for the investigation of nucleotide catabolism. I am aware of only a few references to this as yet (Newby, 1980; Ronca-Testoni and Borghini 1982; Nees and Gerlach, 1983), but investigators should seriously consider that HPLC may offer advantages of speed, precision, economy, or sensitivity over TLC for certain experiments. In addition the realization that the diastereoisomer pairs of certain nucleotide analogs (for example, the S_p and R_p isomers of the phosphorothioate analogs ADPαS and ATPαS) can be resolved by HPLC using reverse-phase separation systems, whereas they are not resolved by other methods, such as TLC, has allowed the detailed characterization of the stereoselectivities of several nucleotide-handling enzymes, notably kinases (see, e.g., Jaffe *et al.*, 1982). We have recently used this approach successfully to discover the stereoselectivities of the ectonucleotidases on cultured vascular cells (Cusack *et al.*, 1983). No prior sample extraction was required, and each reverse phase separation took less than 15 min.

D. Techniques Separating Inorganic Phosphate from Nucleotides or Nucleosides

The methods described here, while of general applicability, will probably be of greatest use for highly replicated nucleotidase assays under optimized conditions.

1. Charcoal

Nucleotides and nucleosides bind quantitatively to charcoal (Fiske, 1934; Crane and Lipmann, 1953). This finding has been used extensively by investigators studying ectonucleotidase catabolism of ATP, ADP, or AMP in which the terminal phosphorus is radiolabeled to yield a simple assay system in which ^{32}P is counted in the supernatant after a charcoal precipitation step (e.g., De Pierre and Karnovsky, 1974a; Stefanovic *et al.*, 1976b; Smith *et al.*, 1980b; Carraway *et al.*, 1980). Adsorbed nucleotides and nucleosides can be recovered from charcoal: Baer and Drummond (1968) used elution with pyridine followed by lyophilization as a method for concentrating samples of perfusion medium.

2. Molybdate

The original colorimetric determination of inorganic phosphorus (Fiske and Subbarow, 1925) is based on the production of phosphomolybdate. Although this method could, in principle, be used to measure phosphate release by ectonucleotidases without the need for separation of the phosphate from the organic phosphorus-containing compounds, it is in practice rarely sensitive enough. When terminally ^{32}P-labeled nucleotides are used, however, a modification of the Fiske and Subbarow assay introduced by Berenblum and Chain (1938) and subsequently improved by Martin and Doty (1949) and Weil-Malherbe and Green (1951), in which the phosphomolybdate is partitioned into organic solvent, has proved useful to several groups studying ectonucleotidases (see, e.g., Harlan *et al.*, 1977; Trams and Lauter, 1974; Widnell, 1972). A more sensitive version of the colorimetric phosphorus assay using malachite green (Itaya and Ui, 1966) has also been used directly in ectonucleotidase assays (Newby *et al.*, 1975; Naito and Lowenstein, 1981). A recent adaptation, four times as sensitive as the method of Itaya and Ui, may therefore also prove useful (De Bruyne, 1983).

E. Measurement of Nucleoside

Several separation methods have been used that are based on the measurement of nucleoside release from 5′-nucleotides rather than phosphate release. Avruch and Wallach (1971) used barium hydroxide to precipitate adenosine and separate it from AMP as the basis of a 5′-nucleotidase assay. It has subsequently been used by others (e.g., Newby *et al.*, 1975; Sun *et al.*, 1975). We found that the method was not reliable in the presence of any adenosine deaminase activity, because inosine was not precipitated satisfactorily. Chatterjee *et al.* (1979) showed that nucleosides and nucleotides can be separated rapidly and quantitatively on disposable alumina columns, which they used as the basis of a radiometric assay for 5′-nucleotidase. Adenosine and inosine have also been separated from AMP and IMP, respectively, by ion-exchange chromatography (Worku and Newby, 1982, 1983). The coupled enzymatic degradation of adenosine to inosine, which is then directly measured by differential UV absorption (Kalckar, 1947), has been used by several laboratories (e.g., Edwards and Maguire, 1970; Burger and Lowenstein, 1970).

A potentially valuable technique for the determination of adenosine is radioimmunoassay. Although highly sensitive, in the first published assay (Schrader *et al.*, 1978) the antibody cross-reacted with other nucleosides or nucleotides, and thus specificity, the main potential advantage of the assay apart from sensitivity, was lacking. An assay based on binding of adenosine to the adenine-analog binding protein of erythrocytes similarly lacked specificity (Olsson *et al.*, 1978). More recently, however, two radioimmunoassays have been published in which the antibodies could detect 1 pmole of adenosine with little or no cross-reactivity with other nucleosides or nucleotides likely to be present in biological samples (Newby and Sala, 1982, Sato *et al.*, 1982), and this assay technique should be increasingly used in future.

F. Cytochemistry

The cytochemical localization of ectonucleotidase activities has been of great importance in defining the cell types within a tissue and even the domains of plasma membrane around a cell that possess such activities. Virtually every paper published on this subject uses the methods of Wachstein and Meisel (1957), who in turn had adapted to various specific phosphatases the Gomori (1941) technique for the localization of non-specific phosphatase. Hydrolysis of substrate yields phosphate, which is immediately precipitated as the lead salt. This reaction is carried out on tissue slices, isolated cells, or organelles (usually after fixation); precipitated lead is viewed by light or (more usually) electron microscopy. There are several potential pitfalls, some general to many cytochemical methods (e.g., whether the localization of reaction product is truly representative of the localization of the enzyme, whether the enzyme is inactivated by the fixatives employed) and some restricted to the detection of nucleotidases (e.g., the specificity of the phosphatase activity, the likelihood of artifactual lead precipitation or phosphate production [discussed in detail by Ganotė *et al.*, 1969]). Biochemical approaches can often substantially improve the usefulness of a cytochemical study by providing confirmatory evidence that the enzyme under study is facing outwards in the plasma membrane or by providing a specific inhibitor for use in controls.

Major early papers demonstrating ectonucleotidase activity, apart from that of Wachstein and Meisel (1957), include those of Wallach and Ullrey (1962) on ecto-ATPase of Ehrlich cells, Marchesi and Barrnett (1963), who noted endothelial ectonucleotidases localized within pinocytic vesicles, Sabatini *et al.* (1963), who investigated the effects of fixatives on enzyme activity, and Borgers *et al.* (1971), who studied the distribution of 5′-nucleotidase in the heart of several mammalian species. Two more recent publications are also noteworthy for their careful attention to optimizing and confirming the specificity of the detection of 5′-nucleotidase (Widnell, 1972; Uusitalo and Karnovsky, 1977a). The particular advantages of cytochemistry were utilized to demonstrate the following findings: changes in the distribution of ectonucleotidase activities within cells or tissue during the onset of malignancy or after drug treatment (Lernmark *et al.*, 1979; Wilson *et al.*, 1981b); changes during the growth of cell monolayers *in vitro* (Ohnishi and Yamaguchi,

1978); the limited distribution of 5′-nucleotidase to subsets of lymphocytes (Uusitalo and Karnovsky, 1977b); and the exposure of granule ATPase in secreting mast cells (Chakravarty and Nielsen, 1981).

IV. 5′-NUCLEOTIDASE: PROPERTIES AND INHIBITORS

The prevalence of 5′-nucleotidase as an ectoenzyme has led to its use as a marker enzyme in the isolation of plasma membranes from many tissues (Riemer and Widnell, 1975), and much more is known of its properties than those of ecto-ADPase or ecto-ATPase. On purification it appears to be a dimer with each subunit of M_r 70,000–80,000 (e.g., Ipata, 1968; Evans and Gurd, 1973; Gutensohn, 1980); it is strongly bound to lipid and its properties are influenced by the nature of its lipid environment (Widnell, 1974; Merisko *et al.*, 1981; Dipple *et al.*, 1982). It is an integral membrane protein, solubilized by detergents such as deoxycholate, and it has recently been shown to span the plasma membrane (Zachowski *et al.*, 1981). The only apparent exceptions to this view are the report by Gibson and Drummond (1972) that 5′-nucleotidase from avian heart is soluble—although the properties of this enzyme make it likely that it is not related to 5′-nucleotidase from other species or sites—and the suggestion that the active site of 5′-nucleotidase in one line of murine plasmacytoma cells faces the cytoplasmic side of the plasma membrane (Zachowski *et al.*, 1977). As noted in Section II.A6, in some cell types latent membrane-bound 5′-nucleotidase activity can be demonstrated intracellularly; in such cases the enzyme appears to be a part of the ectoenzyme that is being recycled as part of the general process of internalization and subsequent reexposure of membrane components (Stanley *et al.*, 1980; Widnell *et al.*, 1982).

5′-Nucleotidase is stimulated by Ca^{2+} or Mg^{2+}. It accepts each of the 5′-nucleoside monosphosphates as substrate, usually with AMP as the most favored, whereas 2′- or 3′-monophosphates are not hydrolyzed (Baer *et al.*, 1966; Burger and Lowenstein, 1970). AMP modified by substitution in the adenine base (e.g., 2-Cl-AMP) is a substrate (Edwards and Maguire, 1970). The enzyme from a wide variety of sources has a K_m value for AMP in the range 5–40 μM (e.g., Baer *et al.*, 1966; Sullivan and Alpers, 1971; De Pierre and Karnovsky, 1974b; Burger and Lowenstein, 1975; Newby *et al.*, 1975; Carraway *et al.*, 1976). The most striking discordance in measured affinity was reported by Frick and Lowenstein (1976) who found a K_m of 13 μM in rat heart homogenates but obtained an apparent K_m of >1mM from perfusion studies with the same tissue. The reason for this discrepancy is not known, although there are several inherent difficulties in attempts to estimate kinetic parametic parameters from perfusion studies: the values obtained depend on flow rate and in general can only be satisfactorily estimated (even then with several assumptions and in a complex manner) from rapid sampling experiments following bolus injections, rather than from steady state clearance values as used by Frick and Lowenstein (see, e.g., Rickaby *et al.*, 1982). Other contributing factors, such as differences in accessibility of the AMP to 5′-nucleotidase in the two systems or the presence of endogenous inhibitors such as ATP (see below) in the perfused heart, have been suggested. Nonetheless, it is clear that in general K_m values for 5′-nucleotidase do not differ by orders of magnitude when determined with intact cells or in membrane preparations; e.g., we have recently found comparable K_m values (150–200 μM) in the pig lung by bolus injection into perfused lungs and by assays on isolated membrane preparations (P. G. Hellewell and J. D. Pearson, unpublished results). Catravas and White (1984), utilizing the mathematical analysis developed by Bronikowski *et al.* (1980) and Ryan and Ryan (1984) have recently reported a K_m value of 2–3 μM for rabbit lung 5′-nucleotidase estimated after bolus injection of AMP *in vivo*. We found very similar K_m values (approximately 20 μM) for 5′-nucleotidase in cultured endothelial cells whether studied in conventional monolayers (Cusack *et al.*, 1983) or in a system in which substrate is perfused through columns of packed cell-bearing microcarrier beads (L. L. Slakey and J. D. Pearson, unpublished results).

As noted in Section II.A5, 5′-nucleotidase can be nonspecifically inhibited by a range of reagents; it is also blocked by high concentrations of cations such as Zn^{2+} or Ni^{2+} (Ipata, 1968). Baer *et al.* (1966) first discovered that 5′-nucleotidase is inhibited by ATP. Burger and Lowenstein (1970) extended this finding, noting that ATP analogs such as adenosine-(α,β)-methylene-triphosphonate (APCPP) and adenosine-(β,γ)-methylene triphosphonate (APPCP) were at least as potent as ATP itself, that ADP was more potent than ATP, and that the ADP analog APCP was more potent than ADP. The mechanism by which these compounds inhibit 5′-nucleotidase, although disputed, seems (at least at low concentrations) to be competitive (Ipata, 1968; Evans and Gurd, 1973; Burger and Lowenstein, 1975). Typical kinetic parameters from the last-cited paper are as follows: K_m (AMP) = 3–6 μM; K_i (ATP) = 0.2 μM; K_i (ADP) = 0.02 μM; K_i (APCP) = 0.002 μM. APCP is not itself catabolized, has negligible effects on other ectonucleotidases, and is thus the usual reagent of choice for the selective inhibition of 5′-nucleotidase.

An AMP analog that may prove to be of interest in distinguishing between 5′-nucleotidases from different cell types is AMPS (where a sulphur atom substitutes for a nonbridging oxygen atom on the phosphate group). It is not hydrolyzed by 5′-nucleotidase on pig aortic endothelial cells (Cusack *et al.*, 1983), whereas it is a substrate for the enzyme from rat heart (Edwards and Maguire, 1970) and pig aortic smooth muscle cells (J. D. Pearson and N. J. Cusack, unpublished results). A separate approach to this problem would be to attempt to raise antibodies that distinguish between 5′-nucleotidase from different cells: conventional and monoclonal antisera that block 5′-nucleotidase have been produced (Newby *et al.*, 1975; Reimer and Widnell, 1975; Siddle *et al.*, 1981), but I am not aware that they have been tested in this way.

Finally, 5′-nucleotidase is strongly and noncompetitively inhibited by the lectin concanavalin A (Riordan and Slavik, 1974; Riemer and Widnell, 1975; Stefanovic *et al.*, 1975; Carraway *et al.*, 1976; Smolen and Karnovsky, 1980). The inhibition is selective (e.g., ecto-ATPase is either unaffected or stimulated; Novogrodsky, 1972; Jarrett and Smith, 1974; Carraway *et al.*, 1980) and has been used as the basis for purification of the enzyme on concanavalin A–sepharose columns (Naito and Lowenstein, 1981).

V. ECTO-ADPASE: PROPERTIES AND INHIBITORS

The distribution and properties of this enzyme have been very poorly studied by comparison with 5′-nucleotidase. The presence of an enzyme that metabolized circulating ADP was first noted by Brashear and Ross (1969). Subsequent studies with perfused tissues or intact cultured vascular cells confirmed the presence of ecto-ADPase activity on endothelium and vascular smooth muscle (Crutchley *et al.*, 1978, 1980; Cooper *et al.*, 1979; Glasgow *et al.*, 1978; Habliston *et al.*, 1978) but did not investigate its substrate specificity. These investigations, stimulated by an interest in whether the vascular wall cells degrade circulating ADP and thus limit blood platelet aggregation, were paralleled by others demonstrating the presence of ADPase in homogenates of vascular tissue (Heyns *et al.*, 1977; Lieberman *et al.*, 1977).

The enzyme has not been purified. Like 5′-nucleotidase, the enzyme is Mg^{2+} or Ca^{2+} stimulated. There is now sufficient evidence, particularly from work with vascular cells, to show that it can be differentiated from other ectoenzymes hydrolyzing nucleotides. We found a K_m of 160 μM for ADP in intact pig aortic endothelial cells in culture and clearly distinguished the enzyme from ecto-(nucleoside triphosphatase) activity: the enzyme is specifically inhibited by ATP analogs (e.g., adenylylimidodiphosphate, APPNP, K_i = 30 μM, or the fluorine-substituted analog, ATPγF, K_i = 60 μM) (Pearson *et al.*, 1980; E. K. Lund and J. D. Pearson, unpublished results), and it shows a characteristic pattern of stereoselectivity when presented with optically active pairs of ADP analogs as substrates (Cusack *et al.*, 1983).

Lieberman *et al.*, (1982) confirmed the plasma membrane location of the enzyme by subfractionation of aortic endothelial cells; their membrane preparation had a K_m for ADP of approximately 50 μM. In parallel cytochemical studies, the enzyme was localized to the apical plasma membrane when fixed monolayers were reacted *in situ* (Wilson *et al.*, 1982). Studies in aortic smooth muscle cells also revealed an exclusive plasma membrane localization of ADPase activity, with a K_m value of 10 μM against ADP in membrane preparations (Leake *et al.*, 1983); our earlier studies with intact cells suggested that the K_m was about 100 μM under these conditions (Pearson *et al.*, 1980).

It seems likely that ecto-(nucleoside diphosphatase) is as widely distributed as 5′-nucleotidase, but it has been investigated in few tissues. In addition to vascular cells, it is known to be present on neutrophils and at least some lymphocytes (De Pierre and Karnovsky, 1974b,c; Smith *et al.*, 1981). A similar enzyme occurs on the membrane bounding neutrophil-specific granules and is translocated to the surface on cell activation (Smith and Peters, 1981, 1982). Although one of the earliest reports of a plasma membrane ADPase was in rat liver (Wattiaux-de Coninck and Wattiaux, 1969), more recent work has suggested that the location of

ADPase in this tissue is exclusively mitochondrial (Smith *et al.*, 1980a; Montague *et al.*, 1984).

VI. ECTO-ATPASE: PROPERTIES AND INHIBITORS

The probability that an ectoenzyme capable of ATP catabolism exists on mammalian cells was first raised by the demonstration that ATP is inactivated on a single passage through the lung (Binet and Burstein, 1950). As noted in Section I, ecto-ATPase activities were detected shortly afterwards on nerve cells and red blood cells (Abood and Gerard, 1954; Herbert, 1956). Ecto-(nucleoside triphosphatase), like the ectodiphosphatase, has not been purified or fully characterized, although its distribution has been somewhat more widely investigated. The Mg^{2+}- or Ca^{2+}-stimulated enzyme is present on cells such as neutrophils, platelets, lymphocytes, macrophages, mast cells, hepatocytes, cardiac myocytes, vascular endothelial cells, vascular smooth muscle cells, and several tumor cells (see, e.g., Wallach and Ullrey, 1962; Ågren *et al*, 1971b; Carraway *et al.*, 1980; Chakravarty and Echetebu, 1978; Chambers *et al.*, 1967; Coetzee and Gevers, 1977; De Pierre and Karnovsky, 1974a,b,c; Pearson *et al.*, 1980). It is entirely unrelated to the Na^+/K^+ transport ATPase, which is potently inhibited by cardiac glycosides (Dunham and Glynn, 1961), in that ouabain has little or no effect on the Ca^{2+}/Mg^{2+}-stimulated ATPase in any cell type. The base specificity of the enzyme is quite broad; e.g., GTP is also a good substrate (Carraway *et al.*, 1980; Pearson *et al.*, 1980). The range of K_m values reported with ATP as substrate is wide (from 20–30 μM up to 2 mM), though most estimates are below 500 μM, and there is evidence that the value obtained depends on whether intact cells or membranes are studied (e.g., Carraway *et al.*, 1980) and on the relative concentrations of Ca^{2+} and Mg^{2+} present (e.g., Ronquist and Ågren, 1975).

Unfortunately, no specific inhibitor of ectotriphosphatase activity has yet been found. Although ADP inhibits the enzyme in some cases (e.g., Chambers *et al.*, 1967; Cooper and Stanworth, 1976), this result is likely to be of little use for work on intact cells where ecto-ADPase activity may be present: nonmetabolized ADP analogs, as noted in Section V, are often potent inhibitors of 5′-nucleotidase, but in general they are less effective inhibitors of ecto-ADPase (Pearson *et al.*, 1980). By analogy, we have tested adenosine tetraphosphate as a possible inhibitor of vascular endothelial ecto-ATPase, but this proved to be a poor inhibitor (K_i approx 1 mM) and a better inhibitor of ecto-ADPase ($K_i \simeq 200$ μM; E. K. Lund and J. D. Pearson, unpublished results). Other potential inhibitors that have proved useful (though their specificity has not been examined) include sulphydryl reagents, such as ethacrynic acid or *N*-ethylmaleimide (Chakravarty and Echetebu, 1978; Smolen and Weissmann, 1978), and phenothiazine drugs (e.g., trifluoperazine) (Medzihradsky *et al.*, 1975). Salem *et al.* (1981) have also shown that in at least three cell types, difluorodinitrobenzene selectively blocked ecto-ATPase rather than 5′-nucleotidase.

VII. OTHER ECTOENZYMES METABOLIZING NUCLEOTIDES

The need to distinguish between specific phosphatases hydrolyzing nucleotides and possible nonspecific phosphatases at the cell surface has already been mentioned (Section II.B). Granulocytes, for example, exhibit significant nonspecific ectophosphatase activity that can degrade ATP or AMP at neutral pH (De Pierre and Karnovsky, 1974b; Newby, 1980). Several other ectoenzymes capable of metabolizing ATP are known, which I will briefly mention below. First, however, it is perhaps worth reminding the reader that the Na^+/K^+ pump ATPase is not an ectoenzyme: it utilizes only intracellular ATP (Sen and Post, 1964).

In our initial experiments characterizing vascular endothelial ectonucleotidases we did not find any evidence of pyrophosphatase activity, i.e., direct catabolism of ATP to AMP (Pearson *et al.*, 1980), but, in our more recent studies, by using APPCP and APPNP as substrates we were able to show that there was a slow degradation of these "nonmetabolizable" substrates to form AMP (Cusack *et al.*, 1983). This is presumably a reflection of ecto-(nucleotide pyrophosphatase) action. This enzyme, which has a preference for substrates such as UDP-glucose or NADH, but which does attack ATP, albeit less efficiently, has been purified from rat liver plasma membrane and shown to be an ectoenzyme (Evans, 1974); on the present very limited evidence it seems unlikely to contribute significantly to the catabolism of extracellular ATP. The pyrophosphate produced could be cleaved by ecto-(pyrophosphate phosphatase), which has been described [although incorrectly named as ecto-(inorganic) pyrophosphatase] on neuronal cells (Stefanovic *et al.*, 1976a).

Exogenous AMP is catabolized by frog muscle to IMP, rather than to adenosine (Dunkley *et al.*, 1966; Manery and Dryden, 1979), suggesting that AMP deaminase, rather than 5′-nucleotidase, may be present as an ectoenzyme on amphibian muscle. In mammalian organ perfusions, there is often formation of inosine or uric acid in addition to adenosine as a product of nucleotide catabolism (Baer and Drummond, 1968; Ronca-Testoni and Borghini, 1982). We have recently presented evidence that adenosine deaminease is present as an endothelial ectoenzyme (Hellewell and Pearson, 1983), although the physiological role of this enzyme (or of plasma adenosine deaminase) is not clear, since the major fate of circulating adenosine is uptake from the plasma followed by intracellular metabolism. It has previously been suggested that in other cell types adenosine deaminase may be present as an ectoenzyme, as well as a cytoplasmic enzyme (e.g., Andy and Kornfeld, 1982).

Several cell types possess protein kinases as ectoenzymes, which can transfer phosphate from ATP to exogenous proteins or to integral membrane proteins (Ågren and Ronquist, 1970; Chang and Cuatrecasas, 1974; Mastro and Rozengurt, 1976; Remold-O'Donnell, 1978; Kang *et al.*, 1979; Sommarin *et al.*, 1981; Kübler *et al.*, 1982, 1983). The function of these enzymes is not clear. They might be involved in receptor-mediated responses to ATP or to other hormones, but it does not seem likely that they will prove to be major regulators of the metabolism of extracellular ATP at the surface of most cells.

Ronquist (1968) and Ågren *et al.* (1971a) found that exogenous ADP could be phosphorylated to ATP at the surface of several cell types when phosphate and a series of cofactors were provided. Later they also found that phosphate transfer from nucleoside triphosphates to nucleoside diphosphates occurred, i.e., that nucleoside diphosphate kinase was present as an ectoenzyme (Ågren *et al.*, 1974). We have found this ectoenzyme on vascular endothelial cells (Pearson *et al.*, 1980). Although we do not yet understand the physiological significance of the presence of such an enzyme, it is clear that it could significantly affect the pattern of nucleotides in the extracellular milieu; for when excess nucleotide triphosphate is present as a phosphate donor, ADP is not catabolized but forms ATP.

VIII. PHYSIOLOGICAL ROLES OF ECTONUCLEOTIDASES

A. Regulation of Biological Responses to Extracellular Nucleotides

This review is primarily concerned with methods, but it is pertinent to summarize here the various areas in which research on ectonucleotidases is being carried out. Even though knowledge of ectonucleotidases, with the possible exception of 5′-nucleotidase, is far from complete, there seems no reason to suppose that these enzymes are not widely distributed among mammalian cells. We have reviewed previously the evidence that ATP can be released into the circulation by various mechanisms, ranging from gross tissue damage to selective cellular stimulation (Pearson *et al.*, 1983); ATP is also released interstitially from nerve endings (White, Chapter 3, this volume). Several other chapters in this volume (in particular that of Burnstock and Buckley, Chapter 11) attest to the fact that extracellular ATP and ADP have potent (and in some cases quite distinct, e.g., in the blood platelet) receptor-mediated biological activities. Thus, a major physiological role of the ectonucleotidases is clearly related to regulating the concentrations of individual extracellular nucleotides to ensure that an appropriate biological resonse occurs, and there is evidence that ectonucleotidase activity modulates the responses of tissues to exogenous nucleotides (see, e.g., Burnstock *et al.*, 1983). Trams *et al.* (1980) have considered a role for the ectonucleotidases in limiting tissue responses to traumatic shock.

Research in our own laboratory and in several others is directed toward a clearer understanding of how the activities of this linked ectoenzyme system are coordinated and controlled. We also intend to define more closely the specificity exhibited by each enzyme for its substrate, with a view to designing analogs that selectively interact with an ectonucleotidase or a nucleotide receptor in the same cell (Cusack *et al.*, 1983).

B. Control of Extracellular Adenosine Production

The discoveries of the diverse biological actions of adenosine, including vasoregulation, modulation of neurotransmission and lipolysis, and definite but as yet poorly understood roles in the regulation of immune function (see Berne *et al.*, 1983), have led to an increasing need to understand how adenosine may be produced extracellularly. There is a longstanding controversy as to the mechanism involved, stemming in part from the fact that 5′-nucleotidase is exclusively an ectoenzyme and thus cannot catabolize intracellular AMP to adenosine (Berne, 1980). We and others (Newby, 1980; Schrader *et al.*, 1982; Pearson *et al.*, 1983) have considered that one pathway by which adenosine is produced extracellularly may be the selective release of ATP from cells (where it is normally present at concentrations approximately 4 orders of magnitude higher than is adenosine), followed by its breakdown to adenosine via the ectonucleotidase system. There is now evidence against this hypothesis in certain experimental situations (Schütz *et al.*, 1981), and the recognition that an intracellular AMPase (with very different properties from ecto-5′-nucleotidase) exists (Van den Berghe *et al.*, 1977; Lowenstein *et al.*, 1983; Worku and Newby, 1982) has partially resolved the problem of intracellular adenosine synthesis from nucleotides. Nonetheless, the possibility of a significant role for ectonucleotidases in the production of extracellular adenosine cannot be ignored.

C. Adenosine Transport and 5′-Nucleotidase

Several authors have noted that adenosine itself is transported into cells more slowly than is adenosine produced from exogenous AMP (Fleit *et al.*, 1975; Frick and Lowenstein, 1978; Dornand *et al.*, 1979). From such data it has been suggested that 5′-nucleotidase vectorially transports the adenosine it produces into the cytoplasm. There is, however, no direct evidence in favor of such a scheme, and the results can be interpreted more easily by supposing a proximity between adenosine carriers and 5′-nucleotidase in the membrane (Sasaki *et al.*, 1983).

D. Intercellular Variations in Ectonucleotidase Activities

There is an increasing body of literature concerning differences in the levels of ectonucleotidases between similar cell types or changes in their levels according to the growth state of the cells concerned. Leukemic lymphocytes seem to lack 5′-nucleotidase (Smith *et al.*, 1982; Sun *et al.*, 1982; Fleit *et al.*, 1975), whereas at least a proportion of normal lymphocytes do possess the ectoenzyme (Rowe *et al.*, 1979; Uusitalo and Karnovsky, 1977b). This lack of 5′-nucleotidase, which may or may not be accompanied by a decline in other ectonucleotidases (Fox *et al.*, 1981; Smith *et al.*, 1982), is also found on some other transformed cells such as the 3T3 cell (Sun *et al.*, 1979). In contrast, although 5′-nucleotidase may decline in early passages after isolation (Hayes *et al.*, 1979; Lieberman *et al.*, 1982), in diploid cells it increases many-fold just before cell replication ceases and population death occurs (Sun *et al.*, 1975, 1979). 5′-nucleotidase levels also selectively drop, while the activities of certain other membrane marker enzymes increase, when macrophages are activated (Bonney *et al.*, 1978; Morahan *et al.*, 1982). Various changes in other ectonucleotidases with malignancy have been found (Wilson *et al.*, 1981a,b; Karasaki *et al.*, 1977; Weiss and Sachs, 1977), and three further striking observations have been reported, although as with all these phenotypic alterations in ectonucleotidase expression, their significance is not yet known. First, the localization of ecto-ATPase on cultured hepatoma cells is preferentially at the area of contact between cells and increases with cell density (Ohnishi and Yamaguchi, 1978). Second, bromodeoxyuridine treatment of cardiac cells *in vitro* raises ecto-ATPase levels without affecting 5′-nucleotidase (Coetzee and Gevers, 1977). Third, the very low level of ecto-ATPase on astroblasts or neuroblasts in culture is dramatically stimulated when the cell types are cocultured (Stefanovic *et al.*, 1977).

XI. CONCLUSION

Ectonucleotidases exist on many cell types. Several assay methods exist, each with its own advantages and disadvantages depending on the type of measurement required. Although the properties of 5′-nucleotidase are now well characterized, those of ecto-(nucleoside diphosphatase) and ecto-(nucleoside triphosphatase) are much less well studied; for example, neither enzyme has been purified from any source, and we do not yet know of a selective inhibitor of the triphosphatase. In this chapter, I have outlined some of the physiological and pathological situations in which the enzyme activities are altered and have discussed what may be the primary function of these enzymes, i.e., the regulation of the concentration of biologically active extracellular nucleotides and nucleosides. Nonetheless, in view of our lack of experimental data, this interpretation may turn out to be at best an oversimplification. I hope that others may be encouraged to use this review as a basis from which to develop methods for the study of these enzymes and thus to gain a clearer understanding of their physiological and pathological roles.

ACKNOWLEDGMENTS

The writing of this review, and thus any defects in it, are my own responsibility, but I wish to thank all those who have contributed conceptually or experimentally to the work from our laboratory mentioned in the text: Sue Carleton, Noel Cusack, John Gordon, Paul Hellewell, Chris Holmquist, Amanda Hutchings, Elizabeth Lund, Andrew Newby, Linda Slakey, and Deborah Wenham.

REFERENCES

Abood, L. G., and Gerard, R. W. 1954. Enzyme distribution in isolated particulates of rat peripheral nerve. *J. Cell Comp. Physiol.*, *43*:379–392.

Ågren, G., and Ronquist, G. 1970. Isolation of ^{32}P-labelled phosphorylserine from Ehrlich mouse-ascites tumour cells suspended in an isotonic medium containing ^{32}P-labelled adenosine triphosphate. *Acta Physiol. Scand.*, *79*:125–128.

Ågren, Pontén, J., Ronquist, G., and Westermark, B. 1971a. Formation of extracellular adenosine triphosphate by normal and neoplastic cells in culture. *J. Cell Physiol.*, *77*:331–336.

Ågren, Pontén, J., Ronquist, G., and Westermark, B. 1971b. Demonstration of an ATPase at the cell surface of intact normal and neoplastic cells in culture. *J. Cell Physiol.*, *78:*171–176.

Ågren, Pontén, J., Ronquist, G., and Westermark, B. 1974. Nucleoside diphosphate kinase at the cell surface of neoplastic human cells in culture. *J. Cell Physiol.*, *83:*91–102.

Andy, R. J., and Kornfeld, R. 1982. The adenosine deaminase binding protein of human skin fibroblasts is located on the cell surface. *J. Biol. Chem.*, *257:*7922–7925.

Avruch, J., and Wallach, D. F. H. 1971. Preparation and properties of plasma membrane and endoplasmic reticulum fragments from isolated rat fat cells. *Biochim. Biophys. Acta.*, *233:*334–337.

Baer, H. P., and Drummond, G. I. 1968. Catabolism of adenosine nucleotides by the isolated perfused rat heart. *Proc. Soc. Exp. Biol. Med.*, *127:*33–38.

Baer, H. P. Drummond, G. I., and Duncan, E. L. 1966. Formation and deamination of adenosine by cardiac muscle enzymes. *Mol. Pharmacol.*, *2:*67–76.

Berenblum, I., and Chain, E. 1938. An improved method for the colorimetric determination of phosphate. *Biochem. J.*, *32:*295–298.

Berg, H. C., 1969. Sulfanilic acid diazonium salt: A label for the outside of the human erythrocyte membrane. *Biochim. Biophys. Acta*, *183:*65–78.

Berne, R. M. 1980. The role of adenosine in the regulation of coronary blood flow. *Circulation Res.*, *47:*807–813.

Berne, R. M., Rall, T. W., and Rubio, R. (eds.) 1983. *Regulatory Function of Adenosine*, Nijhoff, The Hague.

Binet, L., and Burstein, M. 1950. Poumon et action vasculaire de l'adénosine-triphosphate. *Presse Med.*, *58:*1201–1203.

Bonney, R. J., Gery, I., Lin, T.-Y., Meyenhoffer, M. R., Acevedo, W., and Davies, P. 1978. Mononuclear phagocytes from carrageenan-induced granulomas. *J. Exp. Med.*, *148:*261–275.

Borgers, M., Schaper, J., and Schaper, W. 1971. Adenosine-producing sites in the mammalian heart: A cytochemical study. *J. Mol. Cell Cardiol.*, *3:*287–296.

Brashear, R. E., and Ross, J. C. 1969. Disappearance of adenosine diphosphate in vivo. *J. Lab. Clin. Med.*, *73:*54–59.

Bronikowski, T. A., Linehan, J. H., and Dawson, C. A. 1980. A mathematical analysis of the influence of perfusion heterogeneity on indicator extraction. *Math. Biosci.*, *52:*27–51.

Brown, P. R., Krstulovic, A. M., and Hartwick, R. A. 1980. Current state of the art in the HPLC analysis of free nucleotides, nucleosides, and bases in biological fluids. *Adv. Chromatogr.*, *18:*101–138.

Burger, R. M., and Lowenstein, J. M. 1970. Preparation and properties of 5′-nucleotidase from smooth muscle of small intestine. *J. Biol. Chem.*, *245:*6274–6280.

Burger, R. M., and Lowenstein, J. M. 1975. 5′-Nucleotidase from smooth muscle of small intestine and from brain. Inhibition by nucleotides. *Biochemistry*, *14:*2362–2366.

Burnstock, G., Cusack, N. J., Hills, J. M., MacKenzie, I., and Meghji, P. 1983. Studies on the stereoselectivity of the P_2-purinoceptor. *Br. J. Pharmacol.*, *79:*907–913.

Carraway, K. L., Fogle, D. D., Chestnut, R. W., Huggins, J. W., and Carraway, C. A. C. 1976. Ecto-enzymes of mammary gland and its tumors. Lectin inhibition of 5′-nucleotidase of the 13762 rat mammary ascites carcinoma. *J. Biol. Chem.*, *251:*6173–6178.

Carraway, C. A. C., Corrado, F. J., IV, Fogle, D. D., and Carraway, K. L. 1980. Ecto-enzymes of mammary gland and its tumours. Ca^{2+} or Mg^{2+} stimulated adenosine triphosphatase and its perturbation by concanavalin A. *Biochem. J.*, *191:*45–51.

Catravas, J. D., and White, R. E. 1984. Kinetics of pulmonary angiotensin converting enzyme and 5′-nucleotidase in vivo. *J. Appl. Physiol.*, *57.*

Chakravarty, N., and Echetebu, Z. 1978. Plasma membrane adenosine triphosphatases in rat peritoneal mast cells and macrophages—the relation of the mast cell enzyme to histamine release. *Biochem. Pharmacol.*, *27:*1561–1569.

Chakravarty, N., and Nielsen, E. H. 1981. Adenosine triphosphatase in nonsecreting and secreting mast cells. *Agents Actions*, *11:*67–69.

Chambers, D. A., Salzman, E. W., and Neri, L. L. 1967. Characterization of "ecto-ATPase" of human blood platelets. *Arch. Biochem. Biophys.*, *119:*173–178.

Chang, K-J., and Cuatrecasas, P. 1974. Adenosine triphosphate-dependent inhibition of insulin-stimulated glucose transport in fat cells. Possible role of membrane phosphorylation. *J. Biol. Chem.*, *249*:3170–3180.

Chatterjee, S. K., Bhattacharya, M., and Barlow, J. B., 1979. A simple specific radiometric assay for 5′-nucleotidase. *Anal. Biochem.*, *95*:497–506.

Chelliah, R., and Bakhle, Y. S. 1983. The fate of adenine nucleotides in the pulmonary circulation of isolated lung. *Quart. J. Exp. Physiol.*, *68*:289–300.

Chesterman, C. N., Ager, A., and Gordon, J. L. 1983. Regulation of prostaglandin production and ectoenzyme activities in cultured aortic endothelial cells. *J. Cell. Physiol.*, *116*:45–50.

Coetzee, G. A., and Gevers, W. 1977. 5-Bromo-2′-deoxyuridine-stimulated calcium ion- or magnesium ion- dependent ecto-(adenosine triphosphatase) activity of cultured hamster cardiac cells. *Biochem. J.*, *164*:645–652.

Cooper, D. H., and Stanworth, D. R. 1976. Characterisation of calcium-ion-activated adenosine triphosphatase in the plasma membrane of rat mast cells. *Biochem. J.*, *156*:691–700.

Cooper, D. R., Lewis, G. P., Lieberman, G. E., Webb, H., and Westwick, J. 1979. ADP metabolism in vascular tissue, a possible thromboregulatory mechanism. *Thromb. Res.*, *14*:910–914.

Crane, R. K., and Lipmann, R. 1953. The effect of arsenate on aerobic phosphorylation. *J. Biol. Chem.*, *201*:235–243.

Crutchley, D. J., Eling, T. E., and Anderson, M. W., 1978. ADPase activity of isolated perfused rat lung. *Life Sci.*, *22*:1413–1420.

Crutchley, D. J., Ryan, U. S., and Ryan, J. W. 1980. Effects of aspirin and dipyridamole on the degradation of adenosine diphosphate by cultured cells derived from bovine pulmonary artery. *J. Clin. Invest.*, *66*:29–35.

Cummins, J., and Hydén, H. 1962. Adenosine triphosphate levels and adenosine triphosphatases in neurons, glia and neuronal membranes of the vestibular nucleus. *Biochim. Biophys. Acta.*, *60*:271–283.

Cusack, N. J., Pearson, J. D., and Gordon, J. L. 1983. Stereoselectivity of ectonucleotidases on vascular endothelial cells. *Biochem. J.*, *214*:975–981.

De Bruyne, I. 1983. Inorganic phosphate determination: Colorimetric assay based on the formation of a rhodamine B-phosphomolybdate complex. *Anal. Biochem.*, *130*:454–460.

De Pierre, J. W. and Karnovsky, M. L. 1974a. Ecto-enzyme of granulocytes: 5′-nucleotidase. *Science*, *183*:1096–1098.

De Pierre, J. W., and Karnovsky, M. L. 1974b. Ecto-enzymes of the guinea pig polymorphonuclear leukocyte. I Evidence for an ecto-adenosine monophosphatase, -adenosine triphosphatase, and -p-nitrophenylphosphatase. *J. Biol. Chem.*, *249*:7111–7120.

De Pierre, J. W., and Karnovsky, M. L. 1974c. Ecto-enzymes of the guinea pig polymorphonuclear leukocyte. II. Properties and suitability as marker for the plasma membrane. *J. Biol. Chem.*, *249*:7121–7129.

Dieterle, Y., Ody, C., Ehrensburger, A., Stalder, H., and Junod, A. F. 1978. Metabolism and uptake of adenosine triphosphate and adenosine by porcine aortic and pulmonary endothelial cells and fibroblasts in culture. *Circ. Res.*, *42*:869–876.

Dipple, I. M., Gordon, L. M., Houslay, M. D. 1982. The activity of 5′-nucleotidase in liver plasma membranes is affected by the increase in bilayer fluidity achieved by anionic drugs but not by cationic drugs. *J. Biol. Chem.*, *257*:1811–1815.

Dornand, J., Bonnafous, J.-C., Gavach, C., and Mani, J.-C. 1979. 5′-Nucleotidase-facilitated adenosine transport by mouse lymphocytes. *Biochimie*, *61*:973–977.

Dosne, A. M., Legrand, C., Bauvois, B., Bodevin, E., and Caen, J. P. 1978. Comparative degradation of adenylnucleotides by cultured endothelial cells and fibroblasts. *Biochem. Biophys. Res. Commun.*, *85*:183–189.

Dunham, E. T., and Glynn, I. M. 1961. Adenosine triphosphatase activity and the active movement of alkali metal ions. *J. Physiol.*, *156*:274–293.

Dunkley, C R., Manery, J. F., and Dryden, E. E. 1966. The conversion of AMP to IMP by muscle surface enzymes. *J. Cell Physiol.*, *68*:241–248.

Edwards, M. J., and Maguire, M. H. 1970. Purification and properties of rat heart 5′-nucleotidase. *Mol. Pharmacol.* *6*:641–648.

Essner, E., Novikoff, A. B., and Masek, B. 1958. Adenosinetriphosphatase and 5′-nucleotidase activities in the plasma membrane of liver cells as revealed by electron microscopy. *J. Biophys. Biochem. Cytol.*, *4*:711–716.

Evans, W. H. 1974. Nucleotide pyrophosphatase, a sialoglycoprotein located on the hepatocyte surface. *Nature*, *250*:391–394.

Evans, W. H., and Gurd, J. W. 1973. Properties of a 5′-nucleotidase purified from mouse liver plasma membranes. *Biochem. J.*, *133*:189–199.

Fiske, C. H. 1934. The nature of the depressor substance of the blood. *Proc. Natl. Acad. Sci. USA* *20*:25–27.

Fiske, C. H., and Subbarow, Y. 1925. The colorimetric determination of phosphorus. *J. Biol. Chem.*, *66*:375–400.

Fleit, H., Conklyn, M., Stebbins, R. D., and Silber, R. 1975. Function of 5′-nucleotidase in the uptake of adenosine from AMP by human lymphocytes. *J. Biol. Chem.*, *250*:8889–8892.

Fox, R. M., Piddington, S. K., and Tripp, E. H. 1981. Ecto-adenosine triphosphatase deficiency in cultured human T and null leukemic lymphocytes. A biochemical basis for thymidine sensitivity. *J. Clin. Invest.*, *68*:544–552.

Frick, G. P., and Lowenstein, J. M. 1976. Studies of 5′-nucleotidase in the perfused rat heart. *J. Biol. Chem.*, *251*:6372–6378.

Frick, G. P., and Lowenstein, J. M. 1978. Vectorial production of adenosine by 5′-nucleotidase in the perfused rat heart. *J. Biol. Chem.*, *253*:1240–1244.

Ganote, C, E., Rosenthal, A. S., Moses, H. L., and Tice, L. W. 1969. Lead and phosphate as sources of artifact in nucleoside phosphatase histochemistry. *J. Histochem. Cytochem.*, *17*:641–650.

Gibson, W. B., and Drummond, G. I. 1972. Properties 5′-nucleotidase from avian heart. *Biochemistry*, *11*:223–229.

Glasgow, J. G., Schade, R., and Pitlick, F. A. 1978. Evidence that ADP hydrolysis by human cells is related to thrombogenic potential. *Thromb. Res.*, *13*:255–266.

Gomori, G. 1941, The distribution of phosphatase in normal organs and tissues. *J. Cell Comp. Physiol.*, *17*:71–83.

Gurd, J. W., and Evans, W. H., 1974. Distribution of liver plasma membrane 5′-nucleotidase as indicated by its reaction with anti-plasma membrane serum. *Arch. Biochem. Biophys.*, *164*:305–311.

Gutensohn, W. 1980. Human 5′-nucleotidase. Properties and characterisation of the enzyme from placenta, lymphocytes and lymphoblastoid cells in culture. *Adv. Exp. Med. Biol.*, *122B*:295–298.

Habliston, D. L., Ryan, U. S., and Ryan J. W. 1978. Endothelial cells degrade adenosine-5′-diphosphate. *J. Cell Biol.*, *79*:206a.

Harlan, J, de Chatelet, L. R., Iverson, D. B., and McCall, C. E. 1977. Magnesium-dependent adenosine triphosphatase as a marker enzyme for the plasma membrane of human polymorphonuclear leukocytes. *Infect. Immun.*, *15*:436–443.

Hayes, L. W., Goguen, C. A., Stevens, A. L., Magargal, W. W., and Slakey, L. L. 1979. Enzyme activities in endothelial cells and smooth muscle cells from swine aorta. *Proc. Natl. Acad. Sci. USA*, *76*:2532–2535.

Hellewell, P. G., and Pearson, J. D. 1983. Metabolism of circulating adenosine by the porcine isolated perfused lung. *Circ. Res.*, *53*:1–7.

Herbert, E. 1956. A study of the liberation of orthophosphate from adenosine triphosphate by the stromata of human erythrocytes. *J. Cell Comp. Physiol*, *47*:11–36.

Heyns, A. du P., Badenhorst, C. J., and Retief, F. P. 1977. ADPase activity of normal and atherosclerotic human aorta intima. *Thromb. Haem.*, *37*:429–435.

Hoff, H. F., and Graf, J. 1966. An electron microscopy study of phosphatase activity in the endothelial cells of rabbit aorta. *J. Histochem. Cytochem.*, *14*:719–724.

Hoffman, P. C., and Okita, G. T. 1965. Penetration of ATP into the myocardium. *Proc. Soc. Exp. Biol. Med.*, *119*:573–576.

Ipata, P. L. 1968. Sheep brain 5′-nucleotidase. Some enzyme properties and allosteric inhibition by nucleoside triphosphates. *Biochemistry*, *7*:507–515.

Itaya, K., and Ui, M. 1966. A new micromethod for the colorimetric determination of inorganic phosphate. *Clin. Chim. Acta*, *14*:361–366.

Jaffe, E. K., Nick, J., and Cohn, M. 1982. Reactivity and metal-dependent stereospecificity of the phosphorothioate analogs of ADP and ATP and reactivity of Cr(III)ATP in the 3-phosphoglycerate kinase reaction. *J. Biol. Chem.*, *257:*7650–7656.

Jarrett, L., and Smith, R. M. 1974. Stimulation of adipocyte plasma membrane magnesium-stimulated adenosine triphosphatase by insulin and concanavalin A. *J. Biol. Chem.*, *249:*5195–5199.

Kalckar, H. M. 1947. Differential spectrophotometry of purine compounds by means of specific enzymes. II. Determination of adenine compounds. *J. Biol. Chem.*, *167:*445–459.

Kang, E. S., Gates, R. E., Chiang, T. M., and Kang, A. H. 1979. Ectoprotein kinase activity of the isolated rat adipocyte. *Biochem. Biophys. Res. Commun.*, *80:*769–778.

Karasaki, S., Simard, A., and Lamiraude, G. de. 1977. Surface morphology and nucleoside phosphatase activity of rat liver epithelial cells during oncogenic transformation in vitro. *Center Res.*, *37:*3516–3525.

Kübler, D., Pyerin, W., and Kinzel, V. 1982. Protein kinase activity and substrates at the surface of intact Hela cells. *J. Biol. Chem.*, *257:*322–329.

Kübler, D., Pyerin, W., Burow, E., and Kinzel, V. 1983. Substrate-effected release of surface located protein kinase from intact cells. *Proc. Natl. Acad. Sci. USA*, *80:*4021–4025

Leake, D. S., Lieberman, G. S., and Peters, T. J. 1983. Properties and subcellular localization of adenosine diphosphatase in arterial smooth muscle cells in culture. *Biochim. Biophys. Acta*, *762:*52–57.

Lernmark, Å., Söderberg, L.-A., Täljedal, I.-B. 1979. 5′-AMP hydrolysis by suspensions and homogenates of pancreatic islet cells from normal and cortizone-treated rats. *Histochemistry*, *63:*155–161.

Lieberman, G. E., Lewis, G. P., and Peters, T. J. 1977. A membrane-bound enzyme in rabbit aorta capable of inhibiting adenosine-diphosphate-induced platelet aggregation. *Lancet*, *2:*330–332.

Lieberman, G. E., Leake, D. S., and Peters, T. J. 1982. Subcellular localization of adenosine diphosphatase in cultured pig arterial endothelial cells. *Thromb. Haem.*, *47:*249–253.

Lowenstein, J. M., Yu, M.-K., and Naito, Y. 1983. Regulation of adenosine metabolism by 5′-nucleotidases. In: *Regulatory Function of Adenosine*, pp. 117–131. Ed. by Berne, R. M., Rall, T. W., and Rubio, R. Nijhoff, The Hague.

Manery, J. F., and Dryden, E. E. 1979. Ecto-enzymes concerned with nucleotide metabolism. In: *Physiological and Regulatory Functions of Adenosine and Adenine Nucleotides*, pp. 323–339. Ed. by Baer, H. P., and Drummond, G. I. Raven Press, New York.

Marchesi, V. T., and Barrnett, R. J. 1963. The demonstration of enzymatic activity in pinocytic vesicles of blood capillaries with the electron microscope. *J. Cell Biol.*, *17:*547–556.

Martin, J. B., and Doty, D. M. 1949. Determination of inorganic phosphate. Modification of isobutyl alcohol precedure. *Anal. Chem.*, *21:*965–967.

Mastro, A. M., and Rozengurt, E. 1976. Endogenous protein kinase in outer plasma membrane of cultured 3T3 cells. *J. Biol. Chem.*, *251:*7899–7906.

Medzihradsky, F., Lin, H.-L., and Marks, M. J. 1975. Drug inhibitable ecto-ATPase in leukocytes. *Life Sci.*, *16:*1417–1428.

Merisko, E. M., Ojakian, G. K., and Widnell, C. C. 1981. The effects of phospholipids on the properties of hepatic 5′-nucleotidase. *J. Biol. Chem.*, *256:*2983–1993.

Montague, D. J., Peters, T. J. and Baum, H. 1984. Studies on the nature of adenosine diphosphatase activity from rat liver mitochondria. *Biochim. Biophys. Acta*, *771:*9–15.

Morahan, P. S., Rozner, M. A., and Jessee, E. J. 1982. Effect of elicitation on peritoneal macrophage subpopulations: Size distributions, ectoenzyme phenotypes and antitumor activity. *Int. J. Cancer*, *30:*787–794.

Naito, Y., and Lowenstein, J. M. 1981. 5′-Nucleotidase from rat heart. *Biochemistry*, *20:*5188–5194.

Nakatsu, K., and Drummond, G. I. 1972. Adenylate metabolism and adenosine formation in the heart. *Am. J. Physiol.*, *223:*1119–1127.

Nees, S., and Gerlach, E. 1983. Adenine nucleotide and adenosine metabolism in cultured coronary endothelial cells: Formation and release of adenine compounds and possible functional implications. In: *Regulatory Functions of Adenosine*, pp. 347–360. Ed. by Berne, R. M., Rall, T. W., and Rubio, R. Nijhoff, The Hague.

Newby, A. C. 1980. Role of adenosine deaminase, ecto-(5′-nucleotidase) and ecto-(non-specific phosphatase) in cyanide-induced adenosine monophosphate catabolism in rat polymorphonuclear leucocytes. *Biochem. J.*, *186*:907–918.

Newby, A. C., and Sala, G. B. 1982. A new procedure for haptenizing adenosine leading to a more specific radioimmunoassay method. *Biochem. J.*, *208*:603–610.

Newby, A. N., Luzio, J. P., and Hales, CN. 1975. The properties and extracellular location of 5′-nucleotidase of the rat fat-cell plasma membrane. *Biochem. J.*, *146*:625–633.

Norman, G. A., Follett, M. J. and Hector, D. A. 1974. Quantitative thin-layer chromatography of ATP and the products of its degradation in meat tissues. *J. Chromatogr.*, *90*:105–111.

Novogrodsky, A. 1972. Concanavalin A stimulation of rat lymphocyte ATPase. *Biochim. Biophys. Acta*, *226*:343–349.

Ohnishi, T., and Yamaguchi, K. 1978. Effects of db-cAMP and theophylline on cell surface adenosine triphosphatase activity in cultured hepatoma cells, *Exp. Cell. Res.*, *116*:261–268.

Olsson, R. A., Davis, C. J., Gentry, M. K., and Vomacka, R. B. 1978. A radiological binding assay for adenosine in tissue extracts. *Anal. Biochem.*, *85*:132–138.

Pearson, J. D., and Gordon, J. L. 1979. Vascular endothelial and smooth muscle cells in culture selectively release adenine nucleotides. *Nature*, *281*: 384–386.

Pearson, J. D., Carleton, J. S., Hutchings, A., and Gordon, J. L. 1978. Uptake and metabolism of adenosine by pig aortic endothelial and smooth muscle cells in culture. *Biochem. J.*, *170*:265–271.

Pearson, J. D., Carleton, J. S., and Gordon J. L. 1980. Metabolism of adenine nucleotides by ectoenzymes of vascular endothelial and smooth muscle cells in culture. *Biochem. J.*, *190*:421–429.

Pearson, J. D., Hellewell, P.G., and Gordon, J. L. 1983, Adenosine uptake and adenine nucleotide metabolism by vascular endothelium. In: *Regulatory Function of Adenosine*, pp. 333–346. Ed. by Berne, R. M., Rall, T. W., and Rubio, R. Nijhoff, The Hauge.

Pull, I., and McIlwain, H. 1972. Metabolism of [^{14}C]adenine and derivatives by cerebral tissues, superfused and electrically stimulated. *Biochem. J.*, *126*:965–973.

Randerath, K., and Randerath, E. 1964. Ion-exchange chromatography of nucleotides on poly-(ethyleneimine)-cellulose thin layers. *J. Chromatogr.*, *16*:111–125.

Remold-O'Donnell, E. 1978. Protein kinase activity associated with the surface of guinea pig macrophages. *J. Exp. Med.*, *148*:1099–1104.

Rickaby, D. A., Dawson, C. A., and Linehan, J. M. 1982. Influence of blood and plasma flow rate on kinetics of serotonin uptake by lungs. *J. Appl. Physiol.*, *53*:677–684.

Riemer, B. L., and Widnell, C. C. 1975. The demonstration of a specific 5′-nucleotidase activity in rat tissues. *Arch. Biochem. Biophys.*, *171*:343–347.

Riordan, J. R., and Slavik, M. 1974. Interaction of lectins with membrane glycoproteins. Effects of concanavalin A on 5′-nucleotidase. *Biochim. Biophys. Acta.*, *373*:356–360.

Ronca-Testoni, S., and Borghini, F. 1982. Degradation of perfused adenine compounds up to uric acid in isolated rat heart. *J. Mol. Cell. Cardiol.*, *14*:177–180 .

Ronquist, G. 1968. Formation of extracellular adenosine triphosphate by human erythrocytes. *Acta Physiol. Scand.*, *74*:594–605.

Ronquist, G., and Ågren, G. K., 1975, A Mg^{2+} and Ca^{2+} stimulated adenosine triphosphatase at the outer surface of Ehrlich ascites tumor cells. *Cancer Res.*, *35*:1402–1406.

Rothstein, A., and Meier, R. 1948. The relationship of the cell surface to metabolism I Phosphatases in the cell surface of living yeast cells. *J. Comp. Cell Physiol.*, *32*:77–95.

Rowe, M., de Gast, G. C., Platts-Mills, T. A. E., Asherson, G. L., Webster, A. D. B., and Johnson, S. M. 1979. 5′-nucleotidase of B and T lymphocytes isolated from peripheral blood. *Clin. Exp. Immunol.*, *36*:97–101.

Rozengurt, E., and Heppel, L. A. 1979. Reciprocal control of membrane permeability of transformed cultures of mouse liver cells by external and internal ATP. *J. Biol. Chem.*, *254*:708–714.

Ryan, J. W., and Ryan, U. S. 1984. Endothelial surface enzymes and the dynamic processing of plasma substrates. *Int. Rev. Exp. Pathol.*, *26*:1–43.

Ryan, J. W., and Smith, U. 1971. Metabolism of adenosine 5′-monophosphate during circulation through the lungs. *Trans. Assoc. Am. Physicians.*, *84*:297–306.

Sabatini, D. D., Bensch, K., and Barrnett, R. J. 1963. Cytochemistry and electron microscopy. The preservation of cellular structure and enzymatic activity by aldehyde fixation. *J. Cell Biol., 17:*19–58.

Salem, N. Jr., Lauter, C. J., and Trams, E. G. 1981. Selective chemical modification of plasma membrane ectoenzymes. *Biochim. Biophys. Acta, 641:*366–376.

Sasaki, T., Abe, A., and Sakagami, T. 1983 Ecto-5′-nucleotidase does not catalyze vectorial production of adenosine in the perfused rat liver. *J. Biol. Chem., 258:*6947–6951.

Sato, T., Kuninaka, A., Yoshino, H., and Ui, M. 1982. A sensitive radioimmunoassay for adenosine in biological samples. *Anal. Biochem., 121:*409–420.

Schrader, J., Nees, S., and Gerlach, E. 1978. Radioimmunoassay for adenosine in biological samples. *Pflügers Arch., 378:*167–171.

Schrader, J., Thompson, C. I., Hiendlmayer, G., and Gerlach, E. 1982. Role of purines in acetylcholine-induced coronary vasodilation. *J. Mol. Cell Cardiol., 14:*427–430.

Schütz, W., Schrader, J., and Gerlach, E. 1981. Different sites of adenosine formation in the heart. *Am. J. Physiol., 240:*H963–H970.

Sen, A. K., and Post, R. L. 1964. Stoichiometry and localization of adenosine triphosphate-dependent sodium and potassium transport in the erythrocyte. *J. Biol. Chem., 239:*345–352.

Siddle, K., Bailyes, E. M., and Luzio, J. P. 1981. A monoclonal antibody inhibiting rat liver 5′-nucleotidase. *FEBS Lett., 128:*103–107.

Smith, G. P., and Peters, T. J. 1981. Subcellular localization and properties of adenosine diphosphatase activity in human polymorphonuclear leukocytes. *Biochim. Biophys. Acta, 673:*234–242.

Smith, G. P., and Peters, T. J. 1982. The release of granule components from human polymorphonuclear leukocytes in response to both phagocytic and chemical stimuli. *Biochim. Biophys. Acta, 719:*304–308.

Smith, G. P., Smith, G. D., and Peters, T. J. 1980a. Subcellular localization and properties of rat liver adenosine diphosphatase. *Biochem. J., 192:*527–535.

Smith, G. P., Smith, G. D., and Peters, T. J. 1980b. A direct, rapid, radioassay for adenosine diphosphatase. *Clin. Chim. Acta, 101:*287–291.

Smith, G. P., Shah, T., Webster, A. D. B., and Peters, T. J. 1981. Studies on the kinetic properties and subcellular localization of adenosine diphosphatase activity in human peripheral blood lymphocytes. *Clin. Exp. Immunol., 46:*321–326.

Smith, G. P., Shah, T., Webster, A. D. B., and Peters, T. J. 1982. Studies on the kinetic properties and subcellular localization of adenosine nucleotide phosphatases in peripheral blood lymphocytes from control subjects and patients with common variable primary hypogammaglobulinaemia. *Clin. Exp. Immunol., 49:*393–400.

Smith, U., and Ryan, J. W. 1970. An electron microscopic study of the vascular endothelium as a site for bradykinin and ATP inactivation in rat lung. *Adv. Exp. Med. Biol., 8:*249–262.

Smolen, J. E., and Karnovsky, M. L. 1980. Effect of surface modifiers on an ectoenzyme: Granulocyte 5′-nucleotidase. *Infect. Immun., 28:*475–485.

Smolen, J. E., and Weissmann, G. 1978. Mg^{2+}-ATPase as a membrane ecto-enzyme of human granulocytes. *Biochim. Biophys. Acta, 512:*525–538.

Sommarin, M., Henriksson, T., and Jergil, B. 1981. Cyclic AMP-dependent protein phosphorylation on the surface of rat hepatocytes. *FEBS Lett., 127:*285–289.

Stanley, K. K., Edwards, M. R., and Luzio, L. P. 1980. Subcellular distribution and movement of 5′-nucleotidase in rat cells. *Biochem. J., 186:*59–69.

Stefanovic, V., Mandel, P., and Rosenberg, A. 1975. Concanavalin A inhibition of ecto-5′-nucleotidase of intact cultured C6 glioma cells. *J. Biol. Chem., 250:*7081–7083.

Stefanovic, V., Mandel, P. and Rosenberg, A. 1976a. Properties of ecto-(inorganic) pyrophosphatase of nervous system cells in culture. Activation upon partial release of sialic acid from the cell surface. *J. Biol. Chem., 251:*493–497.

Stefanovic, V., Mandel, P., and Rosenberg, A. 1976b. Ecto-5′-nucleotidase of intact cultured C6 rat glioma cells. *J. Biol. Chem., 251:*3900–3905.

Stefanovic, V., Giesielski-Treska, J., and Mandel, P. 1977. Neuroblasts–glia interaction in tissue culture as evidenced by the study of ectoenzymes. Ecto-ATPase activity of mouse neuroblastoma cells. *Brain Res., 122:*313–323.

Sullivan, J. M., and Alpers, J. B. 1971. In vitro regulation of rat heart 5′-nucleotidase by adenosine nucleotides and magnesium. *J. Biol. Chem.*, *246*:3057–3063.

Sun, A. S., Aggarwal, B. B., and Packer, L. 1975. Enzyme levels of normal human cells: aging in culture. *Arch. Biochem. Biophys.*, *170*:1–11.

Sun, A. S., Alvarez, L. J., Reinach, P. S., and Rubin, E. 1979. 5′-Nucleotidase levels in normal and virus-transformed cells: Implications for cellular aging in vitro. *Lab. Invest.*, *41*:1–4.

Sun, A. S., Holland, J. F., Ohnuma, T., and Slankard-Chahinian, M 1982. 5′-Nucleotidase activity in permanent human lymphoid cell lines. Implication for cell proliferation and aging in vitro. *Biochim. Biophys. Acta*, *714*:530–535.

Trams, E. G., and Lauter, C. J. 1974. On the sidedness of plasma membrane enzymes. *Biochim. Biophys. Acta*, *354*:180–197.

Trams, E. G., Kauffman, H., and Burnstock, G. 1980. A proposal for the role of ecto-enzymes and adenylates in traumatic shock. *J. Theoret. Biol.*, *87*:609–621.

Trams, E. G., Lauter, C. J., Salem, N., Jr., and Heine, E. 1981. Exfoliation of membrane ectoenzymes in the form of microvesicles. *Biochim. Biophys. Acta*, *654*:63–70.

Uusitalo, R. J., and Karnovsky, M. J. 1977a. Surface localization of 5′-nucleotidase on the mouse lymphocyte. *J. Histochem. Cytochem.*, *25*:87–96.

Uusitalo, R. J., and Karnovsky, M. J. 1977b. 5′-Nucleotidase in different populations of mouse lymphocytes. *J. Histochem. Cytochem.*, *25*:97–103.

Van Belle, H. 1972. Kinetics and inhibition of alkaline phosphatases from canine tissues. *Biochim. Biophys. Acta*, *289*:158–168.

Van den Berghe, G., Van Pottlesburghe, C., and Hers, H.-G. 1977. A kinetic study of the soluble 5′-nucleotidase of rat liver. *Biochem. J.*, *162*:611–616.

Wachstein, M., and Meisel, E. 1957. Histochemistry of hepatic phosphatases at a physiologic pH. *Am. J. Clin. Pathol.* *27*:13–23.

Wallach, D. F. H., and Ullrey, D. 1962. The hydrolysis of ATP and related nucleotides by Ehrlich ascites carcinoma cells. *Cancer Res.*, *22*:228–234.

Wattiaux-de Coninck, S., and Wattiaux, R. 1969. Nucleosidediphosphatase activity in plasma membrane of rat liver. *Biochim. Biophys. Acta*, *183*:118–128.

Weil-Malherbe, H., and Green, R. H. 1951. The catalytic effect of molybdate on the hydrolysis of organic phosphate bonds. *Biochem. J.*, *49*:286–292.

Weiss, B., and Sachs, L. 1977. Differences in surface membrane ecto-ATPase and ecto-AMPase in normal and malignant cells. *J. Cell. Physiol.*, *93*:183–188.

Widnell, C. C. 1972. Cytochemical localization of 5′-nucleotidase in subcellular fractions isolated from rat liver. I. The origin of 5′-nucleotidase activity in microsomes. *J. Cell Biol.*, *52*:542–558.

Widnell, C. C. 1974. Purification of rat liver 5′-nucleotidase as a complex with sphingomyelin. *Methods Enzymol.*, *32B*:368–374.

Widnell, C. C., Schneider, Y.-J., Pierre, B., Baudhuin, P., and Trouet, A. 1982. Evidence for a continual exchange of 5′-nucleotidase between the cell surface and cytoplasmic membranes in cultured rat fibroblasts. *Cell*, *28*:61–70.

Williamson, J. R., and De Pietro, D. L. 1965. Evidence for extracellular enzymic activity of the isolated perfused rat heart. *Biochem. J.*, *95*:226–232.

Wilson, E. J., and Wormall, A. 1949. Studies on suramin (Antrypol:Bayer 205). Further observations on the combination of the drug with protein. *Biochem. J.*, *45*:224–231.

Wilson, P. D., Rustin, G. J. S., Smith, G. P., and Peters, T. J. 1981a. Electron microscopic cytochemical localization of nucleoside phosphatases in normal and chronic granulocytic leukaemic human neutrophils. *Histochem. J.*, *13*:73–84.

Wilson, P. D., Summerhayes, I. C., Hodges, G. M., Trejdosiewicz, L. K., and Nathrath, W. J. 1981b. Cytochemical markers of bladder carcinogenesis. *Histochem. J.*, *13*:989–1007.

Wilson, P. D., Lieberman, G. E., and Peters, T. J., 1982. Ultrastructural localisation of adenosine diphosphatase activity in cultured aortic endothelial cells. *Histochem. J.*, *14*:215–219.

Worku, Y., and Newby, A. C. 1982. Nucleoside exchange catalysed by the cytoplasmic 5′-nucleotidase. *Biochem. J.*, *205*:502–510.

Worku, Y. and Newby, A. C. 1983. The mechanism of adenosine production inside rat polymorphonuclear leucocytes. *Biochem. J.*, *214*:325–330.

Zachowski, A., Aubry, J., Jonkman-Bark, G., and Lelievre, L. 1977. Localization of the catalytic site of 5′-nucleotidase at the inner surface of murine plasmocytoma plasma membranes. *FEBS Lett.*, *75*:197–200.

Zachowski, A., Evans, W. H., and Paraf, A. 1981. Immunological evidence that plasma-membrane 5′-nucleotidase is a transmembrane protein. *Biochim. Biophys. Acta*, *644*:121–126.

Chapter 6

Adenosine Deaminase

Measurement of Activity and Use of Inhibitors

Ram P. Agarwal

Section of Medical Oncology
Evans Memorial Department of Clinical Research and
Departments of Medicine and Pharmacology, and
Hubert H. Humphrey Cancer Research Center
Boston University Medical Center
Boston, Massachusetts

I. ADENOSINE DEAMINASE AND REGULATION OF ADENOSINE CONCENTRATIONS

The physiologic and pharmacologic importance of purines, adenosine, and their analogs as regulators of blood flow, lipolysis, neurotransmission, and immune functions and their antineoplastic activity has been reviewed in this volume and elsewhere (Burnstock, 1981; Schubert *et al.*, 1979; Suhadolnik, 1970). The enzyme adenosine deaminase (ADA; adenosine aminohydrolase, EC 3.5.4.4), which plays an important role in the regulation of adenosine and its analogs, is the subject of the present discussion.

In most, if not all, tissues, the major source of adenosine is the dephosphorylation of AMP catalyzed by 5′-nucleotidase (EC 3.1.3.5). Other sources, such as *S*-adenosylhomocysteine and dietary purines may also contribute to the adenosine pools. Since free adenosine levels of plasma and cells are very low, adenosine produced, irrespective of its sources, is rapidly metabolized either by deamination to inosine or by phosphorylation to AMP (eqs. 1 and 2).

$$\text{Adenosine} + H_2O \xrightarrow{\text{adenosine deaminase}} \text{inosine} + NH_4^+ \qquad (1)$$

$$\text{Adenosine} + \text{ATP} \xrightarrow{\text{adenosine kinase}} \text{AMP} + \text{ADP} \qquad (2)$$

Thus, the enzymes ADA and adenosine kinase (EC 2.7.1.20) play a crucial role in regulating adenosine concentrations.

Both adenosine deaminase and adenosine kinase are widely distributed in tissues (Anderson, 1973; Arch and Newsholme, 1978; Zielke and Suelter, 1971) and have broad specificity for adenosine analogs (Agarwal *et al.*, 1975; Parks and Brown, 1973). Usually, the activity of ADA is 10- to 100-fold higher than that of adenosine kinase. The K_m of adenosine with ADA is 25–35 μM, whereas for adenosine kinase the values are on the order of 1–2 μ*M*. Activities and the kinetic parameters of the two enzymes suggest that, at low concentrations of adenosine, phosphorylation would be preferred, as might be expected under normal physiological conditions. However, at high concentrations of adenosine, as might occur during cellular breakdown, deamination would be a predominant pathway (Agarwal *et al.*, 1975).

II. ADENOSINE DEAMINASE IN VARIOUS PATHOPHYSIOLOGIC CONDITIONS

Elevated levels of ADA were reported in infectious mononucleosis (Koehler and Benz, 1962), bronchial carcinoma (Nishihara *et al.*, 1970, 1973) and acute leukemia (Scholar and Calabresi, 1973). However, an important event in the history of ADA was the discovery of a genetic deficiency of the enzyme in patients with an autosomal recessive form of severe combined immunodeficiency syndrome (Dissing and Knudsen, 1972; Giblett *et al.*, 1972; Meuwissen *et al.*, 1975; Parkman *et al.*, 1975). These patients have both T-cell and B-cell dysfunctions and are susceptible to fatal infections early in their infancy. Replacement of ADA by transfusion of irradiated normal erythrocytes (with normal ADA content) or a bone marrow transplantation partially ameliorate symptoms of the disease (Parkman *et al.*, 1975; Polmar *et al.*, 1976). The platelets from a patient with combined immunodeficiency that showed markedly diminished response to ADP was restored by the addition of partially purified ADA (Lee *et al.*, 1979). These observations suggested a close relationship between ADA activity and immune dysfunctions.

In addition to these findings, high concentrations of ADA observed in lymphocytes of patients with acute lymphoblastic leukemia (ALL), acute myeloid leukemia (AML), and chronic granulocytic leukemia in blast crisis (CGBLC) and non-T, non-B lymphoblasts (Grever *et al.*, 1983; Koya *et al.*, 1981; Smyth and Harrap, 1975; Smyth *et al.*, 1978) prompted measurements of the enzymic activity in malignant and nonmalignant conditions. B-cells and cells of B-cell origin, including normal lymphocytes transformed by Epstein–Barr virus, multiple myeloma, hairy cell leukemia (Meier *et al.*, 1976), and B-cell ALL and CLL (Ben-Basset *et al.*, 1979; Coleman et al., 1978), have low enzymic activity. In a study of human leukemic cell lines (T-cell, B-cell, and null cells), the T-cell ADA activity was shown to increase during logarithmic growth. The activity then decreased in T-cells but there was no change in activity during the growth cycle of B-cells (Tritsch and Minowada, 1978).

Increased ADA activities have been reported in the lymphocytes of patients with T-cell lymphoma (Kedar *et al.*, 1980), transitional cell carcinoma of bladder (Sufrin *et al.*, 1978), and Waldenstrom's macroglobulinemia (Sidi *et al.*, 1979). But the activity was low in patients with renal cell carcinoma (Sufrin *et al.*, 1977).

Significant differences in ADA activity have been reported in patients who accept or reject renal allografts. The mononuclear cell ADA activity was significantly lower in patients who had maintained their grafts for more than one year than in those who had not (Lum *et al.*, 1978). Furthermore, the patients who had no rejection and no evidence of posttransplant cytomegalovirus infection had normal ADA activity during the first 2 weeks after transplantation; whereas patients who lost their grafts or had the virus infection had significantly higher ADA activity. Thus, ADA levels two weeks after transplantation may serve as a potential useful prognostic indicator of post transplant virus related grafts or patient loss (Lum *et al.*, 1979).

The erythrocytes of autistic children, who may have low cellular immunity, have decreased ADA activity (Stubbs et al., 1982), whereas an overproduction of erythrocytic ADA has been associated with hereditary hemolytic anemia (Miwa *et al.*, 1978).

The correlation of ADA activity with purine nucleoside phosphorylase, ecto-5′-nucleotidase, and the leukemic marker, terminal deoxynucleotidyl transferase, strongly suggests that measurement of this enzyme may offer a biochemical method of distinguishing immunological subsets of lymphoblasts (Barton *et al.*, 1980; Blatt *et al.*, Coleman *et al.*, 1978; Grever *et al.*, 1983; Newby, 1980; Smyth *et al.*, 1978).

III. ASSAY METHODS

The preceeding discussion clearly indicates the present interest in measuring ADA activity under different pathologic and physiologic conditions. Several methods are available for measuring ADA activity, each of which has some limitations. Therefore, the choice of a method depends on the specific requirement and resources available to an investigator. Although different conditions of pH, buffer, incubation time, and temperature have been used, only general conditions are described in this review.

The reaction catalyzed by ADA (eq. 1) is simple: a hydrolytic deamination of adenosine to inosine and ammonia (although the enzyme also catalyzes removal of groups other than ammonia, i.e., halogens, hydroxylamine, and others. these reactions are not relevant here). Therefore, the majority of ADA assay methods are based on the measurement of either the disappearance of substrate or appearance of products. A radioimmunossay has also been developed but is not in common use. Various analytic techniques (high-pressure liquid chromatography spectrophotometery, fluorometry, isotopes, and others) have been employed to quantitate changes in substrate and product concentrations.

Table I. Molar Absorbancy Changes Resulting from Hydrolysis of 6-Substituent of Purine Analogs[a]

Substrate	Wavelength (nm)	A × 10^{-3} *M*
Adenosine	265	−8.6
2′-Deoxyadenosine	265	−8.6
Arabinosyladenine	265	−8.6
8-Aminoadenosine	272	−5.4
8-Azaadenosine	280	−7.2
8-Hydroxyadenosine	272	−4.6
6-Hydroxylaminopurine ribonucleoside	269	−8.2
6-Methoxypurine ribonucleoside	270	+3.9
6-Chloropurine ribonucleoside	246	+6.3
6-Bromopurine ribonucleoside	250	+6.2
6-Iodopurine ribonucleoside	250	+6.4
2,6-Diaminopurine ribonucleoside	256	+3.9
2-Amino-6-methoxypurine ribonucleoside	257	+6.35
2-Amino-6-chloropurine ribonucleoside	264	+9.9
N^6-Methyladenosine	262	−11.2
Formycin A	305	−6.0

[a] Modified from Zielke and Suelter (1971). All values are at pH 7.0–7.4.

A. Methods Based on Disappearance of Adenosine (Substrate)

1. Direct Spectrophotometric Method

Deamination of adenosine to inosine causes a decrease in absorbancy, which is maximum at 265 nm ($-\Delta\epsilon = 8.6 \times 10^{-3}$). Therefore, ADA activity is determined by following the rate of decrease in absorbancy at 265 nm, as described below.

In a quartz cuvette of 1-cm light path are added 0.9 ml of 50 m*M* phosphate buffer, pH 7.4, 10 μl of 10 m*M* adenosine solution, the enzyme and water to make 1 ml. The reaction mixture is usually incubated for 3–5 min at the desired temperature (commonly 30°C or 37°C) and the reaction is then started by addition of the enzyme. The decrease in absorbancy is continuously followed at 265 nm by using a recording spectrophotometer.

This method is the simplest, rapid, and most commonly used for ADA assay. Being a dynamic method, it is very useful for kinetic studies where initial velocity measurement is an important factor. This method is also applicable with other substrates that have large absorbancy differences between them and their products. Molar absorption changes of some interesting adenosine analogs are presented in Table I (Agarwal *et al.*, 1975; Zielke and Suelter, 1971). For an exhaustive list of absorbancy changes, readers are referred to Zielke and Suelter (1971).

A limitation of this method is that it cannot be used in the presence of other materials that have high absorbancy in the region of 265 nm. For example, used in the presence of an inhibitor absorbing at or near 265 nm, with a crude enzyme preparation, or with a large amount of enzyme (particularly with samples of low specific activity), the method would be insensitive. The use of high-substrate concentrations, which might give unacceptably high absorbancy, is limited by this method.

Changes in adenosine and inosine concentrations after a fixed time of incubation of adenosine and ADA may also be followed at 254 nm after their separation by high-pressure liquid chromatography (Agarwal *et al.*, 1982a; Hartwick *et al.*, 1978). However, this is a static method and cannot be used in the presence of substances that absorb and co-elute with the substrate or the product. In addition, it requires expensive equipment.

2. *Fluorometric Method*

Forymcin A, an adenosine analog, is a very good substrate for ADA (Agarwal *et al.*, 1975). Forymcin A exhibits appreciable fluorescence at room temperature, whereas its deaminated product formycin B does not. This property of formycin A has led Wierzchowski and Shugar (1983) to develop a fluorometric assay for ADA as described below.

A mixture of formycin A, ADA, and 20 m*M* phosphate buffer, pH 7.5, is incubated in a spectral cuvette of 1-cm light path. The solution is excited at 295 nm or 305 nm and fluorescence is measured at 338 nm or 354 nm. In order to minimize the contribution of fluorescence from proteins while measuring enzyme levels in cell extracts, excitation wavelengths of 305 nm or 318 nm may be used.

Formycin concentrations are so adjusted that the optical density at excitation wavelength does not exceed 0.3 (4–40 μ*M* at 305 nm and as high as 300 μ*M* at 318 nm).

At substrate concentrations with optical densities ≤ 0.1, the concentration of unchanged substrate is determined by the equation

$$C_t = C_0 \frac{I_t - I_b}{I_0 - I_b} \tag{3}$$

where C_0 and C_t are concentrations at times 0 and t, and I_0, I_t, and I_b are fluorescence intensities at times 0 and t and background fluorescence, respectively. At substrate concentrations of 50 μ*M*, the deamination of formycin is a pseudo-first-order reaction. At high substrate concentrations, resulting high optical density requires introduction of a correction factor (Wierzchowski and Shugar, 1983).

The fluorometric method is more sensitive than the spectrophotometric method, and it may be applied to cell extracts that exhibit a high optical density. The limitation of the method is that one can use only those substrates that have fluorescence and whose products are nonfluorescent.

3. *Radioisotopic Method*

In this method, the ADA activity is measured as the amount of [^{14}C]adenosine deaminated to [^{14}C]inosine. Therefore, isotopic method measures both disappearance of substrate and appearance of products. Since most cellular extracts and crude enzyme preparations may also contain purine nucleoside phosphorylase (PNP; purine nucleoside: orthophosphate ribosyltransferase, EC 2.4.2.1), [^{14}C]inosine formed in the reaction may further be converted to [^{14}C]hypoxanthine. Therefore, any satisfactory chromatographic method that separates substrate from the products may be used in this assay. A general method is described here as an example.

A reaction mixture (100 μl) containing 50 m*M* potassium phosphate, pH 7.4, 1 m*M* EDTA, and 0.1 m*M* [8-^{14}C]adenosine (50 mCi/mmole) is incubated at 37°C. The reaction is started by addition of 10 μl of ADA solution. After 10–30 min of incubation at 37°C the reaction is stopped by heating for 1 min in boiling water bath. A mixture of nonradioactive adenosine, inosine, and hypoxanthine (10 μl) is added as carriers. Ten to twenty microliters of the reaction mixture is applied onto a thin-layer chromatography plate and the compounds are separated by developing the plate in 1-butanol and concentrated ammonium hydroxide (99:1). The spots of adenosine, inosine, and hypoxanthine are visualized by UV light, cut out, and counted by liquid scintillation spectrometry (Nygaard, 1978; Trotta and Balis, 1977). An ultramicroradiochemical method that can measure ADA activity in 5–10 fibroblasts has recently been described (Uitendaal *et al.*, 1978).

The isotopic method is more sensitive than the spectrophotometric method and therefore can be used for samples containing low activity. The method may be used in the presence of components that have high absorptions, crude preparations with optically unclear solutions, cell suspensions, and thin tissue sections. In contrast to the spectrophotometric and fluorometric method, it is a somewhat static method and requires the use of radiochemicals.

B. Methods Based on Measurement of Products of Adenosine Deaminase Reaction

1. Measurement of Inosine

a. Radioisotopic Assay. The isotopic assay for inosine is similar to that described above for adenosine.

b. Coupled Enzymic Assay. Inosine produced during the ADA reaction is determined spectrophotometrically by coupling with purine nucleoside phosphorylase (PNP) and xanthine oxidase (XO)(Hopkinson *et al.*, 1969).

$$\text{Inosine} + \text{phosphate} \xrightarrow{\text{PNP}} \text{hypoxanthine} + \text{ribose-1-phosphate} \qquad (4)$$

$$\text{Hypoxanthine} \xrightarrow{\text{XO}} \text{xanthine} \xrightarrow{\text{XO}} \text{uric acid} \qquad (5)$$

The final product of these reactions, uric acid, which absorbs at 293 nm, is followed by measuring an increase in optical density at this wavelength. In a typical assay, 0.9 ml of 0.22 m*M* adenosine solution in 50 m*M* phosphate buffer, pH 7.4, 10 μl of PNP solution (0.1 U) and 10 μl of xanthine oxidase (0.1 U) are incubated for 3–5 min in a quartz cuvette at 37°C in a recording spectrophotometer. This incubation period permits temperature equilibrium and oxidation of hypoxanthine and xanthine that might be present as contaminants. The reaction is then started by addition of ADA and water to make 1 ml. The rate of uric acid production is monitored by continuous recording of increase in absorbancy at 293 nm. The molar extinction coefficient of uric acid is taken as 12.2×10^3 under these conditions. Commerical preparations of PNP and xanthine oxidase may have ADA activity as a contaminant. Therefore, a similar reaction is repeated without addition of ADA and the appropriate background is substrated from each determination.

Both purine nucleoside phosphorylase and xanthine oxidase are readily available commercially. Appropriate dilutions of these enzymes in 50 m*M* phosphate buffer, pH 7.4, are made fresh each day, whereas adenosine solution may be prepared in bulk and stored frozen.

This is also a dynamic assay and is slightly more sensitive (1.5 times) than the direct spectrophotometric method described above. Another advantage is that the wavelength (293 nm) at which the reaction is followed is far from the absorption (260 nm) of many adenosine analogs; thus, there is less interference from these compounds. A limitation, however, is that the method would not be applicable with ADA substrates whose products do not serve as substrates for PNP and xanthine oxidase reactions. For example, both arabinosyladenine and formycin A are good substrates for ADA but their respective deaminated products, arabinosyl-hypoxanthine and formycin B, are not good substrates of PNP. In addition, if any adenosine analog is a weak substrate for PNP, one might expect high background activity.

2. *Measurement of Ammonia*

a. Coupled Enzymic Assay (Spectrophotometric). The method is a slight modification (Agarwal *et al.*, 1975) of the measurement of ammonia from glutaminase activity (Kvamme *et al.*, 1965). The ammonia liberated during ADA reaction is measured spectrophotometrically in a coupled reaction with glutamate dehydrogenase (GDH), α-ketoglutarate (α-KG), and NADH. The oxidation of NADH to NAD^+ is followed at 340 nm.

$$NH_4^+ + \alpha\text{-KG} + NADH \xrightarrow{GDH} \text{L-glutamate} + NAD^+ + H_2O \quad (6)$$

The assay mixture (1 ml) consisting of 50 m*M* phosphate buffer, pH 7.4, 17 m*M* α-ketoglutarate, 1 m*M* EDTA Na_4, 0.3 m*M* NADH (neutralized), 60 U glutamic dehydrogenase (0.1 ml of stock solution containing 600 U/ml in 50% glycerol), and adenosine deaminase is incubated at 37°C for 3–5 min. The reaction is started by addition of adenosine (0.5 m*M* final concentration). A decrease in absorbancy at 340 n*M* is continuously followed by a recording spectrophotometer. Molar absorbancy change during oxidation of NADH to NAD^+ is 6.22×10^3. The rate of reaction is corrected by subtracting the background rate obtained before addition of substrate.

Caution must be exercised so that no ammonia is present in the vicinity of the reaction and that reagents are free from NH_3. Glutamate dehydrogenase is commercially available either as ammonium sulfate suspension or in a 50% glycerol solution. The latter should be used in present assay methods.

This is also a dynamic assay procedure that permits a direct measurement of the rate of enzymic activity. The substrates and inhibitors absorbing in the vicinity of 260 nm can safely be used in this procedure. (Agarwal *et al.*, 1975). The major disadvantage of the assay is that the K_m of NH_4^+ for glutamate dehydrogenase is relatively high and a lag period of several minutes is usually encountered before a linear reaction rate is achieved. At low concentrations of substrate or in the presence of high ADA activity, all the substrate might be depleted before the linear reaction starts. Other disadvantages of methods based on the measurement of ammonia are that ammonium sulfate precipitates of enzyme (obtained during purification) are unsuitable without prior exhaustive dialysis and that 6-halogenated-, 6-hydroxylamine-, N^6-methylpurine ribonucleosides that do not produce ammonia during ADA reaction cannot be used as substrates.

b. Coupled Enzymic Assay (*Fluorometric*). Loss of fluorescence of NADH on oxidation to NAD^+ (eq. 6) is the basis of two (qualitative and quantitative) fluorometric assay methods of ADA in human blood (Orfanos *et al.*, 1978; Vaca *et al.*, 1979).

In the quantitative assay method (Orfanos *et al.*, 1978) the blood samples are collected on Schleicher and Schuell filter paper (SS #903) and dried. A 6.3 mm in diameter disc is punched out from the dried blood specimen and incubated with 0.3 ml of 13 m*M* adenosine solution in 60 m*M* sodium phosphate buffer, pH 7.2. After incubation at 37°C for 1 hr, the reaction is terminated by addition of 0.2 ml TCA (100 g/liter) and the mixture is centrifuged for 5 min. A blank containing 0.3 ml of phosphate buffer and a standard containing 0.15 μmole ammonium sulfate in 0.3 ml of phosphate buffer are also treated in the same way. The supernatant fluids (250 μl) are transferred to fluorometrica cuvette containing 3 ml of phosphate buffer, pH 7.9. To this mixture are added 0.1 ml of 25 m*M* α-KG and 0.1 ml of 1.4 m*M* NADH (neutralized) solutions, and the contents are mixed by inversion. Initial fluorescence is measured in a flurometer at excitation and emission wavelengths of 365 and 460 nm, respectively. Now 20 μg of GDH (ammonium sulfate free) in 0.05 ml buffer is added and mixed by inversion. Fluorescence is measured again after 15 min. After subtraction of the background fluorescence, the activity is calculated and expressed in terms of units per gram hemoglobin. Hemoglobin is determined from the dried samples by a modified Drabkins solution as described by Orfanos *et al.* (1978).

For the qualitative assay (Vaca *et al.*, 1979), the blood samples are collected either in heparinized tubes or on filter paper as described above and are treated as follows: Ten microliters of heparinized blood or 6.3-cm filter paper with dried blood disc is placed in a test tube (13 × 100 mm). To this is added 100 μl of a mixture containing 0.16 m*M* adenosine and 0.2% saponin in 330 m*M* Tris-HCl buffer, pH 7.0. Following incubation at 37°C for 70 to 90 min, 100 μl of the fluorescent mixture consisting of α-KG (0.08 m*M*), NADH (40 μg), and GDH (about 20 μg, ammonium sulfate free) in 160 m*M* phosphate buffer, pH 6.6 are added. The mixture is shaken gently and allowed to stand for 10–30 min. A few microliters is spotted on Whatman filter paper, dried, and examined for fluorescence under long-wavelength UV light. Blood sample containing ADA loses fluorescence.

This is a qualitative method and may be useful for screening of ADA activity in suspected ADA-deficient patients. However, any negative or doubtful case must be scrutinized more precisely as the method is likely to give both false positive and false negative results. The assay has the advantage that samples collected in areas without laboratory facilities can be sent to laboratories for analysis. Such dried samples have sufficient ADA activity for at least 10 days after collection, which is enough for mailing and analysis. Stability may be increased if samples are stored frozen. Precautions applied are similar to those described for the spectrophotometric assay.

c. Colorimetric Method. The ammonia produced in the reaction is determined by a modification (Rogler-Brown *et al.*, 1978) of the microdiffusion method of Seligson and Seligson (1951) and the colorimetric procedure of Chaney and Marbach (1962).

The reaction mixture containing 50 m*M* phosphate buffer, pH 7.4, 1.0 m*M* adenosine, and the enzyme is incubated at 37°C. Aliquots (0.5 to 1.0 ml) are withdrawn at 0 and specified times (10–30 min intervals) and added to flasks (20-ml serum vials) containing one ml of saturated K_2CO_3 (100 g/100 ml) and are equipped with rubber stoppers holding glass rods with flared ground tips coated with 1 *M* citric acid. The flasks are placed on a rotary mixer (Multipurpose rotator, Scientific Industries, Bohemia, N.Y.) for at least 30 min and the ammonia is allowed to diffuse and to be trapped on the citric acid-coated rods. The ammonia collected is washed into a 1 ml of solution A (phenol, 0.53 *M*, and nitroprusside, 1 m*M*, in water). The color is developed by the addition of 1 ml of solution B (sodium hydroxide, 0.63 *M*, containing sodium hypochlorite, 0.03 *M*, in water). The blue indophenol formed is measured at 625 nm. For standard, 25–100 μl of 1 m*M* ammonium sulfate solution is treated similarly to the reaction aliquots.

Although this method is a static procedure, it has been found very useful for measurement of ADA activity in turbid solutions, intact cells, tissue homogenates, and solutions containing ultraviolet-absorbing materials.

C. Radioimmunoassay of Adenosine Deaminase

This method makes use of antiserum to purified human ADA raised in goat and radioiodinated purified ADA (Wiginton *et al.*, 1981). The assay is carried out at 4°C in a 1.5 ml polypropylene microcentrifuge tube. All components of the assay are diluted with 50 m*M* potassium phosphate, pH 7.2, containing bovine serum albumin (1 mg/ml) and 1 m*M*-β-mercaptoethanol (buffer A). Immunoglobulin G was diluted to precipitate 30–40% of the ^{125}I-labeled adenosine deaminase in the assay in the absence of unlabeled enzyme. In the normal assay, 25 μl of diluted immunoglobulin G is mixed with 50 μl of buffer A containing 0.03–100 ng of unlabeled purified human adenosine deaminase (for standard curve), an appropriate dilution of sample cell extract, or buffer A with no addition (control). The samples are mixed and incubated at 4°C for 16 hr. ^{125}I-labeled adenosine deaminase (25 μl; 15,000 cpm) is added to each tube and samples are further incubated at 4°C for 16 hr. Then 100 μl of a 10% suspension of IgGsorb (heat-killed freeze-dried *Staphylococcus aureus* containing Protein A) is added to each sample, and the samples are incubated at room temperature for 15 min and centrifuged at 8000*g* for 2 min. The resulting pellets are washed twice with buffer A and precipitated ^{125}I radioactivity is determined by gamma counting. The IgGsorb binds 2–3% of the ^{125}I radioactivity in the assay in the absence of the immunoglobulin G. The standard curve for binding competition is determined between unlabeled purified human enzyme and ^{125}I-labeled enzyme. Data for both the standard curve and cell extracts are analysed by the modified logit-log transformation (Rodbard *et al.*, 1969). The least detectable dose (that sample amount statistically different from zero) is taken where the lower 95% confidence limit of the radioactivity bound in the absence of unlabeled enzyme crosses the extrapolated standard line. The least detectable dose determined in this manner was 0.1 ng in a 50 μl sample, or 2 ng/ml.

IV. ADENOSINE DEAMINASE INHIBITORS AND THEIR USE

Because of increasing interest in ADA, several inhibitors of the enzyme have been either synthesized or isolated during the last decade. These inhibitors differ widely in their affinities for ADA, ranging from readily reversible, to semitight, to tight binding (Agarwal *et al.*, 1977). For a recent comprehensive review of these inhibitors, see Agarwal (1982).

A. Synthetic Inhibitors

Based on structure–activity relationships, a large number of compounds were synthesized by a systemic change in the 9-substituent of adenine (Schaeffer, 1971). This procedure had resulted in a number of 9-substituted adenine analogs with wide range of inhibitory potencies including the two very potent inhibitors *erythro*-9-(2-hydroxy-3-nonyl)adenine (EHNA) and *erythro*-9-(2-hydroxy-3-dodecyl)adenine (EHDA) (Schaeffer and Schwender, 1974). EHNA, the best studied of these compounds, is a racemic mixture of *erythro*-(−)-9-(2-*R* hydroxy-3*S* nonyl)adenine and *erythro*-(+)9-(2-*S* hydroxy-3*R* nonyl)adenine (Baker *et al.*, 1981; Bastian *et al.*, 1981). The synthesis of the two *threo* isomers (THNA) has now also been achieved (Bastian *et al.*, 1981).

The isomer (+)-2*S*,3*R* EHNA is 80- to 200-fold more potent as an inhibitor than (−)-2*R*,3*S* EHNA (Baker *et al.*, 1981; Bessodes *et al.*, 1981). Both the isomers of THNA, (+)-2*R*,3*R*-THNA and (−)-2*S*,3*S* THNA were less potent as ADA inhibitors than (+)-2*S*,3*R* EHNA but were more potent than (−)-2*R*,3*S* EHNA (Bessodes *et al.*, 1981).

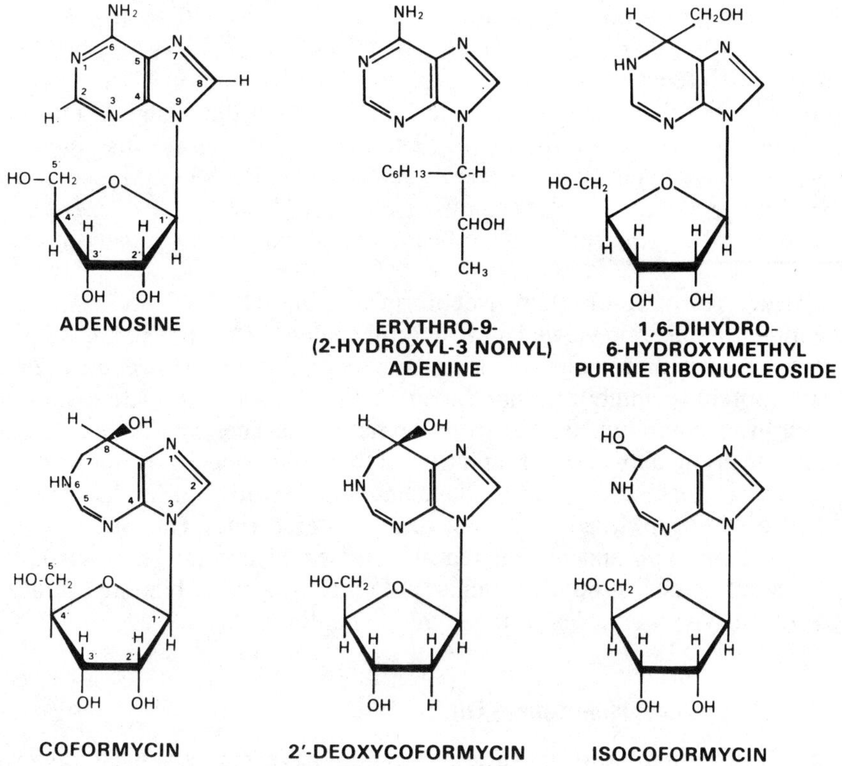

Figure 1. Structures of adenosine and adenosine deaminase inhibitors (from Agarwal, 1982).

A postulated transition-state analog inhibitor (Pauling, 1948) of ADA was synthesized by the photoaddition of methanol to purine ribonucleoside (Evans and Wolfenden, 1970). The photoadduct 1,6-dihydro-6-hydroxymethylpurine ribonucleoside (DHMPR) (Figure 1) was about 100-fold more inhibitory (K_i,1–3 $\times$ $10^{-6}M$) than inosine (K_i,1.2 $\times$ $10^{-4}M$), the product of the reaction (Agarwal *et al.*, 1977; Evans and Wolfenden, 1970).

B. Naturally Occurring Inhibitors

Two antibiotics, coformycin and deoxycoformycin (DCF), resemble the methanol adduct DHMPR and are very potent inhibitors of adenosine deaminase. Coformycin was discovered in the culture filtrates of *Norcardia interforma* and *Streptomyces kaniharaensis* SF-557, and the inhibitory properties of the compound were reported by Sawa *et al.* (1967a,b).The structure of coformycin reported by Nakamura *et al.* (1974) has now been confirmed by X-ray crystallography as 3-(β-D-ribofuranosyl)-6,7,8-trihydroimidazo (4,5-*d*) (1,3)diazepin-8(*R*)-ol (Nakamura *et al.*, 1976). Shimakzaki *et al.* (1979a) have synthesized an isomer of coformycin, 3-β-D-ribofuranosyl-3,6,7,8-tetrahydro-imidazo(4,5-*d*) (1,3)-diazepin-7-ol, isocoformycin. Isocoformycin is also an inhibitor of adenosine deaminase, but its inhibitory potency is much weaker (K_i, 4.5–10.0 × $10^{-8}M$) (Shimazaki *et al.*, 1979b) than coformycin (K_i, $10^{-10}M$) (Cha *et al.*, 1975; Cha, 1976), suggesting that stereospecificity is required for the inhibition of ADA.

Woo *et al.* (1974) isolated an antibiotic, DCF, from the fermentation broth of a strain of *Streptomyces antibioticus*. The aglycon portion of this compound is identical to coformycin, but the sugar moiety of DCF is deoxyribose instead of ribose. DCF is the most potent inhibitor of ADA (K_i, 2.5 × $10^{-12}M$) known to date and its kinetic properties have been studied extensively (Agarwal *et al.*, 1976).

The structures of coformycin, isocoformycin, and DCF are given in Figure 1. These inhibitors may be viewed as structural analogs of the physiological products of the ADA reaction, namely, inosine and deoxyinosine. However, they are much more potent as inhibitors than inosine and represent "transition-state analogs." All three compounds differ from the natural purines by the interposition of a methylene group between N(1) and C(6) of the purine ring. Thus, the structure of the aglycon is not that of a purine base but is a derivative of imidazodiazepin with a hydroxyl group attached to a seven-membered ring. The ring is hydrogenated at C-7 and C-8 and protonated at N-6 (see Figure 1). These structural changes, though minor, produce a remarkable increase in the binding affinity of the coformycin-type molecules to the catalytic center of ADA.

C. Uses of Adenosine Deaminase Inhibitors

Uses of ADA inhibitors in various systems have recently been reviewed (Agarwal, 1982). Therefore, for the sake of brevity only a few examples are presented here.

1. Model for Kinetic Studies of Tight-Binding Inhibitors

The availability of a number of ADA inhibitors ranging in potency from readily reversible, semitight binding, to tight binding has served as an excellent model for testing many new approaches to the study of tight-binding enzyme inhibitors (Agarwal, 1979, 1980; Agarwal *et al.*, 1978; Cha, 1975, 1976; Cha *et al.*, 1975; Rogler-Brown *et al.*, 1978).

2. Modifiers of Metabolism and Disposition of Purine Nucleosides

Many purine nucleoside analogs serve as biochemical antagonists in RNA, DNA, and protein synthesis (Suhadolnik, 1970). Since a majority of these analogs are substrates for ADA, they are rendered ineffective by deamination (Agarwal *et al.*, 1975) and fail to incorporate themselves into the cellular nucleotide pool (Parks and Brown, 1973). Use of ADA inhibitors modifies the metabolism of these analogs and enhances their incorporation into cellular nucleotide pools and subsequent inhibition of RNA and DNA synthesis (Cass and Au-Yeung, 1976; Glazer and Peale, 1978).

3. *Potentiators of Cytotoxicity and Chemotherapeutic Effects*

At the dosages currently used, the ADA inhibitors are not cytotoxic. However, they markedly enhance the cytotoxicity of adenosine analogs. The synergistic antitumor effects of adenosine analogs and ADA inhibitors have been reported in a number of experimental systems both *in vitro* and *in vivo* (Adamson *et al.*, 1977; Caron *et al.*, 1977; Muller *et al.*, 1978).

Since the first demonstration of one complete and two partial remissions in acute lymphoblastic leukemic patients by DCF (Smyth *et al.*, 1979), several investigators have reported selective therapeutic effect of DCF in T-cell malignancies and mycosis fungoides (Major *et al.*, 1981a,b; Koller *et al.*, 1979; Prentice *et al.*, 1980). DCF when used in combination with arabinosyl adenine (Ara-A) caused both the prolongation of half-life of Ara-A as well as enhanced its therapeutic effects (Agarwal *et al.*, 1982b; Major *et al.*, 1983).

The ADA inhibitors coformycin and DCF potentiate the antiviral activity of Ara-A (Conner *et al.*, 1974; Falcon and Jones, 1977; Schroder *et al.*, 1981; Sloan *et al.*, 1977). A high concentration of EHNA (10^{-4} *M*) alone has been reported to cause a significant reduction in herpes simplex virus (North and Cohen, 1978).

4. *Immunosuppressive Agents*

Prolongation of skin and pancreatic islet allografts in mice has been demonstrated by use of EHNA (Lum *et al.*, 1979). Immunosuppression by DCF has also been shown in mouse tumor and skin allografts (Chassin *et al.*, 1977 and Trotta *et al.*, 1980).

REFERENCES

Adamson, R. H., Zaharevitz, D. W., and Johns, D. G. 1977. Enhancement of the biological activity of adenosine analogs by the adenosine deaminase inhibitor 2′-deoxycoformycin. *Pharmacology*, *15*:84–89.

Agarwal, R. P. 1979. Recovery of 2′-deoxycoformycin-inhibited adenosine deaminase of mouse erythrocytes and leukemia L1210 *in vivo*. *Cancer Res.*, *39*:1425–1427.

Agarwal, R. P. 1980. *In vivo* inhibition of adenosine deaminase by 2′-deoxycoformycin in mouse blood and leukemia L1210 cells. *Biochem. Pharmacol.*, *29*:187–193.

Agarwal, R. P. 1982. Inhibitors of adenosine deaminase. *Pharmacol. Ther. 17*:399–429.

Agarwal, R. P., Sagar, S. M., and Parks, R. E., Jr. 1975. Adenosine deaminase from human erythrocytes: Purification and effects of adenosine analogs. *Biochem. Pharmacol.*, *24*:693–701.

Agarwal, R. P., Crabtree, G. W., Parks, R. E., Jr., Nelson, J. A. Keightley, R., Parkman, R., Rosen, R. Stern, R. C., and Polmar, S. H. 1976. Purine nucleoside metabolism in the erythrocytes of patients with adenosine deaminase deficiency and severe combined immunodeficiency. *J. Clin. Invest.*, *57*:1025–1035.

Agarwal, R. P., Spector, T., and Parks, R. E., Jr. 1977. Tight-binding inhibitors IV: Inhibition of adenosine deaminase by various inhibitors. *Biochem. Pharmacol.*, *26*:359–367.

Agarwal, R. P., Major, P. P., and Kufe, D. W. 1982a. Simple and rapid high-performance liquid chromatographic method for analysis of nucleosides in biological fluids. *J. Chromatogr.*, *231*:418–424.

Agarwal, R. P., Blatt, J., Miser, J., Sallan, S., Lipton, J. M., Reaman, G. H., Holcenberg, J., and Poplack, D. G. 1982b. Clinical pharmacology of 9-β-D arabinofuranosyl adenine in combination with 2′-deoxycoformycin. *Cancer Res.*, *42*:3884–3886.

Arch, J. R. S. and Newsholme, E. A. 1978. Activities and some properties of 5′-nucleotidase, adenosine kinase and adenosine deaminase in tissues from vertebrates in relation to the control of the concentration and the physiological role of adenosine. *Biochem. J.*, *174*:965–977.

Anderson, E. P. 1973. Nucleoside and nucleotide kinases. *The Enzymes*, *9*:49–96.

Baker, D. C., Hanvey, J. C., Hawkins, L. D. and Murphy, J. 1981. Identification of the bioactive enantiomer of *erythro*-3-(adenine-9yl)-2-nonanol (EHNA), a semi-tight binding inhibitor of adenosine deaminase. *Biochem. Pharmacol.*, *30*:1159–1160.

Barton, R., Martiniuk, F., Hirschhorn, R., and Goldschneider, I. 1980. Inverse relationship between adenosine deaminase and purine nucleoside phosphorylase in rat lymphocyte population. *Cell. Immunol.*, *49*:208–214.

Bastian, G., Bessodes, M., Panzica, R. P., Abushanab, E., Chen, S. F., Stoeckler, J. D. and Parks, R. E., Jr. 1981. Adenosine deaminase inhibitors. The conversion of a single chiral synthon into *erythro* and *threo*-9-(2-hydroxy-3 nonyl) adenine. *J. Med. Chem.*, *24*:1383–1384.

Ben-Basset, I., Simoni, F., Holtzman, F., and Ramot, B. 1979. Adenosine deaminase activity of normal lymphocytes and leukemic cells. *Israel J. Med. Sci.*, *15*:925–927.

Bessodes, M. D., Bastian, G., Abushanab, E., Panzica, R. P., Berman, S. F., Marcaccio, E. J., Jr., Chen, S. F., Stoeckler, J. D., and Parks, Jr. 1981. Effect of chirality in *erythro*-9-(2-hydroxy-3-nonyl) adenine. *Biochem. Pharmacol.*, *31*:879–882.

Blatt, J., Reaman, G., Poplack, D. G. 1980. Biochemical markers in lymphoid malignancy. *N. Engl. J. Med.*, *303*:918–922.

Burnstock, G. 1981. Neurotransmitters and trophic factors in the autonomic nervous system. *J. Physiol.*, *313*:1–35.

Caron, N., Lee S. H., and Kimball, A. P. 1977. Effect of 2′-deoxycoformycin, 9-β-D-arabinofuranosyladenine-5′-phosphate, and 1-β-D-arabinofuranosylcytosine triple combination therapy on intracerebral leukemia 1210. *Cancer Res.*, *37*:3274–3279.

Cass, C. E., and Au-Yeung, T. H. 1976. Enhancement of 9-β-D-arabinofuranosyl adenine cytotoxicity to mouse leukemia L1210 *in vitro* by 2′-deoxycoformycin. *Cancer Res.*, *36*:1486–1491.

Cha, S. 1975. Tight-binding inhibitors: I. Kinetic behavior. *Biochem. Pharmacol.*, *24*:2177–2185.

Cha, S. 1976. Tight-binding inhibitors: III. A new approach for the determination of competition between tight-binding inhibitors and substrates—inhibition of adenosine deaminase by coformycin. *Biochem. Pharmacol.*, *25*:2695–2702.

Cha, S., Agarwal, R. P. and Parks, R. E., Jr. 1975. Tight-binding inhibitors: II. Non-steady state nature of inhibition of milk xanthine oxidase by allopurinol and alloxanthine and of human erythrocytic adenosine deaminase by coformycin. *Biochem. Pharmacol.*, *24*:2187–2197.

Chaney, A. L., and Marbach, E. P. 1962. Modified reagents for determination of urea and ammonia. *Clin. Chem.*, *8*:130–132.

Chassin, M. M., Chirigos, M. A., Johns, D. G. and Adamson, R. H. 1977. Adenosine deaminase inhibition for immunosuppressive. *N. Engl. J. Med.*, *296*:1232.

Coleman, M. S., Greenwood, M. F., Hutton, J. J., Holland, P., Lampkin, B., Krill, C., and Kastelic, J. E. 1978. Adenosine deaminase, terminal deoxynucleotidyl transferase (TdT), and cell surface markers in childhood acute leukemia. *Blood*, *52*:1125–1131.

Conner, J. D., Sweetman, L., Carey, S., Stuckey, M. A., and Buchanan, R. 1974. Effect of adenosine deaminase upon the antiviral activity *in vitro* of adenine arabinoside for vaccinia virus. *Antimicrob. Ag. Chemother.*, *6*:630–636.

Dissing, J., and Knudsen, B. 1972. Adenosine deaminase deficiency and combined immunodeficiency syndrome. *Lancet*, *2*:1316.

Evans, B., and Wolfenden, R. 1970. A potential transition-state analog for adenosine deaminase. *J. Am. Chem. Soc.*, *92*:4751–4752.

Falcon, M. G., and Jones, B. R. 1977. Antiviral activity in the rabbit cornea of adenine arabinoside, Ara-A 5′-mono-phosphate, and hypoxanthine arabinoside; and interaction with adenosine deaminase inhibitor. *J. Gen. Virol.*, *36*:199–202.

Giblett, E. R., Anderson, J. E., Cohen, F., Pollara, B., and Meuwissen, H. J. 1972. Adenosine deaminase deficiency in two patients with severely impaired cellular immunity. *Lancet*, *2*:1067–1069.

Glazer, R. I., and Peale, A. L. 1978. Cordycepin and xylosyladenine: Inhibitors of methylation of nuclear RNA. *Biochem. Biophys. Res. Commun.*, *81*:521–526.

Grever, M., Coleman, M. S., Balcerzak, S. P. 1983. Adenosine deaminase and terminal deoxynucleotidyl transferase: biochemical markers in the management of chronic myelogeneous leukemia. *Cancer Res.*, *43*:1442–1445.

Hartwick, R., Jeffries, A., Krstulovic, A., and Brown, P. R. 1978. An optimized assay for adenosine deaminase using reverse phase high pressure liquid chromatography. *J. Chromatgr.*, *16*:427–435.

Hopkinson, D. A., Cook, P. J. L., and Harris, H. 1969. Further data on the adenosine deaminase (ADA) polymorphism and a report of a new phenotype. *Ann. Hum. Genet.*, *32*:361–367.

Kedar, A., Tritsch, G. L., Freeman, A. I. 1980. Transient stimulatory adenosine deaminase activity in peripheral lymphocytic lysate from a case of T-cell lymphoma. *Res. Commun. Chem. Pathol. Pharmacol.*, *28*:153–162.

Koehler, L. H., and Benz, E. J. 1962. Serum adenosine deaminase: Methodology and clinical application. *Clin. Chem.*, *8*:133–140.

Killer, C. A., Mitchell, B. S., Grever, M. R., Mejais, E., Malspeis, L., and Metz, E. N. 1979. Treatment of acute lymphoblastic leukemia with 2′-deoxycoformycin: Clinical and biochemical consequences of adenosine deaminase (EC 3.5.4.4) inhibition. *Cancer Treat. Rep.*, *63*:1949–1952.

Koya, M., Kansh, T., Sawada, H., Uchino, H., and Neda, K. 1981. Adenosine deaminase and ecto-5′-nucleotidase activities in various leukemias with special reference to blast crisis of chronic myeloid leukemia. *Blood*, *58*:1107–1111.

Kvamme, E., Tveit, B., and Svennedy, G. 1965. Glutaminase from pig kidney, an allossteric protein. *Biochem. Biophys. Res. Commun.*, *20*:566–572.

Lee, C. H., Evan, S. P., Rosenberg, M. C., Bagnara, A. S., Ziegler, J. B., and Van der Wyden, M. D. 1979. *In vitro* platelet abnormality in adenosine deaminase deficiency and severe combined immunodeficiency. *Blood*, *53*:465–471.

Lum, C. T., Sutherland, D. E. R., Yasmineh, W. G., and Najarian, J. S. 1978. Peripheral blood mononuclear cell adenosine deaminase activity in renal allograft recipients. *J. Surg. Res.*, *24*:388–395.

Lum, C. T., Sutherland, D. E. R., Yashmineh, D. S., Howard, R. J., and Najarian, J. S. 1979. Adenosine deaminase activity in cytomegolovirus related graft and patient loss. *Transplantation Proc.*, *11*:83–88.

Major, P. P., Agarwal, R. P., and Kufe, D. W. 1981a. Deoxycoformycin: Neurological toxicity. *Cancer Chemother. Pharmacol.*, *5*:193–196.

Major, P. P., Agarwal, R. P., and Kufe, D. W. 1981b. Clinical pharmacology of deoxycoformycin. *Blood*, *58*:91–96.

Major, P. P., Agarwal, R. P., and Kufe, D. W. 1983. Clinical pharmacology of arabinosyladenine in combination with deoxycoformycin. *Cancer Chemother. Pharmacol.*, *10*:125–128.

Meier, J., Coleman, M. S., and Hutton, J. J. 1976. Adenosine deaminase activity in peripheral blood cells of patients with hematologic malignancies. *Br. J. Cancer*, *33*:312–319.

Meuwissen, H. J., Pollara, B., and Pickering, R. J. 1975. Combined immunodeficiency disease associated with adenosine deaminase. *J. Pediatr.*, *86*:169–181.

Miwa, S., Fuji, H., Matsumoto, N., Nakatsuji, T., Oda, S., Asano, H., Asano, S., and Miura, Y. 1978. A case of red cell adenosine deaminase over production associated with hereditary hemolytic anemia found in Japan. *Am. J. Hematol.*, *5*:107–115.

Muller, W. E. G., Zahn, R. K., Arendez, J., Maidhof, A., and Umezawa, H. 1978. Influence of coformycin on the cytostatic activity of 9-β-D-Arabinofuranosyladenine and adenosine in mouse L5178Y cells. *Hoppe-Seyler's Z. Physiol. Chem.*, *359*:1287–1295.

Nakamura, H., Koyama, G., Iitaka, Y., Ohno, M., Yagisawa, N., Kondo, S., Maeda, K., and Umezawa, H. 1974. Structure of coformycin, an unusual nucleoside of microbial origin. *J. Am. Chem. Soc.*, *96*:4327–4328.

Nakamura, H., Koyama, G., Umezawa, H., and Iitaka, Y. 1976. The crystal and molecular structure of coformycin. *Acta Cryst.*, *B32*:1206–1212.

Newby, A. C. 1980. Role of adenosine deaminase, ecto (5′-nucleotidase) and ecto (non-specific phosphatase) in cyanide-induced adenosine monophosphate catabolism in rat polymorphonuclear leucocytes. *Biochem. J.*, *186*:907–918.

Nishihara, H., Akedo, H., Okada, H., and Hattori, S. 1970. Multienzyme patterns of serum adenosine deaminase by agar gel electrophoresis. *Clinica. Chim. Acta*, *30*:251–258.

Nishihara, H., Ishikawa, S., Shinkai, K., and Akedo, H. 1973. Multiple forms of human adenosine deaminase. *Biochem. Biophys. Acta*, *302*:429–442.

North, T. W., and Cohen, S. S. 1978. Erythro-9-(2-hydroxy-3-nonyl) adenine as a specific inhibitor of herpes simplex virus replication in the presence and absence of adenosine analogues. *Proc. Nat. Acad. Sci. USA*, *75*:4684–4688.

Nygaard, P. 1978. Adenosine deaminase from *Escherichia coli*. *Methods Enzymol.*, *51*:508–512.

Orfanos, A. P., Nylor, E. W., and Guthrie, R. 1978. Micromethod for estimating adenosine deaminase activity in dried blood spots on filter paper. *Clin. Chem.*, *24*:591–594.

Parkman, R. G., Gelfand, F. W., Rosen, F., Sanderson, A., and Hirschhorn, R. 1975. Severe combined immunodeficiency disease associated with adenosine deaminase deficiency. *N. Engl. J. Med.*, *292*:714–719.

Parks, R. E., Jr., and Brown, P. R. 1973. Incorporation of nucleosides into the nucleotide pools of human erythrocytes, adenosine and its analogs. *Biochemistry*, *12*:3294–3302.

Pauling, L. 1948. Chemical achievement and hope for the future. *Am. Scientist*, *36*:51–58.

Polmar, S. H., Stern, R. C., Schwartz, A. L., Wetzler, E. M., Chase, P. A., and Hirschhorn, R. 1976. Enzyme replacement therapy for adenosine deaminase deficiency and severe combined immunodeficiency. *N. Engl. J. Med.*, *295*:1337–1343.

Prentice, H. G., Smyth, J. F., Ganeshguru, K., Wonk, B., Bradstock, K. F., Janossy, G., Goldstone, A. K., and Hoffbrand, A. V. 1980. Remission induction with adenosine deaminase inhibitor 2′-deoxycoformycin in Thy-lymphoblastic leukemia. *Lancet*. *2*:170–172.

Rodbard, D., Bridson, W., and Rayford, P. L. 1969. Rapid calculation of radioimmunoassay results. *J. Lab. Clin. Med.*, *74*:770–778.

Rogler-Brown, T., Agarwal, R. P., and Parks, R. E., Jr. 1978. Tight-binding inhibitors. VI. Interactions of deoxycoformycin and adenosine deaminase in intact human enthrocytes and Sarcoma 180 cells. *Biochem. Pharmacol.*, *27*:2289–2296.

Sawa, T., Fukagawa, Y., Homma, I., Takeuchi, T., and Umezawa, H. 1967a. Mode of inhibition of coformycin on adenosine deaminase. *J. Antiobiotics* (*Japan*) *Ser.A.*, *20*:227–231.

Sawa, T., Fukagawa, Y., Homma, I., Takeuchi, T., and Umezawa, H. 1967b. Formycin deaminating activity of microorganisms. *J. Antibiotics* (*Japan*) *Ser. A.*, *20*:317–321.

Schaeffer, H. J., 1971. Factors in the design of reversible and irreversible enzyme inhibitors. In: *Drug Design*: pp. 129–159. *Medicinal Chemistry*, Volume 11-Pt. II Ed. by Ariens, E. J. Academic Press, New York.

Schaeffer, H. J., and Schwender, C. F. 1974. Enzyme inhibitors. 26. Bridging hydrophobic regions on adenosine deaminase with some 9-(2-hydroxy-3-alkyl) adenines. *J. Med. Chem.*, *17*:6–8.

Scholar, E. M., and Calabresi, P. 1973. Identification of the enzymic pathway of nucleotide metabolism in human lymphocytes and leukemia cells. *Cancer Res.*, *33*:94–103.

Schroder, H. C. Schuster, D. K., Zahn, R. K., and Muller, W. E. G. 1981. A novel metabolic effect of the adenosine deaminase inhibitor coformycin, a potentiator of antiviral adenosine analogues. *Antiviral Res.*, *1*:383–391.

Schubert, P., Reddington, M., and Kreutzberg, G. W. 1979. On the possible role of adenosine as a modulatory messenger in the hippocampus and other regions of the CNS. *Prog. Brain Res.*, *51*:149–165.

Seligson, D., and Seligson, H. 1951. A microdiffusion method for the determination of nitrogen liberated as ammonia. *J. Lab. Clin. Med.*, *38*:324–330.

Shimazaki, M., Kondo, S., Maeda, K., Ohno, M., and Umezawa, H. 1979a. Synthesis of isocoformycin, an aadenosine deaminase inhibitor of synthetic origin. *J. Antibiotics* (*Japan*), *32*:537–538.

Shimazaki, M., Kumada, Y., Takeuchi, T., Umezawa, H., and Watanabe, K. 1979b. Studies on inhibition of adenosine deaminase by isocoformycin *in vitro* and *in vivo*. *J. Antibiotics* (*Japan*), *32*:654–658.

Sidi, Y., Boer, P. Pick, I., Pinkhas, J., Sperling, O. 1979. Increased adenosine deaminase activity in peripheral lymphocytes in Waldenstrom's macroglubulinaemia. *Lancet*, *1*:500.

Sloan, B. J., Kielty, J. K., and Miller, F. A. 1977. Effect of a novel adenosine deaminase inhibitor (Co-vidarabine, CoV) upon the antiviral activity *in vitro* and *in vivo* of vidarabin (Vira-A^{TM}) for DNA viral replication. *Ann. N.Y. Acad. Sci.*, *284*:60–80.

Smyth, J. F., and Harrap, K. R. 1975. Adenosine deaminase in leukemia. *Br. J. Cancer, 31*:544–549.

Smyth, J. F., Poplack, D. G., Holiman, B. J., and Leventhal, B. G. 1978. Correlation of adenosine deaminase activity with cell surface markers in acute lymphoblastic leukemia. *J. Clin. Invest., 62*:710–712.

Smyth, J. F., Chassin, M. M., Harrap, K. R., Adamson, R. H., and Johns, D. G. 1979. 2′-Deoxycoformycin (DCF): Phase I trial and clinical pharmacology. *Proc. Am. Assoc. Cancer Res., 20*:47.

Stubbs, G., Litt, M., Lis, E., Jackson, R., Voth, W., Lindberg, A., and Litt, R. 1982. Adenosine deaminase activity decreased in autism. *J. Am. Acad. Child. Psych., 21*:71–74.

Sufrin, G., Tritsch, G., Mittleman, A., Moore, R. H., and Murphy, G. P. 1977. Adenosine deaminase activity in patients with renal adenocarcinoma. *Cancer, 40*:796–802.

Sufrin, G., Tritsch, G. L., Mittleman, A., and Murphy, G. P. 1978. Studies of lymphocyte adenosine deaminase activity in patients with renal and transitional cell carcinoma. *Int. Adv. Surg. Oncol., 1*:11–28.

Suhadolnik, R. J. 1970. *Nucleoside Antibiotics*. Wiley, New York.

Tritsch, G. L., and Minowada, J. 1978. Differences in purine metabolizing enzyme activities in human leukemia T-cell, B-cell and null-cell lines. *J. Natl. Cancer Inst., 60*:1301–1304.

Trotta, P. P., and Balis, M. E. 1977. Structural and kinetic alterations in adenosine deaminase associated with the differentiation of rat intestinal cells. *Cancer Res., 37*:2297–2305.

Trotta, P. P., Tedde, A., and Balis, M. E. 1980. Effects on immune function of continuous infusion into mice of 2′-deoxycoformycin (DCF). *Proc. Am. Assoc. Cancer Res., 21*:242.

Uitendaal, M. P., DeBruyn, C. H. M. M., Oei, T. L., Geerts, S. J., and Hosli, P. 1978. Fluctuating adenosine deaminase activities in cultured fibroblasts, *Biochem. Med., 20*:54–62.

Vaca, G., Sanchez-Corona, J., Olivares, N., Medina, C., Ibara, B., and Cantu, J. M. 1979. A simple rapid fluorescent assay for adenosine deaminase activity. *Ann. Genet., 22*:182–184.

Wierzchowski, J., and Shugar, D. 1983. Sensitive fluorimetric assay for adenosine deaminase with formycin as substrate; and substrate and inhibitor properties of some pyrazolopyrimidine and related analogues. *Z. Naturforsch., 38c*:67–73.

Wiginton, D. A., Coleman, M. S., and Hutton, J. J. 1981. Purification, characterization and radioimmunoassay of adenosine deaminase from human leukemic granulocytes *Biochem. J., 195*:389–397.

Woo, P. W. K., Dion, H. W., Lang, S. M., Dahl, L. F., and Durham, L. J. 1974. A novel adenosine and Ara-A deaminase inhibitor (R)-3-(2-deox-β-D-erythropentofuranosyl)-3,6,7,8-tetrahydroimidazo-[4,5-d] [1,3] diazepin-8-ol.

Zielke, C. L., and Suelter, C. H. 1971. Purine nucleoside, and purine nucleotide aminohydrolases. *The Enzymes, 4*:47–78.

Chapter **7**

S-Adenosylhomocysteine Hydrolase

Measurement of Activity and Use of Inhibitors

Peter K. Chiang

Division of Biochemistry
Walter Reed Army Institute of Research
Washington, D.C.

I. INTRODUCTION

S-Adenosylhomocysteine (AdoHcy) is a product in all transmethylation reactions in which *S*-adenosylmethionine (AdoMet) is the methyl donor. In eukaryotes, including plants, the principal pathway for the catabolism of AdoHcy is its hydrolysis to adenosine (Ado) and L-homocysteine (Hcy) by AdoHcy hydrolase (AdoHcyase; EC 3.3.1.1), an enzyme first discovered in rat liver by de la Haba and Cantoni (1959). The reaction (Figure 1) catalyzed by AdoHcyase is reversible, with equilibrium far in the direction of synthesis; the equilibrium constant (K_{eq}) is about 1 μM. Physiologically, however, the reaction proceeds in the hydrolytic direction because both Ado and Hcy are removed efficiently by various enzymes (Figure 1). Adenosine can either be deaminated to inosine by adenosine deaminase or be phosphorylated to AMP by adenosine kinase; homocysteine is either remethylated back to methionine or is converted to cystathionine after condensation with serine.

In bacteria, AdoHcy is metabolized by a different enzyme, AdoHcy nucleosidase, which cleaves AdoHcy irreversibly to yield adenine and *S*-ribosyl-L-homocysteine (Duerre and Walker, 1977; Ferro *et al.*, 1976). The same nucleosidase is also capable of cleaving the glycosyl linkage of 5′-methylthioadenosine to adenine and 5′-methylthioribose. However, 5′-methylthioadenosine nucleosidase from a plant source is incapable of utilizing AdoHcy as substrate (Guranowski *et al.*, 1981a).

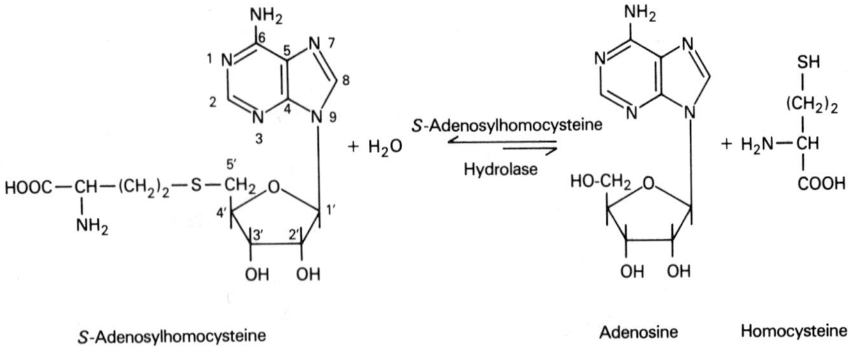

Figure 1. Reaction catalyzed by S-adenosylhomocysteine hydrolase.

Recently, there has been much interest in AdoHcyase because of the importance of transmethylation in biological processes. It has been shown that, *in vivo* and *in vitro*, the accumulation of AdoHcy will lead to feedback inhibition of transmethylation reactions (Chiang *et al.*, 1977; Chiang and Cantoni, 1979; Cantoni and Chiang, 1980; Eloranta *et al.*, 1982; Helland and Ueland, 1982; Cass *et al.*, 1982). Almost without exception, all methyltransferases utilizing AdoMet as the methyl donor are inhibited by AdoHcy competitively and, in most instances, quite potently (Im *et al.*, 1979; Chiang *et al.*, 1980; Pritchard *et al.*, 1982). It also has been postulated that AdoHcy may be involved in the severe combined immunodeficiency disease found in patients with adenosine deaminase deficiency (Hershfield *et al.*, 1979; Palella *et al.*, 1982).

AdoHcyase from various sources has been purified to homogeneity or partially purified (Table I). In general, the native molecular weight of AdoHcyase from mammalian sources is between 180,000–230,000 and, as first reported by Richards *et al.* (1978), mammalian AdoHcyase exists as a tetramer. There are 4 moles of NAD bound per mole of AdoHcyase. Oxidation-reduction of the enzyme-bound NAD as a mechanism of the catalytic cycle has been proposed by Palmer and Abeles (1979). Based on the proposed catalytic mechanism of the enzyme, adenine or an analog of adenine could be released from a nucleoside incubated with AdoHcyase. However, purified AdoHcyase from mouse leukemia L1210 cells failed to release any free adenine upon incubation with adenosine, 9-β-D-arabinofuranosyladenine (Ara-A), or 2-F-Ara-A (White *et al.*, 1982). Furthermore, no free radioactive adenine could be detected when either [^{14}C] adenosine or [^{3}H]-Ara-A was incubated with AdoHcyase purified from hamster liver (I.-K. Kim and P. K. Chiang, unpublished observations). The anomaly exhibited by AdoHcyase isolated from the latter two sources awaits further clarification. Any preparation of purified AdoHcyase should be checked for contamination of adenosine deaminase and adenosine kinase.

II. EXTRACTION OF ADOHCYASE

AdoHcyase is a cytoplasmic enzyme and can readily be extracted from tissues or cells with low ionic buffers, either with a blendor or glass homogenizer. For

Table I. Properties of AdoHcyase Purified from Different Tissues

Enzyme source	K_m (μM) AdoHcy	Ado	Hcy	Reference
Beef liver	6.0[a]	1.9	150.0[a]	Guranowski *et al.* (1981b)
Calf liver	10.5	45.0	—	Palmer and Abeles (1979)
Lupin seed	12.0	45.0	—	Guranowski and Pawełkiewicz (1977)
Mouse liver	0.75	0.2	0.2	Døskeland and Ueland (1982)
Bovine liver	0.75	0.2	—	Døskeland and Ueland (1982)
Bovine arenal	0.75	0.2	—	Døskeland and Ueland (1982)
Human lymphoblast	—	1.0	—	Hershfield and Kredich (1978)
Human placenta	—	1.0	—	Hershfield and Kredich (1978)
Rat brain	36.6	—	—	Schatz *et al.* (1979)
Rat liver	0.9	0.6	60.0	Kajander and Raina (1981)
Rat liver	15.2	1.1	155.0	Fujioka and Takata (1981)
Rat liver	12.3	0.9	164.0	Briske-Anderson and Duerre (1982)
Hamster liver	1.4	1.0	—	Kim *et al.* (1983)
Spinach beet	41.0	13.0	1200.0	Poulton and Butt (1976)

[a] Unpublished observations (P. K. Chiang).

example, AdoHcyase can be extracted from hamster liver with a buffer consisting of 10 m*M* potassium phosphate (pH 7.6), 2 m*M* dithiothreitol, and 1 m*M* EDTA (Kim *et al.*, 1983). Sonic disruption of cells to extract the enzyme has also been used (Cass *et al.*, 1982), and it has been reported that the inclusion of 3 m*M* DL-homocysteine, 20% glycerol, and 0.5% Triton X-100 in the extraction buffer gives maximal yield (Helland and Ueland, 1982).

III. ASSAY METHODS

The present chapter presents only methodology devised or routinely used in the author's laboratory. For a review of other methods used, see Ueland (1983). Since the reaction catalyzed by AdoHcyase is reversible, its activity can be assayed in either direction.

A. Synthetic Direction (Ado + Hcy → AdoHcy)

Determination of AdoHcyase activity in the synthetic direction is simpler because it does not require the laborious synthesis of radioactive AdoHcy. When assaying crude extracts, an inhibitor of adenosine deaminase must be included to prevent the deamination of adenosine in the assay mixture.

1. Sulfopropyl (SP) -Sephadex C-25 Column Method

Assay Conditions (Kim et al., 1983). The standard incubation contains in a final volume of 0.5 ml: 50 m*M* potassium phosphate (pH 7.6), 2 m*M* dithiothreitol,

1 m*M* EDTA, 10% glycerol, 10 m*M* DL-homocysteine, and 20 μ*M* [8-^{14}C]adenosine. An adenosine inhibitor, erythro-9-(2-hydroxy-3-nonyl)adenine (Burroughs Wellcome Company, Research Triangle Park, North Carolina) or 2′-deoxycoformycin (Developmental Therapeutics Program, National Cancer Institute, Bethesda, Maryland) is added at 10 μ*M* when assaying crude enzyme extracts. Alternatively, the substrate can be 3-[8-^{14}C]deaza-adenosine (Southern Research Institute, Birmingham, Alabama), and, in this case, the inclusion of an inhibitor of adenosine deaminase can be omitted because of the unique resistance of a 3-deazapurine nucleoside to deamination (Chiang *et al.*, 1977; Montgomery *et al.*, 1982). The presence of a thiol compound and glycerol stabilizes the enzyme activity.

The reaction is started by the addition of enzyme solution, which should contain no more than 0.1 IU equivalent of purified enzyme activity (about 0.1 nmole AdoHcy formed per minute). After an incubation of 10 min at 30°, the reaction is stopped by the addition of 1 ml of 50 m*M* HCl. The resultant mixture is then poured onto a column (0.8 × 2.5 cm) of SP-Sephadex C-25, equilibrated with 10 m*M* HCl. The column is next washed with 30 ml of 50 m*M* HCl, and the [^{14}C] AdoHcy or 3-deaza-[^{14}C] AdoHcy formed is subsequently eluted with 10 ml of 1 *N* HCl into a scintillation vial. The radioactivity is determined after the addition of 10 ml of a scintillation fluid.

2. *Thin-Layer Chromatography Method*

Assay Conditions (*Guranowski et al., 1981*). The incubation mixture contains the following in 50 μl: 50 m*M* Tris-HCl (pH 8.0), 2 m*M* dithiothreitol, 10 m*M* DL-homocysteine, 10% glycerol, and 20 μ*M* [8-^{14}C]adenosine or [U-^{14}C]adenosine. If [U-^{14}C]adenosine (Amersham Corporation) is used because of its high specific activity, care should be taken to ensure that it is in the β and not the α form since AdoHcyase is stereospecific for the β-pentose configuration, and α-adenosine is neither a substrate nor an inhibitor for the enzyme (Chiang *et al.*, 1977). If necessary, erythro-9-(2-hydroxy-3-nonyl)adenine is added. The enzyme solution to be used is diluted in 50 m*M* Tris-HCl (pH 8.0) containing bovine serum (1 mg/ml). After incubating at 30°C, 15 μl aliquots are transferred at intervals to a small tube containing 5 μl of 0.15 *M* HCl to stop the reaction.

From the resultant mixture, 10 μl is spotted on chromatographic plates (Merck) coated with fluorescent indicator. Two μl of a standard solution of 2 m*M* AdoHcy or 3-deaza-AdoHcy (Southern Research Institute, Birmingham, Alabama) is added to the same spot as carrier. Two types of thin-layer plates and solvent systems can be used. If the chromatographic plate is cellulose, the chromatogram is developed in 5% Na_2HPO_4 for 90 min. If the chromatographic plate is silica gel, the chromatogram is developed for 60 min in 1-butanol/acetic acid/H_2O (12:3:5; v/v/v). After visualization under ultraviolet light, the spots containing the radioactive products are cut and then counted (Table II).

When checking for the ability of any particular nucleoside as an alternative substrate for AdoHcyase, 10 m*M* of DL-[^{35}*S*] homocysteine is used in conjunction with 1 m*M* of the nucleoside to be tested. DL-[^{35}S]Homocysteine is generated by

Table II. Separation by Thin-Layer Chromatography of Adenosine Analogs and Their Corresponding Nucleosidylhomocysteine (NucHcy) Analogs Synthesized by Beef Liver AdoHcyase[a]

Nucleoside	R_f values			
	Cellulose plate[b]		Silica gel plate[c]	
	Nucleoside	NucHcy	Nucleoside	NucHcy
Adenosine	0.43	0.53	0.53	0.23
Adenosine N^1-oxide	0.69	0.74	0.33	0.15
8-Amino-adenosine	0.26	0.33	0.48	0.14
(±)Aristeromycin (carbocyclic adenosine)	0.40	0.40	0.43	0.20
8-Aza-adenosine	0.58	0.65	0.65	0.35
2-Aza-3-deaza-adenosine	0.45	0.52	0.40	0.12
3-Deaza-adenosine	0.41	0.48	0.42	0.12
Formycin A (7-deaza-8-aza-adenosine)	0.50	0.58	0.47	0.17
Inosine	0.69	0.73	0.42	0.17
Nebularine (purine ribonucleoside)	0.71	0.71	0.50	0.24
N^6-Methyl-adenosine	0.52	0.60	0.59	0.30
Pyrazomycin (pyrazofurin)	0.75	0.78	0.54	0.24

[a] Guranowski *et al.* (1981b).
[b] Cellulose plates developed in 5% Na_2HPO_4; R_f for homocysteine is 0.9.
[c] Silica gel plates developed in 1-butanol/acetic acid/H_2O (12:3:5).

incubating DL-[^{35}S]homocystine (Amersham Corporation) in 10 m*M* Tris-HCl (pH 8.0) and a 6-fold excess of dithiothreitol for 30 min at 37°C (Chiang *et al.*, 1977). If standard sample of a nucleosidinylhomocysteine (NucHcy) is required, excess AdoHcyase (about 25 μg of purified enzyme) is added to start the incubation at 30°, which is terminated 16 hr later by heating at 100°C. The denatured protein is removed by filtration and the solution is stored at −20°C. The NucHcy analogs synthesized can be separated from their respective precursor nucleosides by thin-layer chromatography (Table II). Recently, AdoHcyase from beef liver and lupin seeds has been found to catalyze the formation of *S*-nucleosidinylcysteine (NucCys) analogs (Guranowski and Jakubowski, 1983).

3. *Nucleosides That Function as Alternative Substrates*

Table III shows the effectiveness of various nucleosides (Figure 2) that can function as alternative substrates for AdoHcyase of beef liver, using either DL-[^{35}S]homocysteine (Guranowski *et al.*, 1981b) or [3-^{14}C]cysteine (Guranowski and Jakubowski, 1983) as the cosubstrate.

When DL-homocysteine is used as the cosubstrate, 3-deaza-adenosine is the best substrate with an efficiency about 1.5-fold that of adenosine. Next in line is 2-aza-3-deaza-adenosine, which is slightly better than adenosine. In spite of the absence of a 6-amino group, nebularine is 30% as active as adenosine as a sub-

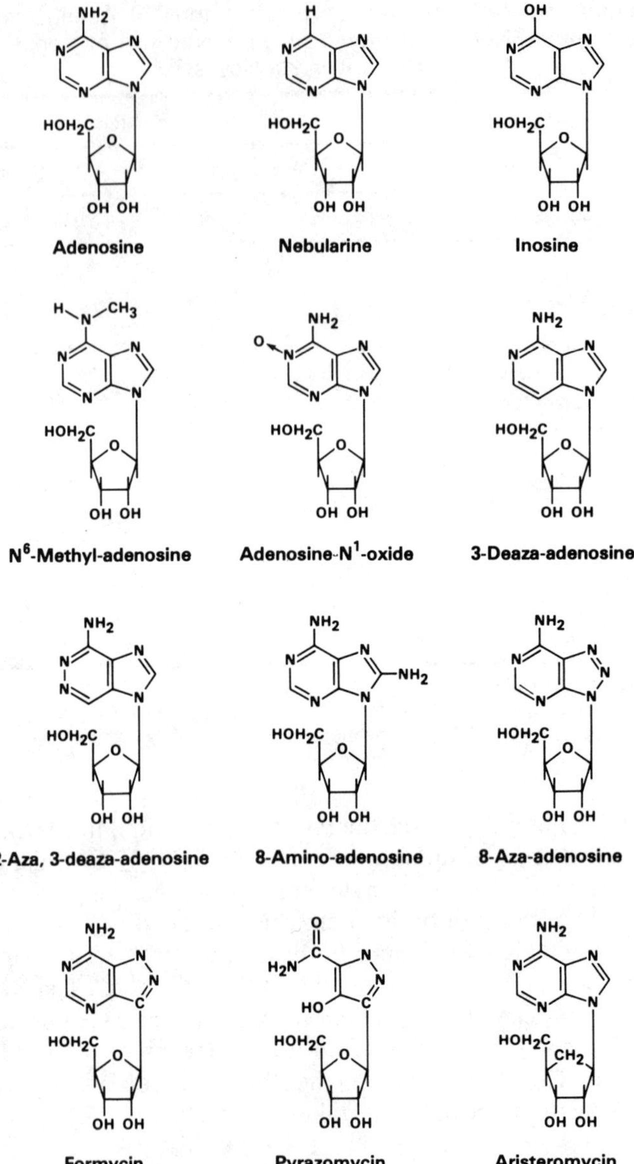

Figure 2. Chemical structures of some adenosine analogues.

strate. Formycin A and N^6-methyl-adenosine are mediocre substrates, whereas 8-aza-adenosine, adenosine N^1-oxide, pyrazomycin, and 8-aminoadenosine are marginally active (10% or less). Inosine can also function as a substrate at only about 1.5% of the rate of adenosine and has a K_m of 1.9 ± 0.3 mM compared to a K_m of 1.8 ± 0.3 μM for adenosine. In addition, 2-amino-adenosine, N^6-hydroxy-adenosine, 2-hydroxy-adenosine, 2-chloro-adenosine and 3-deaza-(±)aristero-

Table III. Relative Effectiveness of Adenosine Analogs in Forming S-Nucleosidylhomocysteines (NucHcy) and S-Nucleosidylcysteines (NucCys) Catalyzed by Beef Liver AdoHcyase

Nucleoside	Relative velocity (%)	
	NucHcy	NucCys[b]
Adenosine	100[a]	100
3-Deaza-adenosine	165[a]	33
2-Aza-3-deaza-adenosine	113[a]	?
Nebularin	34[a]	40
Formycin A	18[a]	12
N^6-Methyl-adenosine	16[a]	12
8-Aza-adenosine	9[a]	0
Adenosine N^1-oxide	5[a]	6
Pyrazomycin	5[a]	0
8-Amino-adenosine	4[a]	0
Inosine	1.5[a]	0
(±)Aristeromycin	0.1[a]	0
2-Amino-adenosine	+[b]	70
N^6-Hydoxy-adenosine	+[b]	70
2-Hydroxy-adenosine	+[b]	0
2-Chloro-adenosine	+[b]	0
3-Deaza-(±)aristeromycin	+[b]	0

[a] Guranowski *et al.* (1981b); assayed at 10 m*M* DL-[^{35}S]homocysteine.
[b] Guranowski and Jakubowski (1983); assayed at 25 m*M* DL-[3-^{14}C]cysteine.

mycin (carbocyclic 3-deaza-adenosine) can also serve as substrates, with efficiencies ranging from good to very poor. Depending on cell types used, 3-deaza-(±)aristeromycin can form small amounts of 3-deaza-(±)aristeromycinylhomocysteine, e.g., in rabbit neutrophils (Garcia-Castro *et al.*, 1983), 3T3-L1 fibroblasts (Guranowski *et al.*, 1981b), and human platelets (P. K. Chiang, unpublished observations). The least effective nucleoside is (±)aristeromycin (carbocyclic adenosine). In contrast to 3-deaza-(±)aristeromycin, no corresponding homocysteine conjugate has ever been found when the 3T3-L1 fibroblasts were incubated with (±)aristeromycin (Guranowski *et al.*, 1981b). This is in agreement with the observation that the 3-deazapurine nucleosides are generally better substrates than the unmodified purine nucleosides (Chiang *et al.*, 1977; Richards *et al.*, 1978; Guranowski *et al.*, 1981b).

With respect to DL-cysteine as a cosubstrate, a narrower spectrum exists for the nucleosides (Guranowski and Jakubowski, 1983). Adenosine is by far the best substrate, followed by 2-amino-adenosine and N^6-hydroxy-adenosine, each of which is about 70% as active. 3-Deaza-adenosine and nebularine have 30–40% efficiency in forming the adducts. Formycin A, N^6-methyl-adenosine, and adenosine N^1-oxide are marginally active (about 10%). The rest of the nucleosides are incapable of forming adducts with cysteine.

The difference between the 2 amino acids, homocysteine and cysteine, in their abilities to react with the same nucleosides to form adducts is hypothesized to be due to the existence of nonidentical catalytic sites for each amino acid (Guranowski and Jakubowski, 1983). One evidence to support this hypothesis is that the reactions with homocysteine and cysteine are not mutually exclusive, i.e., cysteine does not inhibit the synthesis of AdoHcy and homocysteine does not inhibit the synthesis of *S*-adenosylcysteine.

In the presence of erythro-9-(2-hydroxy-3-nonyl)adenine, the formation of NucHcy analogs in mouse lymphocytes was observed for each of the following nucleosides: 3-deaza-adenosine, 8-aza-adenosine, formycin A, 2-amino-adenosine, 2-fluoro-adenosine, N^6-methyl-adenosine, N^6-hydroxy-adenosine, nebularine, and inosine (Zimmerman *et al.*, 1980). Although tubercidin is normally not a substrate for AdoHcyase (Chiang *et al.*, 1977; Guranowski *et al.*, 1981b); *S*-tubercidinylhomocysteine is found in neuroblastoma cells, presumably as a product of the metabolism of *S*-tubercidinylmethionine (Crooks *et al.*, 1979). The report that Ara-A can function as a substrate to form a NucHcy analog (Helland and Ueland, 1981) awaits confirmation by stricter criteria.

B. Hydrolytic Direction (AdoHcy → Ado + Hcy)

Radioactive AdoHcy labeled in either the adenosine or homocysteine portion can be synthesized enzymatically using excess AdoHcyase (de la Haba and Cantoni, 1959). [8-^{14}C]Adenosine or [U-^{14}C]adenosine is preferred over [^{35}S]homocysteine because of the ability of the latter to react readily with other nucleosides present in the assay system to form NucHcy analogs, hence masking the overall picture of hydrolysis.

1. Enzymatic Synthesis of [^{14}C]AdoHcy

A large scale preparation of [^{14}C]AdoHcy can be adapted from the original method described by de la Haba and Cantoni (1959). The incubation contains the following mixture in 100 ml: 5 m*M* potassium phosphate, 10 m*M* [8-^{14}C]adenosine, 40 m*M* L-homocysteine, 800 units of AdoHcyase, and 10 μ*M* of 2′-deoxycoformycin. The latter is added to prevent the deamination of [8-^{14}C]AdoHcy by AMP-deaminase. After incubating at 37°C for 2 hr, 5 ml of ice-cold 70% perchloric acid is added, and the mixture is cooled for 1 hr in ice. After centrifugation of the mixture, 100 ml of 20% phosphotungstic acid is added to the supernatant. After storage at 4° overnight, the precipitate is washed twice with 0.1 *N* H_2SO_4 and then suspended in 50 ml of 0.1 *N* H_2SO_4. This suspension is shaken with 1-butanol and ether (1:1, v/v) at room temperature. The organic layer is discarded after centrifugation, and the acid layer is decanted into a beaker. The remaining precipitate is resuspended in 30 ml of 0.1 *N* H_2SO_4 and again treated as above. After centrifugation and the removal of the organic layer, the acid layer is decanted and combined with the first fraction. After adding 50 μmoles of potassium phosphate buffer (pH 6.5), the solution is adjusted to pH 6.7 with 10 *N* KOH and next lyophilized. The dry powder is dissolved in H_2O to a final volume of 15 ml, and the sulfate is removed by the addition of 0.5 *M* barium iodide dropwise. The barium sulfate precipitate is centrifuged, washed once with H_2O, centrifuged again, and the supernatant is combined with the main fraction. After lyophilization of the solution, the powder is dissolved in H_2O to a final concentration of 0.05 *M* AdoHcy (ϵ = 15.0 cm^2/μmole at pH 7.0). Absolute ethanol is added to a final concentration of 50% and left sitting in ice for a few hours. It is then centrifuged, and the gelatinous precipitate is discarded. Enough ethanol is added to the supernatant to reach 94% saturation and left at 4°C overnight. The amorphous precipitate is centrifuged, washed twice with cold absolute ethanol, and dried in a vacuum. Crystallization of [^{14}C] AdoHcy can be achieved by dissolving the powder in H_2O to a final concentration of about 0.05 *M* and freezing the solution at −20°C. The next day, the solution is placed in a cold room, and crystallization begins after a day or two. Recrystallization can be carried out by centrifuging the crystalline product, which is washed with a small volume of cold H_2O, twice with cold absolute ethanol, and then dried in a vacuum desiccator overnight at room temperature over phosphorous pentoxide.

An easier alternative way to obtain [^{14}C]AdoHcy is by high-pressure liquid chromatography of the enzymatically prepared material. At the end of enzymatic incubation as described in the beginning of the previous paragraph (proportional amount can be adjusted), cold sulfosalicylic acid is added to achieve a final concentration of 5% (Hoffman, 1975). The mixture (normally no more than 2 ml) is filtered by a Whatman GF/C filter, and then is put on a column of Vydac SC cation-exchanger (Separation Group, Hesperia, CA). The exact amount of cation exchanger required per column depends on each particular batch and has to be determined by standard AdoHcy; it varies between 9–30 × 0.6 cm. After washing the column with 100 ml of 10 m*M* ammonium formate (pH 4.0), elution is started by a 100-ml linear gradient of 0.01–0.8 *M* ammonium formate (pH 4.0). [^{14}C]-AdoHcy is eluted in the early fractions, which are combined, lyophilized, dissolved in a small amount of H_2O, and then stored at −20°C.

Another enzymatic synthesis of AdoHcy labeled by L-[2(n)-^{3}H]homocysteine has been described (Trewyn and Kerr, 1977). It is based on the conversion of *S*-adenosyl-L-[2(n)-^{3}H]methionine to *S*-adenosyl-L-[2(n)-^{3}H]homocysteine by glycine *N*-methyltransferase using glycine as the acceptor. The product is purified by a Vydac cation-exchange column with a yield of about 98%. A convenient chemical synthesis of AdoHcy (Borchardt *et al.*, 1976) may also be applied to prepare its radioactive counterpart.

2. *SP-Sephadex C-25 Column Method*

Assay Conditions: The standard incubation contains the following mixture in a final volume of 0.5 ml: 50 m*M* potassium phosphate (pH 7.6) 2 m*M* dithiothreitol, 1 m*M* EDTA, 10% glycerol, 5 IU of calf intestinal adenosine deaminase, and 20 μ*M* [^{14}C]AdoHcy. After 10 min of incubation with AdoHcyase at 30°C, the reaction is stopped by the addition of 100 μl of 5 *M* formic acid. The mixture is next poured onto a column of (0.8 × 2.5 cm) of SP-Sephadex C-25, equilibrated in 0.1 *M* formic acid. Each assay tube is rinsed with 0.5 ml of 0.1 *M* formic acid. [^{14}C]Inosine formed [[^{14}C]adenosine → [^{14}C]inosine (in the presence of adenosine deaminase)] is eluted from the column by 3.5 ml of 0.1 *M* formic acid. The eluate

Table IV. Specific Activities of AdoHcyase in Different Tissues

Tissue	AdoHcyase activity (nmoles/mg per min)	Reference
Beef liver	0.3	Richards *et al.* (1978)
Calf liver	0.8	Palmer and Ables (1979)
Hamster liver	0.7	Kim *et al.* (1983)
Rat brain	0.3	Schatz *et al.* (1979)
Rat liver	44.0	Kajander and Raina (1981)
Rat liver	3.0	Fujioka and Takata (1981)
Rat liver	0.5	Briske-Anderson and Duerre (1982)
Rat liver	24.0	Eloranta *et al.* (1982)
Rat liver	11.0	Chabannes *et al.* (1979)
Rat hepatomas	0.3	Finkelstein *et al.* (1978)
Human blood	0.1	Sacks *et al.* (1982)
Human lymphocytes	2.0	Palella *et al.* (1982)

is collected into a scintillation vial, and the radioactivity is determined after the addition of 10 ml of a scintillation fluid.

IV. SPECIFIC ACTIVITIES OF ADOHCYASE IN TISSUES

Table IV shows the specific activities of AdoHcyase in different tissues. A comparison of the activity of AdoHcyase in the different tissues of rat has been provided by Eloranta (1977). In general, it is the liver and pancreas that have the highest activities of AdoHcyase, and the brain, kidney, adrenal, and spleen have moderate activities of AdoHcyase.

V. L-[^{35}S]HOMOCYSTEINE EXCHANGE REACTION

To check the unknown ability of NucHcy analog to undergo hydrolysis by AdoHcyase, the following radioactive method can be used (Chiang *et al.*, 1977). It utilizes an exchange reaction that measures the incorporation of ^{35}S from [^{35}S]homocysteine into an unlabeled NucHcy in the presence of AdoHcyase:

$$[^{35}\mathrm{S}]\mathrm{Hcy} + \mathrm{NucHcy} \leftrightharpoons [^{35}\mathrm{S}]\mathrm{NucHcy} + \mathrm{Hcy}$$

It has been found by using this exchange method that 3-deaza-AdoHcy and N^6-methyl-AdoHcy undergo hydrolysis catalyzed by AdoHcyase and that *S*-tubercidinyl-homocysteine (7-deaza-AdoHcy) is not a substrate (Chiang *et al.*, 1977).

The assay in 0.5 ml consists of the following mixture: 50 m*M* potassium phosphate (pH 7.6), 2 m*M* dithiothreitol, 1 m*M* EDTA, 10% glycerol, 0.1 m*M* L-[^{35}S]homocysteine, 1 m*M* of a NucHcy analog, and excess AdoHcyase. After incubation at 37°C for a specified time, the reaction products can be checked either by thin-layer chromatography as described (III.A.2), or by SP-Sephadex C-25 column (III.A.1). In the latter method, 1 ml of 50 m*M* HCl is added to stop the reaction. The mixture is then transferred to the SP-Sephadex C-25 column equilibrated in 10 m*M* HCl, and the column is washed with 30 ml of 50 m*M* HCl to remove the unreacted L-[^{35}S]homocysteine. The [^{35}S]NucHcy formed is then eluted directly with 10 ml of 1 *N* HCl into a scintillation vial, and the radioactivity is determined after adding 10 ml of a scintillation fluid.

VI. INHIBITORS OF ADOHCYASE

In view of the different sensitivities of various methyltransferases towards inhibition by AdoHcy, the modulation of AdoHcyase in cells or in animals may be of therapeutic potential. Specifically, an inhibition of AdoHcyase in tissues would lead to an alteration of the cellular ratio of AdoHcy/AdoMet, thus resulting in the inhibition of AdoMet-dependent methyltransferases. Moreover, experimentation with inhibitors of AdoHcyase, *in vitro* and *in vivo*, may establish a hierarchy of different thresholds for the perturbation of transmethylation reactions. A search for specific inhibitors of AdoHcyase was started by Chiang, *et al.* (1977) and led to the discovery of potent and metabolically stable inhibitors that are 3-deazapurine nucleosides (Chiang *et al.*, 1977; Guranowski *et al.*, 1981b; Montgomery *et al.*, 1982).

Inhibitors of AdoHcyase can be divided into four categories: (1) competitive, (2) noncompetitive, (3) irreversible, and (4) competitive and irreversible (mixed). If AdoHcyase is assayed in the hydrolytic direction when studying the inhibitors, the activity of adenosine deaminase [a necessary ingredient in the coupled assay (see Section III.B.2)] should be checked first to insure that it is not inhibitable by the same chemicals. For example, 9-(*S*)-2,3-dihydroxypropyl)-adenine (DHPA) has been reported to be a potent inhibitor of AdoHcyase assayed in the hydrolytic direction (Votruba and Holy, 1982). In contrast, DHPA is a very weak inhibitor of AdoHcyase in our hands (30% inhibited at 1.0 m*M*), and, instead, it is a very powerful inhibitor of adenosine deaminase (P. K. Chiang, unpublished observations).

A. Competitive and Noncompetitive Inhibitors

Table V lists the K_i values for the major competitive inhibitors of AdoHycase. In sharp contrast to their ineffectiveness as substrates, the carbocyclic analogs, (±)aristeromycin and 3-deaza-(±)aristeromycin, are the most potent competitive inhibitors found so far, with K_i values ranging 10^{-6}–$10^{-9}M$. The next most potent analog is 3-deaza-adenosine ($K_i \simeq 10^{-6}$–10^{-7} M). Adenine itself, 3-deaza-adenine and 8-amino-adenosine can inhibit with K_i values around 10^{-5} M. Nucleocidin, adenosylhomocysteine, and 3-deaza-adenosylhomocysteine have K_i values between 3–6 × 10^{-5} M. The K_i values for 3-deaza-Ara-A, N^6-methyl-adenosine, formycin A, and 2-aza-3-deaza-adenosine are in the region of 10^{-4} M. Inosine,

Table V. K_i Values of Major Competitive Inhibitors of Liver AdoHcyase

Inhibitor	K	Enzyme source	Reference
(±) Aristeromycin (carbocyclic adenosine)	5×10^{-9}	Beef	Guranowski *et al.* (1981b)
	1×10^{-8}	Hamster	Kim *et al.* (1983)
3-Deaza-(±)aristeromycin	1×10^{-9}	Hamster	Montgomery *et al.* (1982)
	3×10^{-6}	Beef	Guranowski *et al.* (1981b)
3-Deaza-adenosine	7×10^{-7}	Hamster	Kim *et al.* (1983)
	3×10^{-6}	Beef	Guranowski *et al.* (1981b)
3-Deaza-(±)aristeromycinylhomocysteine	3×10^{-6}	Hamster	Kim *et al.* (1983)
Adenine	9×10^{-6}	Hamster	Kim *et al.* (1983)
3-Deaza-adenine	2×10^{-5}	Hamster	Kim *et al.* (1983)
8-Amino-adenosine	2×10^{-5}	Beef	Guranowski *et al.* (1981b)
Ara-A	2×10^{-5}	Beef	P. K. Chiang (unpublished data)
Nucleocidin	3×10^{-5}	Beef	P. K. Chiang (unpublished data)
Adenosylhomocysteine	5×10^{-5}	Beef	Kim *et al.* (1983)
3-Deaza-adenosylhomocysteine	6×10^{-5}	Hamster	Kim *et al.* (1983)
3-Deaza-Ara-A	9×10^{-5}	Beef	P. K. Chiang (unpublished data)
8-Aza-adenosine	2×10^{-4}	Beef	Guranowski *et al.* (1981b)
N^6-Methyl-adenosine	2×10^{-4}	Beef	Guranowski *et al.* (1981b)
Formycin A	3×10^{-4}	Beef	Guranowski *et al.* (1981b)
2-Aza-3-deaza-adenosine	3×10^{-4}	Beef	Guranowski *et al.* (1981b)

nebularine, and adenosine N^1-oxide are poor inhibitors with K_i values of $1–2 \times 10^{-3}$ *M*. The weakest nucleoside is pyrazomycin ($K_i = 10^{-2}$ *M*).

Substituting the thioether linkage with an amino group yields a noncompetitive inhibitor, N^γ-adenosyl-α,γ-diaminobutyric acid, and the K_i is 3×10^{-4} *M* (Chiang *et al.*, 1978). Two other noncompetitive inhibitors are *S*-isobutyl-3-deazadenosine (3-deaza-SIBA) and *S*-methyl-Ara-A, with a K_i of 4 and 5×10^{-4} *M*, respectively. AdoHcy sulfoxide and AdoHcy sulfone are poor inhibitors, and AdoMet itself is completely inactive.

B. Irreversible Inactivators

There is a large number of irreversible (time-dependent) inactivators of AdoHcyase (Hershfield *et al.*, 1979; Chiang *et al.*, 1981; White *et al.*, 1982); the major ones are shown in Table VI. The K_I values are listed for some of them and are calculated according to the following equation (Borchardt *et al.*, 1977)

$$\frac{1}{K_{\text{app}}} = \frac{K_I}{k_2[I]} + \frac{1}{k_2}$$

The most potent inactivator is Ara-A, the K_I of which is 2 μM. Analogs that have

Table VI. Major Irreversible Inactivators of AdoHcyase

Analog	K_I (μM)	Reference
Ara-A	2	P. K. Chiang (unpublished data)
	19	White *et al.* (1982)
3-Deaza-Ara-A	41	P. K. Chiang (unpublished data)
2-Chloro-3-deaza-adenosine	44	P. K. Chiang (unpublished data)
2-Chloro-adenosine	57	P. K. Chiang (unpublished data)
5′-Methylthio-adenosine	60–120	Fox *et al.* (1982)
2-Fluoro-Ara-A	109	P. K. Chiang (unpublished data)
	122	White *et al.* (1982)
2′-Deoxyadenosine	109	P. K. Chiang (unpublished data)
Nucleocidin	204	P. K. Chiang (unpublished data)
2-Chloro-Ara-A	353	P. K. Chiang (unpublished data)
Adenosine 5′-carboxamide	—	Chiang *et al.* (1981)
S-Isobutyl-adenosine	—	Chiang *et al.* (1981)
S-Isobutyl-3-deaza-adenosine	—	Chiang *et al.* (1981)
D-Eritadenine	—	Votruba and Holý (1982)

halogen substitutions on the purine are modest inactivators. 5′-Substituted analogs can also inactivate the enzyme, and some are quite potent, e.g. adenosine 5′-carboxamide (Chiang *et al.*, 1981).

C. Use of Inhibitors

A multitude of biochemical and biological effects has been observed *in vitro* and *in vivo* when the inhibitors of AdoHcyase are administered (Tables VII and VIII). The most often used inhibitor is 3-deaza-adenosine (Southern Research Institute). It is soluble in water and can be heated by boiling to achieve a concentrated solution. It is stable after repeated freezing and thawing. The new analog, 3-deaza-(±)aristeromycin, is readily soluble in water, but it has not been tested for its effects *in vivo*. The biochemical and biological effects of 3-deaza-adenosine and 3-deaza-(±)aristeromycin are summarized in Tables VII and VIII.

1. In Vivo Use of Inhibitors

Injections of 3-deaza-adenosine will bring about elevations in the tissue levels of AdoHcy and AdoMet, along with the appearance of a novel homocysteine adduct, 3-deaza-AdoHcy (Chiang *et al.*, 1977), which can be assayed by high-pressure liquid chromatography as described in Section IIIB1 or by a newly devised high-pressure liquid chromatography method (Miura *et al.*, 1984).

3-Deaza-adenosine is made up to 10 or 20 mg/ml of saline by heating the solution in a boiling water bath. In order to achieve elevated levels of AdoMet, AdoHcy, and the appearance of 3-deaza-AdoHcy, multiple injections are required (Chiang and Cantoni, 1979). After two injections, AdoHcy increases about 10-fold compared to a 2-fold increase in AdoMet; after three injections, AdoHcy

Table VII. Biochemical Reactions Inhibited by 3-Deaza-adenosine and 3-Deaza-(±)aristeromycin

Inhibition of	3-Deaza-adenosine	3-Deaza-(±)aristeromycin
Transmethylation reactions		
Phospholipid methylation	Yes[a,b,c,d,e,f]	Yes[g]
Protein carboxymethylation	Yes[c,g]	Yes[h]
Nicotinamide methylation	Yes[i]	—
Creatine biosynthesis (guanidoacetate methylation)	Yes[a,j]	—
Perturbation of catecholamine metabolism	Yes[a]	—
DNA methylation	Yes[h]	—
Other biochemical reactions		
AdoMet decarboxylase	Yes[k]	Yes[k]
Thromboxane synthesis (collagen induced)	Yes[l]	—

[a] Chiang *et al.* (1980). [b] Pritchard *et al.* (1982). [c] Garcia-Castro *et al.* (1983).
[d] Shattil *et al.* (1982). [e] Schanche *et al.* (1982). [f] Randon *et al.* (1981).
[g] Zimmerman *et al.* (1979). [h] P. K. Chiang (unpublished). [i] Johnson and Chiang (1981).
[j] Im *et al.* (1979). [k] Gordon *et al.* (1983). [l] Lecompte *et al.* (1982).

Table VIII. Biological Effects of 3-Deaza-adenosine and 3-Deaza-(±)aristeromycin

Biological effects	3-Deaza-adenosine	3-Deaza-(±)aristeromycin
Antiviral	Yes[a,b]	Yes[a]
Antimalarial	Yes[c]	Yes[d]
Chemotaxis	Decreased[e]	Decreased[e]
Phagocytosis	Decreased[f]	Yes[d]
Histamine release from mast cells	Decreased[g]	Yes[d]
Lymphocyte-mediated cytolysis	Decreased[h]	No effect[i]
Platelet aggregation	Enhanced[j]	No effect[j]
Membrane Ig capping	Decreased[k]	?
Differentiation of 3T3-L1 fibroblasts to fat cells	Enhanced[l,m]	Enhanced[d]
HL-60 leukemia cell differentiation	No	Enhanced[n]
tk gene expression in CHO cells	Enhanced[o]	?
Hypotensive	Yes[p]	?
Neutrite extension	Enhanced[q]	?
Aldosterone-stimulated short circuit current in toad bladder cells	Decreased[r]	Yes[d]

[a] Bader *et al.* (1978). [b] Montgomery *et al.* (1982). [c] Trager *et al.* (1980).
[d] P. K. Chiang, unpublished data. [e] Garcia-Castro *et al.* (1983). [f] Leonard *et al.* (1978).
[g] Morita *et al.* (1982). [h] Zimmerman *et al.* (1978). [i] T. P. Zimmerman, personal communication.
[j] Shattil *et al.* (1982). [k] Braun *et al.* (1980). [l] Chiang (1981).
[m] Hyman *et al.* (1982). [n] Lucas *et al.* (1983). [o] Harris (1982).
[p] Phyall *et al.* (1980). [q] Murato and Monard (1982). [r] Chiang *et al.* (1983).

increases 12-fold while AdoMet increases by 3-fold. There is a simultaneous appearance of large amounts of 3-deaza-AdoHcy, up to about 300 nmoles/g liver after 3 injections. The increase in AdoHcy is interpreted as a result of the *in vivo* inhibition of AdoHcyase. The increase in AdoMet is assumed to be the consequence of the inhibition of transmethylation reactions caused by the accumulation of AdoHcy and 3-deaza-AdoHcy.

Each rat tissue responds differently to the administration of 3-deaza-adenosine (Chiang and Cantoni, 1979). Although the spleen can also respond, no other organs seem to exhibit the characteristic increases in AdoHcy and AdoMet. Moreover, in contrast to the rat liver, hamster liver shows a different response to the administration of 3-deaza-adenosine. The increase in the concentration of AdoMet is not accompanied by an increase in AdoHcy, but rather is correlated with the appearance of 3-deaza-AdoHcy. Perturbation of transmethylation reactions has been observed in rats injected with 3-deaza-adenosine.

2. *In Vitro Use of Inhibitors*

Both 3-deaza-adenosine and 3-deaza-(±)aristeromycin have been used extensively to characterize the importance of transmethylation reactions. However, prudence should be exercised when judging the validity of the experiments conducted or the conclusions drawn. Quite often excess amounts of 3-deaza-adenosine are used, and it cannot be shown whether the effect obtained is cytotoxic or cytostatic. Before the experiments are performed, growth properties of the cells should be measured and then dose–response curves should be plotted.

It has become popular to use homocysteine thiolactone in conjunction with 3-deaza-adenosine or even adenosine, with the aim of forcing large amounts of 3-deaza-AdoHcy or AdoHcy to be formed, and any effects obtained are interpreted as a result of the inhibition of transmethylation reactions. However, homocysteine itself can cause a drop in the pH of the assay medium (Shattil *et al.*, 1982), and when used together with [methyl-^{3}H]methionine, the possibility for the remethylation of homocysteine back to methionine (Mudd and Poole, 1975), which then dilutes the specific activity of [methyl-^{3}H]methionine is generally ignored or is not taken into consideration. An apparent inhibition of transmethylation is thus no more than a reflection of the change of the specific activity of the methyl-labeled methionine. Moreover, the acylation of proteins and the formation of diketopiperazine by homocysteine thiolactone can obscure the interpretation of the experiments (Dudman and Wilcken, 1982).

It is increasingly evident that AdoHcyase is a fascinating enzyme with complex properties. The manipulation of this exzyme *in vivo* and *in vitro* can lead to many interesting biological effects. In time, more specific and more potent inhibitors will be developed and may result in the use of AdoHcyase as a biological target for therapeutic purposes. In addition, the development of cell mutants with deficiency of or altered properties of AdoHcyase, as in the work of Kamatani *et al.* (1983), will elucidate the regulation of transmethylation reactions and adenosine toxicity related to AdoHcy.

ACKNOWLEDGMENTS

I thank Drs. Richard K. Gordon and George A. Miura for reading the manuscript.

REFERENCES

Bader, J., Brown, N. R., Chiang, P. K., and Cantoni, G. L. 1978. 3-Deazaadenosine, an inhibitor of adenosylhomocysteine hydrolase, inhibits reproduction of Rous sarcoma virus and transformation of chick embryo cells. *Virology*, *89;*494–505.

Borchardt, R. T., Huber, J. A., and Wu, Y. S. 1976. A convenient preparation of S-adenosylhomocysteine and related compounds. *J. Org. Chem.*, *41:*565–567.

Borchardt, R. T., Wu, Y. S., and Wu, B. S. 1977. S-Adenosyl-L-homocysteine dialdehyde: An affinity labeling reagent for histamine N-methyltransferase. *Biochem. Biophys. Res. Commun.*, *78:*1025–1033.

Braun, J., Rosen, F. S., and Unanue, E. R. 1980. Capping and adenosine metabolism: genetic and pharmacological studies. *J. Exp. Med.*, *151:*174–183.

Briske-Anderson, M., and Duerre, J. A. 1982. S-Adenosylhomocysteine hydrolase from rat liver. *Can. J. Biol. Chem.*, *60:*118–123.

Cantoni, G. L., and Chiang, P. K. 1980. The role of S-adenosylhomocysteine and S-adenosylhomocysteine hydrolase in the control of biological methylation. In: *Natural Sulfur Compounds*, pp. 67–80. Ed. by Cavallini, D., Gaull, G. E., and Zappia, V. Plenum Press, New York.

Cass, C. E., Selner, M., Ferguson, P. J., and Philips, J. R. 1982. Effects of 2′-deoxyadenosine, 9-β-arabinofuranosyladenine, and related compounds on S-adenosyl-L-homocysteine hydrolase activity in synchronous and asynchronous cultured cells. *Cancer Res.*, *42:*4991–4998.

Chabannes, B., Cronenberger, L., and Pacheco, H. 1979. Rat liver S-adenosyl-L-homocysteine hydrolase purification by affinity column chromatography. *Experientia*, *35:*1014–1016.

Chiang, P. K. 1981. Conversion of 3T3-L1 fibroblasts to fat cells by an inhibitor of methylation: effect of 3-deazaadenosine. *Science*, *211:*1164–1166.

Chiang, P. K., and Cantoni, G. L. 1979. Perturbation of biochemical transmethylation by 3-deazaadenosine in vivo. *Biochem. Pharmacol.*, *28:*1897–1902.

Chiang, P. K., Richards, H. H., and Cantoni, G. L. 1977. S-Adenosyl-L-homocysteine hydrolase: Analogues of S-adenosyl-L-homocysteine as potential inhibitors. *Mol. Pharmacol.*, *13:*939–947.

Chiang, P. K., Cantoni, G. L., Bader, J. P., Shannon, W. M., Clayton, S. J., and Montgomery, J. A. 1978. Adenosylhomocysteine hydrolase inhibitors: synthesis of 5′-deoxy-5′-(isobutylthio)-3-deazaadenosine and its effect on Rous sarcoma virus and Gross murine leukemia virus. *Biochem. Biophys. Res. Commun.*, *82:*417–423.

Chiang, P. K., Im, Y. S., and Cantoni, G. L. 1980. Phospholipids biosynthesis by methylations and choline incorporation: Effect of 3-deazaadenosine. *Biochem. Biophys. Res. Commun.*, *94:*174–181.

Chiang, P. K., Guranowski, A., and Segall, J. 1981. Irreversible inhibition of S-adenosylhomocysteine hydrolase by nucleoside analogs. *Archiv. Biochem. Biophys.*, *207:*175–184.

Chiang, P. K., Wiesmann, W. P., and Johnson, J. P. 1983. Aldosterone stimulates methylation reaction and membrane events in cultured toad urinary bladder epithelial cells. *Fed. Proc.*, *42:*717.

Crooks, P. A., Dreyer, R. N., and Coward, J. K. 1979. Metabolism of S-adenosylhomocysteine and S-tubercydinylhomocysteine in neuroblastoma cells. *Biochemistry*, *18:*2601–2609.

de la Haba, G., and Cantoni, G. L. 1959. The enzymatic synthesis of S-adenosyl-L-homocysteine from adenosine and homocysteine. *J. Biol. Chem.*, *234:*603–608.

Døskeland, S. O., and Ueland, P. M. 1982. Comparison of some physical and kinetic properties of S-adenosylhomocysteine hydrolase from bovine liver, bovine adrenal cortex and mouse liver *Biochim. Biophys. Acta.*, *708:*185–193.

Dudman, N. P. B., and Wilcken, D. E. L. 1982. Homocysteine thiolactone and experimental homocysteinemia. *Biochem. Med.*, *27:*244–253.

Duerre, J. A., and Walker, R. D., 1977, Metabolism of adenosylhomocysteine. In: *The Biochemistry of Adenosylmethionine*, pp. 43–57. (Ed. by Salvatore, F., Borek, E., Zappia, V., Williams-Ashman, H. G., and Schlenk, F. Columbia University Press, New York.

Eloranta, T. O. 1977. Tissue distribution of S-adenosylmethionine and S-adenosylhomocysteine in the rat. *Biochem. J.*, *166:*521–529.

Eloranta, T. O., Kajander, E. O., and Raina, A. M. 1982. Effect of 9-β-D-arabinofuranosyladenine and erythro-9-(2-hydroxy-3-nonyl)adenine on the metabolism of S-adenosylhomocysteine, S-adenosylmethionine, and adenosine in rat liver. *Med. Biol.*, *60:*272–277.

Ferro, A. J., Barrett, A., and Shapiro, S. K. 1976. Kinetic properties and the effect of substrate analogues on 5′-methylthioadenosine nucleosidase from *Escherichia coli*. *Biochim. Biophys. Acta*, *438:*487–494.

Finkelstein, J. D., Harris, B. J., Grossman, M. R., and Morri, H. 1978. S-Adenosylhomocysteine metabolism in rat hepatomas (40339). *Proc. Soc. Exp. Biol. Med.*, *159:*313–316.

Fox, I., Palella, T. D., Thompson, D., and Herring, C. 1982. Adenosine metabolism: modification by S-adenosylhomocysteine and 5′-methythioadenosine. *Biochem. Biophys.*, *215:*302–308.

Fujioka, M., and Takata, Y. 1981. S-Adenosylhomocysteine hydrolase from rat liver. *J. Biol. Chem.*, *256:*1631–1635.

Garcia-Castro, I., Mato, J. M., Vasanthakumar, G. I., Wiesmann, W. P., Schiffmann, E., and Chiang, P. K. 1983. Paradoxical effects of adenosine on neutrophil chemotaxis. *J. Biol. Chem.*, *258:*4345–4349.

Gordon, R. K., Brown, N. D., and Chiang, P. K. 1983. Inhibition of adenosylmethionine decarboxylase and perturbation of polyamine metabolism by 3-deaza-(±)aristeromycin. *Biochem. Biophys. Res. Commun.*, *114:*505–510.

Guranowski, A., and Jakubowski, H. 1983. Substrate specificity of S-adenosylhomocysteinase: Cysteine is a substrate of the plant and mammalian enzymes. *Biochim. Biophys. Acta*, *742:*250–256.

Guranowski, A., and Pawełkiewicz, J. 1977. Adenosylhomocysteinase from yellor lupin seeds: Purification and properties. *Eur. J. Biochem.*, *80:*517–523.

Guranowski, A. B., Chiang, P. K., and Cantoni, G. L. 1981a. 5′-Methylthioadenosine nucleosidase: Purification and characterization of the enzyme from *Lupinus luteus* seeds. *Eur. J. Biochem.*, *114:*293–299.

Guranowski, A., Montgomery, J. A., Cantoni, G. L., and Chiang, P. K. 1981b. Adenosine analogues as substrates and inhibitors of S-adenosylhomocysteine hydrolase. *Biochemistry*, *20:*110–115.

Harris, M. 1982. Induction of thymidine kinase in enzyme-deficient Chinese hamster cells. *Cell*, *29:*483–492.

Helland, S., and Ueland, P. M. 1981 The relation between the functions of 9-β-D-arabinofuranosyladenine as inactivator and substrate of S-adenosylhomocysteine hydrolase. *J. Pharmacol. Exp. Ther.*, *218:*758–763.

Helland, S., and Ueland, P. M. 1982. Inactivation of S-adenosylhomocysteine hydrolase by 9-β-D-arabinofuranosyladenine in intact cells. *Cancer Res.*, *42:*1130–1136.

Hershfield, M. S., and Kredich, N. M. 1978. S-Adenosylhomocysteine hydrolase is an adenosine-binding protein: a target for adenosine toxicity. *Science*, *202:*757–760.

Hershfield, M. S., Kredich, N. M., Ownby, D. R., Ownby, H., and Buckley, R. 1979. *In vivo* inactivation of erythrocyte S-adenosylhomocysteine hydrolase by 2′-deoxyadenosine in adenosine deaminase-deficient patients. *J. Clin. Invest.*, *63:*807–811.

Hoffman, J. 1975. A rapid liquid chromatographic determination of S-adenosylmethionine and S-adenosylhomocysteine in subgram amounts of tissue. *Anal. Biochem.*, *68:*522–530.

Hyman, B. T., Stoll, L. L., and Spector, A. A. 1982. Prostaglandin production by 3T3-L1 cells in culture. *Biochim. Biophys. Acta*, *713:*375–385.

Im, Y. S., Chiang, P. K., and Cantoni, G. L. 1979. Guanidoacetate methyltransferase: Purification and molecular properties. *J. Biol. Chem.*, *254:*11047–11050.

Johnson, G. S., and Chiang, P. K. 1981. 1-Methylnicotinamide and NAD metabolism in normal and transformed rat kidney cells. *Archiv. Biochem. Biophys.*, *210:*263–269.

Kajander, E. O., and Raina, A. M. 1981. Affinity-chromatographic purification of S-adenosyl-L-homocysteine hydrolase: Some properties of the enzyme from rat liver. *Biochem. J.*, *193:*503–512.

Kamatani, N., Willis, E. H., and Carson, D. A. 1983. Selection and characterization of a murine lymphoid cell line partially deficient in S-adenosylhomocysteine hydrolase. *Biochim. Biophys. Acta*, *762*:205–214.

Kim, I.-K., Zhang, C.-Y., Chiang, P. K., and Cantoni, G. L. 1983. S-adenosylhomocysteine hydrolase from hamster liver: purification and kinetic properties. *Archiv. Biochem. Biophys.*, *226*:65–72.

Lecompte, T., Randon, J., Chignard, M., Vargaftig, B. B., and Dray, F. 1982. Interference of transmethylation inhibitors with thromboxane synthesis in rat platelets. *Biochem. Biophys. Res. Commun.*, *106*:566–573.

Leonard, E. J., Skeel, A., Chiang, P. K., and Cantoni, G. L. 1978. The action of the adenosylhomocysteine hydrolase inhibitor, 3-deazaadenosine, on phagocytic function of mouse macrophages and human monocytes. *Biochem. Biophys. Res. Commun.*, *84*:102–109.

Lucas, D. L., Chiang, P. K., and Wright, D. 1983. Induction of human promyelocytic leukemia cells by 3-deazaaristeromycin, an inhibitor of methylation. *Fed. Proc.*, *42*:43511.

Miura, G. A., Santangelo, J. R., Gordon, R. K., and Chiang, P. K. 1984. Analysis of S-adenosylmethionine and related sulfur metabolites in animal tissues. *Anal. Biochem.*, *141*:161–167.

Montgomery, J. A., Clayton, S. J., Thomas, H. J., Shannon, W. M., Arnett, G., Bodner, A. J., Kim, I.-K., Cantoni, G. L., and Chiang, P. K. 1982. Carbocyclic analogue of 3-deazaadenosine: a novel antiviral agent-using S-adenosylhomocysteine hydrolase as a pharmacological target. *J. Med. Chem.*, *25*:626–629.

Morita, Y., Siraganian, R. P., Tang, C. K., and Chiang, P. K. 1982. Inhibition of histamine release and phosphatidylcholine metabolism by 5′-deoxy-5′-isobutylthio-3-deazaadenosine. *Biochem. Pharmacol.*, *31*:2111–2113.

Mudd, S. H., and Poole, J. R. 1975. Labile methyl balances for normal humans on various dietary regimens. *Metabolism*, *24*:721–735.

Murato, K., and Monard, D. 1982. Inhibition of S-adenosylmethionine-linked methylation can lead to neurite extension in neuroblastoma cells. *FEBS Lett.*, *144*:321–325.

Palella, T., Schatz, R. A., Wilens, T. E., and Fox, I. H. 1982. S-Adenosylhomocysteine accumulation and selective cytoxicity in cultured T- and B-lymphoblasts. *J. Lab. Clin. Med.*, *100*:269–278.

Palmer, J. L., and Abeles, R. H. 1979. The mechanism of action of S-adenosylhomocysteinase. *J. Biol. Chem.*, *254*:1217–1226.

Phyall, W., Chiang, P., Cantoni, G. L., and Lovenberg, W. 1980. The hypotensive action of 3-deazaadenosine. *Eur. J. Pharmacol.*, *67*:485–488.

Poulton, J. E., and Butt, V. S. 1976. Purification and properties of S-adenosylhomocysteine hydrolase from leaves of spinach beet. *Archiv. Biochem. Biophys.*, *172*:135–142.

Pritchard, P. H., Chiang, P. K., Cantoni, G. L., and Vance, D. E. 1982. Inhibition of phosphatidylethanolamine N-methylation by 3-deazaadenosine stimulates the synthesis of phosphatidylcholine via the CDP-choline pathway. *J. Biol. Chem.*, *257*:6362–6367.

Randon, J., Lecompte, T., Chignard, M., Siess, W., Marlas, G., Dray, F., and Vargaftig, B. B. 1981. Dissociation of platelet activation from transmethylation of their membrane phospholipids. *Nature*, *293*:660–662.

Richards, H. H., Chiang, P. K., and Cantoni, G. L. 1978. Adenosylhomocysteine hydrolase: Crystallization of the purified enzyme and its properties. *J. Biol. Chem.*, *253*:4476–4480.

Sacks, S. L., Merigan, T. C., Kaminska, J., and Fox, I. H. 1982. Inactivation of S-adenosylhomocysteine hydrolase during adenine arabinoside therapy. *J. Clin. Invest.*, *69*:226–230.

Schanche, J.-S., Schanche, T., and Ueland, P. M. 1982. Inhibition of phospholipid methylation in isolated rat hepatocytes by analogues of adenosine and S-adenosylhomocysteine. *Biochem. Biophys. Acta*, *721*:399–407.

Schatz, R. A., Vunnam, C. R., and Sellinger, O. Z. 1979. S-Adenosyl-L-homocysteine hydrolase from rat brain: Purification and some properties. In: *Transmethylation*, pp. 143–153. Ed. by Usdin, E., Borchardt, R. T., and Creveling, C. R. Elsevier, Amsterdam.

Shattil, S. J., Montgomery, J. A., and Chiang, P. K. 1982. The effect of pharmacologic inhibition of phospholipid methylation on human platelet function. *Blood*, *59*:906–912.

Trager, W., Tershakovec, M., Chiang, P. K., and Cantoni, G. L. 1980. Plasmodium falciparum: Antimalarial activity in culture of sinefungin and other methylation inhibitors. *Exp. Parasitol.*, *50*:83–89.

Trewyn, R. A., and Kerr, S. J. 1977. The enzymatic synthesis of S-adenosyl-L-[2(n)-^{3}H]homocysteine. *Anal. Biochem.*, *82*:310–316.

Ueland, P. M. 1983. Pharmacological and biochemical aspects of S-adenosylhomocysteine and S-adenosylhomocysteine hydrolase. *Pharmacol. Rev.*, *34*:223–253.

Votruba, I., and Holy, A. 1982. Eritadenines-Novel type of inhibitors of S-adenosine-L-cysteine hydrolase. *Collect. Czech. Chem. Commun.*, *47*:166–172.

White, E. L., Shaddix, S. C., Brockman, R. W., and Bennett, Jr., L. L. 1982. Comparison of actions of 9-β-D-arabinofuranosyladenine on target enzymes from mouse tumor cells. *Cancer Res.*, *42*:2260–2264.

Zimmerman, T. P., Wolberg, G., and Duncan, G. S. 1978. Inhibition of lymphocyte-mediated cytolysis by 3-deazaadenosine: Evidence by a methylation reaction essential to cytolysis. *Proc. Natl. Acad. Sci. USA*, *75*:6220–6224.

Zimmerman, T. P., Wolberg, G., Stopford, C. R., and Duncan, G. S. 1979. 3-Deazaadenosine as a tool for studying the relationship of cellular methylation reactions to various leukocyte functions. In: *Transmethylation*, pp. 187–196. Ed. by Usdin, E., Borchardt, R. T., and Creveling, C. R. Elsevier, Amsterdam.

Zimmerman, T. P., Wolberg, G., Duncan, G. S., and Elion, G. B. 1980. Adenosine analogues as substrates and inhibitors of S-adenosylhomocysteine hydrolase in intact lymphocytes. *Biochemistry*, *19*:2252–2259.

Chapter **8**

Purine Nucleoside Phosphorylase

Measurement of Activity and Use of Inhibitors

Johanna D. Stoeckler and Robert E. Parks, Jr.

Section of Biochemical Pharmacology
Division of Biology and Medicine
Brown University
Providence, Rhode Island

I. INTRODUCTION

It has long been appreciated that purine nucleoside phosphorylase (PNP; purine nucleoside:orthophosphate ribosyltransferase, EC 2.4.2.1) may play a role in cancer chemotherapy by catalyzing the degradation of potentially cytotoxic purine deoxynucleoside analogs, e.g., 2′-deoxy-6-thioguanosine. More recently, the identification of an immunodeficiency disorder associated with a deficiency in PNP (Giblett *et al.*, 1975) has drawn attention to this enzyme as a possible target for the design of novel immunosuppressive agents. In contrast to the severe combined immunodeficiency disease seen with adenosine deaminase deficiency, where defects occur in both cellular and humoral immunity, patients with PNP deficiency lack cellular, but not humoral, immunity. Also, these individuals excrete the more soluble nucleosides of hypoxanthine and guanine rather than the relatively insoluble end product of purine metabolism, uric acid. Thus it has been proposed that a potent inhibitor of PNP might serve as a biochemical modifier in chemotherapy with purine nucleoside analogs, as a selective immunosuppressive agent, and perhaps in the treatment of secondary gout (Parks *et al.*, 1981; Stoeckler *et al.*, 1980a, 1982; Kazmers *et al.*, 1981).

The authors' laboratory has described many of the structure–activity relationships of human erythrocytic PNP and has identified as inhibitors the substrate analogs, 8-aminoguanine and 8-aminoguanosine (Parks *et al.*, 1981; Stoeckler *et*

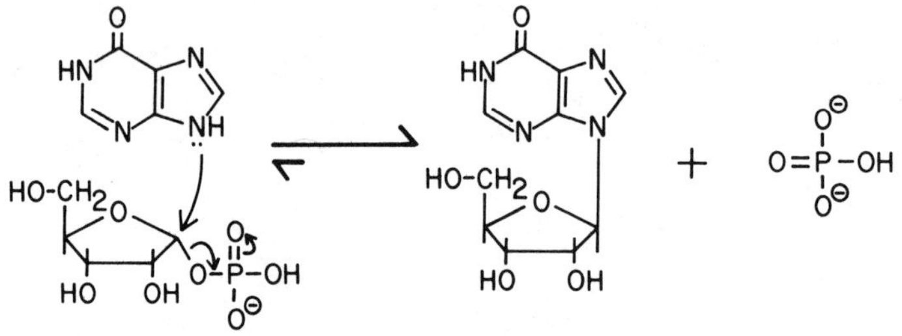

Figure 1. The reaction mechanism of purine nucleoside phosphorylase.

al., 1982), which display immunosuppressant activity (Stoeckler *et al.*, 1980a; Kazmers *et al.*, 1981). The search continues for more potent second-generation inhibitors. For extensive reviews of the literature on PNP, see Parks and Agarwal (1972) and Stoeckler (1984).

PNP is widely distributed in nature, being found in organisms ranging from bacteria to man. This chapter focuses on the properties and assays of the mammalian enzyme, particularly the well-studied human erythrocytic PNP (Stoeckler *et al.*, 1978).

The reaction illustrated in Figure 1 follows an S_N2 mechanism and is readily reversible. The equilibrium favors synthesis of nucleosides, but it is generally believed that the principal metabolic role of PNP involves the degradation of ribonucleosides and deoxyribonucleosides of guanine and hypoxanthine. Adenine has been shown to have substrate activity with PNP, but the kinetic parameters with the mammalian enzyme are so unfavorable (Zimmerman *et al.*, 1971) that it is highly unlikely that this reaction or the phosphorolysis of adenosine plays a role in normal physiology. Instead, PNP rapidly degrades the products of adenosine deaminase (ADA), inosine and 2′-deoxyinosine and can be used as an indicator enzyme for the assay of ADA. The activity of PNP exceeds that of ADA in all human fetal tissues examined except thymus (Carson *et al.*, 1977). The activity in adult human erythrocytes is 10–15 μmoles inosine cleaved per minute per milliliter of packed cells at 30°C, 25- to 80-fold higher than the ADA activity. In contrast, PNP activity is relatively low or absent in the erythrocytes of some laboratory animals, e.g., rats, dogs and cats (Agarwal *et al.*, 1975; Parks and Agarwal, 1972), and this difference must be borne in mind when using such animal models to examine the efficacy of PNP inhibitors.

II. MEASUREMENT OF PNP ACTIVITY

A. Choice of Assay

A number of options are available for assaying PNP. Conditions are easily established for measuring the reaction in either direction, i.e., nucleoside synthesis or phosphorolysis. For example, in the direction of phosphorolysis, the liberation of the purine base may be monitored by a direct or coupled spectro-

Table I. Affinities of Selected Substrates and Inhibitors with Human Erythrocytic PNP[a]

Compound	K_m (μM)	K_i (μM)	Reference[b]
Inosine	30–46		1
Hypoxanthine	19	17	2, 3
Guanosine	32		1
Guanine	20	5	3
6-Thioinosine	70		4
6-Thioguanosine	167		5
8-Aminoguanosine	7	17	3
8-Aminoguanine	11	0.2	3
TCNR[c]		5	6
5′-Deoxy-5′-iodoformycin B		7	3
Formycin B		100	4

[a] The affinity constants reported here were determined at low substrate or inhibitor concentrations.
[b] References: 1. Stoeckler *et al.*, 1980b; 2. Zimmerman *et al.*, 1971; 3. Stoeckler *et al.*, 1982; 4. Sheen *et al.*, 1968; 5. Unpublished data, E. Chu of this laboratory; 6. Willis *et al.*, 1980.
[c] TCNR, 1-β-D-ribofuranosyl-1,2,4-triazole-3-carboxamidine.

photometric assay, by measurement of the formation of radiolabeled purine base, or by high-performance liquid chromatography (HPLC). Such assays are described below. Alternatively, the formation of the pentose phosphate, e.g., ribose 1-phosphate, may be monitored by a radioisotope assay (Milman, 1978) or colorimetrically by the orcinol reaction after removal of the nucleoside with charcoal (Moyer and Fischer, 1976). Finally, a qualitative assay for PNP in spots of dried blood has been developed by Ito *et al.* (1977) as a reliable screen for both ADA and PNP in human blood. This dye-linked assay was originally used to detect PNP in overlay gels for electrophoresis (Edwards *et al.*, 1971).

In the direction of nucleoside synthesis, one may employ a direct spectral assay, a radiolabeled purine base with measurement of the appearance of radiolabeled nucleoside, or high-performance liquid chromatography (HPLC). Also, one may monitor orthophosphate production by a method that distinguishes between orthophosphate and the acid-labile phosphate of the pentose 1-phosphate (Lowry and Lopez, 1946).

Nucleoside or base substrates that are useful for assaying PNP have K_m values in the 10^{-5} M range, as shown in Table I. Therefore, direct spectral assays with saturating substrate concentrations are not feasible because of excessively high initial absorbances. Guanine and guanosine, and other guaninelike base–nucleoside pairs, show large spectral shifts upon reaction with PNP. These substrates are suitable for direct spectrophotometric measurement of their kinetic parameters or the effects of certain inhibitors studied with the substrates at or below their K_m concentrations. Maximal velocities can usually be obtained by extrapolation from kinetic studies. However, an important feature of the reaction of PNP from human erythrocytes (Kim *et al.*, 1968; Agarwal *et al.*, 1975) and certain other mammalian sources is the negative cooperativity, also termed substrate activation, seen at high substrate concentrations. The rates of catalysis at >10 times the K_m concentration are significantly higher than the V_{max} calculated from kinetic studies at low concentrations. With guaninelike substrates those rates can be determined by radioisotope assays, HPLC, or measurements of P_i or the pentose phosphate. Conversely, if kinetic studies are performed only at high substrate concentrations, very high K_m values are determined, i.e., the affinities of the compounds are underestimated, accounting for some of the discrepancies in the literature.

Inosine and inosine analogs, whose base moieties react with xanthine oxidase, can be studied by coupled assays. The urate or urate analog produced absorbs at a wavelength far removed from the λ_{max} of the nucleoside substrate and it is possible to study the PNP reaction over a wide range of substrate concentrations. Inosinelike compounds show very minor spectral changes upon reaction with PNP and therefore are unsuitable for direct spectral assays. The coupled spectrophotometric assay for inosine can detect about 5×10^{-10} moles/min, while radioisotope assays are 100- to 1000-fold more sensitive. An ultramicrochemical assay (Uitendaal *et al.*, 1978) can detect PNP activity in individual cells (see Section C2).

Several of the assays described below can be used with intact cells, but if cell extracts are used, they can be prepared by any standard means. PNP is cytosolic and is fully recovered in the supernatant fraction after centrifugation for 1 hr at 100,000*g*. The enzyme is most stable if frozen in concentrated extracts. PNP may be partially or fully inactivated by heavy metals and thiol-reactive agents such as *p*-hydroxymercuribenzoate (Agarwal and Parks, 1971). In the authors' laboratory, fresh dilutions of purified human erythrocytic PNP are prepared daily in buffer containing 1 m*M* dithiothreitol. Reduction of thiol groups is allowed to take place for 30–60 min at room temperature before the solutions are placed on ice.

B. Dynamic Spectrophotometric Assays

PNP activity can be measured by a number of coupled or direct spectrophotometric assays that employ natural or analog substrates. The choice of assay is dictated by the specific activity of the PNP preparation or the presence of nonprotein UV-absorbing compounds, such as PNP inhibitors and other purines. The initial absorbancy should not greatly exceed 1.0 because solutions that contain proteins or purines, or both, generally deviate from Beer's Law at higher absorbancy values. The assays described below are performed at 30°C because equilibration to this temperature is achieved rapidly.

1. The Coupled Assay with Xanthine Oxidase

The classic assay of PNP was first described by H. M. Kalckar (1947), the discoverer of the enzyme. This method is based on the increase in absorbancy at 293 nm when hypoxanthine is converted to uric acid in the xanthine oxidase reaction.

a. Inosine Phosphorolysis

$$\text{Inosine} + P_i \underset{}{\overset{\text{PNP}}{\rightleftharpoons}} \text{hypoxanthine} + \text{ribose 1-phosphate}$$

$$\text{Hypoxanthine} + 2O_2 \xrightarrow[\text{oxidase}]{\text{xanthine}} \text{uric acid} + 2O_2^-$$

Although the equilibrium of the PNP reaction favors nucleoside synthesis, the use of relatively high concentrations of phosphate and removal of the product, hypoxanthine, shift this equilibrium to favor phosphorolysis. Important advantages of this procedure, in comparison with certain direct spectrophotometric assays, are that the reaction rates are linear for many minutes and that the measurements are made at 293 nm, a wavelength at which background absorbancy from proteins and other substrates is usually low. Under conditions where background absorbancy at this wavelength is high, e.g., in the study of certain inhibitors, inosine may be replaced by the substrate analog, 6-thioinosine, as described in Section b.

This modification of the Kalckar assay has been in use as a standard assay in the authors' laboratory for many years and has proven both convenient and reliable in a variety of studies ranging from enzyme purification to kinetic analyses.

Reagents:

Inosine, 5 m*M*.

Potassium phosphate buffer, 0.5 *M*, pH 7.4.

Xanthine oxidase from buttermilk, 0.2 u/ml water.

Preparations of PNP are diluted in 0.05 to 0.1 *M* Tris, Hepes, or phosphate buffer, pH 7.4, containing 1 m*M* dithiothreitol, so that an appropriate aliquot gives an absorbancy change of 0.005–0.050/min.

Procedure. The reaction is carried out at 30°C in a 1.5-ml quartz cuvette with a 1-cm light path. The reaction mixture contains 0.1 ml each of the potassium phosphate buffer, inosine, and xanthine oxidase reagents plus other additions, e.g., an inhibitor, and sufficient water to yield a final volume of 1.0 ml including the enzyme aliquot. The reaction mixture is preincubated for several minutes to permit temperature equilibration and to degrade any hypoxanthine or xanthine that may contaminate the inosine preparation. The reaction is initiated by addition of the PNP solution and the activity is calculated from the increase in absorbancy at 293 nm ($\epsilon = 1.25 \times 10^4\ M^{-1} \cdot \text{cm}^{-1}$). The enzymic activity is expressed in standard International Units, i.e., 1 u PNP is the amount of enzyme that catalyzes the phosphorolysis of 1 μmole inosine per minute under these standard assay conditions.

Comments. For convenience, the reagents may be combined before being added to the cuvettes. A standard cocktail of 5 m*M* inosine dissolved in 0.5 *M* potassium phosphate buffer (0.1 ml per assay) can be stored indefinitely at −20°C. A mixture containing xanthine oxidase may be stored at 4°C for several days. For typical kinetic studies, inosine is diluted to 0.5 m*M* and added to give a final concentration range of 10–100 μ*M*.

Xanthine oxidase must not be rate-limiting and excess PNP should be added to one cuvette in order to determine the velocity limit. Commercially available xanthine oxidase of specific activity ~1.3 u/mg protein (Grade III, Sigma Chemical Co., St. Louis, MO) is routinely used in our laboratory but preparations of lower purity (e.g. Grade I, specific activity ≅ 0.1 u/mg; Grade IV, specific activity = 0.1 u/mg) are acceptable. Commercial xanthine oxidase suspensions in ammonium sulfate are stable for 6 months to 1 year before reduced activities are noted. Deterioration of the xanthine oxidase is usually associated with a pronounced lag in the reaction rate during the first minutes. The enzyme may be used without prior dialysis unless the kinetics of phosphate are under study, since some preparations contain phosphate buffer.

Xanthine oxidase requires O_2 and is inhibited by cyanide and azide ions. It also reacts with certain hypoxanthine analogs, e.g., 6-mercaptopurine, 8-aminohypoxanthine, and allopurinol, and therefore the coupled assay is unsuitable for studying the inhibition of PNP by such compounds. Significant uricase levels also interfere with this assay.

b. 6-Thioinosine Phosphorolysis. The phosphorolysis of 6-thioinosine (6-mercaptopurine ribonucleoside) yields 6-mercaptopurine, which is also a substrate for xanthine oxidase. 6-Thioinosine absorbs maximally at 320 nm and formation of 6-thiouric acid, the oxidation product of 6-mercaptopurine, is monitored at 348 nm. The advantage of this assay is that neither proteins nor most other purines absorb significantly at this wavelength. The assay is useful for evaluating PNP inhibitors such as 8-aminoguanine or formycin B (see Section III) which absorb strongly at 293 nm, the wavelength at which uric acid formation is detected.

Reagents:

6-Thioinosine, 2 m*M*.

Potassium phosphate buffer, 0.5 *M*, pH 7.4.

Xanthine oxidase from buttermilk, 2 u/ml water.

Dithiothreitol, 100 m*M*.

Preparations of PNP are diluted in 0.05 to 0.1 *M* Tris, Hepes, or phosphate buffer, pH 7.4, containing 1 m*M* dithiothreitol, so that an appropriate aliquot gives an absorbancy change of 0.005–0.050/min.

Procedure. The reagents, 0.35 ml 6-thioinosine, 0.1 ml phosphate buffer, 0.1 ml xanthine oxidase, 0.01 ml dithiothreitol, and sufficient water to give a final volume of 1.0 ml, are mixed in a 1.5-ml cuvette with a 1-cm path length and preincubated at 30°C for several minutes. The reaction is initiated by the addition of PNP and the enzymic activity is calculated from the increase in absorbancy at 348 nm based on $\Delta\epsilon = 2.45 \times 10^4\ M^{-1}\cdot\text{cm}^{-1}$ (Sheen *et al.*, 1968).

Comments. Comments regarding the inosine phosphorolysis assay also apply to this assay. Ten times more xanthine oxidase is required than for the inosine phosphorolysis assay because 6-mercaptopurine is not as good a substrate as hypoxanthine for this enzyme. Dithiothreitol serves to maintain the substrate and enzymic thiol groups in the reduced state.

The concentration of 6-thioinosine in the reaction mixture is 0.7 mM, ten times its K_m concentration with PNP, and contributes <0.5 background absorbancy. Although the $\Delta\epsilon$ for this assay is twice that of the inosine phosphorolysis assay, this procedure has about the same sensitivity because 6-thioinosine reacts with PNP at about one half the rate of inosine.

2. *Direct Spectrophotometric Assays*

These assays exploit the large differences between the spectra of the nucleosides and bases of guanine-type compounds and can be performed in either the phosphorolytic or synthetic direction.

a. Guanosine Synthesis or Phosphorolysis. Partially purified PNP, giving lower background absorbancy, is suitable for these assays.

Reagents for synthesis:

Guanine, 0.8 mM.

Ribose 1-phosphate, dicylohexylammonium salt, 10 mM.

Tris-HCl or Hepes-NaOH buffer, 0.5 M, pH 7.5.

PNP preparations in 0.05 to 0.1 M Tris or Hepes buffer are diluted with the same buffer, pH 7.5, containing 1 mM dithiothreitol, so that an aliquot of 100 μl or less gives an absorbancy change of 0.005–0.040 per minute.

Reagents for phosphorolysis:

Guanosine, 0.8 mM.

Potassium phosphate buffer, 0.5 M, pH 7.5.

PNP preparations are diluted in Tris, Hepes, or phosphate buffer, pH 7.5, containing 1 mM dithiothreitol as above.

Procedure. The appropriate reagents, 0.1 ml of each, and sufficient water to give a final volume of 1.0 ml are mixed in a 1.5-ml quartz cuvette with a 1-cm path length and preincubated at 30°C for several minutes. PNP is added to initiate the reaction and the rate of synthesis or phosphorolysis of guanosine is calculated from the increase or decrease, respectively, in the absorbancy at 258 nm, using $\Delta\epsilon = 5.3 \times 10^3\ M^{-1}\cdot\text{cm}^{-1}$ (Stoeckler *et al.*, 1980b).

Comments. It is important to record the initial reaction because the rates are linear for a much shorter time than with the coupled assays, because of product inhibition. This problem is most pronounced in the phosphorolytic direction since the purine bases have a higher affinity for PNP than the nucleosides.

The stock solution of ribose 1-phosphate (Sigma Chemical Co., St. Louis, MO) is kept on ice and frozen for storage to prevent breakdown. Guanine can be dissolved by addition of 1 N HCl or KOH and heating, avoiding excess acid or base so that the final reaction pH is not altered. PNP preparations in phosphate buffers should be dialyzed against Tris or Hepes before use in the synthetic assay.

b. Assays with Analog Substrates. Guanosine analogs that display good substrate activity with PNP include 6-thioguanosine and 6-selenoguanosine. The assay procedures for synthesis or phosphorolysis are similar to those used for guanosine above except that the reactions are monitored at wavelengths above 300 nm, where there is less interference from protein and non-thiol-containing purines. The spectral parameters at pH 6.5 are as follows: 6-thioguanosine/6-

thioguanine, $\Delta\epsilon = \pm 3.7 \times 10^3 M^{-1} \cdot cm^{-1}$ at 344 nm; 6-selenoguanosine/6-selenoguanine, $\Delta\epsilon = \pm 3.6 \times 10^3 M^{-1} \cdot cm^{-1}$ at 360 nm (Ross *et al.*, 1973). Dithiothreitol (1 m*M*) is added to keep substrate and enzyme thiol groups reduced.

C. Radioisotope Assays

Radiochemical assays provide the most sensitive measure of initial velocity. PNP activity may be determined in either catalytic direction, even in crude extracts or permeabilized cells. If undialyzed extracts are used, 1 m*M* EDTA may be used to block depletion of the purine base by hypoxanthine-guanine phosphoribosyltransferase. The PNP activity of intact cells may also be measured, bearing in mind that the transport and further metabolism of the reactants and products may be rate-limiting. The first assay presented below measures phosphorolysis and further metabolism of nucleoside substrates in intact cells and is useful for evaluating a PNP inhibitor. The second, a procedure reported by Uitendaal *et al.* (1978), is the most sensitive PNP assay in the literature and is used with permeabilized cells. Both these assays could be adapted for use with tissue extracts.

1. Phosphorolytic Assay with Intact Cells

The distribution of radiolabel in nucleoside, base, and nucleotides is determined by chromatography after heat inactivation of the reaction mixture. This assay could be adapted for initial velocity studies with tissue extracts by substituting 50 m*M* phosphate buffer, pH 7.4, for the culture medium and increasing the specific activity of the radiolabeled substrate.

Reagents:

[^{14}C]Nucleoside (guanosine, 2′-deoxyguanosine, or inosine), 0.8 m*M* in medium, 2–10 mCi/mmole.

Growth medium, balanced salt solution or high-phosphate medium (see *Reagents*, Section E).

Cell suspension, approximately $2–10 \times 10^7$ cells/ml medium.

Procedure. The reaction mixture containing 150 μl [^{14}C]nucleoside, 150 μl medium (in which an inhibitor may be present), and 300 μl cell suspension is incubated at 37°C on a shaking water bath (100 oscillations/min). At time intervals ranging from 5 min to several hours, 100 μl aliquots are withdrawn and injected into preheated 12 mm × 75 mm glass tubes and heated for 2 min at 95°C in a heating block. The tubes are centrifuged for 5 min at 1500*g* and 10 or 20 μl of the supernate is analyzed by chromatography. Unlabeled purines are first applied as carriers so that spots can be identified by UV light absorbance at 254 nm. For guanosine nucleoside phosphorolysis, cellulose TLC plates are developed with acetonitrile, 0.1 *M*, ammonium acetate, pH 7.0, and ammonia (60:30:10) for about 50 min (Crabtree and Henderson, 1971), or longer if microcrystalline cellulose is used. The total, acid-soluble nucleotides appear as a streak reaching 2–3 cm up from the origin but are well separated from guanine, guanosine, and 2′-deoxyguanosine. For inosine phosphorolysis, 20 μl aliquots are applied to Whatman 3

MM chromatography paper and subjected to electrophoresis for 30 min at 4000 V and 250 mA in 50 m*M* sodium borate (Fox *et al.*, 1977). Radioactivity is quantitated in hypoxanthine, inosine, and inosine monophosphate (Kazmers *et al.*, 1981). The dried spots are cut out and may be counted in nonaqueous scintillation fluid.

Comments. Alternative chromatographic procedures have been reported. Inosine and hypoxanthine may be separated on CM-cellulose paper (Van der Weyden and Bailey, 1982) or PEI-cellulose TLC plates (Tax and Veerkamp, 1978) with distilled water. If no nucleotide synthesis occurs, guanosine and guanine may be separated on cellulose TLC plates with 1% NH_4OH (Cohen and Sussman, 1975). Ca^{2+} Chelex columns have been employed for isolation of either [^{14}C]ribose 1-phosphate, produced by phosphorolysis of uniformly labeled nucleoside, or [^{14}C]nucleoside synthesized from a radiolabeled base (Milman, 1978).

2. *Ultramicrochemical Assay for PNP Activity in Individual Cells*

For ultramicrochemical determination of PNP, we describe briefly a procedure reported by Uitendaal *et al.* (1978). To prevent evaporation during the incubation, the reaction is carried out in sealed parafilm microcuvettes containing 0.3 μl of incubation mixture delivered with a gauged microconstriction pipette. Cultured fibroblasts grown in plastic dishes are shock-frozen in liquid nitrogen, lyophilized overnight, and selected visually. Small plastic leaflets carrying the cells are cut from the bottoms of the culture dishes and transferred to the parafilm microcuvettes. After addition of the reaction medium, the microcuvettes are sealed and incubated at 37°C. The entire contents of the microcuvettes are subjected to descending chromatography on Whatman 3 MM paper strips with a solvent system of 0.5 *N* ammonia and 0.005 *M* EDTA. In the synthetic direction, the reaction mixture contains the following: Tris-HCl buffer, pH 7.0, 0.17 *M*; bovine serum albumin, 0.5% (w/v), to prevent surface denaturation of the enzyme; penicillin, 0.8‰, streptomycin 0.8‰; EDTA, 3.3 m*M*, to inhibit the hypoxanthine-guanine phosphoribosyltransferase reaction; ribose 1-phosphate, 1.7 m*M*; and [8-^{14}C]hypoxanthine, 0.1 m*M*, specific activity about 50 mCi/mmole. For measurement of the phosphorolytic reaction, a similar reaction mixture is employed with phosphate (4.7 m*M*) replacing the ribose 1-phosphate and [8-^{14}C]inosine (0.27 m*M*, specific activity about 50 mCi/mmole) replacing the hypoxanthine. Depending upon the number of cells examined and the enzymic activities, incubation times of 30–120 min are employed. After separation of the reaction products by paper chromatography, the purine spots are visualized under UV light with the aid of unlabeled hypoxanthine and inosine reference compounds. The spots are cut out and radioactivity is quantitated by liquid scintillation counting.

The above method has been employed to measure the PNP activity in small numbers of fibroblasts, i.e., 1–20. It has been possible to study single normal and immunodeficient B and T lymphocytes with this technique, and with a few hundred cells the K_m values and pH optima of fibroblastic purine nucleoside phosphorylase can be determined.

D. High-Performance Liquid Chromatography Assay

The use of HPLC to separate and quantitate reaction products permits measurement of the PNP activity of intact cells or tissue extracts in both the synthetic and phosphorolytic directions with any natural substrates or substrate analogs. In addition, further metabolism of these reaction products may be monitored, e.g., the accumulation of GTP from 2′-deoxyguanosine (Stoeckler *et al.*, 1982). The conditions below are for cell suspensions, but the assay has been used frequently to study the reaction of purified PNP with analogs at concentrations ranging from 0.05 to 1 m*M*.

Reagents:

2′-Deoxyguanosine, 0.4–4.0 m*M* in medium.

Medium, high-phosphate medium (see *Reagents*, Section E) or any physiological salt solution, such as Puck's saline G or Hank's balanced salts.

Cell suspension, 8–20% in medium.

Procedure. The incubation mixture of 1.0 ml substrate and 2.0 ml medium (containing various inhibitor concentrations, if desired) in a 25-ml plastic vial is preincubated for several minutes at 37°C on a shaking water bath (100 oscillations/min). After addition of 1.0 ml cell suspension, aliquots of 0.8 ml are removed at time intervals ranging from 5 min to 2 hr and mixed with 0.2 ml ice-cold 20% perchloric acid in a 15-ml conical centrifuge tube. The samples are kept on ice for 15 min and vortexed occasionally. Precipitated proteins are sedimented by centrifugation at 1,500*g* for 5 min at 4°C. Most (0.8 ml) of the supernate is transferred to a second tube and neutralized by 0.1–0.2 ml of 5 *N* KOH (exact amount is determined by a trial titration). If low-phosphate medium is used, 0.08 ml of potassium phosphate buffer, 0.5 *M*, pH 7.0, is added before neutralization, making it easier to attain an end point pH between 6.5 and 7.5. The neutralized solution is kept on ice for 15 min and the insoluble potassium perchlorate salt is then removed by centrifugation. The precipitate should be flushed away promptly because perchlorate salts are explosive when dry. The supernatant fluid is stored at −20°C. HPLC analysis for base and nucleoside is carried out on a reversed-phase column. Good separations are achieved in less than 20 min with Waters μBondapak C_{18} analytical columns (30 cm × 4.5 mm) using a linear methanol gradient (0–20% in 11 min; isocratic 20% for 4 min) in 0.01 *M* potassium phosphate, pH 5.5 at a flow rate of 60 ml/hr (Stoeckler *et al.*, 1980b). Nucleotides may be analyzed in less than 60 min by anion-exchange HPLC, e.g., with a Reeve-Angel Partisil-10 SAX column (25 cm × 4.6 mm) using a concave phosphate gradient (low-concentrate eluant, 0.002 *M* KH_2PO_4, pH 4.5; high-concentrate eluant, 0.5 *M* KH_2PO_4, pH 4.5) at a flow rate of 50 ml/hr (Crabtree *et al.*, 1979).

Comments. This procedure employs final concentrations of 0.1 to 1 m*M* substrate and cell suspensions ranging from 2 to 5%. The optimal conditions depend on the PNP activity of a given cell type; higher cell concentrations and lower or higher substrate concentrations may be used. If smaller or larger aliquots are taken, the volumes of the extraction reagents are adjusted accordingly. Although this assay can be used for kinetic studies with isolated PNP, the sensitivity is not suitable for initial velocity studies with intact cells, where factors such as the rate of transport across the plasma membrane and the rate of subsequent metabolism also play important roles. This assay is useful for studying the effects of inhibitors and of cellular environment on PNP activity. The high-phosphate medium gives faster rates of phosphorolysis (see Section IIIB). Complete growth media contain UV-absorbing substances that interfere with the quantitation of purines in the HPLC profiles. Nucleotide analysis can be performed after centrifuging cells through oil into the perchloric acid or washing them with a balanced salt solution before extraction. Nucleosides and bases, which equilibrate rapidly across cell membranes, cannot be quantitated in complete media.

E. Spectrophotometric Point Assay

The PNP activity of intact cells or crude enzyme preparations can be determined by measuring the products of inosine or 6-thioinosine phosphorolysis and the xanthine oxidase reaction after cell lysis or removal of protein by acid precipitation. This assay, with inosine or guanosine as substrate, was the original coupled assay described by Kalckar (1947) for PNP activity in tissue extracts. The technique was adapted for use with inosine or 6-thioinosine in intact cells by Sheen *et al.* (1968). The modification described below (Stoeckler *et al.*, 1980b) gives linear reaction rates for at least 25 min with intact human erythrocytes.

Reagents:

6-Thioinosine, 2 m*M* in medium.

High-phosphate medium (potassium phosphate buffer, 50 m*M* pH 7.4; NaCl, 75 m*M*; $MgSO_4$, 2 m*M*; glucose, 10 m*M*).

Xanthine oxidase, 5 u/ml medium.

Dithiothreitol, 40 m*M* in medium.

Cell suspension, 8% (v/v) in medium.

Procedure. An incubation mixture containing 1.0 ml 6-thioinosine, 1.5 ml medium, 0.4 ml xanthine oxidase, and 0.1 ml dithiothreitol is preincubated for several minutes in a 25-ml plastic vial at 37°C on a shaking water bath (100 oscillations/min). The reaction is started by addition of 1.0 ml cell suspension. Aliquots of 0.8 ml are removed at time intervals ranging from 0 to 20 min and rapidly mixed with 0.2 ml ice-cold 20% perchloric acid in 15-ml conical centrifuge tubes. Extraction and neutralization are performed as described for the HPLC assay (Section D). Finally, 0.8 ml of neutralized extract is allowed to react for 15–30 min at 37°C with 0.1 ml xanthine oxidase to ensure complete oxidation of the 6-thiopurine, and the absorbancy of each solution is then determined at 348 nm in a 1-cm path length cuvette. The enzymic activity is calculated from the rate of increase in absorbancy at 348 nm, $\Delta\epsilon = 2.45 \times 10^4$, after correction for dilution.

Comments. See Comments for the coupled assay and for 6-thioinosine phosphorolysis in Section IIB1. Addition of xanthine oxidase (commercially available) to the incubation medium permits only partial conversion of product to 6-thiouric acid, since the enzyme is excluded from the cells, but helps to reduce product inhibition. Less xanthine oxidase is required during the incubation if inosine is used as the substrate.

III. THE USE OF PNP INHIBITORS

A. Currently Available Inhibitors

A potent inhibitor of PNP could be used to simulate the suppression of cellular immunity that occurs in PNP deficiency, as well as to test the hypothesis that analogs of 2′-deoxyguanosine might have unique chemotherapeutic activities if their phosphorolytic cleavage were prevented. The competitive inhibitors identified to date have affinity constants ranging from 10^{-4} to 10^{-7} *M* and in general might be expected to cause only partial blockage of PNP activity.

Table I lists the C-nucleosides, formycin B ($K_i = 1 \times 10^{-4}$ *M*) and 5′-chloro-5′-deoxyformycin B ($K_i = 1 \times 10^{-5}$ *M*) and TCNR (1-β-D-ribofuranosyl-1,2,4-triazole-3-carboxamidine, $K_i = 5 \times 10^{-6}$ *M*), which resembles 5-amino-4-imidazole carboxamide ribonucleotide, an intermediate of purine biosynthesis *de novo*. These compounds are true inhibitors of PNP and are fully resistant to phosphorolysis (Sheen *et al.*, 1968; Stoeckler *et al.*, 1982; Willis *et al.*, 1980). It is important to note that formycin B and TCNR can also be converted to nucleotides and have cytotoxic actions unrelated to the inhibition of PNP (Cowan *et al.*, 1981; Willis *et al.*, 1980). 5′-Chloro-5′-deoxyformycin B, in which the 5′-halogen prevents phosphorylation, may be a pure PNP inhibitor but further testing with purine-metabolizing enzymes is required.

8-Aminoguanine ($K_i = 1\text{–}2 \times 10^{-7}$ *M*) and 8-aminoguanosine ($K_i = 1.7 \times 10^{-5}$ *M*) are alternative substrates for PNP. The phosphorolysis of 8-aminoguanosine itself results in spectral changes at 256 and 290 nm and may interfere with spectrophotometric assays at wavelengths below 300 nm (Stoeckler *et al.*, 1982). The more soluble nucleoside reacts intracellularly with PNP to generate the more potent inhibitor 8-aminoguanine (Stoeckler *et al.*, 1982). These compounds appear to function as pure inhibitors because they lack substrate or inhibitor activity with the other enzymes of purine metabolism, namely, hypoxanthine-guanine phosphoribosyltransferase, guanase, xanthine oxidase (Stoeckler *et al.*, 1982), adenosine deaminase, and *S*-adenosylhomocysteine hydrolase (Kazmers *et al.*, 1981). 8-Aminoguanosine alone has been found to be nontoxic at 100 μ*M* concentration to human lymphocytic cell lines and other cultured human tumor cells (Kazmers *et al.*, 1981; unpublished observations of E. N. Spremulli, Roger Williams Cancer Center).

A new competitive inhibitor, 9-deaza-5′-deoxy-5′-iodoinosine, has been developed by R. S. Klein, Sloan-Kettering Memorial Institute. Preliminary tests in our laboratory indicate that it has an affinity comparable to that of 8-aminoguanine. This compound is a C-nucleoside that cannot be phosphorylated at the 5′-position and may prove to be a highly specific PNP inhibitor.

B. Effects of PNP Inhibition

PNP deficiency *per se* does not appear harmful to cells in the absence of exogenous purine nucleosides. Symptoms of the deficiency do not appear in patients until several months to several years after birth and are chiefly related to severely defective T-cell immunity, although neurological disorders and anemias are sometimes also seen (for a review, see Ammann, 1978). The symptoms of PNP deficiency are milder in patients who have as little as 1% or less of normal enzymic activity (Gelfand *et al.*, 1978). The biochemical effects of PNP deficiency include the following: hypouricemia and hypouricosuria; appearance of purine deoxyribonucleosides and highly elevated ribonucleosides in body fluids; high levels of dGTP in erythrocytes; and low activity of *S*-adenosylhomocysteine hydrolase (see Martin and Gelfand, 1981, for a review).

Effects on the immune system have been attributed to the generation of toxic deoxynucleotides from 2′-deoxyguanosine in T lymphoblasts (Chan, 1978; Gudas *et al.*, 1978). Intraerythrocytic deoxyguanosine nucleotides may be responsible for the observed hemolytic anemia (Simmonds *et al.*, 1982). The reduction in *S*-adenosylhomocysteine hydrolase activity may be caused by the 100-fold increase in the plasma concentration of inosine, which is an irreversible inhibitor of this enzyme (Hershfield, 1981). Thus, the effects of PNP deficiency appear to be caused primarily by the elevated concentrations of its nucleoside substrates. Evidence from a study with mice suggests that the primary source of the deoxynucleosides is the catabolism of nucleotides from nuclei extruded during normal erythrocytic maturation (Smith and Henderson, 1982).

In the absence of exogenous 2′-deoxyguanosine, PNP deficiency or inhibition is not toxic to cultured cells. PNP-deficient mouse T-lymphoma cells grow normally in tissue culture but are inhibited by 2′-deoxyguanosine, with $ID_{50} \cong 10^{-5}$ *M* (Ullman *et al.*, 1979). As noted above (Section IIIA) the PNP inhibitor 8-aminoguanosine does not impair the growth of a variety of human tumor lines. 8-Aminoguanosine does significantly potentiate the cytotoxicity of 2′-deoxyguanosine in some T-cell lymphoblast lines (Kazmers *et al.*, 1981).

Since infusion of small amounts of irradiated erythrocytes has elicited a partial recovery of T-cell functions in two PNP-deficient patients (Ammann, 1978), an effective systemic PNP inhibitor would have to inhibit completely the high PNP activity of human red cells. Our laboratory has examined the effects of 8-aminoguanosine on human erythrocytes. The erythrocyte suspensions (5%, v/v) were incubated in Puck's saline G with 100 μ*M* 8-aminoguanosine and 200 μ*M* 2′-deoxyguanosine, as described under the HPLC assay (Section D). More than 80% of the deoxyguanosine was cleaved after 1 hr and none remained after 2 hr. Earlier studies (Stoeckler *et al.*, 1982) of human erythrocytes with guanosine (100 μ*M*) and 8-aminoguanine (100 μ*M*) showed that in high-phosphate medium (50 m*M* phosphate, as described in Section D), which favors the phosphorolytic PNP reaction as well as 5-phosphoribosyl-1-pyrophosphate synthesis, over 90% of the nucleoside was cleaved within 30 min but only 25% was converted to GTP during that time and 60% after 1 hr. This finding indicates that the metabolic removal of the purine base is unnecessary for complete phosphorolysis of the nucleoside in intact erythrocytes. Our recent unpublished studies have shown that nucleotide synthesis from 2′-deoxyguanosine is slower than from guanosine. 8-Aminoguanosine, while slowing the phosphorolysis of the nucleoside, actually stimulates the GTP synthesis, presumably because its own cleavage provides ribose 1-phosphate which is a precursor of 5-phosphoribosyl-1-pyrophosphate. This effect is most pronounced in high-phosphate media.

A radioisotope assay was used by Kazmers *et al.* (1981) to study the inhibition of PNP in human T and B lymphoblasts in RPMI 1640 medium. They reported 98% inhibition of the phosphorolysis of 200 μM inosine and no depletion of 100 μM 8-aminoguanosine from the medium during a 1-hr incubation.

Although 8-aminoguanosine significantly potentiated the cytotoxicity of deoxyguanosine in MOLT-4 T-lymphoblast cells in culture (Kazmers *et al.*, 1981) and showed dose-dependent inhibition of mouse spleen cell blastogenesis (Stoeckler *et al.*, 1980a), the results with human erythrocytes and mouse tumor cell lines (Stoeckler *et al.*, 1982) indicate that a more potent inhibitor of PNP is needed to achieve good *in vivo* inhibition.

ACKNOWLEDGMENTS

This work was supported by a grant from the American Cancer Society, ACS CH-7V, and is a publication from the Roger Williams Cancer Center, USPHS grants CA 13943 and 20892. We thank Lorraine DeFusco and Joyce Rose for typing the manuscript.

REFERENCES

Agarwal, R. P., and Parks, R. E., Jr. 1971. Purine nucleoside phosphorylase from human erythrocytes. V. Content and behavior of sulfhydryl groups. *J. Biol. Chem., 246:*3763–3768.

Agarwal, K. C., Agarwal, R. P., Stoeckler, J. D., and Parks, R. E., Jr. 1975. Purine nucleoside phosphorylase. Microheterogeneity and comparison of kinetic behavior of the enzyme from several tissues and species. *Biochemistry, 14:*79–84.

Ammann, A. J. 1978. Immunological aberrations in purine nucleoside deficiencies. *Ciba Found. Symp., 68:*55–75.

Carson, D. A., Kaye, J., and Seegmiller, J. E. 1977. Lymphospecific toxicity in adenosine deaminase deficiency and purine nucleoside phosphorylase deficiency: possible role of nucleoside kinase(s), *Proc. Natl. Acad. Sci. USA, 74:*5677–5681.

Chan, T. 1978. Deoxyguanosine toxicity on lymphoid cells as a cause for immunosuppression in purine nucleoside phosphorylase deficiency. *Cell, 14:*523–530.

Cohen, A., and Sussman, M. 1975. Guanosine metabolism and regulation of fruiting body construction in *Dictyostelium discoideum. Proc. Natl. Acad. Sci. USA, 72:*4479–4482.

Cowan, M. J., Cashman, D., and Ammann, A. J. 1981. Effects of formycin B on human lymphocyte deoxyribonucleic acid synthesis. *Biochem. Pharmacol., 30:*2651–2656.

Crabtree, G. W., and Henderson, J. F. 1971. Rate-limiting steps in the interconversion of purine ribonucleotides in Ehrlich ascites tumor cells *in vitro. Cancer Res., 31:*985–991.

Crabtree, G. W., Agarwal, R. P., Parks, R. E., Jr., Lewis, A. F., Wotring, L. L., and Townsend, L. B. 1979. N-Methylformycins. Reactivity with adenosine deaminase, incorporation into intracellular nucleotides of human erythrocytes and L1210 cells and cytotoxicity in L1210 cells. *Biochem. Pharmacol., 28:*1491–1500.

Edwards, Y. H., Hopkinson, D. A., and Harris, H. 1971. Inherited variants of human nucleoside phosphorylase. *Ann. Hum. Genet. Lond., 34:*395–408.

Fox, I. H., Andres, C. M., Gelfand, E. W., and Biggar, D. 1977. Purine nucleoside phosphorylase deficiency: Altered kinetic properties of a mutant enzyme. *Science, 197:*1084–1086.

Gelfand, E. W., Dosch, H.-M., Biggar, W. D., and Fox, I. H. 1978. Partial purine nucleoside phosphorylase deficiency. Studies of lymphocyte function. *J. Clin. Invest., 61:*1071–1080.

Giblett, E. R., Ammann, A. J., Wara, D. W., Sandman, R., and Diamond, L. K. 1975. Nucleoside-phosphorylase deficiency in a child with severely defective T-cell immunity and normal B-cell immunity. *Lancet 1:*1010–1015.

Gudas, L. J., Ullman, B., Cohen, A., and Martin, D. W., Jr. 1978. Deoxyguanosine toxicity in a mouse T lymphoma: Relationship to purine nucleoside phosphorylase-associated immune dysfunction. *Cell, 14:*531–538.

Hershfield, M. D. 1981. Proposed explanation for S-adenosylhomocysteine hydrolase deficiency in purine nucleoside phosphorylase and hypoxanthine-guanine phosphoribosyltransferase-deficient patients. *J. Clin. Invest., 67:*696–701.

Ito, K., Sakura, N., Usui, T., and Uchino, H. 1977. Screening for primary immunodeficiencies associated with purine nucleoside phosphorylase deficiency or adenosine deaminase deficiency. *J. Lab. Clin. Med., 90:*844–848.

Kalckar, H. M. 1947. Differential spectrophotometry of purine compounds by means of specific enzymes I. Determination of hydroxypurines. *J. Biol. Chem., 167:*429–443.

Kazmers, I. S., Mitchell, B. S., Dadonna, P. E., Wotring, L. L., Townsend, L. B., and Kelley, W. N. 1981. Inhibition of purine nucleoside phosphorylase by 8-aminoguanosine: Selective toxicity for T lymphoblasts. *Science, 214:*1137–1139.

Kim, B. K., Cha, S., and Parks, R. E., Jr. 1968. Purine nucleoside phosphorylase from human erythrocytes. II. Kinetic analysis and substrate-binding studies. *J. Biol. Chem., 243:*1771–1776.

Lowry, O. H., and Lopez, J. A. 1946. The determination of inorganic phosphate in the presence of labile phosphate esters. *J. Biol. Chem., 162:*421–428.

Martin, D. W., Jr., and Gelfand, E. W. 1981. Biochemistry of diseases of immunodevelopment. *Ann. Rev. Biochem., 50:*845–877.

Milman, G. 1978. Chinese hamster purine nucleoside phosphorylase. *Methods Enzymol., 51:*538–543.

Moyer, T. P., and Fischer, A. G. 1976. Purification and characterization of a purine-nucleoside phosphorylase from bovine thyroid. *Arch. Biochem. Biophys., 174:*622–629.

Parks, R. E., Jr., and Agarwal, R. P. 1972. Purine nucleoside phosphorylase. In: *The Enzymes*, 3rd ed., Volume 7, pp. 483–514. Ed. by Boyer, P. D. Academic Press, New York.

Parks, R. E., Jr., Stoeckler, J. D., Cambor, C., Savarese, T. M., Crabtree, G. W., and Chu, S.-H. 1981. Purine nucleoside phosphorylase and 5′-methylthioadenosine phosphorylase: targets of chemotherapy. In: *Molecular Actions and Targets for Cancer Chemotherapeutic Agents*, pp. 229–252. Ed. by Sartorelli, A., Lazo, J. S., and Bertino, J. R. Academic Press, New York.

Ross, A. F., Agarwal, K. C., Chu, S.-H., and Parks, R. E., Jr. 1973. Studies on the biochemical actions of 6-selenoguanine and 6-selenoguanosine. *Biochem. Pharmacol., 22:*141–154.

Sheen, M. R., Kim, B. K., and Parks, R. E., Jr. 1968. Purine nucleoside phosphorylase. III. Inhibition by the inosine analog formycin B of the isolated enzyme and of nucleoside metabolism in intact erythrocytes and Sarcoma 180 cells. *Mol. Pharmacol., 4:*293–299.

Simmonds, H. A., Watson, A. R., Webster, D. R., Sahota, A., and Perrett, D. 1982. GTP depletion and other erythrocyte abnormalities in inherited PNP deficiency. *Biochem. Pharmacol., 31:*941–946.

Smith, C. M., and Henderson, J. F. 1982. Deoxyadenosine triphosphate accumulation in erythrocytes of deoxycoformycin-treated mice. *Biochem. Pharmacol., 31:*1545–1551.

Stoeckler, J. D. 1984. Purine nucleoside phosphorylase: A target for chemotherapy. In: *Developments in Cancer Chemotherapy*, pp. 35–60. Ed. by Glazer, R. I. CRC Press, Boca Raton.

Stoeckler, J. D., Agarwal, R. P., Agarwal, K. C., and Parks, R. E., Jr. 1978. Purine nucleoside phosphorylase from human erythrocytes. In: *Methods Enzymol., 51:*530–538.

Stoeckler, J. D., Cambor, C., Burgess, F. W., Erban, S. B., and Parks, R. E., Jr. 1980a. Purine nucleoside phosphorylase inhibitors as potential chemotherapeutic and immunosuppressive agents. *Pharmacologist, 22:*99.

Stoeckler, J. D., Cambor, C., and Parks, R. E., Jr. 1980b. Human erythrocytic purine nucleoside phosphorylase: Reaction with sugar-modified nucleoside substrates. *Biochemistry, 19:*107.

Stoeckler, J. D., Cambor, C., Kuhns, V., Chu, S.-H., and Parks, R. E., Jr. 1982. Inhibitors of purine nucleoside phosphorylase. C(8) and C(5′) substitutions. *Biochem. Pharmacol., 31:*163–171.

Tax, W. J. M., and Veerkamp, J. H. 1978. Activity of adenosine deaminase and purine nucleoside phosphorylase in erythrocytes and lymphocytes of man, horse and cattle. *Comp. Biochem. Physiol., 61B:*439–441.

Uitendaal, M. P., deBruyn, C. H. M., Oei, T. L., Hösli, P., and Griscelli, C. 1978. A new ultramicrochemical assay for purine nucleoside phosphorylase. *Anal. Biochem., 84:*147–153.

Ullman, B., Gudas, L. J., Clift, S. M., and Martin, D. W., Jr. 1979. Isolation and characterization of purine-nucleoside phosphorylase-deficient T-lymphoma cells and secondary mutants with altered ribonucleotide reductase: genetic model for immunodeficiency. *Proc. Natl. Acad. Sci. USA, 76:*1074–1078.

Van der Weyden, M. B., and Bailey, L. 1982. A micromethod for determining adenosine deaminase and purine nucleoside phosphorylase activity in cells from peripheral blood. *Clin. Chim. Acta., 82:*179–184.

Willis, R. C., Robins, R. K., and Seegmiller, J. E. 1980. An *in vivo* and *in vitro* evaluation of 1-β-D-ribofuranosyl-1,2,4-triazole-3-carboxamidine. *Mol. Pharmacol., 18:*287–295.

Zimmerman, T. P., Gersten, N. B., Ross, A. F., and Miech, R. P. 1971. Adenine as substrate for purine nucleoside phosphorylase. *Can. J. Biochem., 49:*1050–1054.

III

Adenosine Transport

Chapter 9

Measurement and Inhibition of Membrane Transport of Adenosine

Alan R. P. Paterson, Eric R. Harley, and Carol E. Cass

Cancer Research Group
McEachern Laboratory
University of Alberta
Edmonton, Alberta, Canada

I. INTRODUCTION

The effects of adenosine on a variety of physiological processes in cells and tissues have been widely interpreted in terms of regulatory roles for adenosine. These effects are mediated by the presence of adenosine (or certain related compounds) on extracellular adenosine receptors on the responsive cells. An understanding of such apparent regulatory actions of adenosine will require not only knowledge of the biochemical events linking receptor occupancy and the cellular response, but also an understanding of the source and delivery of adenosine molecules to receptors and of their clearance from the immediate vicinity of the receptors. Cellular utilization appears to be a principal means of clearing of extracellular adenosine from the vicinity of receptors. Because adenosine and other physiological nucleosides leave and enter cells mainly by way of nucleoside-specific transport* mechanisms, transport is a primary step both in the formation and in the disposition of extracellular adenosine. This chapter is concerned with the measurement of adenosine transport in cell suspensions and with the potent inhibition of this process by several agents. Because of the emphasis of this volume on methodology, the material presented is selective rather than comprehensive.

* We define transport as the transporter-mediated passage of permeant molecules across the plasma membrane of cells. Transporters are permeant-specific, transmembrane polypeptide elements that catalyze the movement of particular molecular species into or out of cells.

II. GENERAL ASPECTS OF NUCLEOSIDE TRANSPORT

In many types of animal cells, movements of nucleoside molecules across the plasma membrane are transporter mediated (for reviews, see Plagemann and Wohlhueter, 1980; Paterson *et al.*, 1981a, 1983b). Cellular nucleoside transport mechanisms are recognizable by their catalysis of nucleoside fluxes many times larger than those attributable to simple diffusion. These fluxes are recognized as mediated by their concentration dependence and saturability, by competitive inhibition by related permeants, and by their ability to catalyze exchanges between intracellular and extracellular nucleoside molecules. These properties distinguish transporter-mediated fluxes from diffusional fluxes, which proceed at rates directly proportional to permeant concentrations and are not influenced by related permeants or inhibitors.

Nucleoside transport is a reversible, nonconcentrative process termed "facilitated diffusion." Nucleoside transport mechanisms exhibit low specificity with respect to the aglycone portion of their substrates in that a variety of pentofuranosides with (1) physiological purine and pyrimidine nucleobases and (2) variously substituted nucleobases and other heterocyclic structures in place of the latter are transported (Cass and Paterson, 1972; Cohen *et al.*, 1979; Paterson *et al.*, 1979; Sirotnak *et al.*, 1983). Adenosine and deoxyadenosine may be the "preferred" substrates for the nucleoside transporter of human erythrocytes and some types of cultured cells since a number of workers have reported K_m values for inward transport of adenosine (Taube and Berlin, 1972; Strauss *et al.*, 1976, 1977; Green, 1980; Harley *et al.*, 1982; Paterson *et al.*, 1984*) and deoxyadenosine (Paterson *et al.*, 1984) that are lower than those of the other physiological nucleosides (Paterson *et al.*, 1981a).

A number of potent inhibitors of nucleoside transport have been recognized and certain of these are proving to be valuable probes of transporter function and biology (Cass *et al.*, 1981; Paterson *et al.*, 1983a,b; Jarvis *et al.*, 1982, 1983; Young *et al.*, 1983). For example, members of two families, pentofuranosides of S^6-substituted 6-thiopurines and of N^6-substituted adenine derivatives (Paterson *et al.*, 1981a, 1983a,b), are potent inhibitors of nucleoside transport. Of these, the most extensively studied is NBMPR†, which binds tightly (K_D 0.1–1 n*M*) to plasma membrane sites, occupancy of which correlates with loss of transporter function (Cass *et al.*, 1974). Several members of these two inhibitor families compete with NBMPR at the high-affinity binding sites on cultured cells (Paterson *et al.*, 1983a). In addition, several vasoactive compounds (dipyridamole, dilazep, hexobendine, and lidoflazine), which are not nucleosides and are well known as inhibitors of adenosine transport, inhibit the transport of nucleosides and the site-specific binding of NBMPR (Van Belle, 1970; Pohl and Brock, 1974; Kolassa *et al.*, 1978; Lum *et al.*, 1979; Paterson *et al.*, 1980, 1984).

* Our values for the K_m of adenosine transport in several cell types, determined by two methods (see below), are consistently 4- to 5-fold lower than those reported by Plagemann and Wohlhueter (1980). These differences may have a methodological basis.

† NBMPR, 6[(4-nitrobenzyl)thio]-9-β-D-ribofuranosylpurine (nitrobenzylthioinosine).

III. NUCLEOSIDE TRANSPORT AND FLUXES

Cellular uptake of most nucleosides proceeds in two consecutive, separate steps, transport across the plasma membrane and intracellular metabolic transformation. The reversible transport step is rapid in many cell types and, under some conditions, may be faster than the subsequent metabolic transformations of the permeant. The latter state leads to complex time courses of nucleoside accumulation in cells (Heichal *et al.*, 1978b). In measurement of nucleoside transport rates, we and others have used the concept that, regardless of the complexity of the time course, the initial rate of a cellular uptake process is intrinsically a transport rate (Harley *et al.*, 1982). Because of the rapidity of nucleoside transport, it has been technically difficult, particularly in studies of adenosine permeation, to obtain time courses of cellular uptake that are definitive of initial rates.

A cell suspension is essentially a two-compartment system and rates of permeant movement (fluxes) between the compartments are most simply quantitated in terms of accumulation in an initially empty compartment, which may be the medium if an efflux process is to be followed, or the cellular compartment if influx is under study. "Empty" means the absence of permeant and, in the case of equilibrium exchange* experiments, the absence of isotopically labeled permeant from one compartment. Initial rates of movement of labeled permeant under such conditions are unidirectional fluxes.

IV. MEASUREMENT OF INFLUX

A. General

Inward fluxes of nucleosides in suspended cells may be measured from time courses of their accumulation. In cells that metabolize permeant, such time courses are complex because (1) the permeation step is reversible and may be faster under some conditions than subsequent metabolic steps, and (2) the metabolic fate of influent nucleoside molecules is usually complex, as is that of adenosine (Figure 1). Insight into the considerable influence of cellular anabolism of influent nucleoside molecules on the kinetics of their net accumulation in cells has come through the work of Heichal *et al.* (1978b), Koren *et al.* (1979), Wohlhueter *et al.* (1979), and of Wohlhueter and Plagemann (1980).

B. Nonmetabolized Permeants

Transport becomes the principal, if not the sole, determinant† of the time course of cellular nucleoside accumulation if the permeating species is not me-

* The transporter-mediated exchange between nucleoside molecules in the two compartments when their nucleoside concentrations are at equilibrium.

† Rates of diffusional entry of nucleosides into cells may be very low, as indicated by the protection of cells in culture by (1) NBMPR and (2) mutational impairment of transporter function against otherwise lethal concentrations of cytotoxic nucleosides in the culture medium (Cohen *et al.*, 1979; Paterson *et al.*, 1979; Cass *et al.*, 1981). Plagemann and Wohlheuter (1980) have commented on this issue.

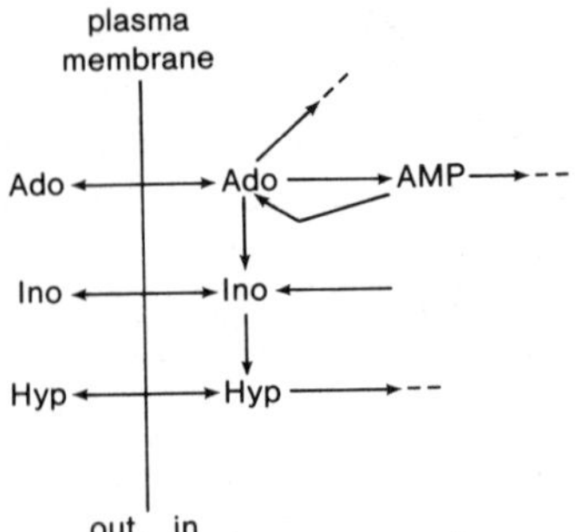

Figure 1. The metabolic fate of influent adenosine.

tabolized. This condition is realized naturally in the permeation of uridine and thymidine in human erythrocytes (Oliver and Paterson, 1971) and has been approached in kinetic studies of nucleoside permeation in ATP-depleted and kinase-deficient cells, circumstances in which anabolism of some permeating species is reduced or eliminated [for example, see Kessel and Shurin (1968) and Wohlhueter *et al.* (1979)]. Wohlhueter *et al.* (1979) have developed integrated rate equations based on the "simple carrier" model* of Lieb and Stein (1974) that describe the time course of cellular accumulation of nucleosides under conditions in which cellular metabolism of the nucleoside permeant is impaired. By fitting these equations to progress curves for cellular accumulation of adenosine, uridine and thymidine, kinetic constants for the transport process have been deduced (Plagemann *et al.*, 1978; Wohlhueter *et al.*, 1979; Lum *et al.*, 1979).

C. Metabolized Permeants

In cells that metabolize adenosine, initial rates of adenosine accumulation (which, by definition, are transport rates) change to steady state values that are the resultant of (1) rates of inward and outward transport and (2) rates of metabolic removal of intracellular adenosine from transport equilibria. Significant departures from initial rates may occur within a few seconds of influx initiation, particularly at permeant concentrations approaching those that saturate the transporter (Lum *et al.*, 1979).

Plagemann and Wohlhueter (1980) have reviewed the nucleoside transport literature prior to the advent of the rapid sampling technologies and have concluded that, in most of that early work, assays purporting to measure nucleoside transport failed to do so because intervals of permeant uptake were sufficiently long that the flux measurements obtained were influenced by cellular metabolism. However, current rapid sampling methods for the measurement of nucleoside accumulation in cells that metabolize the permeating species yield time courses

* "Simple" in this term means that the transporter protein (in loading or unloading conformation) interacts with only one molecule of permeant at a time. "Carrier" refers to a transporter protein which must exist in at least two conformations, each enabling interaction with permeant from one membrane face only (Lieb, 1982).

that are definitive of initial uptake rates for adenosine and other nucleosides. Plagemann and Wohlhueter (1980) cite examples demonstrating that nucleoside transport rates in cultured Novikoff hepatoma and leukemia P388 cells are similar whether or not the permeant is metabolized.

V. MEASUREMENT OF EFFLUX

Kinetic studies of the operation of the nucleoside transporter in the efflux direction have the limitation that intracellular concentrations of free nucleoside are ordinarily very small. The loading of cells with nucleosides in concentrations that enable study of outward fluxes requires that the intracellular permeant is not subject to enzymatic transformations. For example, because uridine and thymidine are not metabolized in human erythrocytes, substantial intracellular concentrations of these physiological nucleosides may be developed simply by allowing cells to equilibrate with permeant-containing medium. ATP depletion and use of kinase-deficient mutants have also been tactics employed to impair cellular metabolism of adenosine (Lum *et al.*, 1979) and of other physiological nucleosides (Plagemann *et al.*, 1978; Wohlhueter *et al.*, 1979) to allow intracellular concentrations of the latter to approach those of the loading medium. Moreover, certain nucleoside analogs are so poorly metabolized in some cell types that substantial intracellular concentrations may be developed (Kessel and Shurin, 1968; Kessel, 1978; Dahlig-Harley *et al.*, 1984). Kinetic characterization of outward fluxes of uridine and thymidine in nonmetabolizing experimental systems have been employed to test the conformity of transporter kinetic behavior with the predictions of the simple carrier model (Cabantchik and Ginsburg, 1977; Plagemann *et al.*, 1978; Wohlhueter *et al.*, 1979). The general conclusion is that uridine transport in nonmetabolizing cells conforms to the predictions of a simple carrier mechanism and is directionally symmetric in fresh human erythrocytes and several lines of cultured cells (Plagemann and Wohlhueter, 1980; Wohlhueter and Plagemann, 1982; Jarvis *et al.*, 1983) but is directionally asymmetric in stored erythrocytes (Cabantchik and Ginsburg, 1977).

The inhibition of nucleoside efflux by NBMPR and congeners, and by the transport-inhibiting vasodilators, has received scant attention. Cass and Paterson (1972) reported that HNBTGR* rapidly blocked equilibrium exchange diffusion of uridine in human erythrocytes measured in the efflux direction. Jarvis *et al.* (1982) demonstrated that in human erythrocytes, NBMPR was a competitive inhibitor of uridine influx, but a noncompetitive inhibitor of zero-*trans* uridine efflux, and concluded that NBMPR binds preferentially to the external membrane face of the erythrocyte.

* HNBTGR, 2-amino-6-[(2-hydroxy-5-nitrobenzyl)thio]-9-β-D-ribofuranosylpurine (hydroxynitrobenzylthioguanosine).

VI. INHIBITORS OF NUCLEOSIDE TRANSPORT AS "STOPPERS" IN FLUX ASSAYS

The tightly bound inhibitors of nucleoside transport, NBMPR and HNBTGR, have been employed as "stoppers" in studies of nucleoside permeation kinetics (for example, Cass and Paterson, 1972; Cabantchik and Ginsburg, 1977; Harley *et al.*, 1982). The "instantaneous" character of NBMPR inhibition of adenosine permeation in cultured L5178Y cells was demonstrated by comparing time courses of adenosine uptake in (1) cells exposed to medium containing both adenosine and NBMPR, and (2) cells exposed first to adenosine and then to NBMPR. These time courses intersected virtually at time zero, indicating that the blockade of adenosine permeation was "instantaneous."

Because nucleoside transport mechanisms are known to differ markedly in NBMPR sensitivity from one cell type to another (Belt, 1983; Paterson *et al.*, 1983a), it is apparent that the response of particular cells to inhibitors of this class must be evaluated before their use as transport stoppers.

Among the vasodilators recognized as inhibitors of adenosine transport (dipyridamole [Lum *et al.*, 1979], dilazep [Pohl and Brock, 1974], hexobendine [Kolassa *et al.*, 1978], and lidoflazine [Van Belle, 1970]), dipyridamole and dilazep have been employed as stopping agents in assays of nucleoside fluxes (Bowen *et al.*, 1979, Paterson *et al.*, 1984). The applicability to cell types other than S49 cells and human erythrocytes (Paterson *et al.*, 1984) of transport quenching by dilazep has not been reported.

VII. APPROACHES TO MEASUREMENT OF ADENOSINE TRANSPORT RATES

This discussion will address current experimental approaches to the measurement of cellular accumulation of adenosine during brief, carefully timed intervals. While the kinetics of uptake may also be studied by measuring changes in permeant concentration in the medium (Oliver and Paterson, 1971), this tactic is better employed in the measurement of efflux.

Much of the present methodology for measurement of cellular accumulation rates has developed with suspended cells and depends heavily upon modern fluid-dispensing technology and the fast starting microcentrifuges of the Eppendorf type. Short interval methods with cell monolayers, although intrinsically slower and less versatile than those employing suspended cells, increase the range of cell types in which adenosine transport may be studied. Only a few studies demonstrating inward transport of nucleosides in tissues have been reported (for example, Oliver, 1971; Kolassa and Paterson, 1982).

It is common practice in short-interval permeation experiments to employ replicate assay mixtures that differ only in experimental variables such as permeant concentration or uptake time. Timing is usually started by completion of assay mixtures (addition of permeant to replicate monolayer cultures or mixing of cell suspension with permeant solution). In measuring transport in suspended cells by the oil-layer centrifugation method assay mixtures are often assembled in plastic centrifuge tubes (often in the centrifuge) above a quantity of oil in the tube tip. Centrifuges (such as the Eppendorf model 5412) that achieve gravitational forces approaching 15,000*g* within a few seconds of starting are usually employed. In some procedures, incubation mixtures are completed by the simple addition of cells or permeant, while in others, cell suspension and permeant solutions are brought together in dispensing-mixing devices during addition to the centrifuge tube (Wohlhueter *et al.*, 1978; Chello *et al.*, 1983).

In the procedures discussed below, intervals of adenosine uptake are ended by (1) separation of cells from permeant (rinsing of monolayers, pelleting of suspended cells under oil), (2) cooling, (3) addition of transport inhibitor, or (4) combinations of these. While stopping method (3) is rapid, it should be appreciated that stopping with NBMPR and congeners is not of general applicability. The dilazep-quenched-flow procedure (see below) recently used to measure adenosine accumulation in S49 cells during decisecond intervals (Paterson *et al.*, 1983a,b, 1984) is a special case of method (3). The use of transport inhibitors as stoppers in uptake assays must be justified with each cell-permeant system. Although isotopic dilution (Strauss *et al.*, 1980) would probably stop cellular accumulation of isotopically labeled permeant molecules as rapidly as addition of transport inhibitors, transporter-mediated exchange of intracellular free nucleoside (isotopically labeled) with the extracellular nonisotopic diluent would probably occur. Stopping by isotopic dilution alone would not be a sound tactic with cells that do not metabolize the permeant, particularly in cells with a nucleoside transport system subject to *trans* acceleratory effects, such as human erythrocytes (Lieb, 1982). Combinations of stopping techniques have been employed, as in (1) rinsing of monolayers with cold, inhibitor-containing medium (Rozengurt *et al.*, 1978) and (2) rapid pelleting of cells under oil after blocking permeation with transport inhibitor (Harley *et al.*, 1982).

Although the starting and stopping procedures in the above assays are usually manual, considerable precision in timing may be achieved by performing these operations in response to counted signals from a metronome. In the quenched-flow procedure, timing of the interval of permeant uptake is an intrinsic characteristic of the system and, therefore, timing is precise.

VIII. MEASUREMENT OF ADENOSINE TRANSPORT RATES

In this section, we review briefly methods recently used (Table I) to measure adenosine accumulation in cells during short intervals and we comment on the application of these methods to the assay of adenosine transport rates.

A. Monolayers

Monolayers of cells on cover slips (Taube and Berlin, 1972), in culture dishes (Heichal *et al.*, 1978a), and in bottles (Paterson *et al.*, 1977) may be exposed to

Table I. Kinetic Studies of Adenosine Transport in Nucleated Cells

Cells	Assay of adenosine uptake rate		Kinetic constants	References
	Stopping method	Uptake interval		
Rabbit polymorphonuclear leukocytes (monolayers)	Cold rinse	45 sec, 37°	K_m, 10 μ*M* V_{max}, 0.22 pmoles/10^6 cells per sec	Taube and Berlin (1972)
Mouse splenic lymphocytes	Oil-layer pellet	20 sec, 37°	K_m, 12 μ*M*	Strauss *et al.* (1976)
P388 mouse leukemia[a]	Oil-layer pellet	2.8 sec, 24°	K_m, 176 ± 59 μ*M* V_{max}, 49 ± 8 pmoles/μl cell H_2O per sec	Lum *et al.* (1979)
ATP-depleted P388 mouse leukemia	Oil-layer pellet	Time course, 24°	K_m, 123 ± 8.9 μ*M* V_{max}, 29.2 ± 0.7 pmoles/μl cell H_2O per sec	Lum *et al.* (1979)
C1300 murine neuroblastoma[a]	Oil-layer pellet	10 sec, 22°	K_m, 24.3 ± 25 μ*M* V_{max}, 5.6 ± 0.4 pmoles/μl cell H_2O/sec	Green (1980)
L1210 mouse leukemia	Oil-layer pellet	Time course (5, 7.5, 10 sec), 25°	K_m, 13.4 ± 1.4 μ*M* V_{max}, 48.1 ± 5.2 nmoles/g dry weight per sec	Chello *et al.* (1983)
L5178Y mouse lymphoma[a]	NBMPR + oil-layer pellet	Time course, 22°	K_m, 21 ± 2^b μ*M* V_{max}, 18 ± 1^b pmoles/μl cell H_2O/sec	Harley *et al.* (1982)
L5178Y mouse lymphoma[a]	Dilazep, quenched flow, oil-layer pellet	Time course, 22°	K_m, 29 ± 4^b μ*M* V_{max}, 20.5 ± 1.4^b pmoles/μl cell H_2O/sec	Paterson *et al.* (1984)

[a] Cultured.
[b] ± S.E.

medium containing labeled permeant for brief intervals that are ended by flooding (dishes and bottles) or dipping (cover slips) the drained monolayers in cold medium. Minimum intervals of permeant uptake with these procedures are 5–10 sec. Uptake intervals may also be ended by flooding monolayers with medium containing inhibitors of nucleoside transport, as Rozengurt *et al.* (1978) have done with NBMPR. Dilazep (see below) might well be used for this purpose also. The inclusion of an appropriate transport inhibitor in rinsing media may reduce transporter-mediated loss of permeant during washing of monolayers. For assays of their isotopic content, the washed monolayers may be lysed in known volumes of detergent, sodium or potassium hydroxide, or protein solubilizer solutions.

B. Suspended Cells: Oil-Layer Centrifugation

In this procedure, transport assay mixtures are assembled above an oil layer in centrifuge tubes and intervals of labeled adenosine uptake are ended by starting the centrifuge. With cultured cells, the oils are usually silicone oil mixtures (Strauss *et al.*, 1976; Wohlhueter *et al.*, 1978) with specific gravities intermediate between those of the medium and the cells, which, under centrifugal force, pellet under the oil layer carrying only minor amounts of medium. Dibutyl phthalate has been used in oil-layer centrifugation of erythrocytes (Oliver and Paterson, 1971). Extracellular space in 15,000*g* cell pellets is usually estimated with isotopically labeled inulin or sucrose and represents 10–20% of the pellet water space. The latter parameter is measured as the ^{3}H content of the cell pellet acquired from ^3H_2O in the medium. The intracellular water space in cell pellets is calculated as the difference between the water content and the extracellular space of the cell pellet. An alternative means of correcting for the presence of extracellular medium in the pellet is that of Strauss *et al.* (1977, 1980) who, in kinetic studies of radiolabeled adenosine uptake, included assay mixtures in which high concentrations (10 m*M*) of nonisotopic adenosine rendered the mediated incorporation of radioisotope insignificant, yet operationally defined the permeant content of the extracellular compartment in cell pellets.

In the applications of simple oil-layer centrifugation procedures listed in Table I, the amounts of cell-associated adenosine at time zero can not be determined. The use of transport inhibitor-treated cells might possibly provide appropriate time zero ordinate values for the simple oil-layer centrifugation procedures, as in the inhibitor-stopped assay systems (below). Such time-zero values would include both nonspecific adsorption and binding of adenosine to cell receptors. The absence of experimental time-zero values in the procedures of Table I is a considerable disadvantage in the estimation of initial rates in a process as rapid as adenosine accumulation. As Lum *et al.* (1979) noted, time courses of adenosine uptake by P388 cells were appreciably curved at the earliest sampling time (2.8 sec) achieved in their oil-layer centrifugation procedure.

Advantages of the oil-layer centrifugation procedure are (1) the extracellular medium in the cell pellet is a highly consistent fraction, (2) tube walls above the oil layer are easily washed, and (3) cells are removed from the medium by about 2 sec after switch-on in the Eppendorf 5412 centrifuge (Wohlhueter *et al.*, 1978;

Strauss *et al.*, 1980; Harley *et al.*, 1982). The pelleting time is properly added to the nominal uptake interval (elapsed clock time at centrifuge switch-on).

In the oil-layer centrifugation procedures listed in Table I, fluxes were determined from the cellular accumulation of adenosine during the intervals listed. Some evidence was presented in most of the studies listed that time courses were approximately linear during these intervals, and data analysis by conventional methods yielded the kinetic constants listed (Table I). In the study by Chello *et al.* (1983), rates were estimated from the cellular uptake of adenosine during 5, 7.5, and 10 sec of exposure. Using replicate assay mixtures and a conventional oil-layer procedure for ending intervals of cellular uptake of [^{3}H]adenosine, Lum *et al.* (1979) (1) measured rates of adenosine transport by cultured P388 mouse leukemia cells from the cellular uptake during the first 2.8 sec of adenosine exposure and (2) determined time courses of adenosine accumulation by ATP-depleted P388 cells in the presence of deoxycoformycin, a potent inhibitor of adenosine deaminase. The adenosine fluxes measured in procedure (1) saturated as adenosine concentrations were increased, yielding the kinetic constants listed. Kinetic constants, extracted from the time course data of procedure (2) by fitting an integrated rate equation, agreed with those determined by procedure (1). While analysis of time course data for uridine and thymidine permeation in ATP-depleted cells has yielded kinetic constants that agree with those determined by conventional initial rate methods with ATP-replete cells (Plagemann and Wohlhueter, 1980), K_m values for adenosine transport in these and other experiments (Plagemann and Wohlhueter, 1980) are somewhat higher than contemporary values obtained by other methods (Table I and Table II). The reasons for this discrepancy are not apparent.

C. Suspended Cells: NBMPR as Stopper

Harley *et al.* (1982) demonstrated that the accumulation of adenosine and its metabolites by certain types of suspended cells was ended virtually instantaneously by the rapid addition of NBMPR-containing medium (final concentration 5–10 μM) to assay mixtures. In their method, cells were pelleted under oil immediately after addition of NBMPR to the assay mixtures. In the experiment cited in Table I, time courses of adenosine uptake by cells were obtained by allowing adenosine accumulation to proceed in replicate assay mixtures for graded intervals of 2 sec or more. Time courses were begun with time zero values for cell-associated adenosine that were obtained by simultaneous addition of NBMPR and adenosine, followed immediately by oil-layer centrifugation. The time courses yielded initial rates of adenosine uptake that were concentration dependent.

D. Suspended Cells: Dilazep Quenched-Flow Procedure

Two factors, (1) the rapidity of adenosine transport and (2) our complete dependence in determining transport rates on initial rates of accumulation in adenosine-metabolizing cells, have focussed attention on the technology of measuring adenosine uptake during short intervals. The virtually instant blockade of aden-

Table II. Kinetic Constants of Adenosine Influx at 22–24 and 37°C

Cells	Assay procedure			Kinetic constants[a]	
	Method	Stopping method	Temperature (°C)	K_m	V_{max}
S49 mouse lymphoma	Manual timing	Inhibitor[b] + oil-layer pellet	22–24	27 ± 15	8.4 ± 3.3 (7)[c]
	Quenched flow[c]	Dilazep + oil-layer pellet	37	103 ± 46	57 ± 15 (3)
Human erythrocytes[d]	Quenched flow	Dilazep + oil-layer pellet	22	25 ± 14	15 ± 5 (8)
	Quenched flow	Dilazep + oil-layer pellet	37	98 ± 17	80 ± 9 (3)
Walker 256 carcinosarcoma[e]	Manual timing	Isotope dilution[f] + oil-layer pellet	22–24	19.5 ± 38[g]	5.8 ± 0.5[g]
Novikoff hepatoma	Manual timing	Isotope dilution[f] + oil-layer pellet	22–24	35 ± 8	9.6 ± 0.1 (2)
P388 mouse leukemia[h]	Manual timing	NBMPR + oil-layer pellet	22–24	21 ± 3[g]	12 ± 1[g]

[a] Unless otherwise noted, values are expressed as the mean ± S.D. Where more than one experiment was conducted, the number of determinations is indicated in parentheses.
[b] Dilazep or NBMPR.
[c] Data are those of Figure 1.
[d] Data are from Paterson *et al.* (1984).
[e] Data are from Paterson *et al.* (1983a).
[f] Uptake reactions were quenched by addition of nonisotopic adenosine to a final concentration of 5 m*M*.
[g] Means ± S.E.
[h] Data are from Paterson *et al.* (1981b).

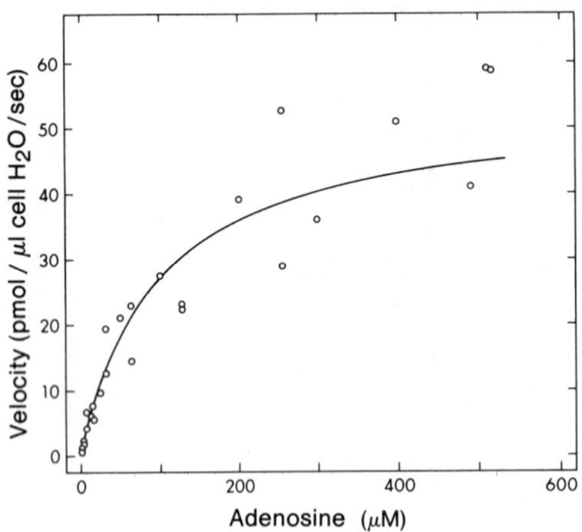

Figure 2. Use of the quenched-flow procedure in a kinetic study of adenosine transport at 37°C by cultured mouse lymphoma S49 cells. Rates of uptake of [2-^{3}H]adenosine were determined at 37°C using the quenched-flow procedure as described in Paterson *et al.* (1984). Logarithmically growing cells were harvested by centrifugation and resuspended in 37°C "transport" medium ($NaHCO_3$-free Fischer's medium with 20 m*M* HEPES, pH 7.4) at 1.1–2.2 × 10^7 cells/ml. Cell suspensions were used for transport assays within 20 min of preparation. Intervals of permeant uptake were initiated by the mixing of streams of cell suspensions and [2-^{3}H]adenosine-containing transport medium and were terminated by mixing with 1 m*M* cold dilazep. The quenched stream was sampled, after discarding the first 1.3 ml of effluent, by collecting 0.7 ml of effluent and pelleting cells from two 0.3-ml portions under oil. The ^{3}H content of the cell pellets was determined as described elsewhere (Harley *et al.*, 1982). Velocities were obtained by least square linear fits of time courses, and kinetic constants (presented in Table II) were obtained as described previously (Harley *et al.*, 1982). Data from three separate experiments are presented, each value representing a velocity calculated from a three-point time course (0.05, 0.3, and 0.5 sec; two determinations/point).

osine permeation in L5178Y cells by 333 μ*M* dilazep (Paterson *et al.*, 1984) has been applied to the quenching of adenosine permeation in a simple quenched-flow system, enabling (1) measurement of adenosine uptake during intervals between 0.05 and 0.5 sec and (2) construction of definitive, early time courses of uptake (Paterson *et al.*, 1984). The time courses had time zero intercepts that were independent of concentration and similar to those measured in Section C, reflecting an "adenosine space" greater than the "sucrose space".* The concentration dependence of initial rates measured from these time courses yielded kinetic constants (Table I) that were similar to those measured with the NBMPR stopping method (Section C). Use of the dilazep quenched-flow technology with other cell-permeant systems should be preceded by testing for effectiveness of permeation blockade.

The quenched-flow technique, which has been useful in following rapid biochemical reactions, has been adapted to the measurement of adenosine transport in cultured cells and erythrocytes through the use of dilazep as a quencher (Table II; Figure 2). A rapidly flowing stream of medium containing labeled adenosine was mixed with another stream containing cells to initiate an interval of adenosine uptake and the resulting cell-permeant mixture was then mixed with a third stream containing 333 μ*M* dilazep to terminate uptake. The length of the reaction line and the velocity of flow in that line determine the uptake interval, which, in the procedure of Paterson *et al.* (1984), was varied between 0.05 and 0.5 sec by

* In experiments with cultured cells and erythrocytes, values for the adenosine space have been 1.2 to 2.4 times the size of the sucrose space (mean ± S.D., 1.7 ± 0.4).

changing line lengths. Cells from the quenched mixture were immediately pelleted under oil for assay of adenosine content.

Time courses of adenosine uptake obtained by the quenched-flow procedure define initial rates of uptake. In the cases presented in Table II, assay intervals were sufficiently short that linear time courses were obtained, and curve-fitting procedures (other than linear least squares) were not required for calculation of initial rates. The kinetic constants for adenosine transport by cultured L5178Y mouse lymphoma cells at room temperature (22–24°C), measured by the quenched-flow procedure, agreed with those obtained by conventional methods with manual timing. The quenched-flow procedure has allowed measurement of adenosine transport at 37°C in cultured S49 lymphoma cells (Figure 1) and in human erythrocytes (Paterson *et al.*, 1984; data summarized in Table II). In both cell types, the K_m and V_{max} values for zero-*trans* influx were higher at 37°C than at room temperature.

IX. CONCLUSIONS

Current methods for measuring rates of inward transport of adenosine in adenosine-metabolizing cells depend upon determination of initial rates of cellular accumulation of the nucleoside. Time courses used to define initial rates of adenosine accumulation (or to establish that cellular uptake of adenosine during a specific interval measures initial rates) must be obtained at very early times (a few seconds) after flux initiation and, ideally, should begin with experimental time-zero values for cell-associated adenosine.

Several current methods allow measurement of adenosine uptake by suspended cells during brief, graded intervals and enable construction of time courses that define initial accumulation rates. These methods have particular limitations that require careful assessment of their applicability to one cell type or another. While the centrifugal pelleting of cells under oil layers has been widely used as a means of ending intervals of permeant uptake, the shortest first interval after initiation of influx will be almost 3 sec because of manipulation time plus that required for the pelleting process (about 2 sec). Depending upon cell type and conditions (particularly temperature), accumulation rates may not be constant during this interval. Stopping by oil-layer centrifugation and by isotope dilution would appear to be the principal means of ending uptake intervals in cells with inhibitor-insensitive nucleoside transporters.

With the use of nucleoside transport inhibitors such as NBMPR and dilazep to end intervals of adenosine accumulation, the initial intervals after influx initiation may be brief (e.g., 1 sec in manual procedures or 0.05 sec with quenched-flow procedures), and time-zero values may be determined. Inhibitor addition with immediate oil-layer centrifugation as a means of ending intervals of adenosine uptake is recommended. The use of NBMPR, dilazep, or other inhibitors as transport stoppers is not of general applicability, as the existence of NBMPR-insensitive nucleoside transport mechanisms in some cell types has demonstrated.

Demonstration of inhibitor effectiveness is an essential part of each application to an uptake assay.

The quenched-flow procedure might employ quenchers other than dilazep. The particular advantage of this procedure is that very brief, precise intervals of permeant uptake may be obtained. The need for substantial quantities of cells in quenched-flow assays will constrain use of this procedure to conditions that require decisecond intervals of permeant uptake to define initial rates of fast permeation processes.

Dilution with nonisotopic permeant has the same potential as the nucleoside transport inhibitors for rapid termination of uptake intervals and may be of value in measuring transport rates in cells with inhibitor-insensitive transporters, providing it can be shown that cellular efflux of the permeant is not significant under the assay conditions.

ACKNOWLEDGMENTS

A.R.P.P and C.E.C. are Research Associates of the National Cancer Institute of Canada.

REFERENCES

Belt, J. A. 1983. Heterogeneity of nucleoside transport in mammalian cells. Two types of transport activity in L1210 and other cultured neoplastic cells. *Mol. Pharmacol., 24:*479–484.

Bowen, D., Diasio, R. B., and Goldman, I. D. 1979. Distinguishing between membrane transport and intracellular metabolism of fluorodeoxyuridine in Ehrlich ascites cells by application of kinetic and high performance liquid chromatographic techniques. *J. Biol. Chem., 254:*5333–5339.

Cabantchik, Z. I., and Ginsburg, H. 1977. Transport of uridine in human red blood cells: Demonstration of a simple carrier mechanism. *J. Gen. Physiol., 69:*75–96.

Cass, C. E., and Paterson, A. R. P. 1972. Mediated transport of nucleosides in human erythrocytes: Accelerative exchange diffusion of uridine and thymidine and specificity toward pyrimidine nucleosides as permeants. *J. Biol. Chem., 247:*3314–3320.

Cass, C. E., Gaudette, L. A., and Paterson, A. R. P. 1974. Mediated transport of nucleosides in human erythrocytes. Specific binding of the inhibitor nitrobenzylthioinosine to nucleoside transport sites in the erythrocyte membrane. *Biochim. Biophys. Acta, 345:*1–10.

Cass, C. E., Kolassa, N., Uehara, Y., Dahlig-Harley, E. R., and Paterson, A. R. P. 1981. Absence of binding sites for the transport inhibitor nitrobenzylthioinosine on nucleoside transport-deficient mouse lymphoma cells. *Biochim. Biophys. Acta, 649:*769–777.

Chello, P. L., Sirotnak, F. M., Dorick, D. M., Yang, C.-H., and Montgomery, J. A. 1983. Initial rate kinetics and evidence for duality of mediated transport of adenosine, related purine nucleosides, and nucleoside analogues in L1210 cells. *Cancer Res., 43:*97–103.

Cohen, A., Ullman, B., and Martin, D. W., Jr. 1979. Characterization of a mutant mouse lymphoma cell with deficient transport of purine and pyrimidine nucleosides. *J. Biol. Chem., 254:*112–116.

Dahlig-Harley, E., Paterson, A. R. P., Robins, M. J., and Cass, C. E. 1984. Transport of uridine and 3-deazauridine in cultured human lymphoblastoid cells. *Cancer Res., 42:*161–165.

Green, R. D. 1980. Adenosine transport by a variant of C1300 murine neuroblastoma cells deficient in adenosine kinase. *Biochim. Biophys. Acta, 598:*366–374.

Harley, E. R., Paterson, A. R. P., and Cass, C. E. 1982. Initial rate kinetics of the transport of adenosine and 4-amino-7-(β-D-ribofuranosyl)pyrrolo[2,3-*d*]pyrimidine (tubercidin) in cultured cells. *Cancer Res., 42:*1289–1295.

Heichal, O., Bibi, O., Katz, J., and Cabantchik, Z. I. 1978a. Nucleoside transport in mammalian cell membranes. III. Kinetic and chemical modification studies of cytosine-arabinoside and uridine transport in hamster cells in culture. *J. Membr. Biol., 39:*133–157.

Heichal, O., Ish-Shalom, D., Koren, R., and Stein, W. D. 1978b. The kinetic dissection of transport from metabolic trapping during substrate uptake by intact cells. Uridine uptake by quiescent and serum-activated N1L8 hamster cells and their murine sarcoma virus-transformed counterparts. *Biochim. Biophys. Acta, 551:*169–186.

Jarvis, S. M., Hammond, J. R., Paterson, A. R. P., and Clanachan, A. S. 1982. Species differences in nucleoside transport: A study of uridine transport and nitrobenzylthioinosine binding by mammalian erythrocytes. *Biochem. J., 208:*2202–2208.

Jarvis, S. M., Hammond, J. R., Paterson, A. R. P., and Clanachan, A. S. 1983. Nucleoside transport in human erythrocytes: A simple carrier with directional symmetry in fresh cells, but with directional assymetry in cells from outdated blood. *Biochem. J., 210:*457–461.

Kessel, D. 1978. Transport of a nonphosphorylated nucleoside, 5′-deoxyadenosine, by murine leukemia L1210 cells. *J. Biol. Chem., 253:*400–403.

Kessel, D., and Shurin, S. B. 1968. Transport of two non-metabolized nucleosides, deoxycytidine and cytosine arabinoside, in a subline of the L1210 murine leukemia. *Biochim. Biophys. Acta, 163:*179–187.

Kolassa, N., and Paterson, A. R. P. 1982. Uptake of cytidine by isolated, perfused mouse liver. *Can. J. Physiol. Pharmacol., 60:*167–173.

Kolassa, N., Stengg, R., and Turnheim, K. 1978. Influence of hexobendine, dipyridamole, dilazep, lidoflazine, inosine and purine riboside on adenosine uptake by the isolated epithelium of guinea pig jejunum. *Pharmacology, 16:*54–60.

Koren, R., Shohami, E., and Yeroushalmi, S. 1979. A kinetic analysis of cytosine-β-D-arabinoside by rat B77 cells: Differentiation between transport and phosphorylation. *Eur. J. Biochem., 95:*333–339.

Lieb, W. R. 1982. A kinetic approach to transport studies, in *Red Cell Membranes—A Methodological Approach*, pp. 135–164. Ed. by Ellory, J. C., and Young, J. D. Academic Press, London.

Lieb, W. R., and Stein, W. D. 1974. Testing and characterizing the simple carrier. *Biochim. Biophys. Acta, 373:*178–196.

Lum, C. T., Marz, R., Plagemann, P. G. W., and Wohlhueter, R. M. 1979. Adenosine transport and metabolism in mouse leukemia cells and in canine thymocytes and peripheral blood leukocytes. *J. Cell. Physiol., 101:*173–200.

Oliver, J. M. 1971. The effects of oestradiol on nucleoside transport in rat uterus. *Biochem. J., 121:*83–88.

Oliver, J. M., and Paterson, A. R. P. 1971. Nucleoside transport: 1. A mediated process in human erythrocytes. *Can. J. Biochem., 49:*262–270.

Paterson, A. R. P., Babb, L. R., Paran, J. H., and Cass, C. E. 1977. Inhibition by nitrobenzylthioinosine of adenosine uptake by asynchronous HeLa cells. *Mol. Pharmacol., 13:*1147–1158.

Paterson, A. R. P., Yang, S., Lau, E. Y., and Cass, C. E. 1979. Low specificity of the nucleoside transport mechanism of RPMI 6410 cells. *Mol. Pharmacol., 16:*900–908.

Paterson, A. R. P., Lau, E. Y., Dahlig, E., Cass, C. E. 1980. A common basis for inhibition of nucleoside transport by dipyridamole and nitrobenylthioinosine? *Mol. Pharmacol., 18:*40–44.

Paterson, A. R. P., Kolassa, N., and Cass, C. E. 1981a. Transport of nucleoside drugs in animal cells. *Pharmacol. Ther., 12:*515–536.

Paterson, A. R. P., Kolassa, N., Lynch, T. P., Jakobs, E. S., and Cass, C. E. 1981b. Transport of nucleosides in animal cells. In: *Nucleosides and Cancer Treatment*, pp. 3–17. Ed. by Tattersall, M. H. N., and Fox, R. M. Academic Press, Sydney.

Paterson, A. R. P., Jakobs, E. S., Harley, E. R., Cass, C. E., and Robins, M. J. 1983a. Inhibitors of nucleoside transport as probes and drugs. In: *Development of Target-Oriented Anticancer Drugs*, pp. 4–56. Ed. by Cheng, Y.-C., Goz, B., and Minkoff, M. Raven Press, New York.

Paterson, A. R. P., Jakobs, E. S., Harley, E. R., Fu, N.-W., Robins, M. J., and Cass, C. E. 1983b. Inhibition of nucleoside transport. In: *Regulatory Function of Adenosine*, pp. 203-220. Ed. by Berne, R. M., Rall, T. W., and Rubio, R. Martinus Nijhoff, The Hague.

Paterson, A. R. P., Harley, E. R., and Cass, C. E. 1984. Inward fluxes of adenosine in erythrocytes and cultured cells measured by a quenched-flow method. *Biochem. J., 224:*1001–1008.

Plagemann, P. G. W., and Wohlhueter, R. M. 1980. Permeation of nucleosides, nucleic acid basis and nucleotides in animal cells. *Curr. Top. Membr. Transp., 14:*225–330.

Plagemann, P. G. W., Marz, R., and Wohlhueter, R. M. 1978. Uridine transport in Novikoff rat hepatoma cells and other cell lines and its relationship to uridine phosphorylation and phosphorolysis. *J. Cell. Physiol., 97:*49–72.

Pohl, J., and Brock, N. 1974. Vergleichende Untersuchungen zur Hemmung des Adenosinabbaus in vitro durch Dilazep. *Arzneim Forsch., 24:*1901–1905.

Rozengurt, E., Mierzejewski, K., and Wigglesworth, N. M. 1978. Uridine transport and phosphorylation in mouse cells in culture: Effect of growth-promoting factors, cell cycle transits and oncogenic transformation. *J. Cell Physiology, 97:*241–252.

Sirotnak, F. M., Chello, P. L., Dorick, D. M., and Montgomery, J. A. 1983. Specificity of systems mediating transport of adenosine, 9-β-D-arabinofuranosyl-2-fluoroadenine, and other purine nucleoside analogues in L1210 cells. *Cancer Res., 43:*104–109.

Strauss, P. R., Sheehan, J. M., and Kashket, E. R. 1976. Membrane transport by murine lymphocytes. *J. Exp. Med., 144:*1009–1021.

Strauss, P. R., Sheehan, J. M., and Kashket, E. R. 1977. Membrane transport by murine lymphocytes. II. The appearance of thymidine transport in cells from concanavalin A-stimulated mice. *J. Immunol., 118:*1328–1334.

Strauss, P. R., Sheehan, J. M., and Taylor, J. 1980. Plasma membrane mediated thymidine transport in AKR spleen cells. *Can. J. Biochem., 58:*1405–1413.

Taube, R. A., and Berlin, R. D. 1972. Membrane transport of nucleosides in rabbit polymorphonuclear leukocytes. *Biochim. Biophys. Acta, 225:*6–18.

Van Belle, H. 1970. The disappearance of adenosine in blood. Effect of lidoflazine and other drugs. *Eur. J. Pharmacol., 11:*241–248.

Wohlhueter, R. M., and Plagemann, P. G. W. 1980. The roles of transport and phosphorylation in nutrient uptake in cultured animal cells. *Int. Rev. Cytol., 64:*171–240.

Wohlhueter, R. M., and Plagemann, P. G. W. 1982. On the functional symmetry of nucleoside transport in mammalian cells. *Biochim. Biophys. Acta, 689:*249–260.

Wohlhueter, R. M., Marz, R., Graff, J. C., and Plagemann, P. G. W. 1978. A rapid-mixing technique to measure transport in suspended animal cells: Applications to nucleoside transport in Novikoff hepatoma cells. *Methods Cell Biol., 20:*211–236.

Wohlhueter, R. M., Marz, R., and Plagemann, P. G. W. 1979. Thymidine transport in cultured mammalian cells: Kinetic analysis, temperature dependence and specificity of the transport system. *Biochim. Biophys. Acta, 553:*261–268.

Young, J. D., Jarvis, S. M., Robins, M. J., and Paterson, A. R. P. 1983. Photoaffinity labeling of the human erythrocyte nucleoside transporter by N^6-(p-azidobenzyl)adenosine and nitrobenzylthioinosine. *J. Biol. Chem., 258:*2202–2208.

Chapter **10**

The Use of Ligands in the Study of the Nucleoside-Transport Complex

Nitrobenzylthioinosine

James D. Young and Simon M. Jarvis*

Department of Biochemistry, Faculty of Medicine
The Chinese University of Hong Kong
Shatin, N.T., Hong Kong
and *Department of Physiology, University of Alberta
Edmonton, Alberta, Canada

I. INTRODUCTION

Permeation of physiological and cytotoxic nucleosides across the plasma membrane of animal cells is mediated largely by nucleoside-specific transporters sensitive to inhibition by nanomolar concentrations of nitrobenzylthioinosine (NBMPR) and related 6-thiopurine ribonucleosides. Transport inhibition by NBMPR results from reversible high-affinity binding of ligand to cell membranes, an association that represents a specific interaction with functional nucleoside transport proteins. The commercial availability of high-specific activity [^{3}H]-NBMPR within the last few years has led to significant advances in our knowledge of the kinetic and molecular properties of this carrier system. In the present chapter we detail and discuss the methodologies associated with the use of this ligand.

We first briefly review what is known about the nucleoside transporter and its inhibition by NBMPR. A generally applicable method for the measurement of *reversible* high-affinity binding of NBMPR to membrane preparations using glass-fiber filters is then presented together with representative results for NBMPR binding to a crude membrane preparation from guinea pig cardiac muscle. Other methods available for the measurement of NBMPR binding activity are also discussed. We also describe how NBMPR can be used a *covalent* photoaffinity probe of the nucleoside transporter. In this case we illustrate the technique using human erythrocyte "ghosts" and purified plasma membranes from guinea pig liver. Finally, we discuss future prospects for the use of NBMPR and related inhibitors of nucleoside transport.

II. NUCLEOSIDE TRANSPORT IN ANIMAL CELLS

Before considering the methodologies involved in using ligands to study the nucleoside transporter, we briefly outline the chemical, kinetic, and molecular properties of the transport system and its interaction with NBMPR. For more comprehensive reviews of nucleoside transport in animal cells, readers should refer to recent articles by Plagemann and Wohlhueter, (1980), Paterson *et al.* (1981), and Young and Jarvis (1983).

A. Properties of the Nucleoside Transporter

Most mammalian erythrocytes and a variety of other cell types possess a common broad-specificity transport system for both purine and pyrimidine nucleosides (apparent K_m for influx 25–2000 μM) (for references see Plagemann and Wohlhueter, 1980; Paterson *et al.*, 1981; Young and Jarvis, 1983). Transport is by a nonconcentrative facilitated diffusion process, the properties of which are consistent with a simple carrier mechanism (Cabantchik and Ginsburg, 1977; Wohlhueter *et al.*, 1979; Harley *et al.*, 1982; Wohlhueter and Plagemann, 1982; Jarvis *et al.*, 1983a). Interestingly, the carrier is asymmetric in cells from outdated stored blood (Jarvis *et al.*, 1983a). A comparison of the effects of thiol reagents and trypsin on nucleoside transport activity in intact erythrocytes and disrupted membranes has provided evidence that the erythrocyte nucleoside transporter exhibits chemical asymmetry (Jarvis and Young, 1982a). Transport activity in other cell types is also inhibited by some organomercurials (Eilam and Cabantchik, 1977; Dahlig-Harley *et al.*, 1981).

The development of NBMPR as a specific probe for the nucleoside transporter (see Section IIB) has been exploited to explore the molecular properties of the transport system. Detergent extraction of human erythrocyte membranes in combination with DEAE-cellulose ion-exchange chromatography results in substantial purification of NBMPR binding activity (Jarvis and Young, 1981). This preparation contains only two detectable protein bands, band 4.5 and a trace of band 7 (nomenclature of Steck, 1974), and is capable of catalyzing NBMPR-sensitive uridine transport when reconstituted into phospholipid vesicles (Belt *et al.*, 1984). Studies aimed at covalently labeling the NBMPR binding site of the human erythrocyte carrier using either a photoaffinity analogue of NBMPR, $[^3H]N^6$-(*p*-azidobenzyl) adenosine (ABA), or $[^3H]$-NBMPR itself following exposure to UV light, have resulted in selective incorporation of radioactivity into band 4.5 polypeptides (Young *et al.*, 1983; Jarvis *et al.*, 1983b; Wu *et al.*, 1983a,b). No incorporation occurs in membranes prepared from nucleoside-impermeable sheep

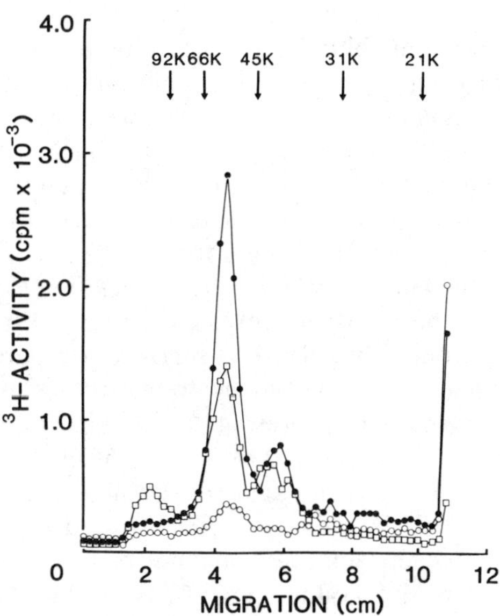

Figure 1. Photoaffinity labeling of nucleoside transport proteins in membranes isolated from human erythrocytes and guina pig liver. Purified plasma membranes from guinea pig liver were prepared from a crude P_2 membrane fraction by centrifugation (10,000*g* for 15 min) in a self-generating Percoll density gradient (17.5% [v/v] Percoll, starting density 1.05) using a fixed-angle rotor. The plasma membrane fraction that formed a band just below the surface of the gradient was collected and washed twice in 50 m*M* Tris-Hcl, pH 7.4. Human erythrocyte "ghosts" were prepared as described previously (see, e.g., Jarvis and Young, 1981). Photolysis with [^{3}H]-NBMPR in the presence and absence of NBTGR was performed as described in the text. Liver membranes (0.75 mg protein) in the presence (○) and absence (●) of NBTGR. Erythrocyte membranes (0.3 mg protein) in the absence of NBTGR (□). Data points for photolysis of erythrocyte membranes in the presence of NBTGR essentially coplotted with the liver NBTGR results and are not shown. Molecular weight standards (Bio-Rad) are from the same slab gel (J. S. Wu and J. D. Young, unpublished data).

erythrocytes and covalent attachment of [^{3}H]-NBMPR is blocked by transported nucleosides and by nitrobenzylthioguanosine (NBTGR) and dipyridamole (Jarvis *et al.*, 1983b; Wu *et al.*, 1983b). These experiments strongly implicate bank 4.5 membrane proteins(s) (apparent molecular weight 45,000–65,000) in erythrocyte nucleoside permeation. In the native membrane, the size of the functional transporter, determined by radiation inactivation analysis of reversible NBMPR binding activity and uridine transport, was estimated to be 120,000 (Jarvis *et al.*, 1980, 1983c), suggesting that the transporter may exist in the membrane as a dimer. Initial experiments suggest that the nucleoside transporters from rat and guinea pig lung and liver, guinea pig cardiac muscle and brain, and mouse S49 lymphoma cells have similar molecular weights on SDS–polyacrylamide gels to that of the erythrocyte system (see Figure 1).

B. Nitrobenzylthioinosine: A Specific Probe of the Nucleoside Transporter

The best characterized and most useful ligand in the study of the nucleoside-transport complex to date has been the *S*-substituted 6-thiopurine ribonucleoside, NBMPR. NBMPR is a potent inhibitor of nucleoside transport in many cell types and inhibition is associated with tight, but reversible, high-affinity binding of inhibitor to functional specific sites on the cell membrane (apparent K_d 0.1–1.0 n*M*) (Cass *et al.*, 1974, 1981; Jarvis and Young, 1980, 1982a; Jarvis *et al.*, 1982a,b). Transported nucleosides are competitive inhibitors of high-affinity NBMPR binding with apparent K_i values similar to the apparent K_m values for equilibrium exchange transport (Cass and Paterson, 1976; Jarvis *et al.*, 1982a, 1983d). Kinetic studies with erythrocytes have demonstrated that NBMPR is an apparent competitive inhibitor of uridine influx and uridine equilibrium exchange efflux but an apparent noncompetitive inhibitor of uridine efflux (Eilam and Cabantchik, 1977; Jarvis *et al.*, 1982a). Recently, we have proposed that much of the above evidence favors the simple view that the erythrocyte NBMPR binding site is identical to the nucleoside permeation site of the carrier and that the NBMPR binding site is largely located on the outer surface of the erythrocyte cell membrane (Jarvis and Young, 1982a). Results from the effects of nucleoside substrates and inhibitors on the kinetics of NBMPR dissociation from the erythrocyte carrier are consistent with the above model (Jarvis *et al.*, 1983d). We cannot, however, exclude the possibility that NBMPR binds to a separate allosteric inhibitor site.

The inference from the above studies that high-affinity NBMPR binding activity in membranes represents a specific interaction with functional nucleoside transporters is supported by studies of nucleoside transporter variants. For example, AE_1 mouse lymphoma cells, a nucleoside transport deficient clone derived from S49 cells (Cohen *et al.*, 1979), and erythrocytes from nucleoside-impermeable type sheep lack functional nucleoside transport systems and do not bind inhibitor (Jarvis and Young, 1980; Cass *et al.*, 1981). In contrast to erythrocytes and S49 lymphoma cells, NBMPR inhibition of nucleoside transport by many cultured cells appears to be complex (for examples see Slaughter *et al.*, 1981; Eilam and Cabantchik, 1977; Wohlhueter *et al.*, 1978; Paterson *et al.*, 1980). It has been shown that some lines of cultured cells possess to a varying degree nucleoside transporters with a low sensitivity to NBMPR (IC_{50} 1–10 μM) (Slaughter *et al.*, 1981; Wohlhueter *et al.*, 1978; Belt, 1983). The mechanism of this low sensitivity remains to be determined.

III. EXPERIMENTAL

A. Reversible Nitrobenzylthioinosine Binding: Filtration

In this section we describe the method used to study the reversible binding of NBMPR to a crude membrane preparation from guinea pig cardiac muscle. In typical experiments, membrane preparations are incubated simultaneously in buffer with labeled and unlabeled NBMPR for a time sufficient to reach a steady-state of binding. The membrane-bound [^{3}H]-NBMPR is then separated from the free inhibitor in the medium by filtration, a rapid and simple procedure that can be used with membrane preparations from a wide range of cell types and tissues.

Equilibrium binding assays (final volume 1 ml) are initiated by adding membrane suspensions (0.2 mg protein in 50 mM Tris-HCl buffer, pH 7.4) to medium containing graded concentrations of [^{3}H]-NBMPR (0.05–5.0 nM) in the presence and absence of excess nonradioactive NBMPR (or nitrobenzylthioguanosine (NBTGR) (10 μM–added from a 10 mM stock solution stored in dimethylsulfoxide at −20°C). When inhibitors of binding activity are to be evaluated, incubation mixtures also contain test compounds. Nonradioactive NBMPR is available from both Aldrich Chemical Co., WI 53201, USA and Calbiochem-Behring, San Diego, CA 92112, USA. [G-^{3}H]NBMPR (specific radioactivity ~16 Ci/mmole) can be

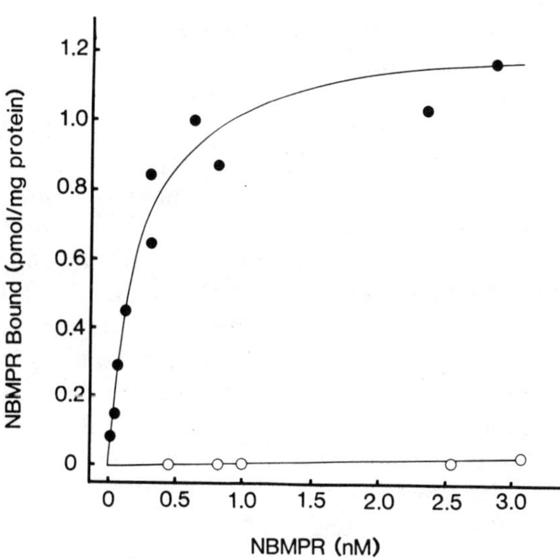

Figure 2. Binding of [^{3}H]nitrobenzylthioinosine to guinea pig cardiac membranes. Atrial and ventricular tissue was homogenized in ice-cold isotonic sucrose (Polytron, 20 sec at setting 5), centrifuged at 1000*g* for 10 min, and the supernatant recentrifuged at 20,000*g* for 20 min to obtain a crude membrane pellet (P_2) which was resuspended in 50 m*M* Tris-HCl, pH 7.4. [^{3}H]-NBMPR binding to this membrane fraction in the presence (○) and absence of NBTGR (●) was measured as described in the text. Values are means of duplicate estimates (K. F. Kwan and S. M. Jarvis, unpublished data).

purchased from Moravek Biochemicals, Brea, CA 92621, USA. Incubations (30 min at room temperature) are terminated by filtering 0.95 ml aliquots through glass fiber filters (Whatman GF/C, which are washed with ice-cold buffer before sample filtration) under suction. The filters are washed twice with 5 ml aliquots of ice-cold buffer. It is essential that ice-cold buffer is used to ensure that bound counts are not lost during washing. The entire procedure is completed within 10 sec. Control experiments have established that free [^{3}H]-NBMPR does not bind to glass fiber filters. The filters are dried and counted for radioactivity with 10 ml of scintillation fluid. This represents the bound radioactivity. Free radioactivity is found by subtracting bound from total. Total radioactivity is usually measured by counting the radioactivity contained in suitably sized aliquots of the [^{3}H]-NBMPR solutions. Care must be taken to ensure that the degree of quenching for both the bound and total radioactive samples is either the same or normalized by using quench correction techniques.

The binding of [^{3}H]-NBMPR to guinea pig cardiac membranes in this filtration technique is shown in Figure 2, where membrane-associated binding is plotted against the equilibrium free concentration of the inhibitor. Binding in the absence of NBTGR can be resolved into two components: (1) a saturable association responsible for the binding of 1.23 pmoles/mg protein with an apparent K_d of 0.23 n*M* and (2) a nonsaturable component responsible for the binding of 0.019 pmoles/mg protein at 1 n*M*. The saturable component of binding is abolished in the presence of NBTGR and the difference in binding in the presence and absence of NBTGR is defined as specific binding.

In addition to the wide application of the filtration methodology to the study of equilibrium binding of [^{3}H]-NBMPR to membrane preparations from various sources, the technique can also be applied to investigations of the kinetics of [^{3}H]-NBMPR binding (see, e.g., Jarvis *et al.*, 1983d). The technique has the distinct advantage of permitting the rapid termination of the reaction, a necessary prerequisite for kinetic studies. A disadvantage of filtration techniques is the inability to measure directly the concentrations of unbound ligand. Although it is possible to collect the free radioactivity not bound to the filter, this activity is diluted due to the washing steps. Measurement of the free radioactivity is especially important under circumstances of severe inhibitor depletion, which are most likely to occur at low inhibitor concentrations. A technique that overcomes this difficulty is to separate bound from free inhibitor by centrifugation to yield a cell or membrane-free supernatant and a pellet containing both bound and free ligand. Aliquots of the supernatant can be retained to determine the free radioactivity. Unbound inhibitor in the pellet can be estimated using an appropriate space markers (e.g., inulin) or be removed be repeated washings with ice-cold medium. Control experiments with [^{3}H]-NBMPR have established that no significant binding activity is lost during washing (Jarvis and Young, 1980). However, binding of other ligands may be reversible at 0°C and therefore control experiments must be carried out to ensure that bound counts are not lost during washing. [^{3}H]-NBMPR bound to cultured intact cells has been separated from free inhibitor by centrifugation (Eppendorf microcentrifuge 5412 or equivalent for 30 sec) of the cell suspension through a silicone oil-paraffin oil solution (specific gravity 1.03 g/ml) contained in 1.5 ml polypropylene microcentrifuge tubes (Cass *et al.*, 1981).

A disadvantage of standard centrifugation techniques is the possible loss of membrane material due to incomplete sedimentation, a problem also encountered with filtration of small membrane fragments. This difficulty can be overcome by using a higher gravitational force, such as that achievable with the Beckman Airfuge, which can reach speeds of up to 95,000 rpm within 60 sec. Such forces (150,000*g*) should be capable of sedimenting membrane vesicles, e.g., protein preparations reconstituted into phospholipid liposomes, that do not sediment or bind to filters under normal circumstances. An alternative technique for measuring ligand binding that alleviates the above difficulty is equilibrium dialysis (see, e.g., Jarvis and Young, 1981). This technique has the added advantage that it can be used to measure binding to solubilized fractions. However, the long times (15–20 hr) employed for equilibration in this procedure have the intrinsic disadvantage that denaturation of binding activity may occur during the equilibration. For specific details on how to measure NBMPR binding using centrifugation and equilibrium dialysis methods, readers are referred to a recent article by the authors (Jarvis and Young, 1982b).

B. Covalent Radiolabeling of the Nucleoside Transporter

Binding of NBMPR to the transporter is normally fully reversible. In this section we describe the use of NBMPR as a *covalent* photoaffinity probe of the nucleoside transporter. The procedure of exposing site-bound [^{3}H]-NBMPR to high-intensity UV light under equilibrium binding conditions in the presence of dithiothreitol as a free-radical scavenger was orginally developed using human erythrocyte "ghosts" (Jarvis *et al.*, 1983b; Wu *et al.*, 1983a,b; Young *et al.*, 1983) but can, as shown below, be readily adapted to membranes prepared from other sources. Highly purified membrane fractions are not essential for these experiments.

Freshly prepared human erythrocyte "ghosts" and plasma membranes from guinea pig liver in 50 mM Tris-HCl, pH 7.4 (~2 mg protein per milliliter) are equilibrated at room temperature for 30 min with a saturating concentration of [^{3}H]-NBMPR (final concentration, 50 n*M*) in the presence and absence of 20 μ*M* NBTGR as competing ligand. Membrane suspensions are then cooled to 4°C and supplemented with 50 m*M* dithiothreitol (final concentration). Photolysis is carried out in conventional 3-ml silica spectrophotometer cuvettes (10 mm light path) with continuous stirring at 4°C. Samples are exposed to high-intensity UV light at a distance of 6.5 cm from a 450-watt mercury arc lamp (Conrad-Hanovia Inc., Newark, New Jersey, USA) for 45 sec (for erythrocyte membranes the optimal exposure time is between 30 and 120 sec). Samples are then diluted 10-fold with buffer containing 10 μ*M* NBTGR and allowed to stand at room temperature for 10 min before recovery of the membrane fraction by centrifugation. The membrane pellets are washed twice more with NBTGR-containing buffer and dissolved in gel electrophoresis buffer at room temperature (see below). If necessary, insoluble material can be removed by centrifugation before application of the sample to the gel. The solubilized membranes are relatively stable at this stage and can be stored at −70°C for several days.

In our laboratories, SDS–polyacrylamide gel electrophoresis is carried out in 1- or 1.5-mm-thick slab gels by the method of Thompson and Maddy (1982) using the Laemmli buffer system (Laemmli, 1970). Bio-Rad Laboratories, Richmond, CA 94804, USA and Raven Scientific Ltd., Haverhill, Suffolk, UK manufacture suitable slab-gel electrophoresis equipment. Samples in the gel sample buffer are not heated before application to the gel in order to avoid protein aggregation (Wu *et al.*, 1983b). Radioactivity in the various regions of the gel is determined by slicing the gel into 2-mm fractions using a Bio-Rad gel slicer. The ^{3}H content of these slices is measured by liquid scintillation counting in toluene containing 0.4% (w/v) Omnifluor and 3% (v/v) Protosol (New England Nuclear). Vials are allowed to stand at 37°C for 36 hr before counting. Recoveries of applied radioactivity are typically in the range 75–80%, provided that the gel slices are given sufficient time to swell. Omnifluor-Protosol scintillation fluid gives very low background counts, an important consideration when working with low activity samples.

Representative electropherograms for erythrocyte and liver membranes are shown in Figure 1. In agreement with previously published results, the major peak of radiolabeling in human erythrocyte membranes migrates as a broad peak in the band 4.5 region of the gel (apparent molecular weight 45,000–65,000). Minor high- and low-molecular-weight peaks are also apparent. These correspond to aggregates of the transporter and degradation products, respectively. Covalent labeling of membrane protein is abolished when photolysis is carried out in the presence of NBTGR. The electropherogram of guinea pig liver membranes exhibits a similar symmetrical peak of radioactivity in the band 4.5 region of the gel, suggesting that the nucleoside carriers from the two sources have similar molecular weights.

Membranes also usually exhibit nonspecific (NBTGR-insensitive) labeling in the lipid region of the gel.

It is important to emphasize that the above technique can be applied directly to a wide variety of cell types and tissues using membranes of variable purity. Approximately 10–20% of available high-affinity NBMPR binding sites are covalently labeled under these conditions. It should be noted that sample volumes as small as 0.1–0.2 ml can be successfully photoaffinity-labeled using microcuvettes with a 1-mm light path. We have also been able to photoaffinity-label the nucleoside carrier in intact human erythrocytes using dilute cell suspensions in rectangular uncovered perspex dishes (Wu *et al.*, 1983b). [^{3}H]-ABA, a conventional photoaffinity analog of NBMPR, can also be used to label the erythrocyte nucleoside transporter, yielding a similar radioactivity profile on SDS–polyacrylamide gels to that obtained with NBMPR (Young *et al.*, 1983). The possibility of artifactual proteolysis of carrier protein during and after membrane isolation should always be considered. Appropriate precautions include the use of membranes soon after preparation and the addition of protease inhibitors to membrane buffers.

IV. FUTURE PROSPECTS

Studies of reversible NBMPR binding activity have provided important insights into the functioning of the nucleoside transporter in erythrocytes and other cells and tissues. We anticipate that experiments of this type will continue to provide useful information on the properties of the carrier. It is, however, the recent development of NBMPR in its new role as a specific photolabile ligand that offers the most exciting prospects for the future. As shown in this chapter, it is now a relatively simple task to identify the carrier protein on SDS–polyacrylamide gels and to compare the radiolabeled transporters from different tissues. The availability of a covalent label for the transporter has important implications for solubilization and isolation studies. It is to be anticipated that our understanding of the cell biology, physiology and biochemistry of the nucleoside transporter will increase dramatically over the next few years.

ACKNOWLEDGMENTS

S.M.J. is a Scholar of the Alberta Heritage Foundation for Medical Research (AHFMR). We thank the Cancer Research Campaign (UK), the Medical Research Council of Canada, and the AHFMR for financial support.

REFERENCES

Belt, J. A. 1983. Nitrobenzylthioinosine-insensitive uridine transport in human lymphoblastoid and murine leukemia cells. *Biochem. Biophys. Res. Commun.*, *110*:417–423.

Belt, J. A., Jarvis, S. M., Paterson, A. R. P., Tse, C. M., Wu, J. S. and Young, J. D. 1984. Reconstitution of the human erythrocyte nucleoside transporter into liposomes. *J. Physiol., 353:*87P.

Cabantchik, Z. I., and Ginsburg, H. 1977. Transport of uridine in human red blood cells. Demonstration of a simple carrier mechanism. *J. Gen. Physiol., 69:*75–96.

Cass, C. E., and Paterson, A. R. P. 1976. Nitrobenzylthioinosine binding sites in the erythrocyte membrane. *Biochim. Biophys. Acta, 419:*285–294.

Cass, C. E., Gaudette, L. A., and Paterson, A. R. P. 1974. Mediated transport of nucleosides in human erythrocytes. Specific binding of the inhibitor nitrobenzylthioinosine to nucleoside transport sites in the erythrocyte membrane. *Biochim. Biophys. Acta, 345:*1–10.

Cass, C. E., Kolassa, N., Uehara, Y., Dahlig-Harley, E., Harley, E. R., and Paterson, A. R. P. 1981. Absence of binding sites for the transport inhibitor nitrobenzylthioinosine on nucleoside transport-deficient mouse lymphoma cells. *Biochim. Biophys. Acta, 649:*769–777.

Cohen, A., Ullman, B., and Martin, D. W. Jr. 1979. Characterization of a mutant mouse lymphoma cell with deficient transport of purine and pyrimidine nucleosides. *J. Biol. Chem., 254:*112–116.

Dahlig-Harley, E., Eilam, Y., Paterson, A. R. P., and Cass, C. E. 1981. Binding of nitrobenzylthioinosine to high affinity sites on the nucleoside transport mechanism of HeLa cells. *Biochem. J., 200:*295–305.

Eilam, Y., and Cabantchik, Z. I. 1977. Nucleoside transport in mammalian cell membranes: a specific inhibitory mechanism of high affinity probes. *J. Cell Physiol., 92:*185–202.

Harley, E. R., Paterson, A. R. P., and Cass, C. E. 1982. Initial rate kinetics of the transport of adenosine and 4-amino-7-(β-D-ribofuranosyl) pyrimidine (tubercidin) in cultured cells. *Cancer Res., 42:*1289–1295.

Jarvis, S. M., and Young, J. D. 1980. Nucleoside transport in human and sheep erythrocytes: evidence that nitrobenzylthioinosine binds specifically to functional nucleoside transport sites. *Biochem. J., 190:*377–383.

Jarvis, S. M., and Young, J. D. 1981. Extraction and partial purification of the nucleoside transport system from human erythrocytes based on the assay of nitrobenzylthioinosine binding activity. *Biochem. J., 194:*331–339.

Jarvis, S. M., and Young, J. D. 1982a. Nucleoside translocation in sheep reticuloytes and erythrocytes from newborn lambs. A proposed model for the nucleoside transporter. *J. Physiol. (Lond.), 324:*47–66.

Jarvis, S. M., and Young, J. D. 1982b. Inhibitor binding studies. Nitrobenzylthioinosine, a specific high-affinity inhibitor of nucleoside transport. In: *Red Cell Membranes—A Methodological Approach*, pp. 263–273. Ed. by Ellory, J. C., and Young, J. D. Academic Press, London.

Jarvis, S. M., Ellory, J. C., and Young, J. D. 1980. Nucleoside transport in human erythrocytes: Apparent molecular weight of the nitrobenzylthioniosine binding complex estimated by radiation inactivation analysis. *Biochem. J. 190:*373–376.

Jarvis, S. M., McBride, D., and Young, J. D. 1982a. Erythrocyte nucleoside transport: Asymmetrical binding of nitrobenzylthioinosine to nucleoside permeation sites. *J. Physiol. (Lond.), 324:*31–46.

Jarvis, S. M., Hammond, J. R., Paterson, A. R. P., and Clanachan, A. S. 1982b. Species differences in nucleoside transport: a study of uridine transport and nitrobenzylthioinosine binding. *Biochem. J., 208:*83–88.

Jarvis, S. M., Hammond, J. R., Paterson, A. R. P., and Clanachan, A. S. 1983a. Nucleoside transport in human erythrocytes. A simple carrier with directional symmetry in fresh cells but with directional asymmetry in cells from outdated blood. *Biochem. J., 210:*457–461.

Jarvis, S. M., Kwong, Y. P., Wu, J. S., and Young, J. D. 1983b, Nitrobenzylthioinosine, a specific photoaffinity probe of the erythrocyte nucleoside transporter. *J. Physiol. (Lond.), 343:*93P.

Jarvis, S. M., Fincham, D. A., Ellory, J. C., Paterson, A. R. P., and Young, J. D. 1983c. Nucleoside transport in human erythrocytes. Nitrobenzylthioinosine binding and uridine transport activities have similar radiation target sizes. *Biochim. Biophys. Acta, 772:*227–300.

Jarvis, S. M., Janmohamed, S. N., and Young, J. D. 1983d. Kinetics of nitrobenzylthioinosine binding to the human erythrocyte nucleoside transporter. *Biochem. J., 216:*661–667.

Laemmli, U. K. 1970. Cleavage of structural proteins during the assembly of the head of bacteriophage T4, *Nature (Lond.), 227:*680–685.

Paterson, A. R. P., Lau, E. Y., Dahlig, E., and Cass, C. E. 1980. A common basis for inhibition of nucleoside transport by dipyridamole and nitrobenzylthioinosine? *Mol. Pharmacol., 18:*40–44.

Paterson, A. R. P., Kolassa, N., and Cass, C. E. 1981. Transport of nucleoside drugs in animal cells. *Pharmacol. Ther., 12:*515–536.

Plagemann, P. G. W., and Wohlhueter, R. M. 1980. Permeation of nucleosides and nucleic acid bases and nucleotides in animal cells. *Curr. Top. Membr. Transp., 14:*225–330.

Steck, T. L. 1974. The organization of proteins in the human red blood cell membrane. *J. Cell Biol., 62:*1–19.

Slaughter, R. S., Fenwick, R. G., Jr., and Barnes, E. M. 1981. Hypoxanthine and thymidine compete for transport in Chinese hamster fibroblasts. *Arch. Biochem. Biophys., 211:*494–499.

Thompson, S., and Maddy, A. H. 1982. Gel electrophoresis of erythrocyte membrane proteins. In: *Red Cell Membranes—A Methodological Approach*, pp. 67–94. Ed. by Ellory, J. C., and Young, J. D. Academic Press, London.

Wohlhueter, R. M., and Plagemann, P. G. W. 1982. On the functional symmetry of nucleoside transport in mammalian cells. *Biochim. Biophys. Acta, 689:*249–260.

Wohlhueter, R. M., Marz, R., and Plagemann, P. G. W. 1978. Properties of the thymidine transport system of Chinese hamster ovary cells as probed by nitrobenzylthioinosine. *J. Membr. Biol., 42:*247–264.

Wohlhueter, R. M., Marz, R., and Plagemann, P. G. W. 1979. Thymidine transport in cultured mammalian cells. Kinetic analysis, temperature dependence and specificity of the transport system. *Biochim. Biophys. Acta, 553:*261–268.

Wu, J. S., Jarvis, S. M., and Young, J. D. 1983a. The human erythrocyte nucleoside and glucose transporters are both band 4.5 membrane polypeptides. *Biochem. J., 214:*995–997.

Wu, J. S., Kwong, F. Y. P., Jarvis, S. M., and Young, J. D. 1983b. Identification of the erythrocyte nucleoside transporter as a band 4.5 polypeptide. Photoaffinity labelling studies using nitrobenzylthioinosine. *J. Biol. Chem., 258:*13745–13751.

Young, J. D., and Jarvis, S. M. 1983. Nucleoside transport in animal cells. Review. *Bioscience Reports, 3:*309–322.

Young, J. D., Jarvis, S. M., Robins, M. J., and Paterson, A. R. P. 1983. Photoaffinity labelling of the human erythrocyte nucleoside transporter by N^6-(ρ-Azidobenzyl) adenosine and nitrobenzylthioinosine. Evidence that the transporter is a band 4.5 polypeptide. *J. Biol. Chem., 258:*2202–2208.

IV

Classification and Identification of Receptors for Adenosine and Adenine Nucleotides

Chapter **11**

The Classification of Receptors for Adenosine and Adenine Nucleotides

Geoffrey Burnstock and Noel J. Buckley

Department of Anatomy and Embryology
Center for Neuroscience
University College, London
London, England

I. INTRODUCTION

Adenosine and adenine nucleotides exert potent extracellular actions on a wide range of physiological systems, including the nervous, cardiovascular, gastrointestinal, urogenital, respiratory and lymphatic systems (Drury and Szent-Györgi, 1929; Green and Stoner, 1950; Burnstock, 1972, 1975, 1981; Phillis and Wu, 1982; Berne *et al.*, 1983; Daly *et al.*, 1983b). Many of these actions are mediated via purinergic receptors, and since the introduction of the P_1/P_2, A1/A2, and R_i/R_a classification systems for purinoceptors (Burnstock, 1978; Van Calker *et al.*, 1979; Londos *et al.*, 1980), much attention has focussed on the characterization of these receptor types in a range of tissues. By way of introduction, we present a brief overview of the means by which receptors may be classified before considering the application of these techniques to the classification of purinoceptors into P_1 and P_2 subtypes followed by an appraisal of the proposed A1/A2 subclassification of the P_1 purinoceptor. A more detailed consideration of these individual aspects may be found in accompanying chapters. We conclude the chapter with a brief assessment of the validity of the existing classification systems and the prospects for future developments in this expanding field of research.

II. RECEPTOR CLASSIFICATION

Receptors may be conceived as consisting of essentially two components: a recognition component lying at the surface of the cell that is responsible for the binding of receptor ligands and a catalytic component that mediates the physiological response. Various transducers and cofactors may also be necessary in order to provide an integrated linkage between receptor occupation and the elicited response.

Attempts at classifying receptors can be divided into two categories: pharmacological studies that categorize a response in relation to a series of agonists or antagonists and biochemical studies that characterize the association of a receptor ligand with its recognition site. Both strategies can offer different types of information on the nature of the receptor and both have unique theoretical and experimental constraints imposed upon their interpretations. It is unfortunate that, on many occasions, little attempt has been made to correlate the results drawn from these two approaches. Before consideration of specific examples of the application of such methodologies applied to purinergic receptors, a brief overview of the principles underlying these different approaches is given. Comprehensive treatments of the analysis of drug receptor interactions may be found in several contemporary texts (see Triggle and Triggle, 1976; Boeynaems and Dumont, 1980).

A. Pharmacological Classification

The pharmacological characterization of a receptor on the basis of agonist activity rank orders involves the generation of dose–response curves with a series of agonists and relies on the assumption that agonists that act on the same receptor display similar activity ratios in all preparations containing the receptor. However, the analysis of such dose–response curves may be complicated by several factors:

1. The measured response may not be directly proportional to receptor occupancy due to the multiciplicity of intermediate steps between receptor occupation and transduction of the final response:

$$L + R \xrightleftharpoons{\text{recognition}} LR \overset{\text{transduction}}{\rightarrow \rightarrow \rightarrow \rightarrow} \text{Response}$$

Many examples exist of "spare receptors" whereby only a small fractional occupancy of the receptor population is necessary in order to elicit a full pharmacological response.

2. Agonists acting on the same receptor may not show similar agonist activity orders at all such receptors since the activity of an agonist is a product of both its affinity for the receptor and its intrinsic activity (efficacy), hence an agonist may act on the same receptor and produce the same fractional response, but at a different receptor occupancy in different preparations.

3. The receptors may interact with others, thus exhibiting positive or negative cooperative behavior and thereby causing deviations from the regular hyperbolic dose–response curves.

4. The sensitivity of a receptor may change in response to the continued presence of an agonist (e.g., desensitization).

5. Agonists may produce a response by acting at more than one receptor.

6. The concentration of agonists in the local environment of the receptor may differ from that in the bulk phase because of differences in solubility, rates of diffusion, rates of loss, and other factors.

Despite these limitations, agonist activity rank orders have been used successfully to distinguish between several receptor classes, for example α- and β-adrenoceptors (Ahlquist, 1948) and also the further division of the β-adrenoceptor into β_1 and β_2 subclasses (Lands *et al.*, 1967). The classification of the purinoceptor into P_1 and P_2 purinoceptors (Burnstock, 1978) and the subdivision of the P_1 adenosine receptor into A1/R_i and A2/R_a subclasses (Van Calker *et al.*, 1979; Londos *et al.*, 1980) also rely heavily on the use of agonist activity rank orders. The relative stereoselectivity of a pair of stereoisomers is often used as a diagnostic tool in receptor classification since their similarity of chemical structure would be expected to minimise differences in solubility, diffusion, and so on (for example, the relatively greater potency of the *l*-stereoisomers of many β-agonists and β-antagonists at the β-adrenoceptor). However, the same limitations apply to stereoisomers as to any other pair of agonists. This is especially pertinent to the use of the diastereomers L-PIA and D-PIA in the A1/A2 classification, since differences in lipid solubility and sites of action for the two compounds have been reported (see below).

The use of selective/specific competitive antagonists offers a preferable means of distinguishing receptor types as many of the problems incurred in the use of agonists are obviated, such as the relationship between occupancy and response, thus enabling the affinity of an antagonist to be determined with relative ease. The only assumptions made are that the same agonist occupancy produces the same response and that the affinity of competitive antagonists for a receptor is the same in all tissues and does not vary when tested against a series of agonists acting on the same receptor. The recent subclassification of muscarinic receptors into M1 and M2 receptors was based on the discovery of a unique selective antagonist, pirenzepine (Hammer *et al.*, 1980). The methylxanthines have been used to specifically antagonize the P_1 purinoceptor, although for some of these compounds, doubts have been expressed about the competitive nature of their inhibition and their specificity of action.

Attempts have also been made to classify receptors according to the cellular response that they elicit, even though there is no prerequisite for a given receptor to be linked exclusively to any particular effector/transduction mechanism. An example is provided by the α-adrenoceptor, which appears to be linked to an inhibitory adenylate cyclase unit, whilst the β-adrenoceptor is linked to a stimulatory adenylate cyclase unit (see Rodbell, 1980). P_1 purinoceptors (both A1 and A2), in many instances, appear to be linked to adenylate cyclase while in other systems the actions of adenosine seem to be transduced by other means, such as by the opening of Ca^{2+} channels.

B. Biochemical Classification

The relatively recent introduction of radioligand binding techniques has permitted the direct investigation of the interaction of a receptor ligand with its recognition site and its application has greatly enhanced our understanding and classification of a wide variety of receptor types. The technique essentially consists of measuring either the association of a radiolabeled ligand with its binding site or its displacement from the binding site by a series of unlabeled ligands. By such means, it is possible to ascertain the affinity constants of a wide variety of ligands. However, ligand binding studies can be sterile unless attempts are made to correlate the rank order of affinity constants so obtained with their rank order of pharmacological activity. Such comparisons are obviously facilitated by the use of radiolabeled antagonists as ligands. Other arguments that favor the choice of antagonists include the fact that antagonists frequently exhibit higher affinities and less complex binding behavior than agonists. On the other hand, the latter point can also be used to advocate the choice of radiolabeled agonists in order to demonstrate a greater degree of receptor heterogeneity. Ideally, both types of ligand should be employed.

The use of the radiolabeled methylxanthines as adenosine receptor antagonists has met with limited success in characterization of the P_1 site because of their low affinity and equivocal specificity. The A1 purinoceptor has received most attention since a variety of high affinity, highly specific, and metabolically stable radiolabeled agonists are available (lately an A1-selective antagonist has also been introduced; Bruns *et al.*, 1983), but relatively few attempts have been made to correlate the agonist binding site with the pharmacological receptor.

III. P_1/P_2 CLASSIFICATION OF RECEPTORS

A basis for distinguishing two types of purinergic receptor was proposed by Burnstock in 1978, based largely on an analysis of the voluminous literature about the actions of purine nucleotides and nucleosides on a wide variety of tissues (Burnstock, 1978). Since that time, many experiments have been carried out that support and extend this proposal (see Burnstock, 1981; Daly *et al.*, 1983b; Berne *et al.*, 1983).

The original classification into P_1 and P_2 purinoceptors was based on four criteria: the relative potencies of ATP, ADP, AMP, and adenosine; the selective actions of antagonists, particularly methylxanthines; the activation of adenylate cyclase by adenosine, but not by ATP; the introduction of prostaglandin synthesis by ATP, but not by adenosine (see Table I).Thus the following classification was proposed: P_1 purinoceptors are more responsive to adenosine and AMP than to ATP and ADP; methyxanthines such as theophylline and caffeine are selective competitive antagonists, and occupation of these receptors leads to inhibition or activation of an adenylate cyclase system with resultant changes in levels of intracellular cyclic AMP. P_2 purinoceptors are more responsive to ATP and ADP than to AMP and adenosine, are not antagonized by methylxanthines, do not act via an adenylate cyclase system, and their occupation may lead to prostaglandin synthesis.

Evaluation and expansion of this classification has taken several directions, including studies of the stereoselectivity of P_1 and P_2 purinoceptors (Cusack *et al.*, 1979; Brown *et al.*, 1982a; Burnstock *et al.*, 1983), analysis of the influence of ectoenzymatic breakdown of nucleotides and uptake of adenosine in measurement of relative agonist potencies (Collis and Pettinger, 1982; Moody *et al.*, 1984), development of more potent and selective P_1- and P_2-purinoceptor antagonists (Hogaboom *et al.*, 1980; Griffith *et al.*, 1981; Fredholm and Persson, 1982; Bruns *et al.*, 1983), and selective desensitization of the P_2 purinoceptor by the slowly degradable analog α,β-methylene ATP (Kasakov and Burnstock, 1983; Meldrum and Burnstock, 1983; Sneddon and Burnstock, 1984).

A. Stereospecificity

Evidence for stereospecificity of the P_1 purinoceptor has been presented recently (Brown *et al.*, 1982a). The potency of the D enantiomers for producing inhibitory effects on the driven left atria, the trachea and cholinergic excitatory (twitch) responses of the ileum of the guinea pig was as follows: 5′-*N*-ethylcarboxamidoadenosine (NECA) > 2-chloroadenosine > 2-azidoadenosine > adenosine. The L enantiomers of adenosine and these analogs did not produce inhibitory responses in the atrium and transmurally stimulated ileum, and they were considerably less potent in the trachea.

D-Methylthio ATP has been shown recently to be about 200 times more potent than ATP and 700 times more potent than the L-methylthio ATP enantiomer in producing relaxation of the guinea-pig taenia coli, suggesting that the inhibitory P_2 purinoceptors are probably stereospecific (Burnstock *et al.*, 1983). However, significant differences in the excitatory responses of the guinea pig bladder and frog ventricle to the D and L enantiomers were not found.

B. Antagonists

Whereas theophylline and caffeine are effective competitive antagonists to P_1 purinoceptors in a wide variety of tissues (see Daly, 1983), 8-phenyltheophylline has been shown to be substantially more potent than theophylline in antagonizing adenosine-induced accumulation of cyclic AMP in slices of guinea pig cerebral cortex (Smellie *et al.*, 1979) and in human fibroblasts (Bruns, 1980), as well as antagonizing the responses elicited by adenosine of the guinea pig atrium, rabbit basilar artery, cholinergic nerve terminals in the guinea pig ileum (Griffith *et al.*, 1981) and adrenergic terminals in the rat vas deferens (Clanachan, 1981). Diethyl-8-phenyl-theophylline was more potent than 8-phenyltheophylline in fat cells and brain cells (Fredholm and Persson, 1982), and a compound claimed to be 70,000 times more potent than theophylline in bovine brain, namely 1,3-dipropyl-8-(2-amino-4-chlorophenyl)-xanthine (PACPX), has also been reported (Bruns *et al.*, 1983).

Several compounds, including quinidine, 2-substituted imidazolamines, and 2,2′ pyridylisatogen tosylate, have been shown during the past 10 years to antagonize responses to ATP in various preparations, but none of these compounds are competitive antagonists and all have nonspecific actions (Burnstock and Brown, 1981). When low concentrations of apamin were shown by Schuba and Vladimirova (1980) to block ATP, but not adenosine, the possibility that this substance acted as a P_2-purinoceptor antagonist was considered. However, it was subsequently shown to act by blocking K^+ channels rather than as a competitive ATP antagonist (Banks *et al.*, 1979); nevertheless, it is a useful agent to distinguish P_1- and P_2-purinoceptor inhibitory actions in the gut (Brown and Burnstock, 1981).

A most promising development is the claim that amylazido aminopropronyl ATP ($ANAPP_3$) is a specific P_2 antagonist. However, it is a difficult compound to use, because it must be incubated with the tissues in the dark before exposure to light in order to be effective and its action is irreversible (Hogaboom *et al.*, 1980); further, it may be more effective against the excitatory than the inhibitory actions of ATP (Frew and Lundy, 1982).

A useful technique for producing selective block of P_2 purinoceptors has been developed, namely, by desensitization with the slowly degradable analog of ATP, α,β-methylene ATP. Low concentrations of this drug have been shown to selectively block responses to P_2-purinoceptor agonists in the bladder (Kasakov and Burnstock, 1983) and vas deferens (Meldrum and Burnstock, 1983; Sneddon and Burnstock, 1984).

C. Ectoenzymatic Breakdown of ATP

Extracellular breakdown of ATP is rapid and involves a number of different enzymes (see Manery and Dryden, 1979). This finding means that some of the actions of ATP and ADP might be mediated via P_1 purinoceptors following breakdown to AMP and adenosine. It is not a problem to distinguish these actions where P_1 and P_2 purinoceptors mediate opposite effects, as, for example, in the bladder and pulmonary arteries where ATP contracts, while adenosine relaxes, the smooth muscle. However, it is more difficult to distinguish these actions in tissues where adenine nucleotides and nucleosides both produce relaxation, e.g., intestine or portal vein. Several studies have been carried out to try to resolve which effects of ATP are due to the direct and indirect actions of ATP (Collis and Pettinger, 1982; Moody *et al.*, 1984). Several experimental tests are useful to resolve this question. If ATP is less potent than adenosine this is the first indication of a possible indirect action; if the responses to ATP are blocked by methylxanthines and if the slowly degradable analog of ATP, α,β-methylene ATP has no action, then this is confirmation of indirect action. The use of a combination of 5′-nucleotidase and adenosine deaminase, which convert AMP and adenosine to inosine, respectively, to test whether ATP responses are reduced as well as those to AMP and adenosine is problematical since ATP is known to inhibit the action of 5′ nucleotidase (Burger and Lowenstein, 1970).

IV. SUBCLASSIFICATION OF THE P_1 PURINOCEPTOR

A. A1/A2 and R_i/R_a Receptor Subclasses

Table I summarizes the two principal criteria that have been used to distinguish between A1- and A2-type receptor characteristics: the order of potency of a series of adenosine receptor agonists (either as agonists of a pharmacological response or as displacing agents in radioligand binding assays) and stereoselectivity with respect to the diastereomers L-N^6-phenylisoproprop yladenosine (N^6-

[R(−)-L-methyl-2-phenethyl]adenosine)(L-PIA) and D-N^6-phenylisopropyladenosine (D-PIA). The original classifications of adenosine receptors into the A1/R_i and A2/R_a subtypes were based purely on the relative potency of three agonists, namely, L-PIA, NECA, and adenosine, on the adenylate cyclase systems of several cell types. Londos *et al.* (1980) examined the actions of these adenosine analogs on the adenylate cyclase of three cell types: rat liver cells, I-10 Leydig cells, and rat adipocytes. The analogs stimulated the adenylate cyclase in membrane preparations of rat liver and I-10 Leydig cells and inhibited the enzyme in adipocyte membranes. The potency series NECA > AD > PIA was observed for the stimulatory actions, whereas the converse was found for the inhibitory action, i.e., PIA > AD > NECA. These agonist potency series were also observed when the corresponding physiological responses of steroidogenesis and lipolysis were measured in whole cells. The terms R_a and R_i were proposed to describe the receptors mediating the stimulatory and inhibitory actions on adenylate cyclase, respectively.

Van Calker *et al.* (1979) similarily concluded from studies on cultured glial cells from mouse brain that adenosine acted at two cell surface receptors: one high affinity and inhibitory to adenylate cyclase and the other low affinity and stimulatory to adenylate cyclase. They named these sites A1 and A2 respectively. At the inhibitory A1 site, L-PIA was more potent than adenosine, whereas the converse was true at the excitatory A2 site. We have adopted the A1/A2 convention in favor of the R_i/R_a classification, as the former system is in keeping with the nomenclatures used in other recent receptor subclassifications, e.g., histamine H1 and H2 receptors, dopamine D1 and D2 receptors, serotonin S1 and S2 receptors, and muscarinic M1 and M2 receptors.

The use of stereoselectivity in the A1/A2 classification is a more recent addition. L-PIA [N^6-[*R*(−)-1-methyl-2-phenethyl]adenosine] was shown to be 70-fold more potent than its diastereomer D-PIA in inhibiting lipolysis in rats, but both diastereomers were equipotent in inhibiting corticosterone synthesis in rat adrenal slices (Vapaatojo *et al.*, 1971). Smellie *et al.* (1979) showed that the adenosine receptor mediated accumulation of cAMP by rat brain slices displayed little stereoselectivity, whereas the EPSP in such slices was a 100-fold more sensitive to inhibition by L-PIA than by D-PIA. Both the inhibition of lipolysis and the depression of the EPSP are both believed to be A1 receptor-mediated actions, whereas the accumulation of cAMP is thought to be an A2 action (Londos *et al.*, 1980; Trost and Schwabe, 1981; Reddington *et al.*, 1982; Dunwiddie and Fredholm, 1982). Hence, the idea evolved that stereoselectivity was an exclusive property of the A1 receptor. Since then L-PIA and D-PIA have been used in a wide range of systems (see Table I).

An extensive array of adenosine analogs has been used on many different tissue preparations in order to characterize adenosine receptors both biochemically and pharmacologically. Examination of Table I, however, shows such agonist potency orders to be extremely variable. Whereas the N^6-substituted derivatives are generally the most active analogs at A1 sites, there appears to be little consensus on the order of potency within this group of compounds. On the other hand, the stereoselective nature of the A1 site appears to offer a more consistent criterion for classification. Thus the A1 receptor seems to be best characterized

Table I. Subclassification of Adenosine Receptors[a]

	Potency order of adenosine analogs[b]	L-PIA/ D-PIA ratio	A1/A2[c]	References
	Central nervous system			
Rat brain membranes				
Binding of [^{3}H]-PIA	L-PIA > D-PIA > CADO > AD	40	A1	Schwabe and Trost (1980)
Binding of [^{3}H]-CADO	L-PIA > CADO > NCPCA > D-PIA > NECA	25	A1	Williams and Risley (1980)
Binding of [^{3}H]-CADO	CADO > AD > L-PIA > CHA > D-PIA, NECA	500	A1	Wu and Phillis (1982)
Inhibition of adenylate cyclase	L-PIA, CHA > NECA	—	A1	Cooper *et al.* (1980)
Rat striatal membranes				
Stimulation of adenylate cyclase	NECA > CADO, NECA	—	A2	Wojcik and Neff (1983)
Inhibition of adenylate cyclase	L-PIA > CADO, NECA	—	A1	Wojcik and Neff (1983)
Rat brain sections				
Binding of [^{3}H]-CHA	L-PIA > D-PIA	100	A1	Goodman and Snyder (1982)
Rat hippocampal slice				
Binding of [^{3}H]-CHA	CHA > L-PIA > CADO > D-PIA	50	A1	Reddington *et al.* (1982)
Depression of EPSP	CHA > L-PIA > CADO > D-PIA	100	A1	Reddington *et al.* (1982)
Rat hippocampal slice				
Binding of [^{3}H]-CHA, [^{3}H]-PIA, [^{3}H]-NECA	CHA, L-PIA > NECA	—	A1	Dunwiddie and Fredholm (1982)
Depression of EPSP	L-PIA > CHA > NECA > CADO	—	A1	Dunwiddie and Fredholm (1982)
Stimulation of adenylate cyclase	NECA > L-PIA > CADO	—	A2	Dunwiddie and Fredholm (1982)
Rat hippocampal slice				
Binding of [^{3}H]-CHA	L-PIA > D-PIA	>100	A1	Fredholm *et al.* (1982)
Stimulation of adenylate cyclase	NECA > L-PIA, D-PIA, CADO > AD	1	A2	Fredholm *et al.* (1982)
Rat hippocampal slice				
Depression of evoked response	L-PIA > D-PIA	100	A1	Smellie *et al.* (1979)
Stimulation of adenylate cyclase	L-PIA > D-PIA	5	A2	Smellie *et al.* (1979)
Guinea-pig cortical membranes				
Binding of [^{3}H]-CHA	L-PIA > CHA > CADO, NCPCA > D-PIA	37	A1	Bruns *et al.* (1980)
Stimulation of adenylate cyclase	NCPCA > CADO > L-PIA > CHA > D-PIA	5	A2	Bruns *et al.* (1980)
Guinea-pig cortical slice				
Stimulation of adenylate cyclase	L-PIA > D-PIA	5	A2	Smellie *et al.* (1979)
Bovine brain membranes				
Binding of [^{3}H]-CHA	L-PIA > CHA > D-PIA > CADO	33	A1	Gavish *et al.* (1982)
Solubilized bovine brain membranes				
Binding of [^{3}H]-CHA	L-PIA > CHA > D-PIA > CADO	14	A1	Gavish *et al.* (1982)
Rat cortical neurones				
Depression of cortical firing	NECA > NCPCA, CADO > L-PIA, CHA	—	A2	Phillis and Wu (1983)
Rat cortical synaptosomes				
Depression of K^+-evoked Ca^{2+} uptake	NECA > CHA, CADO > L-PIA > D-PIA	5	A2	Wu *et al.* (1982)
	Peripheral tissues			
Guinea-pig atria				
Negative inotropic effect	NECA > CADO > AD	—	—	Brown *et al.* (1982a)

Table I. *Continued*

	Potency order of adenosine analogs[b]	L-PIA/D-PIA ratio	A1/A2[c]	References
Guinea-pig atria Negative inotropic effect	NECA > CHA > L-PIA, CADO > AD > D-PIA	100	A1	Collis (1983)
Guinea pig atria Negative inotropic and chronotropic effect	L-PIA > CHA > NECA > CADO > D-PIA	100	A1	Evans and Schenden (1982)
Guinea pig heart Increase in coronary flow	L-PIA > D-PIA	20	A1	Vapaatolo *et al.* (1975)
Rat atria Negative inotropic effect	L-PIA > NCPCA > D-PIA	100	A1	Paton and Kurahashi (1981)
Guinea pig trachea Relaxation	NECA > CADO > AD	—	—	Brown *et al.* (1982a)
Guinea pig trachea Relaxation	NCPCA > NECA > CADO > L-PIA > AD > D-PIA	5	A2	Brown and Collis (1982)
Guinea pig taenia coli Relaxation	NECA > CADO > L-PIA > CHA > D-PIA	2	A2	Burnstock *et al.* (1984)
Guinea pig taenia coli Relaxation	AD > PIA > CADO > NECA	—	—	Baer and Muller (1983)
Guinea pig aorta Relaxation	NCPCA > NECA > CADO > AD > L-PIA > D-PIA > CHA	3	A2	Collis and Brown (1983)
Rat superior cervical ganglion Hyperpolarising after-potential	L-PIA > CADO > AD	—	A1	Henon and McAfee (1983)
Guinea pig ileum Inhibition of twitch	NECA > CADO > AD	—	—	Brown *et al.* (1982a)
Guinea pig ileum Inhibition of twitch	NCPCA > L-PIA > AD > D-PIA	88	A1	Paton (1981)
Rat vas deferens Inhibition of twitch	NCPCA > L-PIA > AD > D-PIA	91	A1	Patron (1981)
Rat portal vein Inhibition of twitch	NECA > CADO, L-PIA > D-PIA, CHA, AD	3	A2	Kennedy and Burnstock (1984)
Rabbit portal vein Inhibition of twitch	L-PIA, CHA, NCPCA, NECA > CADO > AD D-PIA	100	A1	Brown *et al*. (1982b)
Dog coronary myocytes	NECA, NCPCA > L-PIA, CHA > AD	10	A2	Kusachi *et al.* (1983)
Rabbit anococcygeus muscle Inhibition of twitch	L-PIA > NECA > CADO > AD	—	A1	Stone (1983)
Rabbit kidney Inhibition of noradrenaline release	L-PIA > NECA, CADO > AD	—	A1	Fredholm *et al.* (1983)
Rat liver Binding of [^{3}H]-CHA	CHA > L-PIA > D-PIA > AD > NECA	2	A2	Schütz *et al.* (1982b)
Stimulation of adenylate cyclase	NECA > CHA > AD	—	A2	
Rat liver membranes Stimulation of adenylate cylcase	NECA > AD > L-PIA	—	A2	Londos *et al.* (1980)
Mouse Leydig cells Stimulation of adenylate cyclase	NECA > AD > L-PIA	—	A2	Londos *et al.* (1980)
Stimulation of steroidogenesis	NECA > AD > L-PIA	—	A2	London *et al.* (1980)

(*Continued*)

Table I. *Continued*

	Potency order of adenosine analogs[b]	L-PIA/D-PIA ratio	A1/A2[c]	References
Rat adipocytes				
Inhibition of adenylate cyclase	L-PIA > AD > NECA	—	A1	Londos *et al.* (1980)
Inhibition of lipolysis	L-PIA > NECA	—	A1	Londos *et al.* (1980)
Rat adipocytes				
Binding of [^{3}H]-PIA	L-PIA > CHA > CADO > D-PIA	11	A1	Trost and Schwabe (1981)
Rat				
Inhibition of lipolysis	L-PIA > D-PIA	70	A1	Vapaatolo *et al.* (1971)
Y-1 adrenal tumor				
Inhibition of adenylate cyclase	L-PIA > AD > NECA	—	A1	Londos *et al.* (1980)
Rat				
Inhibition of corticesterone synthesis	L-PIA = D-PIA	1	A2	Vapaatolo *et al.* (1971)
Cultured glial cells from mouse brain				
Inhibition of adenylate cyclase	L-PIA > AD	—	A1	Van Calker *et al.* (1979)
Stimulation of adenylate cyclase	AD > L-PIA	—	A2	Van Calker *et al.* (1979)
Rat brain microvessels				
Stimulation of adenylate cyclase	NECA > AD, CADO > L-PIA > D-PIA	5	A2	Schütz *et al.* (1982a)
Rat testes membrane				
Binding of [^{3}H]-CHA	CHA, L-PIA > D-PIA	79	A1	Murphy and Snyder (1981)
Human platelet membranes				
Binding of [^{3}H]-NECA	NECA > CADO> AD > L-PIA, CHA, D-PIA	1	A2	Lenschow *et al.* (1982)
Calf thymocytes				
Binding of [^{3}H]-NECA	NECA > CADO > AD > L-PIA > CHA > D-PIA	1	A2	Ukena *et al.* (1982)
Mouse				
Inhibition of locomotor activity	L-PIA > D-PIA	—	A1	Snyder *et al.* (1981)
Rat				
Disruption of operant behavior	L-PIA, CHA > CADO > D-PIA	167	A1	Coffin and Carney (1983)

[a] The examples cited here are not exhaustive.
[b] L-N^6-phenylisopropyladenosine (N^6-[*R*(−)-1-methyl-2-phenethyl]adenosine) (L-PIA); D-N^6-phenylisopropyladenosine (D-PIA); 2-chloroadenosine (CADO); N^6-cyclohexyladenosine (CHA); 5′-*N*-ethylcarboxamide adenosine (NECA); 5′-*N*-cyclopropropylcarboxamide adenosine (NCPCA); adenosine (AD).
[c] For the purpose of clarity the nomenclature proposed by Van Calker *et al.* (1979) is used throughout.

by the greater relative potency of L-PIA and N^6-cyclohexyladenosine (CHA) compared with the 5′-substituted compounds NECA and 5′-*N*-cyclopropropylcarboxamide adenosine (NCPCA) and by a marked degree of stereoselectivity with regard to the diastereomers L-PIA and D-PIA. Conversely, at the A2 site, NECA and NCPCA are more potent than or equipotent with L-PIA and CHA and very little stereoselectivity is displayed. However, certain peripheral actions appear to be mediated by a receptor type that shows mixed characteristics. The negative inotropic response of guinea pig atria (Brown *et al.*, 1982a; Collis, 1983) and rat atria (Paton and Kurahashi, 1981; Paton, 1983) and the inhibition of twitch

Table II. Summary of A1/A2 Receptor Classification[a]

Receptor type	Location	Potency order of adenosine analogs	Stereoselectivity
A1	Brain, atria, superior cervical ganglion, adipocytes, cultured glia	L-PIA, CHA > NECA, NCPCA	L-PIA > D-PIA
	Prejunctional sites in peripheral nervous system, atria	NECA, NCPCA ≥ L-PIA, CHA	L-PIA > D-PIA
A2	Brain, trachea, taenia coli, aorta, liver, I-10 Leydig cells, microvessels, thymocytes, cultured glia, platelets	NECA, NCPCA ≥ L-PIA, CHA	L-PIA ≃ D-PIA

[a] Abbreviations as in Table I.

in the guinea pig ileum and rat vas deferens (Paton, 1981; Brown *et al.*, 1982; Paton, 1983) and rabbit portal vein (Brown *et al.*, 1982b) all appear to be mediated by a receptor that shows an A2-type agonist potency order while retaining a marked degree of stereoselectivity indicative of an A1-type receptor. In these cases, the stereoselectivity was chosen to be the definitive characteristic and the receptor was hence classified as A1, although for the present they are probably best left out of the A1/A2 schemata (see Table II).

B. Variability of Agonist Potency Profiles

In addition to the theoretical limitations imposed on the interpretation of agonist potency orders outlined above, there are several possible sources of the variability seen in such profiles. In the pharmacalogical studies there is the possibility of a contribution to the overall response being measured by non-receptor-mediated effects. For instance, 2-chloroadenosine (CADO) may act partially via an intracellular site, at least in guinea pig trachea, since blockade of the adenosine receptor with theophylline did not antagonize the response to CADO and inhibition of the adenosine transport system with dipyridamole or dilazep produced a decrease in the maximal response (Brown and Collis, 1982). Another problem relates to the use of D-PIA, which in guinea pig atrium has an amphetamine-like action, thereby causing release of catecholamines and inhibiting their reuptake into nerve terminals (Collis, 1983). Caution should also be exercised in interpreting stereoselective actions of L-PIA and D-PIA in whole organ and in *in vivo* studies, as such stereoselective effects could also be explained by the greater lipid solubility of L-PIA (Vapaatalo *et al.*, 1975). Some of the variation seen in the radioligand binding studies may be due to the use of different experimental protocols. Most such studies necessitate the inclusion of adenosine deaminase in the incubation medium in order to reduce the levels of endogenous adenosine that would otherwise compete with the radioligand for occupation of the receptor (Bruns *et al.*, 1980; Schwabe and Trost, 1980; Williams and Risley, 1980). However, two studies investigated the binding of [^{3}H]-CADO to rat brain membranes in the absence of adenosine deaminase and at 0°C (Wu *et al.*, 1980; Wu and Phillis, 1982). Under such conditions, although high affinity, highly stereoselective sites were described, the specific binding was nevertheless displaced by relatively low concentrations of pharmacologically inactive compounds such as adenine and inosine. However, when the assay was conducted at 23°C in the presence of adenosine deaminase, then adenine and inosine were ineffective at displacing the bound [^{3}H]-CADO (Williams and Risley, 1980). The two studies also showed marked differences in the regional distribution of [^{3}H]-CADO binding in various brain regions. The temperature at which the assay is conducted was also seen to be important when using [^{3}H]-PIA as a radioligand. Many agonists were more potent in competing with [^{3}H]-PIA in assays on fat cell membranes conducted at 37°C than on similar assays conducted on brain cell membranes at 0°C, whereas, conversely the antagonist theophylline was more effective as a displacing agent at 0°C (Schwabe and Trost, 1980; Trost and Schwabe, 1981).

C. Limitations of Ligand Binding Studies

The use of [^{3}H]adenosine in classification studies of adenosine receptors is problematic because of to its uptake, metabolism, and the multiplicity of non-receptor binding sites to which it can bind. In pharmacological studies these effects can be minimized by using compounds such as dipyridamole or 6-(*p*-nitrobenzyl) thioguanosine (NBTG) to inhibit the uptake process (Turnheim *et al.*, 1978; Paterson *et al.*, 1980) and 2-deoxycoformycin or erythro-9-(2-hydroxy-3-nonyl) adenine (EHNA) to inhibit the adenosine deaminase (Skolnick *et al.*, 1978; Plunkett *et al.*, 1979). Early attempts to characterize the adenosine receptor by radioligand binding techniques using [^{3}H]adenosine met with little success (Malbon *et al.*, 1978; Dutta and Mustafa, 1979; Schwabe *et al.*, 1979; Dutta and Mustafa, 1980; Newman *et al.*, 1981; Ghai and Mustafa, 1982; Newman and Levitzki, 1982; Schütz and Brugger, 1982; Schwabe, 1983). All these studies revealed a multiplicity of binding sites that showed displacement profiles inconsistent with those expected for adenosine receptors, such as antagonism of binding by pharmacologically inactive compounds such as adenine and 2′,5′-dideoxyadenosine, whereas pharmacologically potent compounds such as PIA and theophylline had little or no effect. In addition to these problems, even though many of the assays were conducted at 0°C in the presence of adenosine deaminase inhibitors, substantial metabolism of adenosine still occured (Schwabe *et al.*, 1979).

Hence, although an extensive array of adenosine analogs may provide useful information, it is only necessary to use a limited number of adenosine analogs in order to characterize a pharmacological response or binding site as A1, A2, or otherwise, namely, L-PIA, D-PIA and NECA (see Table II).

The potent vasodilatory actions of adenosine have been the focus of much interest (for review, see Su, 1981) since they were first reported over half a century ago (Drury and Szent-Györgi, 1929) and it is therefore somewhat surprising that very few studies have been directed towards classifying the receptor mediating this response. Microvessels from rat brain (Schütz *et al.*, 1982a) and rabbit heart (Mistry and Drummond, 1983) possess a receptor that is stimulatory to adenylate cyclase and displays an A2-type agonist potency, and the coronary relaxation produce in dog by adenosine and its analogs also shows characterics of an A2 receptor (Olsson and Kusachi, 1983; Kusachi *et al.*, 1983). Attempts at characterizing the adenosine receptor of vascular smooth muscle by radioligand binding techniques have met with little success, undoubtedly for the most part owing to the use of [^{3}H]adenosine as the radioligand, which incurs the problems of non-specific binding discussed previously (Dutta and Mustafa, 1980; Ghai and Mustafa, 1982; Schütz and Brugger, 1982). Our knowledge of adenosine receptor subclasses would be greatly extended if more vascular tissues were characterized both pharmacologically and by ligand binding studies using metabolically stable adenosine analogs. If, as the initial studies have indicated, the vascular adenosine receptor transpires to be an A2 type, then such studies would provide a valuable counterpoint to the better characterised A1 type receptors of the central nervous system.

Equally useful would be characterization of other peripheral adenosine receptors by radioligand binding techniques. Several studies have failed to demonstrate significant levels of specific binding of tritiated analogs to tissues such as heart, lung, small intestine, kidney, vas deferens, thyroid, submandibular gland, adrenal gland, pancreas, ovary, and fat, where pharmacological studies have provided abundant evidence of adenosine receptors (Williams and Risley, 1980; Murphy and Snyder, 1981). These findings could conceivably be due to either a low concentration of receptors or a low affinity of the receptors for the analogs used in these studies, or both. In an attempt to circumvent these limitations, autoradiographic procedures have been used to localize the binding sites for adenosine receptor ligands ([^{3}H]-NECA, [^{3}H]-CHA and [^{3}H]-PIA) in frozen sections of guinea pig intestine and rabbit lung (Buckley and Burnstock, 1983a,b). In the case of the guinea pig intestine, the label was seen to be predominantly associated with the enteric ganglia, whereas in the rabbit lung the label was associated with the respiratory epithelium. The enteric ganglia and respiratory epithelium represent only a small proportion of the total weight in these tissues and binding studies performed on homogenates of whole intestine or lung would presumably be unable to detect such small fractions of specific binding. Although these sites showed certain characteristics of adenosine receptors, such as antagonism by CADO and CHA, they were not blocked by theophylline. The uptake blockers, dipyridamole and dilazep, and the P-site antagonist 2′,5′-dideoxyadenosine were without effect. The failure of theophylline to antagonize the binding was also observed to apply to the sites originally visualized autoradiographically in sections of rat brain by Goodman and Snyder (1982). One possible explanation for this discrepancy is that the receptors in frozen tissue have characteristics different from those in whole tissue or membrane homogenates. Preparations of enteric synaptosomes or bovine sympathetic ganglia may provide an adequate source of peripheral material in which the amount and concentration of adenosine receptors would be sufficient to permit conventional radioligand binding assays to be performed.

D. cAMP and Purinoceptor Classification

The original classification of adenosine receptors into A1/R_i and A2/R_a subtypes was based largely on the ability of adenosine and its analogs to stimulate or inhibit the production of cAMP. However, as pointed out by Daly (1983), few actions of adenosine have been shown unequivocally to be mediated via changes in the level of cAMP. Although, in many cases, adenosine receptor agonists have been shown to alter the levels of cAMP, the involvement of such changes in the production of the final response is unclear.

Several studies have indicated differences in the receptors mediating the pharmacological response and the receptor mediating changes in cAMP levels. One of the best characterized systems in which such correlative studies have been performed is the rat hippocampal slice (see Table I). These studies have revealed an A1-receptor binding site by radioligand-binding techniques (Dunwiddie and Fredholm, 1982; Fredholm *et al.*, 1982; Reddington *et al.*, 1982), an A1 receptor responsible for the depression of the excitatory postsynaptic potential (EPSP) (Smellie *et al.*, 1979; Dunwiddie and Fredholm, 1982; Fredholm *et al.*, 1982; Reddington *et al.*, 1982), and an A2 receptor mediating increases in the levels of cAMP (Reddington and Schubert, 1979; Smellie *et al.*, 1979; Dunwiddie and Freholm, 1982). Clearly, the receptors mediating the electrophysiological response and the rise in cAMP must be different. However, other studies have shown that the depression of cortical firing and the depression of K^+-evoked Ca^{2+} uptake into cortical synaptosomes to be mediated via a receptor with A2 characteristics (Wu *et al.*, 1982; Phillis and Wu, 1983).

The involvement of cAMP has also been questioned in tissues where the response to adenosine can be overcome by raising the extracellular Ca^{2+} concentration. Such systems include the presynaptic inhibition of neurotransmitter release and the adenosine-induced relaxation of smooth and cardiac muscle. The possibility is raised that, in these tissues, the adenosine receptor is linked to a Ca^{2+} channel, since a rise in intracellular Ca^{2+} levels is known to accompany neurotransmitter secretion (Rubin, 1970), cardiac muscle contraction (Schrader *et al.*, 1975), and smooth muscle contraction (Fenton *et al.*, 1982). The relationship, if any, between cAMP levels and intracellular Ca^{2+} levels remains unclear, however.

These points serve to underline the concept that a receptor is best conceived as being constructed of two units: a recognition component and a catalytic component. It is entirely possible that the same recognition component (e.g., A1 or A2) could be linked to a variety of catalytic components (e.g., stimulatory or inhibitory regulatory units of adenylate cyclase or Ca^{2+} channels) in the same or different cell types (see Triggle and Triggle, 1976, for a discussion of these concepts). Hence, it is preferable not to classify adenosine receptors according to their effect on adenylate cyclase, at least until the linkage between receptor occupation and cAMP levels is understood more thoroughly. As a corollary, it would be prudent to accept the possibility that an A1-type receptor may be found that is linked to a stimulatory unit of adenylate cyclase and, conversely, that an A2-type receptor may prove to be coupled to inhibition of adenylate cyclase. Equally plausible is the possibility that a receptor may have an A1-type or A2-type character but not be linked to adenylate cyclase.

A recent study has reported the synthesis of a potent xanthine antagonist (1,3-dipropyl-8-(2-amino-4-chlorophenyl)xanthine that is highly specific for the A1 receptor (Bruns *et al.*, 1983). This compound represents a very significant advance and its use should help greatly in clarifying some of the ambiguities accompanying the use of agonists in defining adenosine receptor subclasses. In addition, the reported high affinity (K_i 22 pM) of this compound should also make it an ideal candidate for use in ligand binding studies.

V. CONCLUDING REMARKS

Experiments reported since 1978 are consistent with the P_1/P_2 classification, although it has been pointed out that care must be taken to distinguish direct and indirect actions of ATP. Some of the anomalies revealed in recent experiments may be explicable in terms of the possibility of the existence of different types of P_2 purinoceptor. For example, marked differences have been revealed between the responses of the bladder, vas deferens, and frog heart, on the one hand, and the taenia coli and portal vein, on the other, to 2-methylthio ATP, α,β-methylene ATP, apamin, UV light, and $ANAPP_3$; stereoselectivity has been shown for one group, but not the other. Further studies are needed to investigate this question.

The P_1 purinoceptor has been sub-divided according to two criteria: (1) The potency orders of adenosine analogs distinguishes three types of adenosine receptor (see Table II); (2) the effect of receptor stimulation on the levels of cAMP distinguishes two, and perhaps three, types of receptor. However, in most cases there has been little attempt to correlate purinoceptors classified according to these two criteria. Clarification of these subclassifications must await the development of specific, high-affinity antagonists for each subclass.

The nature and distribution of the various purinoceptor subclasses is of potential therapeutic importance, since such knowledge would assist in the design of drugs selectively targeted at specific cell and tissue types.

REFERENCES

Ahlquist, R. P. 1948. A study of adrenotropic receptors. *Am. J. Physiol., 153*:586–599.

Baer, H. P., and Muller, M. J. 1983. Adenosine receptors in smooth muscle. In: *Regulatory Functions of Adenosine* p. 500. Ed. by Berne, R. M., Rall, T. W., and Rubio, R. Martinus Nijhoff, Boston.

Banks, B. E. C., Brown, C., Burgess, G. M., Burnstock, G., Claret, M., Cocks, T., Jenkinson, D. H., and Parson, H. 1979. Some peripheral activities of apamin, *Toxicon, 17* (Suppl. 1):4.

Berne, R. M., Rall, T. W., and Rubio, R. (eds.). 1983. *Regulatory Functions of Adenosine*. Martinus Nijhoff, Boston.

Boeynaems, J. M., and Dumont, J. E. (eds) 1980. *Outlines of Receptor Theory*. Elsevier, Amsterdam.

Brown, C., and Burnstock, G. 1981. Evidence in support of the P_1/P_2 purinoceptor hypothesis in the guinea-pig taenia coli. *Br. J. Pharmacol., 73:*617–624.

Brown, C. M., and Collis, M. G. 1982. Evidence for an A_2/R_a adenosine receptor in the guinea-pig trachea. *Br. J. Pharmacol., 76:*381–387.

Brown, C., Burnstock, G., Cusack, N. J., Meghji, P., and Moody, C. J. 1982a. Evidence for stereospecificity of the P_1-purinoceptor. *Br. J. Pharmacol., 75:*101–107.

Brown, C. M., Collis, M. G., and Titley, K. 1982b. Evidence for a presynaptic A_1 adenosine receptor in the rabbit portal vein. *Br. J. Pharmacol., 77:*537P.

Bruns, R. F. 1980. Adenosine receptor activation in human fibroblasts: nucleoside agonists and antagonists. *Can. J. Physiol. Pharmacol., 58:*673–691.

Bruns, R. F., Daly, J. W., and Snyder, S. H. 1980. Adenosine receptors in brain membranes: Binding of N^6-cyclohexyl[^{3}H]adenosine and 1,3-diethyl-8-[^{3}H]phenylxanthine. *Proc. Natl. Acad. Sci. USA, 77:*5547–5551.

Bruns, R. F., Daly, J. W., and Snyder, S. H. 1983. Adenosine receptor binding: Structure-activity analysis generates extremely potent xanthine antagonists. *Proc. Natl. Acad. Sci. USA, 80:*2077–2080.

Buckley, N., and Burnstock, G. 1983a. Autoradiographic localisation of peripheral adenosine binding sites using ^{3}H-NECA. *Brain Res., 269:*374–377.

Buckley, N., and Burnstock, G. 1983b. Autoradiographic localisation of binding sites for muscarinic and adenosine receptor ligands. *Neurosci. Letts.* (*Suppl.*)*, 14:*546.

Burger, R. M., and Lowenstein, J. M. 1970. Preparation and properties of 5′-nucleotidase from smooth muscle of small intestine. *J. Biol. Chem., 245:*6274–6280.

Burnstock, G. 1972. Purinergic nerves. *Pharmacol. Rev., 24:*509–581.

Burnstock, G. 1975. In: *Handbook of Psychopharmacology*, Vol. 5, *Synaptic modulators*, pp. 131–194. Ed. by Iversen, L. L., Iversen, S. D., and Snyder, S. H. Plenum Press, New York.

Burnstock, G. 1978. A basis for distinguishing two types of purinergic receptor. In: *Cell Membrane Receptors for Drugs and Hormones*, pp. 107–118. Ed. by Straub, R. W., and Bolis, L. Raven Press, New York.

Burnstock, G. (ed.). 1981. *Purinergic Receptors.* Chapman and Hall, London.

Burnstock, G., and Brown, C. 1981. An introduction to purinergic receptors: history, classification and future developments. In: *Purinergic Receptors*, pp. 1–45. Ed. by Burnstock, G. Chapman and Hall, London.

Burnstock, G., Cusack, N. J., Hills, J. M., MacKenzie, I., and Meghji, P. 1983. Studies on the stereoselectivity of the P_2-purinoceptor. *Br. J. Pharmacol., 79:*907–913.

Burnstock, G., Hills, J. M., and Hoyle, C. H. W. 1984. Evidence that the P_1-purinoceptor in the guinea-pig taenia coli is an A_2 subtype. *Br. J. Pharmacol., 81:*533–541.

Clanachan, A. S. 1981. Antagonism of presynaptic adenosine receptors by theophylline 9-beta-D-riboside and 8-phenyltheophylline. *Can. J. Physiol. Pharmacol., 59:*603–606.

Coffin, V. L., and Carney, J. M. 1983. Behavioral pharmacology of adenosine analogs. In: *Physiology and Pharmacology of Adenosine Derivatives*, pp. 267–274 Ed. by Daly, J. W., Kuroda, Y., Phillis, J. W., Shimizu H., and Ui, M. Raven Press, New York.

Collis, M. G. 1983. Evidence for an A_1-adenosine receptor in the guinea-pig atrium. *Br. J. Pharmacol., 78:*207–212.

Collis, C., And Brown, C. 1983. Adenosine relaxes the aorta by interacting with an A_2 receptor and an intracellular site. *Br. J. Pharmacol., 79:*256P.

Collis, M. G., and Pettinger, S. J. 1982. Can ATP stimulate P_1-receptors in guinea-pig atrium without conversion to adenosine? *Eur. J. Pharmacol., 81:*521–529.

Cooper, D. M. F., Londos, C., and Rodbell, M. 1980. Adenosine receptor-mediated inhibition of rat cerebral cortical adenylate cyclase by a GTP-dependent process. *Mol. Pharmacol., 18:*598–601.

Cusack, N. J., and Planker, M. 1979. Relaxation of isolated taenia coli of guinea-pig by enantiomers of 2-azido analogues of adenosine and adenine nucleotides. *Br. J. Pharmacol., 67:*153–158.

Cusack, N. J., Hickman, M. E., and Born, G. V. R. 1979. Effects of D- and L-enantiomers of adenosine, AMP and ADP and their 2-chloro- and 2-azido-analogues on human platelets. *Proc. R. Soc. B., 206:*139–144.

Daly, J. W. 1983. Role of ATP and adenosine receptors in physiologic processes: Summary and prospectus. In: *Physiology and Pharmacology of Adenosine Derivatives* pp. 275–290. Ed. by Daly, J. W., Kuroda, Y., Phillis, J. W., and Ui, M. Raven Press, New York.

Daly, J. W., Bruns, R. F., and Snyder, S. H. 1983a. Adenosine receptors in the central nervous system: Relationship to the central actions of methylxanthines. *Life Sci., 28:*2083–2097.

Daly, J. W., Kuroda, Y., Phillis, J. W., and Ui, M. (eds.). 1983b. *Physiology and Pharmacology of Adenosine Derivatives*. Raven Press, New York.

Drury, A. N., and Szent-Györgi, A. 1929. The physiological activity of adenine compounds with especial reference to their action upon the mammalian heart. *J. Physiol. (Lond.), 28:*213–237.

Dunwiddie, T. V., and Fredholm, B. B. 1982. Adenosine receptors in the rat hippocampus. *Proc. Scand. Brit. Pharmac. Soc.* P8.

Dutta, P., and Mustafa, S. J. 1979. Saturable binding of adenosine to the dog heart microsomal fraction: competitive inhibition by aminophylline. *J. Pharmacol. Exp. Ther., 211:*496–501.

Dutta, P., and Mustafa, S. J. 1980. Binding of adenosine to the crude plasma membrane fraction isolated from dog coronary and carotid arteries. *J. Pharmacol. Exp. Ther., 214:*496–502.

Evans, D. B., and Schenden, J. A. 1982. Adenosine receptors mediating cardiac depression. *Life Sci., 31:*2425–2432.

Fenton, R. A., Bruttig, S. P., Rubio, R., and Berne, R. M. 1982. Effect of adenosine on calcium uptake by intact and cultured vascular smooth muscle. *Am. J. Physiol., 242:*H797–H804.

Fredholm, B. B., and Persson, C. G. A. 1982. Xanthine derivatives as adenosine receptor antagonists. *Eur. J. Pharmacol., 81:*673–676.

Fredholm, B. B., Jonzon, B., Lindgren, E. and Lindström, K. 1982. Adenosine receptors mediating cyclic AMP production in the rat hippocampus, *J. Neurochem., 39:*165–175.

Fredholm, B. B., Gustafsson, L. E., Hedqvist, P., and Sollevi, A. 1983. Adenosine in the regulation of neurotransmitter release in the peripheral nervous system. In: *Regulatory Functions of Adenosine*, p. 479–493 Ed. by Berne, R. M., Rall, T. W., and Rubio, R. Martinus Nijhoff, Boston.

Frew, R., and Lundy, P. M. 1982. Effect of arylazido aminopropionyl ATP ($ANAPP_3$), a putative ATP antagonist, on ATP responses of isolated guinea-pig smooth muscle. *Life Sci., 30:*259–267.

Gavish, M., Goodman, R. R., and Snyder, S. H. 1982. Solubilized adenosine receptors in the brain: Regulation by guanine nucleotides. *Science, 215:*1633–1635.

Ghai, G., and Mustafa, S. J. 1982. Demonstration of a putative adenosine receptor in rabbit aorta. *Blood Vessels, 19:*117–125.

Goodman, R. R., and Snyder, S. H. 1982. Autoradiographic localization of adenosine in rat brain using [^{3}H]cyclohexyladenosine. *J. Neurosci., 2:*1230–1241.

Green, H. N., and Stoner, H. B. 1950. *Biological Actions of the Adenine Nucleotides*. Lewis, London.

Griffith, S., Meghji, P., Moody, C. J., and Burnstock, G. 1981. 8-Phenyltheophylline: A potent adenosine antagonist. *Eur. J. Pharmacol., 75:*61–64.

Hammer, R., Berrie, C. P., Birdsall, N. J. M., Burgen, A. S. V., and Hulme, E. C. 1980. Pirenzepine distinguishes between different subclasses of muscarinic receptors. *Nature, 283:*90–92.

Haslam, R. J., and Cusack, N. J. 1981. Blood platelet receptors for ADP and for adenosine. In: *Purinergic receptors*, pp. 221–285. Ed. by Burnstock, G. Chapman and Hall, London.

Henon, B. K., and McAfee, D. A. 1983. The ionic basis of adenosine receptor actions on postganglionic neurones in the rat. *J. Physiol. (Lond.), 336:*607–620.

Hogaboom, G. K., O'Donnell, J. P., and Fedan, J. S. 1980. Purinergic receptors: Photoaffinity analog of adenosine triphosphate is a specific adenosine triphosphate antagonist. *Science, 208:*1273–1276.

Kasakov, L., and Burnstock, G. 1983. The use of the slowly degradable analog, α, β-methylene ATP, to produce desensitization of the P_2-purinoceptor: Effect on non-adrenergic, non-cholinergic responses of the guinea-pig urinary bladder. *Eur. J. Pharmacol., 86:*291–294.

Kennedy, C., and Burnstock, G. 1984. Evidence for an inhibitory pre-junctional P_1-purinoceptor, with characteristics of the A_2-subtype, in the rat portal vein. *Eur. J. Pharmacol., 100:*363–368.

Kusachi, S., Thompson, R. D., and Olsson, R. A. 1983. Ligand selectivity of dog coronary adenosine receptors resembles that of adenylate cyclase stimulatory (R_a) receptors. *J. Pharmacol. Exp. Ther., 227:*316–321.

Lands, A. M., Arnold, A., McAuliff, J. P., Ludena, F. P., and Brown, T. G. 1967. Differentiation of receptor systems activated by sympathomimetic amines. *Nature, 214:*597–598.

Lenschow, V., Hüttemann, E., Ukena, D., and Schwabe, U. 1982. Study of R_a adenosine receptors in human platelets by radioligand binding. *Naunyn-Schmiedebergs Arch. Pharmacol., 321* (Suppl.): R31.

Londos, C., Cooper, D. M. F., and Wolff, J. 1980. Subclasses of external adenosine receptors, *Proc. Natl. Acad. Sci. USA, 77:*2551–2554.

Malbon, C. C., Hert, R. C., and Fain, J. N. 1978. Characterization of [^{3}H]adenosine binding to fat cell membranes. *J. Biol. Chem., 253:*3114–3122.

Manery, J. F., and Dryden, E. E. 1979. Ecto-enzymes concerned with nucleotide metabolism. In: *Physiology and Regulatory Functions of Adenosine and Adenine Nucleotides*, pp. 323–339. Ed. by Baer, H. P., and Drummond, G. I. Raven Press, New York.

Meldrum, L., and Burnstock, G. 1983. Evidence that ATP acts as a co-transmitter with noradrenaline in sympathetic nerves supplying the guinea-pig vas deferens. *Eur. J. Pharmacol., 92:*161–163.

Mistry, G., and Drummond, G. I. 1983. Effects of adenosine, its analogs, adrenergic agents, and prostaglandins on adenylate cyclase of heart microvessels. In: *Regulatory Functions of Adenosine*, p. 529. Ed. by Berne, R. M., Rall, T. W., and Rubio, R. Martinus Nijhoff, Boston.

Moody, C. M., Meghji, P., and Burnstock, G. 1984. Stimulation of P_1-purinoceptors by ATP depends partly on its conversion to AMP and adenosine and partly on direct action. *Eur. J. Pharmacol., 97:*55–65.

Murphy, K. M. M., and Snyder, S. H. 1981. Adenosine receptors in rat testes: Labeling with [^{3}H]cyclohexyladenosine. *Life Sci., 28:*917–920.

Newman, M., and Levitzki, A. 1982. Characteristics of high-affinity binding to rat brain synaptosomes and turkey erythrocyte membranes. *Biochim. Biophys. Acta, 685:*129–136.

Newman, M. E., Patel, J., and McIlwain, H. 1981. The binding of adenosine to synaptosomal and other preparations from the mammalian brain. *Biochem. J., 194:*611–620.

Olsson, R. A., and Kusachi, S. 1983. Adenosine (Ado) initiates coronary relaxation via adenylate cyclase-associated stimulatory (R_a) receptors In: *Regulatory Functions of Adenosine*, p. 532. Ed. by Berne, R. M., Rall, T. W., and Rubio, A. Martinus Nijhoff, Boston.

Paterson, A. R. P., Lau, E. Y., Dahlig, E., and Cass, C. E. 1980. A common basis for inhibition of nucleoside transport by dipyridamole and nitrobenzylthioninosine? *Mol. Pharmacol., 18:*40–44.

Paton, D. M. 1981. Structure-activity relations for presynaptic inhibition of noradrenergic and cholinergic transmission by adenosine: evidence for action on A_1 receptors. *J. Auton. Pharmacol., 1:*287–290.

Paton, D. M. 1983. Evidence for A_1 receptors for adenosine in heart and in adrenergic and cholinergic nerves. In: *Physiology and Pharmacology of Adenosine Derivatives*, pp. 275–290 Ed. by Daly, J. W., Kuroda, Y., Phillis, J. W., and Ui, M. Raven Press, New York.

Paton, D. M., and Kurahashi, K. 1981. Structure-activity relations for negative chronotropic action of adenosine in isolated rat atria: Evidence for an action on A_1 receptors. *IRCS Med. Sci., 9:*447.

Phillis, J. W., and Wu, P. H. 1982. The role of adenosine and its nucleotides in central synaptic transmission. *Progr. Neurobiol., 16:*187–239.

Phillis, J. W., and Wu, P. H. 1983. Roles of adenosine and adenine nucleotides in the central nervous system. In: *Physiology and Pharmacology of Adenosine Derivatives*, pp. 219–236. Ed. by Daly, J. W., Kuroda, Y., Phillis, J. W., Shimizu, H., and Ui, M. Raven Press, New York.

Plunkett, W., Alexander, L., Chubb, S., and Loo, T. L. 1979. Comparison of the activity of 2′-deoxycoformycin and etythro-9-(2-hydroxy-3-nonyl) adenine *in vivo*. *Biochem. Pharmacol., 28:*201–206.

Reddingon, M., and Schubert, P. 1979. Parallel investigations of the effects of adenosine on evoked potentials and cyclic AMP accumulation in hippocampus slices of the rat. *Neurosci. Lett., 14:*37–42.

Reddington, M., Lee, K. S., and Schubert, P. 1982. An A_1-adenosine receptor, characterized by [^{3}H]cyclohexyladenosine binding, mediates the depression of evoked potentials in a rat hippocampal slice preparation. *Neurosci. Lett., 28:*275–279.

Rodbell, M. 1980. The role of hormone receptors and GTP regulatory proteins in membrane transduction. *Nature, 284:*17–22.

Rubin, R. P. 1970. The role of Ca^{2+} in the release of neurotransmitter substances and hormones. *Pharmacol. Rev., 22:*389–428.

Schrader, J., Rubio, R., and Berne, R. M. 1975. Inhibition of slow action potentials of guinea-pig atrial muscle by adenosine: A possible effect on Ca^{2+} influx. *J. Mol. Cell Cardiol., 7*:427–433.

Schuba, M. F., and Vladimirova, I. A. 1980. Effect of apamin on the electrical responses of smooth muscle to adenosine-5′-triphosphate and to non-adrenergic, non-cholinergic nerve stimulation. *Neuroscience, 5*:853–859

Schütz, W., and Brugger, G. 1982. Characterization of [^{3}H]adenosine binding to media membranes of hog carotid arteries. *Pharmacology, 24*:26–34.

Schütz, W., Steurer, G., and Tuisl, E. 1982a, Functional identification of adenylate cyclase-coupled adenosine receptors in rat brain microvessels. *Eur. J. Pharmacol., 85*:177–184.

Schütz, W., Tuisl, E., and Kraupp, O. 1982b. Adenosine receptor agonists: Binding and adenylate cyclase stimulation in rat liver plasma membranes. *Naunyn Schmiedebergs Arch. Pharmacol., 319*:34–39.

Schwabe, U. 1983. General aspects of binding of ligands to adenosine receptors. In: *Regulatory Functions of Adenosine*, pp. 77–96. Ed. by Berne, R. M., Rall, T. W., and Rubio, R. Martinus Nijhoff, Boston.

Schwabe, U., and Trost, T. 1980. Characterization of adenosine receptors in rat brain by (−)[^{3}H]N^6-phenylisopropyladenosine. *Naunyn Schmiedebergs Arch. Pharmacol., 313*:179–187.

Schwabe, U., Kiffe, H., Puchstein, C., and Trost, T. 1979. Specific binding of [^{3}H]adenosine to rat brain membranes. *Naunyn Schmiedebergs Arch. Pharmacol., 310*:59–67.

Skolnick, P., Nimitkitpaison, Y., Stalvey, L., and Daly, J. W. 1978. Inhibition of brain adenosine deaminase by 2′-deoxycoformycin and erythro-9-(2-hydroxy-3-nonyl)adenine. *J. Neurochem., 30*:1579–1582.

Smellie, F. W., Daly, J. W., Dunwiddie, T. V., and Hoffer, B. J. 1979. The dextro and laevorotatory isomers of *N*-phenylisopropyladenosine: Stereospecific effects on cyclic AMP formation and evoked responses in brain slices, *Life Sci., 25*:1739–1748.

Sneddon, P., and Burnstock, G. 1984. Inhibition of excitatory junction potentials in guinea-pig vas deferens by α,β-methylene-ATP: Further evidence for ATP and noradrenaline as cotramsmitters. *Eur. J. Pharmacol., 100*:85–90.

Snyder, S. H., Katims, J. J., Annau, Z., Bruns, R. F., and Daly, J. W. 1981. Adenosine receptors and behavioral actions of methylxanthines. *Proc. Natl. Acad. Sci. USA, 78*:3260–3264.

Stone, T. W. 1983. Purine receptors in the rat annococcygeus muscle. *J. Physiol. (Lond.), 335*:591–608.

Su, C. 1981. Purinergic receptors in blood vessels. In: *Purinergic Receptors*, pp. 93–117. Ed. by Burnstock, G. Chapman and Hall, London.

Triggle, D. J., and Triggle, C. R. 1976. The molecular basis of neurotransmitter–receptor interactions. In: *Chemical Pharmacology of the Synapse*, pp. 431–594. Ed. by Triggle, D. J. and Triggle, C. R. Academic Press, London.

Trost, T., and Schwabe, U. 1981. Adenosine receptors in fat cells. Identification by (−)-N^6-[^{3}H]phenylisopropyladenosine binding. *Mol. Pharmacol., 19*:228–235.

Turnheim, K., Plank, B., and Kolassa, N. 1978. Inhibition of adenosine uptake in human erythrocytes by adenosine-5′-carboxamides, xylosyladenine, dipyridamole, hexobendine and p-nitrobenzylthioguanosine. *Biochem. Pharmacol., 27*:2191–2197.

Ukena, D., Martens, D., and Schwabe, U. 1982. Specific binding of 5′-N-ethylcarboxamide[^{3}H]adenosine to calf thymocyte membranes. *Naunyn-Schmiedeberg's Arch. Pharmacol., 321 (Suppl.)*:R38.

Van Calker, D., Muller, M., and Hamprecht, B. 1979. Adenosine regulates via two different types of receptors, the accumulation of cyclic AMP in cultured brain cells. *J. Neurochem., 33*:999–1005.

Vapaatalo, H., Bieck, P., and Westerman, E. 1971. Action of phenylisopropyladenosine (PIA) on the synthesis of corticosterone. *Naunyn Schmiedebergs Arch. Pharmacol., 269*:465–466.

Vapaatalo, H., Onken, D., Neuvonen, P. J., and Westermann, E. 1975. Stereospecificity in some central and circulatory effects of phenylisopropyladenosine (PIA), *Arzneimittelforsch., 25*:407–410.

Williams, M., and Risley, E. A. 1980. Biochemical characterization of putative central purinergic receptors by using 2-chloro[^{3}H]adenosine, a stable analog of adenosine. *Proc. Natl. Acad. Sci. USA, 77*:6892–6896.

Wojcik, W. J., and Neff, N. H. 1983. Differential location of adenosine A_1 and A_2 receptors in striatum. *Neurosci. Lett., 41*:55–60.

Wu, P. H., and Phillis, J. W. 1982. Adenosine receptors in rat brain membranes: characterization of high affinity binding of [^{3}H]-2-chloroadenosine. *Int. J. Biochem., 14*:399–404.

Wu, P. H., Phillis, J. W., Balls, K., and Rinaldi, B. 1980. Specific binding of 2-[^{3}H]chloroadenosine to rat brain cortical membranes. *Can. J. Physiol. Pharmacol., 58*:576–579.

Wu, P. H., Phillis, J. W., and Thierry, D. L. 1982. Adenosine receptor agonists inhibit K^+-evoked Ca^{2+} uptake by rat brain cortical synaptosomes. *J. Neurochem., 39*:700–708.

Chapter **12**

The Pharmacologic Estimation of Potencies of Agonists and Antagonists in the Classification of Adenosine Receptors

Terry P. Kenakin and H. J. Leighton

Department of Pharmacology
The Wellcome Research Laboratories
Burroughs Wellcome Company
Research Triangle Park, North Carolina

I. THE STUDY OF ADENOSINE RECEPTORS IN ISOLATED TISSUES

A. Receptor Classification

This chapter outlines some of the methods used to quantitate drug effects in isolated tissues for the purposes of adenosine receptor classification. There are advantages and disadvantages to studying adenosine receptors in isolated tissues. The disadvantages are that numerous pharmacokinetic factors and reflex mechanisms make extrapolation of isolated tissue data to whole animals and man hazardous. Also, the quantitative parameters for drugs are calculated from models assuming an equilibrium between the drugs and the receptors, which is a condition often not obtained in intact tissues. However, these factors are balanced by two major advantages. If it is assumed that the independent variable in pharmacologic experiments is drug concentration and the dependent variable is tissue response, experiments in isolated tissues allow adequate control of the independent variable (under careful experimental conditions) such that meaningful dependent variables can be obtained. Also, quantitative estimates of agonist efficacy, a quantity currently inaccessible in biochemical binding studies, can be obtained from experiments in isolated tissues. Thus, drug affinity and efficacy can be quantified and used in the classification of adenosine receptors.

The circular nature of this classification process should not be forgotten, i.e., new experimental purine receptor subtypes are discovered only after the discovery of new experimental selective drugs for purine receptors. Thus, the criteria for definition of selective drugs should be stringent to avoid the proliferation of bogus receptor subtypes that may only reflect differences between tissues. The quantitation of parameters that reflect drug–receptor interaction (affinity, efficacy) rather than drug–tissue interaction (potency, intrinsic activity) are required for the orderly classification of purine receptors. The null methods devised to measure affinity and efficacy are specifically designed to cancel tissue factors and yield receptor-related parameters.

B. Receptor and Tissue Factors

As a starting point, the definition of what is meant by tissue and receptor factors will given. Tissue factors are considered to be (1) any uptake, degradation process that produces a disparity between the concentration of drug in the organ bath and that at the drug receptor, (2) the number of viable drug receptors in the tissue, and (3) the efficiency of the stimulus–response mechanisms that translate the stimulus from the receptors into tissue response. The parameters reflecting the molecular interactions of drugs with receptors are (1) K_A, the equilibrium dissociation constant of the drug for the drug receptor and (2) intrinsic efficacy (ϵ, Furchgott, 1966), a measure of the ability of an agonist to produce a stimulus (Stephenson, 1956) from a single drug receptor. Tissue factors can be variable between organs that have identical purine receptors. This variability can profoundly affect the outcome of attempts to obtain meaningful estimates of parameters which reflect drug and receptor interaction.

The control of tissue factors is a prerequisite to the effective quantification of drug receptor effects; therefore, as a preface to the discussion of K_A and ϵ, the controllable aspects of these tissue factors will be considered. Foremost among these are the uptake and degradation processes for purines in isolated tissues.

II. AGONIST REMOVAL MECHANISMS

A. Tissue Sensitization to Agonists

If there is a removal mechanism for the agonist in a tissue, then the steady-state concentration of the agonist at the receptor is controlled by the rate of diffusion into the receptor compartment and the rate of uptake (or removal) out of the receptor compartment. Various models have been devised that allow calculation of the effects of agonist-uptake processes on the observed potency of agonists (Waud, 1969a; Furchgott, 1972; Furchgott *et al.*, 1973; Ebner and Waud, 1978; Kenakin, 1980a, 1981, 1982a; Ebner, 1981). In general these models, which are similar, equate the rate of entry of drug into the receptor compartment (a bulk diffusion phenomenom) to the rate of removal from the receptor compartment (assumed to be a process following Michaelis–Menten kinetics). Thus, the rate of entry (R_{in}) equals (Waud, 1969a; Furchgott, 1972)

$$R_{\text{in}} = k_t([A]_o - [A]_i) \tag{1}$$

where k_t is a bulk diffusion constant, $[A]_o$ and $[A]_i$ refer to the molar concentrations of agonist in the organ bath and receptor compartment, respectively, and R_{out} equals

$$R_{\text{out}} = \frac{[A]_i \cdot V_{\max}}{[A]_i + K_m\left(1 + \frac{[I]}{K_I}\right)} \tag{2}$$

where $V_{\max}$ and K_m describe the maximal velocity of uptake and Michaelis–Menten constant for uptake of the agonist and $[I]$ and K_I refer to the molar concentration of uptake inhibitor and equilibrium dissociation constant of the inhibitor for the site of uptake. It can be shown that (Kenakin, 1980a, 1981)

$$x = \frac{[A]}{[A']} = \frac{y\left(1 + \frac{[I]}{K_I}\right)}{y + \frac{[I]}{K_I}} \tag{3}$$

where $[A]$ and $[A']$ refer to equiactive agonist concentrations before and after uptake inhibitors and x is the observed sensitization of a tissue to the agonist. The maximal sensitization (y) to the agonist, which would be observed if the uptake process was completely inhibited, is defined as (Furchgott, 1972)

$$y = \frac{V_{\max}}{k_t \cdot K_m} \cdot \frac{1}{\left(1 + \frac{[A]_i}{K_m}\right)} + 1 \tag{4}$$

The dependence of maximal sensitization on $V_{\max}$ *and* k_t, and hence the maximal effect of uptake on any agonist in a tissue, is shown by equation 4. Figure 1 shows the theoretical effects of uptake in two tissues, both with identical uptake processes with respect to K_m and $V_{\max}$ but with different kinetics of diffusion (the diffusion agonist into tissue I is 10 times faster than into tissue II; k_t tissue I = 10 × k_t tissue II). Comparing curves A and C in Figure 1, it can be seen that the inhibition of uptake produces 10 times the sensitization in the tissue with the slower diffusion. Such disparities in diffusion could be the result of muscle geometry, the mathematical expression of which has variously been expressed as a tortuosity factor λ (diffusion rate = rate of free diffusion ÷ λ^2 [Venter, 1978]) and V/S, the volume-to-surface ratio of an isolated tissue preparation (Ebner and

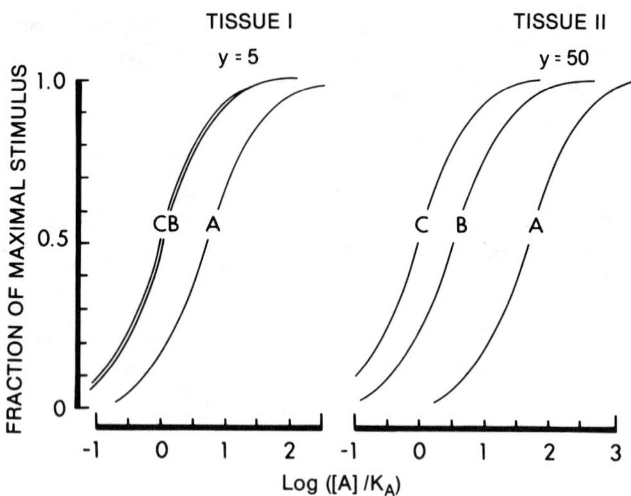

Figure 1. Effects of uptake inhibition on concentration–response curves to agonists. Ordinates: responses as a fraction of the maximal response. Abscissae: logarithms of molar concentration of agonist expressed as a fraction of the equilibrium dissociation constant of the agonist for the receptor. The maximal sensitization obtainable in tissue I is 5 and in tissue II is 50. (A) Concentration–response curve in the absence of uptake inhibitor, (B) in the presence of $[I]/K_I = 30$, and (C) when uptake is completely inhibited.

Waud, 1978). Differences in these factors are encompassed by the general term k_t in equation 4.

It would be predicted that in a tissue with restricted diffusion, even a weak uptake process could produce a sizable disparity between $[A]_i$ and $[A]_o$. An example of how important diffusion and uptake, working in concert, can be in the control of observed agonist response is shown in Figure 2. In guinea pig ileum, 2′-deoxyadenosine is converted from a partial agonist to a full agonist by inhibition of uptake. Clearly, the effects of uptake and degradation processes on purine agonists can vary between tissue types and even within the same tissue type if differences in animal weight or age lead to heterogeneity in the V/S of tissues. For example, Ebner and Waud (1978) have shown a correlation between V/S and β-adrenoceptor agonist potency within cat papillary muscles that reflects differences in the effect of an uptake process as a function of diffusion of agonist.

B. The Effective Inhibition of Agonist Uptake Processes

A prediction of this model, supported by experiment, is the dependence of sensitization of tissues to agonists upon two factors: the concentration of uptake inhibitor and the magnitude of y, the maximal sensitization of the tissue to the agonist. Specifically, the larger is y, the more uptake inhibitor is required to effectively neutralize the uptake process. This can be illustrated by calculations using equation 3. Figure 1 shows that for tissue I ($y = 5$) and tissue II ($y = 50$), the effects of the same concentration of uptake inhibitor ($[I]/K_I = 30$) differ considerably. Thus, for tissue I, this concentration of uptake inhibitor is sufficient

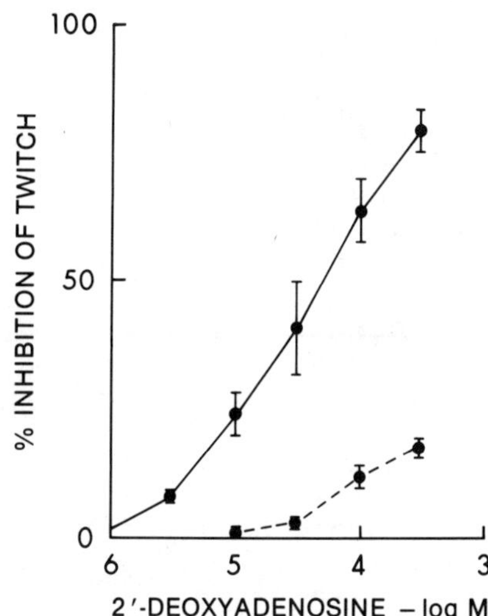

Figure 2. Effect of 2′-deoxyadenosine in the absence (●– – –●) and presence of dipyridamole (0.2 μm, ●——●) on twitch response of the guinea ileum elicited by a 0.1-Hz stimulus.

to produce very near maximal sensitization while submaximal sensitization is produced in tissue II. Given a range of tissues with different uptake and diffusion characteristics such that y varies from 2 to 50, Figure 3A shows the dependence of sensitization upon the concentration of uptake inhibitor. This has relevance to drug receptor classification if agonist potency ratios (*see below*) are used quantitatively when one or both of the agonists is taken up by the tissue. Figure 3B shows the dependence of the potency ratios for two agonists, only one of which is taken up by the tissue, on the concentration of uptake inhibitor. The differences observed as a function of the maximal sensitization serve as a caveat to the extrapolation of effective concentations of inhibitors for purine uptake and degradation mechanisms from one tissue to another.

A logarithmic metameter of equation 3 can be used to calculate the K_I for an uptake inhibitor in an isolated tissue (Kenakin, 1981):

$$\log\left[\frac{y(x-1)}{y-x}\right] = \log[I] - \log K_I \tag{5}$$

This equation is based on the premise that since sensitization of tissues to agonists (x) is dependent upon $[I]/K_I$ and since $[I]$ is known, then K_I can be calculated from the observed sensitization as a function of $[I]$ and the maximal sensitizations. Figure 4 shows an example of the use of this method to quantify the inhibition of adenosine uptake in guinea pig atria by diazepam.

C. Mechanisms of Purine Uptake

To discuss the effective inhibition of agonist uptake processes for adenosine and related derivatives requires a consideration of the mechanism of uptake and its relationship to the purine riboside metabolizing enzymes. As discussed in gen-

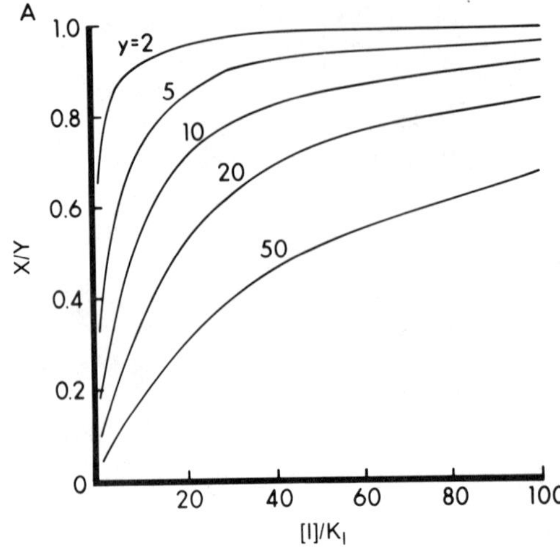

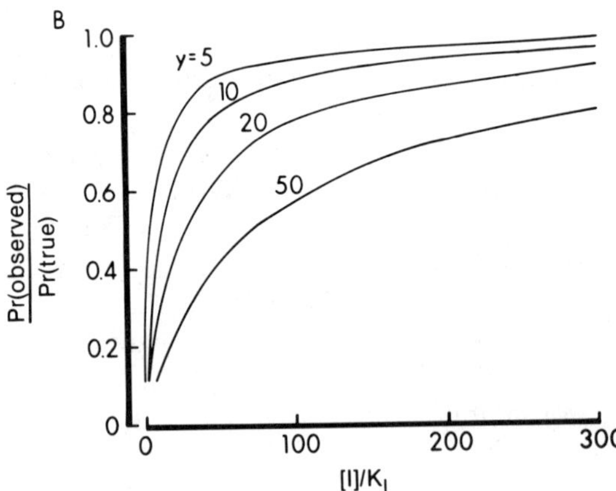

Figure 3. Tissue sensitization and potency ratios as functions of uptake inhibition. (A) Ordinates: fraction of total sensitization of tissues to an agonist. Abscissae: molar concentrations of uptake inhibitor as multiples of the equilibrium dissociation constant of the uptake inhibitor for the site of uptake. Sensitization shown for tissues for which the maximal sensitization varies from 2 to 50. (B) Ordinates: potency ratios for two agonists, one of which is removed from the receptor compartment by an uptake process, expressed as fractions of the true potency ratio obtained in the absence of uptake. Abscissae: as for 3A. Ratios of potency ratios in tissues for which the maximal sensitization varies from 5 to 50. From Kenakin (1980a) with permission.

eral terms above, the first step in the process of accurately estimating potencies and classifying purine receptor types in a tissue is to inhibit the uptake and metabolism of the purine agonist. Although some species differences exist, most tissues have a very effective transport system for adenosine and related nucleotides. Adenosine nucleotide transport has the characteristics of facilitated diffusion; the uptake process proceeds because of the ensuing metabolism of adenosine by adenosine deaminase (EC 3.5.4.6) to inosine, adenosine kinase (EC 21.1.20) to adenosine monophosphate, and *S*-adenosylhomocysteine hydrolase (EC 3.3.1.1) to *S*-adenosylhomocysteine. The V_{max} for adenosine uptake will in part depend on the activity of these enzymes in the particular cell type, as well as on the complicated further metabolism of these products to hypoxanthine, xanthine, uric acid, ADP, ATP, dADP, dATP, and IMP whose production results in various positive and negative biochemical feedback factors on the primary metabolism enzymes. V_{max} will also depend on the number of transport carrier molecules. A

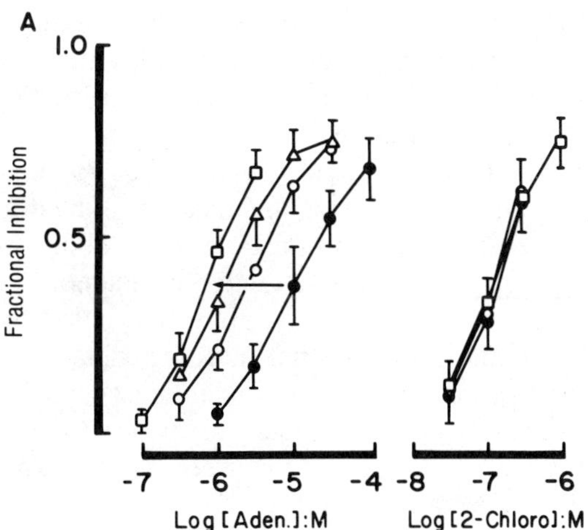

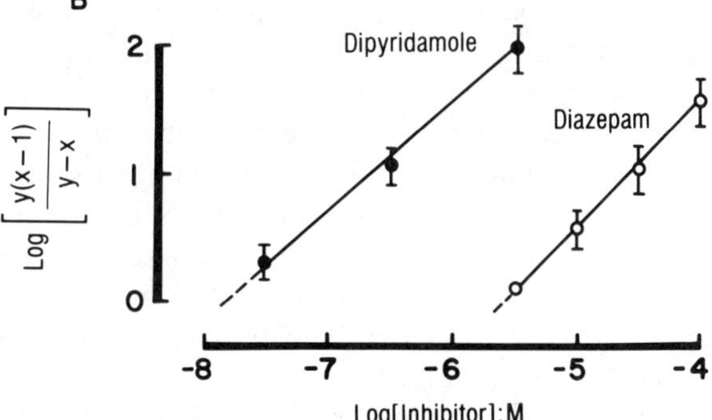

Figure 4. Inhibition of adenosine uptake in guinea pig left atria by diazepam and dipyridamole. (A) Ordinates: Depression of electrically stimulated contractions of left atria expressed as fractions of basal contractions. Abscissae: logarithms of molar concentrations of either adenosine or 2-chloradenosine. Responses in the absence (●, n = 6) and presence of diazepam 10 μM (○, n = 5), 30 μM (△, n = 4), and 100 μM (□, n = 5). Corresponding symbols and values of n for 2 chloroadenosine (2-Chloro). Arrow represents direction of movement of concentration–response curves to adenosine with increasing concentrations of diazepam. (B) Ordinates: sensitization to adenosine expressed as in equation 5. Abscissae: logarithms of molar concentrations of either dipyridamole or diazepam. Regressions for dipyridamole (●, n = 8) and diazepam (○, n = 15). Broken lines are extensions of regression lines to intercept indicating the pK_I. Bars represent S.E.M. From Kenakin (1981) with permission.

single carrier is thought to transport all purine nucleosides, although each purine has its own K_m for the carrier. Thus, when we consider inhibition of agonist removal from the receptor compartment, several important factors come into play, e.g., number of carrier molecules, maximal velocity of agonist metabolism by enzymes, and the K_m of the agonist for the carrier. Since these are multiplicative processes, an agonist may appear very weak or very potent depending on the importance of these mechanisms in the tissue.

The above-mentioned tissue factors associated with uptake (i.e., number of carrier molecules, activity of metabolizing enzymes) contribute to the degree of sensitization seen with an agonist that is a substrate for uptake/metabolism. These factors probably contribute to the species differences and tissue differences on uptake. For example, the apparent uptake (or capacity for metabolism) is very negligible in the following preparations: guinea pig taenia coli (Maguire and Satchell, 1979), rat heart (Stafford, 1966; Hopkins and Goldie, 1971; Kolassa *et al.*, 1971), and rabbit intestine (Stafford, 1966). In other preparations (e.g., guinea pig ileum and atria), apparent uptake is very important and may alter order of potency measurements. *In vivo* uptake and metabolism varies greatly: Uptake was found to be greatest in the chicken, less in humans and pigs, much less in dogs, rats, guinea pigs, sheep and goats, and essentially insignificant in cows and horses (Van Belle, 1969). Although all cells are believed to remove adenosine from the extracellular space, the actual inhibition of uptake may be secondary to the inhibition of the metabolizing enzymes that drive the diffusion process. Inhibition of uptake may be secondary to blockade of metabolizing enzymes. For example, Hopkins and Goldie (1971) suggest that dipyridamole blocks uptake of adenosine in guinea pig hearts by inhibiting its phosphorylation by membrane-bound kinase.

Another enzyme that may contribute to the various differences noted with purine agonists is ecto-5′-nucleotidase (EC 3.1.3.5), an enzyme that degrades 5′-phosphate to purine ribosides. In some tissues, this enzyme is very active and has greatly complicated the assessment of whether 5′-purine riboside phosphates, e.g., ATP, can function as direct agonists or must first be degraded to purine ribosides. This issue is complicated further by the fact that in certain tissues, ATP may be taken up intact (Chaundry, 1982). Thus it may be concluded that order of potency studies or potency ratio studies would be expected to produce disparate data if uptake and metabolism factors are not carefully controlled.

Two approaches have been used to account for the vagaries of uptake and metabolism. One is to use agonists that are not substrates for uptake, a factor determined indirectly from studies comparing the potency of the agonist in the presence and absence of uptake inhibitors. Thus, lack of tissue sensitization in the presence of an uptake inhibitor implies poor uptake characteristics for the agonist. It is interesting to note that most agonists that are not substrates for uptake are also very poor substrates for metabolism. Thus *N*-6-substituted adenosine derivatives (e.g., *N*-6–phenylisopropyladenosine; PIA) are generally potent agonists, unaffected by uptake inhibitors and poor substrates for adenosine deaminase. Adenosine derivatives substituted with a 2-halo-derivatives (e.g., 2-chloroadenosine) are poor substrates for adenosine kinase, unaffected by uptake inhibitors and potent agonists. The other major structural modification that improves potency are 5′-substitutions (e.g., NECA). In the latter case, NECA is a poor substrate for adenosine kinase. Therefore, potency ratios or order of potency measurements may often be a measure of enzymatic metabolism as much as affinity for the uptake carrier.

Ideally, one would want to employ a purine nucleotide uptake inhibitor that functioned only to block the carrier involved in uptake. An analogy to the catecholamine system is appropriate. The use of cocaine to block uptake 1 and estradiol to block uptake 2 are preferred over tricyclics and metanephrine because the latter two inhibitors also antagonize α, β, muscarinic, histamine H_1, and, possibly, H_2 receptors and in the case of amitriptylene inhibit phosphodiesterase. Depending on the degree of sensitization, one may need to use up 100 times the K_I for uptake to effectively eliminate uptake in some tissues. Therefore, the choice of purine uptake inhibitor should be the one which has the least secondary actions relative to its K_I for uptake.

D. Inhibitors of Purine Uptake

Agents commonly used to block uptake include the coronary vasodilators dipyridamole, lidoflazine, and hexobendine and nitrobenzylthioguanosine (NBG) and nitrobenzylthioinosine. Less commonly used agents include *p*-chloromercuribenzoate, *N*-ethylmaleimide (suggesting that sulfhydryl groups are involved in the uptake mechanism), papaverine, flurazepam, and morphine (Bender *et al.*, 1981), and diazepam (Clanachan and Marshall, 1980; Kenakin, 1981; and Phillis *et al.*, 1980) and a variety of purines including cytidine, inosine, guanosine, uridine, thymidine, formycin, and tubercidin (Bender *et al.*, 1981). Of the above uptake inhibitors, dipyridamole and nitrobenzylthioguanosine are the most commonly used inhibitors in receptor studies. However, their selectivity and potency for uptake inhibition are not comparable. The nitrobenzylthioinosines and guanosines have reported K_I values ranging between 0.15 nM and 0.97 nM (Cass *et al.*, 1974; Marangos *et al.*, 1982; Jarvis and Young, 1980). The K_I value for dipyridamole has been reported to be lower (0.85 μM; Marangos *et al.*, 1982). Relative to the K_I for uptake inhibition, dipyridamole appears to have the most secondary side effects.

Dipyridamole inhibits cyclic nucleotide phosphodiesterase (PDE) and adenosine deaminase with K_I values of 16 μM for PDE (Kukovetz and Pöch, 1970) and approximately 100 μM for deaminase (Gerlach and Deuticke, 1963). Additionally, dipyridamole inhibits particulate adenosine kinase, K_I approximately 5 μM (Hopkins and Goldie, 1971), as well as monosaccharide transport (Renner *et al.*, 1972) and choline transport (Plagemann and Roth, 1969). In addition to being more potent, the nitrobenzylthio derivatives apparently have fewer side effects, i.e., are not inhibitors of base of glucose transport (Paterson *et al.*, 1983) and do not directly affect nucleotide metabolism.

The secondary actions of dipyridamole occur in some cases at less than 10 times the apparent K_I for uptake inhibition. Although the mechanism of uptake inhibition does appear to be independent of purine riboside metabolism, certain secondary effects, i.e., PDE inhibition and inhibition of purine base and glucose transport may make this inhibitor unsuitable for quantitative receptor analysis in tissues where PDE inhibition affects the response of the tissue (e.g., heart, various vascular tissues, and catecholamine release). The effects on choline uptake may also alter cholinergic mechanisms. Several investigators have reported an apparent sensitizaton of the purine receptor to dipyridamole. For example, Dowdle and Maske (1980) suggested that dipyridamole/adenosine followed a pattern of facilitated agonist competition. A similar suggestion was made by Paton (1981). Based on the available side effect data, the nitrothiobenzyl derivatives seem to be the best agents to specifically block uptake. Unfortunately, until recently much of the work in the literature has employed dipyridamole as the uptake inhibitor of choice because the other agents were not commercially available.

Assuming that uptake is effectively neutralized and $[A]_i = [A]_o$, then concentration–response curves to a purine agonist should reflect the interaction of these agonists with receptors and the subsequent interaction of the resulting stimulus with the stimulus–response mechanism of the tissue. However, when dealing with partial agonists, other tissue factors become important.

III. COMPARISON OF RECEPTORS BY AGONISTS

A. General Considerations

To derive information strictly pertaining to the interaction of the agonist with the receptor (essential for drug receptor classification), null techniques must be used that eliminate influences of different receptor number and efficiency of coupling of receptors between various tissue types. For example, the intrinsic activity of an agonist (maximal response) is critically dependent upon these tissue factors and should not be used in receptor classification. Differences in these tissue factors alone can cause drugs to be full agonists, partial agonists, or antagonists in various tissues. This fact should essentially preclude the comparison of maximal responses of partial agonists between different tissues for receptor classification.

The potency ratio of a full and partial agonist is not independent of tissue factors such as receptor number and the efficiency of the coupling between stimulus and response and therefore should not be used to classify receptors. Specifically, differences in the efficiency of stimulus–response relationships will produce lateral shifts of the concentration–response curves along the concentration axis to full agonists and little shift but rather a change in the maximal responses to partial agonists. Thus, since the potency ratio is derived from the relative positions of concentration–response curves to agonists along the concentration axis, more than one potency ratio can be obtained for a full and partial agonist in two tissues with identical receptors but differences in receptor reserve for the full agonist (for example, see Fig. 1 in Furchgott, 1972).

Thus, the comparison of full agonists offers the most unambiguous method of receptor classification by agonists. Assuming that there is a receptor reserve for two agonists A_1 and A_2 ($K_{A1} > [A_1]$ and $K_{A2} > [A_2]$), and that response is a single valued function of stimulus, and stimulus $S = \epsilon \cdot \rho \, [R_t]$ where ϵ is the intrinsic efficacy (Furchgott, 1966), ρ the fractional receptor occupancy, and $[R_t]$ the total receptor number, then

$$S_1 = \frac{\epsilon_1[A_1]}{K_{A1}} \text{ and } S_2 = \frac{\epsilon_2[A_2]}{K_{A2}} \tag{6}$$

Therefore, the potency ratio (pr) of the two full agonists is given in

$$pr = \frac{[A_1]}{[A_2]} = \frac{\epsilon_2 \cdot K_{A1}}{\epsilon_1 \cdot K_{A2}} \tag{7}$$

Thus the potency ratio reflects agonist receptor parameters that are independent of tissue factors. This is contingent upon the fact that there be a receptor reserve in the tissues and $[A] < K_A$. Under these circumstances, the magnitude of the potency ratio is unique for agonist–receptor combinations and is a valuable drug receptor parameter. As such, PR should be utilized quantitatively rather than order of potency, which is a crude and possibly misleading quantity.

B. Classification of Purine Receptors with Agonists

Although the quantitative comparison of potency ratios of full agonists offers the most theoretically sound approach to purine receptor classification to date, a great deal of literature presents data on rank order of potency of full and partial agonists (often with no regard to uptake and metabolism). The caveats regarding these approaches should be kept in mind when this data is reviewed in terms of receptor classification.

The first attempt to classify purine receptors was made by Burnstock (1978), who based his classification of purine receptors on rank order of potency. The majority of isolated tissue studies to date have continued to use this technique. Although of a general qualitative and descriptive value, this approach is subject to numerous errors. More sophisticated approaches such as measurement of agonist affinity and efficacy have not been studied in isolated tissues.

The present state of the art suggests that there are two cell surface purine receptors: one receptor site has the rank order adenosine $>$ 5′-substituted phosphates (ATP); the other has the rank order ATP $>$ ADP $\simeq$ AMP $\simeq$ adenosine. Activation of the receptor defined as adenosine $>$ ATP generally leads to inhibition (i.e., relaxation, negative inotropy and chronotropism, and inhibition of adrenergic and cholinergic transmission). These responses are antagonized in a qualitative fashion by theophylline and derivatives. Activation of the other putative receptor is associated with excitatory effects (e.g., contraction of the trachea, bladder, parts of the intestine, and uterus and increases in chronotropism). The latter effects apparently are not antagonized by theophylline.

The following examples serve to illustrate how rank order of potency studies may lead to confusion in the literature. In studies using the guinea pig fundus Okwuasaba *et al.* (1977) ranked purine agonists in the following order: ATP $>$ ADP $>$ adenosine. The rank order suggests a P_2 or A_2 receptor, but all agonists were antagonized by theophylline, suggesting a P_1 or A_1 receptor. On the other hand Jager and Schevers (1980) using the guinea pig taenia caecum ranked the purine agonist in the following order of potency: ATP $\geq$ ADP $\geq$ AMP $>$ adenosine. They suggested that on this basis the taenia caecum effects were due to P_2-receptor activation. Potential errors and confusion in the literature could be greatly reduced by appropriate use of purine uptake inhibitors and converting rank order studies into potency ratio studies.

Although blockade of uptake greatly reduces potential errors in rank order of potency measurements, which are the result of metabolism, it does not eliminate metabolism as a consideration in the case of 5′-phosphates. Ecto-5′-nucleotidase (EC 3.1.3.5), a cell surface enzyme that degrades 5′-phosphates to purine ribosides, may cause tissue-dependent errors when agonist activity is assessed. In some tissues, this enzyme is very active and has greatly complicated the assessment of whether purine ribosides like ATP can function as direct agonists or must first be degraded to adenosine. The possibility also exists that ATP can be taken up directly into cells (Chaundry, 1982). When the latter case is dominant, uptake inhibitors would be expected to potentiate the action of ATP. Therefore, the observed activity with ATP or a derivative of ATP may depend on uptake and cell surface metabolism to other active purine agonists.

Most commonly, when ATP has been shown to produce inhibitory effects or is antagonized by theophylline, it has been argued that adenosine is the active agonist due to metabolism by ecto-5′-nucleotidase or pyrophosphorylases. Clearly, what is needed is a potent inhibitor of ecto-5′-nucleotidase, which is not a purine agonist. The best alternatives to date are 5′-modified phosphates, which are agonists and inhibitors of ecto-5′-nucleotidase. One of the most impressive of these agonists is α, β-methylene-ADP. Since this purine is not easily hydrolyzed to adenosine, data generated with this compound suggest that certain 5′-modified compounds may activate cell surface purine receptors.

The use of stable analogs of ATP and studies utilizing adenosine deaminase suggest that ATP can activate cell surface purine receptors without prior degradation. Maguire and Satchell (1979) found that the α,β-methylene isoteres of ATP and ADP, as well as 6′-deoxyhomoadenosine 6′-phosphonylpyrophosphate, were agonists in the guinea pig taenia coli and were not potentiated by dipyridamole. However, the βγ-methylene isosteres of ATP were potentiated by dipyridamole suggesting that ATP pyrophosphohydrolase can inactivate βγ derivatives in certain tissues. The studies have led to the use of α,β and βγ isosteres to classify purine receptors as "ATP" or "adenosine"-like. For example, α,β-methylene-ATP is inactive in the guinea pig trachea. The authors (Christie and Satchell, 1980) conclude from this study that receptors for adenosine, but not ATP, are present in the trachea. Perhaps the absence of a response does not necessarily mean absence of binding to a receptor. As an alternative explanation, α,β-methylene-ATP may be considered a weak agonist that cannot translate a response (due to efficiency of coupling) in the trachea, i.e., α,β-methylene-ADP is an antagonist in this preparation.

Another approach to the study of whether ATP or its analogs can directly activate purine receptors prior to hydrolysis is to study these compounds in the presence of adenosine deaminase. In the rat urinary bladder preparation, Dahlen and Hedqvist (1980) used this technique to compare ATP and βγ-methylene-ATP. Because exogenous adenosine deaminase blocked the inhibition by adenosine, but not ATP or βγ-methylene-ATP, the authors conclude that ATP was a direct-acting agonist. Thus, it would appear that in some tissues, ATP can directly activate purine receptors. However, the question remains whether ATP activates the same purine receptor as adenosine.

Perhaps the most compelling data suggesting that ATP and ADP activate receptors distinct from the adenosine receptor are the opposing effects (relaxation/contraction) that are observed in certain tissues. ATP and ADP have been shown to directly contract a number of preparations while inhibiting transmural stimulation. This action of ATP and ADP is usually resistant to theophylline antagonism and antagonized noncompetitively by quinidine and 2,2′-dipyridylisatogen. The contractile effects have been observed in the rat urinary bladder

(Brown *et al.*, 1979), rabbit intestine (Frew *et al.*, 1976; Frew and Baer, 1979), guinea pig urinary bladder (Burnstock *et al.*, 1972), guinea pig uterus (Moritoki *et al.*, 1979), rat portal vein (Sjöberg and Wahlström, 1975), rabbit detrusor (Jhamandas *et al.*, 1980), guinea pig vas deferens (Kazíc and Milosavlgevic 1980; Fedan *et al.*, 1981; Holck and Marks, 1978), and frog atria (Burnstock and Maghji, 1981). In general, these secondary effects tend to occur at higher concentrations than the relaxant and negative chronotropic effects. Obviously, these contractile effects complicate receptor analysis, just as, for example, α-receptor analyses with NE as an agonist without a β-adrenoceptor antagonist.

These secondary effects probably result from the stimulation of prostaglandin synthesis. As early as 1974, Needleman *et al.* noted that ATP stimulated prostaglandin synthesis. In the rabbit intestine indomethacin and the prostaglandin antagonist 7-oxa-13-prostyndic acid antagonized the contractile response of α,β-methylene-ADP (Frew and Baer, 1979). In the guinea pig uterus, the prostaglandin antagonist polyphloretin phosphate and SC 19220 blocked the contractile effects of ATP. On the other hand, the biphasic effects on heart rate noted in atrial preparations and the theophylline-resistant relaxations of the rabbit ileum probably result from the release of catecholamines. These secondary effects of ATP and its analogs, as well as the question of direct vs indirect action of ATP, have clearly hindered careful receptor analysis in various tissues. For quantitative receptor studies, we suggest that an indomethacin pretreatment be employed when studying 5′-modified adenosine phosphates. One also wonders if this secondary effect on prostaglandin synthesis could account for the stimulation of adenylate cyclase; i.e., are prostaglandins responsible for increases in cAMP accumulation after treatment with purines?

While potency ratios for full agonists are valuable quantitative parameters, it is preferable to measure K_A and relative efficacy for agonists if possible since these values are thought to reflect the molecular interactions of the agonist for purine receptors and serve as unique quantities for receptor classification.

C. Measurement of the Affinity of a Full Agonist

The method of partial alkylation of the receptors allows the estimation of K_A for a full agonist. Equiactive concentrations of full agonists before $[A]$ and after $[A']$ partial alkylation of the receptor pool (to produce partial depression of the maximal response of the full agonist) are compared in a double reciprocal regression according to the following equation (Furchgott, 1966):

$$\frac{1}{[A]} = \frac{1}{[A']}\cdot\frac{1}{q} + \frac{1}{K_A}\cdot\frac{(1-q)}{q} \tag{8}$$

Thus, the K_A can be calculated from:

$$K_A = \frac{\text{Slope} - 1}{\text{Intercept}} \tag{9}$$

It should be noted that values near the top of the concentration–response curves have been shown to give the most reliable estimate of K_A with this method (Thron, 1970).

The method for the estimation of K_A was derived strictly in terms of a reduction in receptor number by an alkylating agent. For purines, some promising photoactive alkylating agents could allow for this method to be used (Fedan *et al.*, 1983). Alternatively, functional antagonism of the responses to full agonists has been employed to estimate K_A by equation 8, the rationale for this being the similarity of effect observed with physiological antagonists and alkylating agents (Buckner and Saini, 1975; Buckner *et al.*, 1978). Although there is no theoretical justification for the use of fuctional antagonism for this purpose, recent evidence suggests that valid estimates of K_A for agonists can result (Su and Leighton, 1983).

D. Measurement of Relative Efficacy of Two Full Agonists

A comparison of the concentration–response curves to two full agonists can yield an estimate of the relative magnitude of the intrinsic efficacies of the two agonists by the method of MacKay (1966a,b). By this method, a double reciprocal plot of equiactive concentrations of the two agonists can be applied to the following equation:

$$\frac{1}{[A_1]} = \frac{1}{[A_2]} \cdot \left(\frac{K_2}{K_2} \cdot \frac{\epsilon_1}{\epsilon_2}\right) + \frac{\epsilon_1}{\epsilon_2 \cdot K_2}\left(1 - \frac{\epsilon_2}{\epsilon_1}\right) \tag{10}$$

The arthmetic sign of the intercept will indicate the relative magnitude of ϵ_2 and ϵ_1, i.e., if negative, $\epsilon_2 > \epsilon_1$ and if positive, $\epsilon_2 < \epsilon_1$. The technical difficulty of this method arises when the curves are parallel and the intercept tends towards the origin.

From this analysis it can be seen that if the equilibrium dissociation constant for one of the agonists is known, then the relative magnitudes of the intrinsic efficacies of the two agonists can be calculated from

$$\frac{\epsilon_2}{\epsilon_1} = (1 + \text{Intercept} \cdot K_1)^{-1} \tag{11}$$

Given reliable estimates of K_A for two full agonists, then the relative intrinsic efficacy of these two agonists can readily be calculated by the method of Furchgott (1966). Assuming

$$S_1 = \epsilon_1 \cdot \rho_1[R_t] \quad \text{and} \quad S_2 = \epsilon_2 \cdot \rho_2[R_t]$$

in a tissue ($[R_t]$ constant) then comparison of receptor occupancy (calculated by the adsorption isotherm and K_A) at equal responses (equal stimuli assumed) yields relative intrinsic efficacy as the relative fractions of receptor occupancy required for the two agonists to yield equal responses (Furchgott, 1966):

$$\frac{\rho_1}{\rho_2} = \frac{\epsilon_2}{\epsilon_1} \tag{12}$$

This can be achieved by plotting response as a function of logarithm of the receptor occupancy of each agonist; the separation between the curves along the abscissal scale is the logarithm of the ratio of the relative efficacy of the two agonists.

E. Measurement of the Affinity of a Partial Agonist

If it is assumed that there is a receptor reserve for the full agonist (i.e., $[A] < K_A$), then an equation analogous to that given by MacKay (equation 10) can be devised that relates equiactive concentrations of full and partial agonist (Barlow *et al.*, 1967; Waud, 1969b):

$$\frac{1}{[A]} = \frac{\epsilon_A}{\epsilon_P} \cdot \frac{K_P}{K_A} \cdot \frac{1}{[P]} + \frac{\epsilon_A}{\epsilon_P} \cdot \frac{1}{K_A} \tag{13}$$

Thus, K_P can be calculated by K_P = slope ÷ intercept.

If the assumption about a receptor reserve for the full agonist is incorrect (i.e., if $[A] \nless K_A$), then the estimate yields (Kenakin and Black, 1978):

$$K_P = \frac{\text{Slope}}{\text{Intercept}} \left(1 - \frac{\epsilon_P}{\epsilon_A}\right) \tag{14}$$

and the procedure will overestimate K_P. This error diminishes to zero if $\epsilon_A \gg \epsilon_P$. While equation 13 (and equation 8) can be used to estimate K_P and K_A conveniently by linear regressional analysis, they may not yield the best estimate of these parameters. Parker and Waud (1971) have shown that a computer fitting of the data directly to a hyperbola gives more accurate estimates.

Another way to estimate the equilibrium dissociation constant of a partial agonist is by comparing equiactive concentrations of the full agonist in the absence $[A]$ and presence $[A']$ of the partial agonist. Thus, assuming a receptor reserve for the full agonist (Stephenson, 1956; Colquhoun 1973):

$$[A] = \frac{[A']}{\left(1 + \frac{[P]}{K_P}\right)} + \frac{\epsilon_P}{\epsilon_A} \cdot \frac{[P]}{K_P} \cdot \frac{K_A}{\left(1 + \frac{[P]}{K_P}\right)} \tag{15}$$

Thus

$$K_P = \frac{[P] \cdot \text{Slope}}{1 - \text{Slope}} \tag{16}$$

If a receptor reserve is not present (i.e., $[A] \nless K_A$), then the method will yield an overestimation of K_P (MacKay, 1966a,b; Kenakin and Black, 1978):

$$K_P = \frac{[P] \cdot \text{Slope}}{(1 - \text{Slope})} \left(1 - \frac{\epsilon_P}{\epsilon_A}\right) \tag{17}$$

which tends toward the true K_P if $\epsilon_A \gg \epsilon_P$. This method utilizes a regression of $[A']$ upon $[A]$ which can be improved by weighting factors (Marano and Kaumann, 1976). As initially described, this method yields one estimate of the K_P for every one concentration of partial agonist. A range of partial agonist concentrations can be utilized to yield as estimate of K_P from a larger sample (Kaumann and Marano, 1982). Thus, a logarithmic form of equation 17 yields a function of the slopes of regressions according to equation 16 on log $[P]$ and log K_P as a linear regression (Kaumann and Marano, 1982):

$$\log\left(\frac{1}{\text{Slope}} - 1\right) = \log[P] - \log K_P \quad (18)$$

In the presence of a partial agonist, the concentration–response curves to a full agonist will be shifted to the right of the control (obtained in the absence of partial agonist) and the resulting dose ratios can be utilized in the Schild equation (equation 21, *see below*). There are a number of factors that must be considered in the estimation of antagonist affinity by the Schild method that will be dealt with in the following section. However, there are specific theoretical problems raised by the use of this method for partial agonists concerning the relative efficacy of the full and partial agonist that are appropriate for discussion here. The Schild method, when applied to the antagonism of a full agonist by a partial agonist, yields an unambiguous estimate of the K_P for the partial agonist only if response is a linear function of stimulus (Van Rossum, 1963; Jenkinson, 1979). When stimulus and response are not linearly related, the efficacy of the partial agonist complicates interpretation of the estimate of the K_P given by a Schild regression. This complication stems from the required assumption about the nature of the function that relates stimulus and response. For example, it can be shown that it the tissue response is a rectangular hyperbolic function of stimulus, then the observed K_P from a Schild regression yields (Jenkinson, 1979):

$$\text{Intercept} = \log K_P(1 - \alpha)^{-1} \quad (19)$$

where α is the intrinsic activity (Ariens, 1954) of the partial agonist. The weaker is the partial agonist (lower α), the closer will be the estimate to the true K_P.

The complication of the efficacy of the partial agonist can be eliminated if a fraction of the receptors are alkylated to a point where the partial agonist produces no response (Furchgott and Bursztyn, 1967; Waud, 1969b; Parker and Waud, 1971; Parker, 1972; Kenakin, 1981). Under these circumstances, the partial agonist can be utilized as a simple competitive antagonist and a K_P estimate made by the Schild method. Alternatively, physiological antagonism can be used to achieve the same end. Thus, the responses to a weak partial agonist can be suppressed by an appropriate physiologic stimulus such that the partial agonist can be utilized as a competitive antagonist (Buckner and Saini, 1975; Buckner *et al.*, 1978; Kenakin and Beek, 1980).

F. Measurement of Relative Efficacy of a Full and Partial Agonist

The relative efficacy of a full and partial agonist can be measured, given reliable estimates of the K_A and K_P of the drugs, by the method of Furchgott (1966) (see equation 12). Alternatively, if the K_A for the full agonist is known then an estimate of ϵ_P/ϵ_A can be made from the method of Barlow *et al.* (1967) and Waud (1969b). Thus, from equation 13 can be derived (Ruffolo *et al.*, 1979):

$$\frac{\epsilon_P}{\epsilon_A} = (\text{Intercept} \cdot K_A)^{-1} \tag{20}$$

IV. COMPETITIVE ANTAGONISTS

A. The Schild Regression

The equilibrium dissociation constant of a competitive antagonist for a drug receptor is a fundamental parameter in drug receptor classification. The common method for estimating this parameter is by a regression of log (dose ratio − 1) upon the logarithm of the molar concentration of the antagonist according to the Schild equation (Arunlakshana and Schild, 1959):

$$\log(dr - 1) = n \cdot \log[B] - \log K_B \tag{21}$$

A linear Schild regression with a slope of unity indicates the pK_B ($-\log K_B$) from the Schild equation at the point where log(dr − 1) = 0. The slope of a Schild regression is the criterion by which the judgment is made as to whether or not a drug is a simple competitive antagonist. If the slope of the Schild regression is not unity, then either the antagonist is not competitive or the experiments have not been carried out under equilibrium conditions. This latter point can be an additional useful feature of Schild regression, since slopes not equal to unity for known competitive antagonists can be sensitive indicators of nonequilibrium experimental conditions. If portions of a Schild regression for an antagonist are less than unity, it could mean that an uptake mechanism for the agonist is affecting the position of the concentration–response curves along the concentration axis (Furchgott, 1972). Therefore, some cancellation of the receptor antagonism could be observed if the concentrations of agonist are elevated to levels that saturate agonist uptake (Blinks, 1967; Furchgott, 1972; Furchgott *et al.*, 1973), if the receptor antagonist inhibits agonist uptake (Furchgott, 1966, 1972), or if the antagonist potentiates the agonist responses by some other mechanism (Kenakin, 1982b). These effects have been observed for the inhibition of adenosine responses by theophylline (Clanachan and Muller, 1980). Alternatively, the slope of the Schild regression may be greater than one, suggesting an inadequate time of equilibration of the antagonist with the receptors (Kenakin, 1980b). Therefore, the slope of the Schild regression is a valuable parameter in studies aimed at drug and drug receptor classification.

The pA_2 ($-$log of the molar concentration of antagonist that produces a dose ratio of 2) is an empirical constant often used for receptor classification, but it should be pointed out that theoretically this is unsound. Since antagonist potency is subject to nonequilibrium experimental conditions, reliance on a single pA_2 is hazardous as a measure of antagonist potency; there is no way of knowing, without a full Schild regression and an estimate of slope, whether or not the pA_2 reflects the true pK_B.

Theoretically, if two agonists yield the same pK_B for a given antagonist in a tissue, this suggests that the two agonists activate the same receptor (Schild, 1947). The converse assumption has been used to delineate heterogeneous receptor populations in tissues. If antagonists display agonist-dependent pK_B values (assuming uptake processes are adequately inhibited), it is possible that the tissue possesses a mixture of receptors subserving the same response for which the agonist has differing affinities and efficacy and the antagonist differing affinity.

Theoretical modeling shows that the Schild regressions under these types of circumstances may be linear with a slope of unity over a large range of antagonist concentrations (Lemoine and Kaumann, 1983; Kenakin, 1984). There is experimental evidence for such effects in guinea pig trachea where agonist-dependent pK_B estimates for various β-adrenoceptors antagonists are obtained from Schild regressions with slopes of unity (Furchgott, 1978; O'Donnell and Wanstall, 1979). The importance of the agonist dependency of the pK_B lies in the fact that a tissue factor, namely, the relative concentrations of the two receptor types, and not a receptor factor, controls the resulting pK_B estimate. Thus, three separate pK_B estimates for one antagonist made with three agonists may not imply three receptor subtypes, but rather a mixture of two receptor subtypes for which the agonists have varying degrees of affinity and efficacy.

B. Classification of Purine Receptors with Antagonists

The Schild regression, with caveats mentioned above, is the most valuable technique to classify receptors. The most important requirement of the technique is to have at hand potent (high-affinity) antagonists that have no secondary effects beyond the receptor surface. As will be obvious from the comments below, this is the major and most pressing difficulty to overcome if careful, quantitative classification of purine receptors is to be undertaken.

To date, three families of adenosine antagonists have been found: xanthines, benzo[g] pteridines, and 9-substituted purines. As exemplified by theophylline (1,3-dimethylxanthine), the alkylxanthines have been the most widely studied. Based primarily on binding studies, Bruns *et al.* (1980, 1983) have shown that 1,3-dipropyl substitutions and 8-phenyl substitutions enhance potency. Thus, 8-phenyltheophylline is more potent than theophylline. Unfortunately, this compound is not very soluble in solvents that are compatible with isolated tissues. As a result, the compound has not been widely used. It has the advantage of being a very weak phosphodiesterase inhibitor relative to theophylline. Recently Bruns *et al.* (1983) have described a theophylline derivative, 1,3-dipropyl-8-(2-amino-4-chlorophenyl)xanthine, with extraordinary binding potency. This compound has

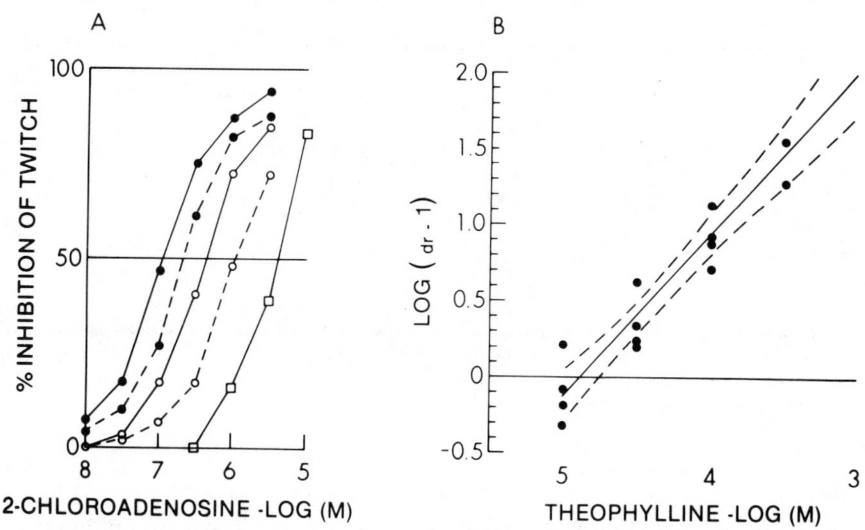

Figure 5. Antagonism of 2-chloroadenosine inhibition of twitch response in the guinea pig ileum by theophylline. Panel A: concentration–response curves for 2-chloroadenosine in the absence (●——●) and presence of theophylline 10 μM (●---●), 30 μM (○——○), 100 μM (○---○), and 300 μM (□——□). Panel B: Schild regression for theophylline. Regression computed from 14 data points, yielding a pK_B of 4.9 (4.5–5.3) and slope of 1.08 (0.88–1.29). Taken from Leighton and Parmeter (1982).

a K_I for adenosine receptors of .022 nM or approximately 70,000 times more potent than theophylline. This agent may prove very valuable in the classification of purine receptors because it offers the needed potency to distinguish multiple receptor sites that have different affinities for the same antagonist.

As indicated, theophylline has been the most widely used antagonist to date to classify P_1 or A_1 purine receptor mechanisms. Figure 5 shows the effect of theophylline on 2-chloroadenosine inhibition of guinea pig ileum response to field stimulation. Although weak in this tissue, theophylline is a competitive antagonist (slope not different from unity), yielding a pK_B of 4.9 (4.7–5.6). Similar results in terms of pA_2 have been obtained by Colman (1980) and Karlsson *et al.* (1982) in the guinea pig trachea and by Clanachan and Muller (1980) in the rat vas deferens, but the slopes of regressions were less than unity. Thus, in addition to low potency, various secondary effects of theophylline may complicate the receptor analysis.

It is well known that theophylline is a phosphodiesterase inhibitor with IC_{50} values of 500, 950, and 1000 μM for calcium-dependent, calcium-independent, and membrane-bound phosphodiesterase, respectively (Smellie *et al.*, 1979). At 500 μM, theophylline is an inhibitor of 5′-nucleotidase Tsuzuki and Newburgh, 1975; Fredholm *et al.*, 1978). In cardiac muscle, theophylline produces positive inotropic and chronotropic effects that are thought to result from a direct effect

Table I. Antagonism of Guinea Pig Atrial Responses to 2-Chloroadenosine by Theophylline

Conditions	p*A*2	Slope
Spontaneously beating atria		
Theophylline alone[a]	—	—
Theophylline in the presence of isoproterenol, 0.1 μ*M*	4.9	1.6
Theophylline in the presence of SQ20,009, 10 μ*M*	4.4	1.2
Theophylline in the presence of SQ20,009 10 μ*M* and isoproterenol 0.1 μ*M*	4.8	1.3
Electrically driven atria[b]		
Theophylline alone	4.8	0.8

[a] Measurement not possible due to 50–100% increases in spontaneous rate in the presence of theophylline (10–300 μ*M*).
[b] Atria were stimulated at 0.5 Hz at 34°C.

on the contractile elements and indirectly via catecholamine release (Marcus *et al.*, 1972). Both of these effects may reflect alterations in calcium utilization.

These side effects limit the utility of theophylline for classifying purine receptors. This is exemplified by Table I, which shows the results in guinea pig atria of theophylline antagonism of 2-chloroadenosine. Presumably, most of the difficulties with the use of theophylline in cardiac tissues are due to PDE inhibition, but even under conditions designed to negate the PDE effect (non-xanthine PDE inhibition and elevation of cAMP with isoproterenol), a proper Schild regression could not be obtained. However, the data suggest that purines activate a single site in cardiac tissue.

Theophylline may also present problems for studying purine inhibition of adrenergic transmission. For example, theophylline (Leighton and Parmeter, 1982) antagonizes the effects of 2-chloroadenosine in the field stimulated rat vas deferens, but the calculated pA_2 is frequency dependent (Figure 6). A characteristic of a proper Schild analysis is that the calculated pK_B for antagonist is independent of the agonist or the conditions of the preparation (ionic contents of physiologic buffer, field stimulation, and so on). Studies in the vas deferens suggest caution when one interprets the results of theophylline antagonism of an adrenergically mediated response. Further advances in purine receptor classification may be expected as more potent and selective antagonists become available.

V. DRUG SELECTIVITY AND RECEPTOR DIFFERENCES

The classification of drug receptors in isolated tissues depends upon the observation of unique profiles of agonism and antagonism of drugs on these tissues. With respect to agonism, care should be taken in interpreting the meaning of response (or absence of response) to selective agonists. Absence of a response to an agonist does not necessarily imply the absence of receptors for that agonist; it is possible that the agonist does not have sufficient intrinsic efficacy to allow

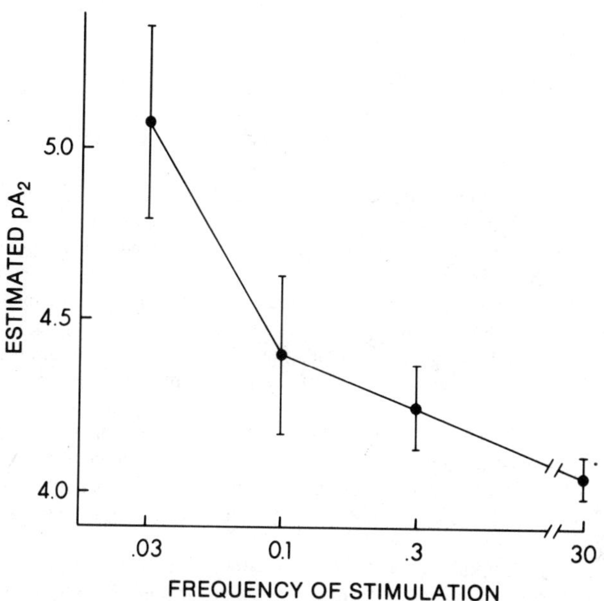

Figure 6. Effect of frequency of stimulation (0.03, 0.1, and 0.3 Hz, continuous; or 30 Hz, 200-msec duration at 100-sec intervals) on estimated pA_2 for theophylline, 30 μM, in the rat vas deferens. The agonist employed was 2-chloroadenosine.

sufficient stimulus to produce an observable response. Under these circumstances, it should be determined whether or not the "agonist" that produces no obvious response in a given tissue produces antagonism of a more powerful agonist. Likewise, the observation of a response to a selective agonist does not necessarily imply presence of the receptor for which the agonist has been shown to be selective. This conclusion assumes no other properties for the agonist, i.e., specificity as opposed to selectivity.

Assuming that drug receptor parameters for a series of drugs has been found to be different in two different tissues, what governs the decision that the receptors are different? A useful guideline, with respect to differences in K_B, has been the suggestion of Furchgott (1972) that a 3-fold difference in the K_B constitutes evidence to suggest differences in receptors. Wherever linear regressions are utilized to obtain drug receptor data, analyses of covariance of regression lines provides a useful method for comparing differences in slope and elevation of these lines (Kenakin and Black, 1978). Thus, all of the data, for example, in a Schild regression can be utilized, rather than only the pK_B.

In general, there are sufficient null techniques available for the orderly classification of purine receptors in isolated tissues. While the lack of potent and selective drugs has hampered the effective utilization of these techniques, the discovery of these tools should provide new opportunities for achieving unambiguous quantitation of purine receptor effects.

REFERENCES

Arunlakshana, O., and Schild, H. O. 1959. Some quantitative uses of drug antagonists. *Br. J. Pharmacol., 14*:48–58.

Barlow, R. B., Scott, N. C., and Stephenson, R. P. 1967. The affinity and efficacy of onium salts on the frog rectus abdominis. *Br. J. Pharmacol., 31*:188–196.

Bender, A. S., Wu, P. H., and Phillis, J. W. 1981. Some biochemical properties of the rapid adenosine uptake system in rat brain synaptosomes. *J. Neurochem., 37*:1282–1290.

Blinks, J. R. 1967. Evaluation of the cardiac effects of several beta adrenergic blocking agents. *Ann. N.Y. Acad. Sci., 139*(3):673–685.

Brown, C., Burnstock, G., and Cocks, T. 1979. Effects of adenosine 5′-triphosphate (ATP) and β,γ-methylene ATP on rat urinary bladder. *Br. J. Pharmacol., 65*:97–102.

Bruns, R. F., Daly, J. W., and Snyder, S. H. 1980. Adenosine receptors in brain membranes: Binding of N^6-cyclohexyl [^{3}H]adenosine and 1,3-diethyl-8-[^{3}H]phenylxanthine. *Proc. Natl. Acad. Sci., 77*:5547–5551.

Bruns, R. F., Daly, J. W., and Snyder, S. H. 1983. Adenosine receptor binding: Structure–activity analysis generates extremely potent xanthine antagonists. *Proc. Natl. Acad. Sci., 80*:2077–2080.

Buckner, C. K., and Saini, R. K. 1975. On the use of functional antagonism to estimate dissociation constants for β-adrenergic receptor agonists in isolated guinea pig trachea. *J. Pharmacol. Exp. Ther., 194*:565.

Buckner, C. K., Torphy, T., and Costa, D. J. 1978. Studies on β-adrenergic mediating changes in mechanical events and adenosine 3′,5′-monophosphate levels. Rat atria. *Eur. J. Pharmacol., 47*:259–271.

Burnstock, G. 1978. A basis for distinguishing two types of purinergic receptors. In: *Cell Membrane Receptors for Drugs and Hormones*, pp. 107–118. Ed. by Straub, R. S., and Bolis, L. Raven Press, New York.

Burnstock, G., and Meghji, P. 1981. Distribution of P_1- and P_2-purinoceptors in guinea pig and frog heart. *Br. J. Pharmacol., 73*:879–885.

Burnstock, G., Dumselay, B., and Smythe, A. 1972. Atropine resistant excitation of the urinary bladder: The possibility of transmission via nerves releasing a purine nucleotide. *Br. J. Pharmacol., 44*:451–461.

Cass, C. E., Gaudette, L. A., and Paterson, A. R. P. 1974. Mediated transport of nucleosides in human erythrocytes. Specific binding of the inhibitor nitrobenzyl thioinosine to nucleoside transport sites in the erythrocyte membrane. *Biochim. Biophys. Acta, 345*:1–10.

Chaundry, I. H. 1982. Does ATP cross the plasma cell plasma membrane? *Yale J. Biol. Med., 55*:1–10.

Christie, J., and Satchell, D. G. 1980. Purine receptor in the trachea: Is there a receptor for ATP? *Br. J. Pharmacol., 70*:512–514.

Clanachan, A. S., and Marshall, R. J. 1980. Potentiation of the effects of adenosine on isolated cardiac and smooth muscle by diazepam. *Br. J. Pharmacol., 71*:459–466.

Clanachan, A. S., and Muller, M. J. 1980. Effect of adenosine uptake inhibition on the nature and potency of theophylline as a presynaptic adenosine receptor antagonist. *Can. J. Physiol. Pharmacol., 58*:805–809.

Colman, R. A. 1980. Purine antagonists in the identification of adenosine receptors in guinea pig trachea and the role of purines in non-adrenergic inhibitory neurotransmission. *Br. J. Pharmacol., 69*:359–366.

Colquhoun, D. 1973. The relation between classical and cooperative models for drug action. In: *Drug Receptors*, pp. 149–182. Ed. by Rang, H. P. University Park Press, Baltimore.

Dahlen, S.-E., and Hedqvist, P. 1980. ATP, β,γ-methylene ATP and adenosine inhibit non-cholinergic non-adrenergic transmission in rat urinary bladder. *Acta Physiol. Scand., 109*:137–142.

Dowdle, E. B., and Maske, R. The effects of dipyridamole on guinea pig ileum longitudinal muscle-myenteric plexus preparation. *Br. J. Pharmacol., 71*:235–244.

Ebner, F. 1981. The inhibition by (±)-Propanolol of the positive inotropic effects of (±)-isoprenaline and (−)-noradrenaline, *Naunyn-Schmeidebergs Arch. Pharmacol., 316*:96–107.

Ebner, F., and Waud, D. R. 1978. The role of uptake of noradrenaline for its positive inotropic effect in relation to muscle geometry. *Naunyn-Schmeidebergs Arch. Pharmacol., 303:*1–6.

Fedan, J. S., Hogaboom, G. K., O'Donnell, J. P., Colby, J., and Westfall, D. P. 1981. Contribution of purines to the neurogenic response of the vas deferens of the guinea pig. *Eur. J. Pharmacol., 69:*41–53.

Fedan, J. S., Hogaboom, G. K., Westfall, D. P., and O'Donnell, J. P. 1983. Photoaffinity labeling of P_2-purinergic and H_1-histamine receptors in smooth muscle. *Proc. Fed. Am. Soc. Exp. Biol., 42:*2846–2850.

Fredholm, B. B., Hedqvist, P., and Vernet, L. 1978. Effect of theophylline and other drugs on rabbit renal cyclic nucleotide phosphodiesterase, 5′-nucleotidase and adenosine deaminase. *Biochem. Pharmacol., 27:*2845–2850.

Frew, R., And Baer, H. P. 1979. Adenosine-α,β-methylene diphosphate effects in intestinal smooth muscle: Sites of action and possible prostaglandin involvement. *J. Pharmacol. Exp. Ther., 211:*525–530.

Frew, R., McKenzie, S. G., Bär, H. P., and Hutchison, K. J. 1976. The relaxant effects of adenosine-5′-α,β-methylene diphosphonate on the longitudinal smooth muscle of the rabbit ileum. *Can. J. Physiol. Pharmacol., 54:*626–629.

Furchgott, R. F. 1966. The use of β-haloalkylamines in the differentiation of receptors and in the determination of dissociation constants of receptor–agonist complexes. In: *Advances in Drug Research*, Volume 3, pp. 21–55. Ed. by Harper, N. J., and Simmonds, A. B. Academic Press, London.

Furchgott, R. F. 1972. The classification of adrenoceptors (adrenergic receptors). An evaluation from the standpoint of receptor theory. In: *Catecholamines Handbook of Experimental Pharmacology*, Volume 33, pp. 283–335. Ed. by Bloschko, H., and Muscholl, E. Springer-Verlag, Berlin.

Furchgott, R. F. 1978. Pharmacological characterization of receptors: Its relation to radioligand-binding studies. *Proc. Fed. Am. Soc. Exp. Biol., 37:*115–120.

Furchgott, R. F., and Bursztyn, P. 1967. Comparison of dissociation constants and of relative efficacies of selected agonists acting on parasympathetic receptors. *Ann. N.Y. Acad. Sci., 144:*882–889.

Furchgott, R. F., Jurkiewicz, A., and Jurkiewicz, N. H. 1973. Antagonism of propanolol to isoproterenol in guinea pig trachea: Some cautionary findings. In: Frontiers in Catecholamine Research, pp. 295–300. Ed. by Usdin, E., and Snyder, S. H. Pergamon Press, Elmsford, New York.

Gerlach, E., and Deuticke, B. 1963. Adenosine deaminase inhibition with dipyridamole. *Arzneim-Forsch., 13:*48–54.

Holck, M. I., and Marks, B. H. 1978. Purine nucleoside and nucleotide interactions on normal and subsensitive alpha adrenoceptor responsiveness in guinea pig vas deferens. *J. Pharmacol. Exp. Ther., 205:*104–117.

Hopkins, S. V., and Goldie, R. G. 1971. A species difference in the uptake of adenosine by heart. *Biochem. Pharmacol., 20:*3359–3365.

Jager, L. P., and Schevers, J. A. M. 1980. A comparison of effects evoked in guinea pig taenia caecum by purine nucleotides and by purinergic nerve stimulation. J. Physiol., 299:75–83.

Jarvis, S. M., and Young, J. D. 1980. Nucleoside transport in human and sheep erythrocytes: Evidence that nitrobenzylthioinosine binds specifically to functional nucleoside transport sites. *Biochem. J., 190:*377–383.

Jenkinson, D. H. 1979. Partial agonists in receptor classification. In Proceeding of the VII Congress of Medicinal Chemistry, pp. 373–383. Ed. by Simpkins, M. A. Cotswold Press, Oxford..

Jhamandas, K., Nakatsu, K., Downie, J. W., Bartlett, V., and Elliott, J. 1980. Action of coenzyme A on adenine derivative receptors in isolated tissues. *Eur. J. Pharmacol., 62:*247–252.

Karlsson, J.-A., Kjellin, G., and Persson, C. G. A. 1982. Effects on tracheal smooth muscle of adenosine and methylxanthines and their interaction. *J. Pharm. Pharmacol., 34:*788–793.

Kaumann, A. J., and Marano, M. 1982. On equilibrium dissociation constants for complexes of drug-receptor subtypes. Selective and non-selective interactions of partial agonists with two plausible β-adrenoceptor subtypes mediating positive chronotropic effects of (−)-isoprenaline in kitten atria. *Naunyn-Schmeidebergs Arch. Pharmacol., 318:*192–201.

Kazic, T., and Milosavlgevic, D. 1980. Interaction between adenosine triphosphate and noradrenaline in the isolated vas deferens of the guinea pig. *Br. J. Pharmacol., 71:*93–98.

Kenakin, T. P. 1980a. Errors in the measurement of agonist potency ratios produced by uptake processes: A general model applied to β-adrenoceptor agonists. *Br. J. Pharmacol., 71:*407–417.

Kenakin, T. P. 1980b. Effects of equilibration time on the attainment of equilibrium between antagonists and drug receptors. *Eur. J. Pharmacol., 66:*295–306.

Kenakin, T. P. 1981. A pharmacological method to estimate the pK_I of competitive inhibitors of agonist uptake processes in isolated tissues. *Naunyn-Schmeidebergs Arch. Pharmacol., 316:*89–95.

Kenakin, T. P. 1982a. The potentiation of cardiac responses to adenosine by benzodiazepine. *J. Pharmacol. Exp. Ther., 222:*752–758.

Kenakin, T. P. 1982b. The Schild regression in the process of receptor classification. *Can. J. Physiol. Pharmacol., 60:*249–265.

Kenakin, T. P. 1984. The classification of drugs and drug receptors in isolated tissues. *Pharmacol. Rev., 36:*165–222.

Kenakin, T. P., and Beek, D. 1980. Is prenalterol (H133/80) really a selective beta-adrenoceptor agonist? Tissue selectivity resulting from differences in stimulus-response relationships. *J. Pharmacol. Exp. Ther., 213:*406–412.

Kenakin, T. P., and Black, J. W. 1978. The pharmacological classification of practolol and chloropractolol. *Mol. Pharmacol., 14:*607–623.

Kolassa, N., Pfleger, K., and Träm, M. 1971. Species difference in action and elimination of adenosine after dipyridamole and hexobendine. *Eur. J. Pharmacol., 13:*320–325.

Kukovetz, W. R., and Pöch, G. 1970. Inhibition of cyclic-3′,5′-nucleotide-phosphodiesterase as a possible mode of action of papavarine and similarly acting drugs. *Naunyn Schmeidebergs Arch. Pharmacol., 267:*189–194.

Leighton, H. J., and Parmeter, L. L. 1982. Schild analysis of purinergic receptors in various isolated tissues. *Pharmacologist 24:*686.

Lemoine, H., and Kaumann, A. J. 1983. A model for the interaction of competitive antagonists with two receptor-subtypes characterized by a Schild-plot with apparent slope unity. *Naunyn Schmeidebergs Arch. Pharmacol., 322:*111–120.

Maguire, M. H., and Satchell, D. G. 1979. The contribution of adenosine to the inhibitory actions of adenine nucleotides on the guinea pig taenia coli: Studies with phosphate-modified adenine nucleotide analogs and dipyridamole. *J. Pharmacol. Exp. Ther., 211:*626–633.

MacKay, D. 1966a. A general analysis of the receptor–drug interaction. *Br. J. Pharmacol., 26:*9–16.

MacKay, D. 1966b. A new method for the analysis of drug-receptor interactions. In: *Advances in Drug Research,* Volume 3, pp. 1–20. Ed. by Harper, N. J., and Simmonds, A. B. Academic Press, London.

Marangos, P. J., Patel, J., Clark-Rosenberg, R., and Martino, A. M. 1982. [^{3}H]Nitrobenzylthioinosine binding as a probe for the study of adenosine uptake sites in brain. *J. Neurochem., 39:*184–188.

Marano, M., and Kaumann, A. J. 1976. On the statistics of drug-receptor constants for partial agonists. *J. Pharmacol. Exp. Ther., 198:*518–525.

Marcus, M. L., Skelton, C. L., Graver, L. E., and Epstein, S. E. 1972. Effects of theophylline on myocardial mechanics. *Am. J. Physiol., 222:*1361–1365.

Moritoki, H., Takei, M., Kasai, T., Matsumura, Y., and Ishida, Y. 1979. Possible involvement of prostaglandins in the action of ATP on guinea pig uterus. *J. Pharmacol. Exp. Ther., 211:*104–111.

Needleman, P., Minkes, M. S., and Douglas, J. R. 1974. Stimulation of prostaglandin biosynthesis by adenine nucleotides. *Circ. Res., 34:*455–461.

O'Donnell, R. S., and Wanstall, J. C. 1979. The importance of choice of agonist in studies designed to predict β_2:β_1 adrenoceptor selectivity of antagonists from pA_2 values on guinea pig trachea and atria. *Naunyn-Schmeidebergs Arch. Pharmacol., 308:*183–190.

Okwuasaba, F. K., Hamilton, J. T., and Cook, M. A. 1977. Relaxations of guinea pig fundic strip by adenosine, adenine nucleotides and electrical stimulation: Antagonism by theophylline and desensitization to adenosine and its derivatives. *Eur. J. Pharmacol., 46:*181–198.

Parker, R. B. 1972. Measurement of drug-receptor dissociation constants of muscarinic agonists on intestinal smooth muscle. *J. Pharmacol. Exp. Ther., 180:*62–70.

Parker, R. B., and Waud, D. R. 1971. Pharmacological estimation of drug-receptor dissociation constants. Statistical evaluation. 1. Agonists. *J. Pharmacol. Exp. Ther., 177:*1–12.

Paterson, A. R. P., Jakobs, E. S., Harley, E. R., Fu, N.-W., Robins, M. J., and Cass, C. E. 1983. Inhibition of nucleoside transport In: *Regulatory Function of Adenosine*, Volume 2, pp. 203–220. Ed. by Berne, R. M., Rall, T. W., and Rubio, A. Martinus Nijhoff, Boston.

Paton, D. M. 1981. Structure-activity relations for presynaptic inhibition of noradrenergic and cholinergic transmission by adenosine: Evidence for action on A_1 receptors. *J. Auton. Pharmacol., 1:*287–290.

Phillis, J. W., Siemens, R. K., and Wu, P. H. 1980. Effects of diazepam on adenosine and acetylcholine release from rat cerebral cortex: Further evidence for a purinergic mechanism in action of diazepam. *Br. J. Pharmacol., 70:*341–348.

Plagemann, P. G. W., and Roth, M. F. 1969. Permeation as the rate limiting step in the phosphorylation of uridine and choline and their incorporation into macromolecules by Novikoff hepatoma cells. *Biochemistry, 8:*4782–4789.

Renner, E. D., Plagemann, P. G. W., and Bernlohr, R. W. 1972. Permeation of glucose by simple and facilitated diffusion by Novikoff rat heptatoma cells in suspension culture and its relationship to glucose metabolism. *J. Biol. Chem., 247:*5765–5776.

Ruffolo, R. R. Jr., Dillard, R. D., Waddell, J. E., and Yaden, E. L. 1979. Receptor interactions of imidazolines. III. Structure-activity relationships governing alpha adrenergic receptor occupation and receptor activation of mono- and dimethoxy-substituted tolazoline derivatives in rat aorta. *J. Pharmacol. Exp. Ther., 211:*733–738.

Schild, H. O. 1947. pA, a new scale for the measurement of drug antagonism. *Br. J. Pharmacol., 2:*189–206.

Sjöberg, B., and Wahlström, B. A. 1975. The effort of ATP and related compounds on spontaneous mechanical activity in the rat portal vein. *Acta Physiol. Scand., 94:*46–53.

Smellie, F. W., Davis, C. W., Daly, J. W., and Wells, J. N. 1979. Alkylxanthines: Inhibition of adenosine-elicited accumulation of cyclic AMP in brain slices and of brain phosphodiesterase activity. *Life Sci., 24:*2475–2482.

Stafford, A. 1966. Potentiation of adenosine and the adenine nucleotides by dipyridamole. *Br. J. Pharmacol., 28:*218–227.

Stephenson, R. P. 1956. A modification of receptor theory. *Br. J. Pharmacol., 11:*379–393.

Su, Y. F., and Leighton, H. J. 1983. Functional antagonism to determine dissociation constants of presynaptic α-2adrenoceptor agonists. *Pharmacologist, 25:*196.

Thron, C. D. 1970. Graphical and weighted regression analyses for the determination of agonist dissociation constants. *J. Pharmacol. Exp. Ther., 175:*541–553.

Tsuzuki, J., and Newburgh, R. W. 1975. Inhibition of 5′-nucleotidase in rat brain by methylxanthines. *J. Neurochem., 25:*895–896.

Van Belle, H. 1969. Uptake and deamination of adenosine by blood. Species differences, effect of pH, ions, temperature, and metabolic inhibitors. *Biochim. Biophys. Acta, 192:*124–132.

Van Rossum, J. M. 1963. Cumulative dose-response curves. II. Technique for the making of dose–response curves in isolated organs and the evaluation of drug parameters. *Arch. Int. Pharmacodyn. Ther., 143:*299–330.

Venter, J. C. 1978. Cardiac sites of catecholamine action: Diffusion models for soluble and immobilized catecholamine action or isolated cat papillary muscles. *Mol. Pharmacol., 14:*562–574.

Waud, D. R. 1969a. A quantitative model for the effect of a saturable uptake on the slope of the dose-response curve. *J. Pharmacol. Exp. Ther., 167:*140–141.

Waud, D. R. 1969b. On the measurement of the affinity of partial agonists for receptors. *J. Pharmacol. Exp. Ther., 170:*117–122.

Chapter **13**

Use of Radioligands in the Identification, Classification, and Study of Adenosine Receptors

Ulrich Schwabe

Pharmakologisches Institut
der Universität Heidelberg
Federal Republic of Germany

I. INTRODUCTION

Pharmacologically important adenosine receptors can be divided into two subtypes, namely, R_i (A_1) and R_a (A_2). The distinction between these two subtypes was first achieved in adenylate cyclase studies of several different cellular systems (Van Calker *et al.*, 1979; Londos *et al.*, 1980). The R_i adenosine receptor has a high affinity for adenosine and mediates inhibition of adenylate cyclase activity. The R_a adenosine receptor has a lower affinity and mediates stimulation of enzyme activity. In addition to these external receptors, nearly all cyclase preparations contain a third adenosine-sensitive site that is located at the internal side of the cell membrane and mediates inhibition of enzyme activity (Londos and Wolff, 1977).

Both R-type adenosine receptors have been further characterized in adenylate cyclase studies by the use of selected adenosine analogs. N^6-substituted adenosine

Abbreviations used in this chapter: ACTH, adrenocorticotropic hormone; ADP, adenosine 5′-diphosphate; ATP, adenosine 5′-triphosphate; CHA, N^6-cyclohexyladenosine; CPCA, 5′-*N*-cyclopropylcarboxamidoadenosine; cyclic AMP, adenosine cyclic 3′,5′-monophosphate; DPX, 1,3-diethyl-8-phenylxanthine; EDTA, ethylenediaminetetraacetic acid; GTP, guanosine 5-triphosphate; HPIA, (−)N^6-*p*-hydroxyphenylisopropyladenosine; IBMX, 3-isobutyl-1-methylxanthine; IHPIA, (−)N^6-iodo-p-hydroxyphenylisopropyladenosine; NECA, 5′-*N*-ethylcarboxamidoadenosine; PIA, (−)N^6-phenylisopropyladenosine.

analogs such as (–)N^6-phenylisopropyladenosine (PIA) and cyclohexyladenosine (CHA) are more potent at the R_i adenosine receptor than 5′-substituted adenosine derivatives such as 5′-*N*-ethylcarboxamidoadenosine (NECA) and 5′-*N*-cyclopropylcarboxamidoadenosine (CPCA) (Londos *et al.*, 1980). The reverse order of potency has been observed at the R_a adenosine receptor. Although many adenosine effects appear to involve adenylate cyclase, it should be mentioned that not all effects of adenosine are mediated via cyclic AMP (Schütz and Tuisl, 1981).

The prototypical adenosine antagonists are the xanthine derivatives, such as theophylline, caffeine, and 3-isobutyl-1-methylxanthine (IBMX). Their adenosine antagonist properties were first discovered in studies on cyclic AMP formation in brain, where they inhibit the adenosine-induced rise in cyclic AMP levels (Sattin and Rall, 1970). Methylxanthines have been shown to competitively antagonize the stimulation of adenylate cyclase by adenosine in R_a-subtype selective cells such as human platelets (Haslam and Lynham, 1972) and the inhibition of cyclase by adenosine in R_i-subtype selective cells, such as rat fat cells (Londos *et al.*, 1978). It is important to mention that methylxanthines are more potent as adenosine antagonists than as inhibitors of cyclic AMP phosphodiesterase (Fredholm, 1980; Londos *et al.*, 1981). Although a large number of xanthine derivatives has been evaluated as adenosine antagonists at both receptor subtypes (Londos *et al.*, 1980; Bruns, 1981; Bruns *et al.*, 1983), none of these compounds appears to be a selective antagonist at R_i or R_a adenosine receptors.

The inhibitory adenosine P site is probably associated with the catalytic component of adenylate cyclase. 2′,5′-Dideoxyadenosine is the most potent analog at this additional adenosine-sensitive site (Londos and Wolff, 1977). The above mentioned N^6-substituted and 5′-substituted analogs of adenosine are inactive, whereas adenosine itself is considerably effective as inhibitor. For this reason, the subtype-selective analogs of adenosine are usually preferred in adenosine receptor studies. Methylxanthines do not antagonize P-site effects of adenosine, and other antagonists have not yet been described. A physiological role of the adenosine P site still remains to be elucidated.

II. GENERAL METHODOLOGICAL APPROACH TO RADIOLIGAND-BINDING STUDIES OF ADENOSINE RECEPTORS

The characterization of adenosine receptors was first achieved by adenylate cyclase studies in which the relative potencies of agonists and antagonists were compared. An alternative method of estimating receptor affinities for adenosine and related compounds is to measure their competition for receptor binding of radiolabeled compounds termed radioligands. These radioligand-binding techniques have first been developed for the study of polypeptide hormone receptors using ^{125}I-labeled hormones, such as ACTH, insulin, and glucagon (Lefkowitz *et al.*, 1970; Freychet *et al.*, 1971; Cuatrecasas, 1971; Rodbell *et al.*, 1971). In the next decade, the investigation of a great variety of receptor systems by radioligand binding rapidly expanded and has fundamentally changed the area of receptor research. The main advantage of the radioligand binding technique over the classic pharmacologic approach of measuring the biological response is the determination of the initial physicochemical interaction of the radioligand with the receptor located on the plasma membrane. Thus, the receptor sites can be identified directly with less interference by subsequent steps mediating the biological response to the ligand. The receptor sites can be quantitated by measuring the maximal number of binding sites. The specificity can be rapidly identified by evaluating the structure–activity relationship of relevant compounds. The kinetics of the interaction with the radioligand can be determined and the receptor protein can be purified by solubilization and affinity chromatography.

A. Radioligands

The first attempts to identify adenosine receptors by radioligand binding were carried out with radioactively labeled adenosine. Although [^{3}H]adenosine binding was rapid and reversible, it did not have the binding characteristics expected of adenosine receptors, as shown by low affinities, high-capacity binding sites, and deviating structure–activity profiles (Malbon *et al.*, 1978; Schwabe *et al.*, 1979; Newman *et al.*, 1981; Schütz and Brugger, 1982). A further difficulty emerged from the considerable metabolism of [^{3}H]adenosine even at low temperatures and in the presence of adenosine deaminase inhibitors (Schwabe *et al.*, 1979; Newman *et al.*, 1981). From these results it has been concluded that it is necessary to use radiolabeled adenosine analogs that are resistant to adenosine-metabolizing enzymes and exhibit a higher receptor specificity than adenosine.

In 1980, specific high-affinity radioligands were developed independently by four different groups. R_i adenosine receptors with the appropriate characteristics could now be labeled with both agonist and antagonist ligands. The agonist radioligands were 2-chloro[^{3}H]adenosine (Williams and Risley, 1980a; Williams and Risley, 1980b; Wu *et al.*, 1980), N^6-cyclohexyl[^{3}H]adenosine ([^{3}H]-CHA) (Bruns *et al.*, 1980) and (–)N^6-phenylisopropyl[^{3}H]adenosine ([^{3}H]-PIA) (Schwabe and Trost, 1980). In addition, 1,3-diethyl-8-[^{3}H]phenylxanthine ([^{3}H]-DPX) has been introduced as the first antagonist radioligand that appeared to label both R_i and R_a adenosine receptors in brain membrane preparations (Bruns *et al.*, 1980). Two years later, two additional radioligands were developed to study adenosine receptors. 5′-*N*-Ethylcarboxamido[^{3}H]adenosine ([^{3}H]-NECA) was utilized as a radioligand for R_a adenosine receptors in rat liver (Schütz *et al.*, 1982a). In the same year (±) [^{125}I]N^6-*p*-hydroxyphenylisopropyladenosine ([^{125}I]-HPIA) was synthesized as the first radioiodinated ligand and used for the characterization of R_i adenosine receptors in brain (Munshi and Baer, 1982; Schwabe *et al.*, 1982). The structure of all these radioligands is shown in Figure 1.

Attempts to develop a radioligand for the adenosine P site associated with adenylate cyclase were not successful (Nimit *et al.*, 1982). Although 2′,5′-dideoxy[^{3}H]adenosine bound with relatively high affinity to rat brain membranes, profiles for inhibition of binding by various compounds did not correlate with the potencies as agonists at the P site.

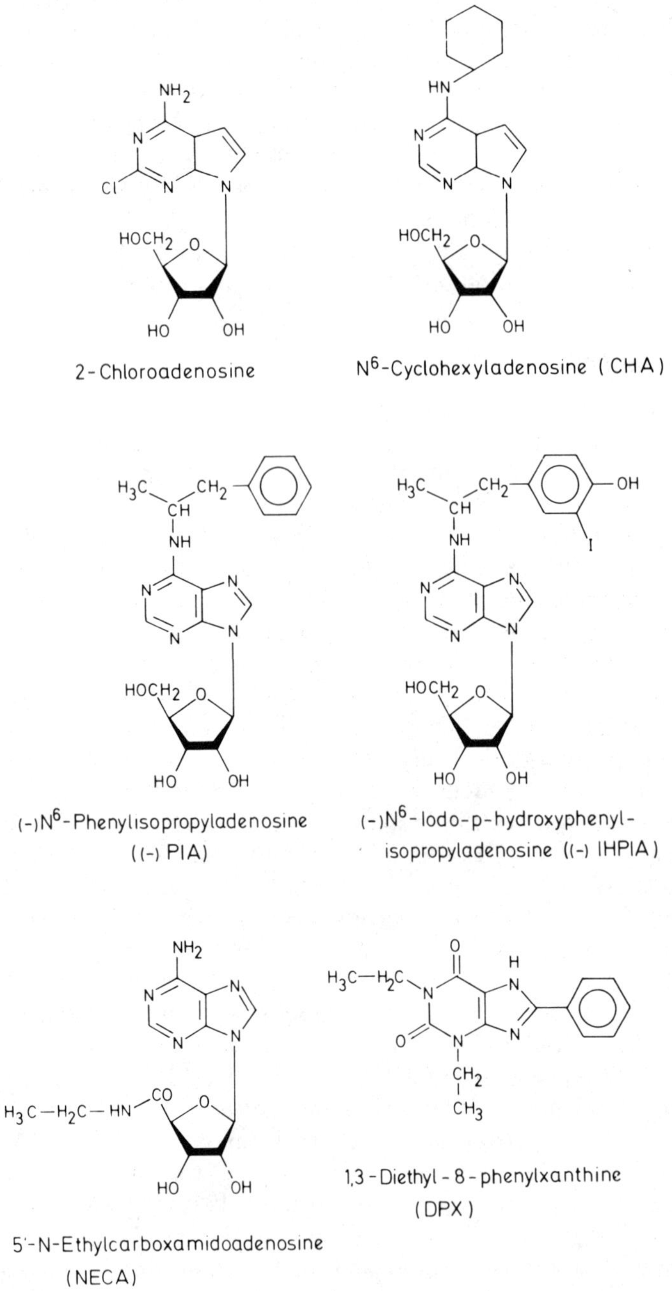

2-Chloroadenosine

N^6-Cyclohexyladenosine (CHA)

(-)N^6-Phenylisopropyladenosine
((-) PIA)

(-)N^6-Iodo-p-hydroxyphenyl-
isopropyladenosine ((-) IHPIA)

1,3-Diethyl-8-phenylxanthine
(DPX)

5'-N-Ethylcarboxamidoadenosine
(NECA)

Figure 1. Structures of adenosine and xanthine derivatives used for radioligand binding studies of adenosine receptors.

B. Tissue Preparations

The initial radioligand binding studies of adenosine receptors were performed with membrane preparations from mammalian brain that contain both R_i and R_a adenosine receptors linked to adenylate cyclase (Bruns *et al.*, 1980; Schwabe and Trost, 1980; Williams and Risley, 1980b). The results obtained with the various radioligands in different laboratories were in reasonable agreement. Subsequently, these techniques have been extended to many other tissues.

Receptors for adenosine appear to be widely distributed in all tissues, since numerous physiological functions are modulated by adenosine. Under these conditions, it is always essential to define the cell type responsible for the observed binding in order to correlate the binding data to distinct cellular functions. Obviously, this general requirement cannot be met in complex organs such as brain, heart, or liver. In each of these organs the various tissue components deserve attention, in particular the large portion of vascular tissue that is highly responsive to adenosine. There are, however, sources of adenosine receptors that consist of single cell types such as isolated fat cells for R_i adenosine receptors and human platelets for R_a adenosine receptors. These cell types should be preferred if the selectivity of radioligands for subtypes of adenosine receptors is examined.

The great majority of radioligand binding studies is carried out with particulate fractions of tissue homogenates that have previously been used for assay of adenylate cyclase activity. Thus, radioligand binding and adenosine receptor-induced response of adenylate cyclase can easily be evaluated under identical conditions. The membrane preparations should always be free of residual amounts of endogenous adenosine, which even in repeatedly washed membrane preparations interferes considerably with radioligand binding to R_i adenosine receptors, whereas R_a adenosine receptors are less sensitive to low endogenous concentrations of adenosine. Removal of adenosine is achieved by treatment of the membrane preparation with adenosine deaminase resulting in a 3- to 4-fold increase of specific binding as compared to untreated membranes (Bruns *et al.*, 1980; Schwabe and Trost, 1980; Williams and Risley, 1980b). The same observation was made with a purified plasma membrane preparation (Trost and Schwabe, 1981). These results indicate an additional formation of adenosine after the washing procedure, possibly by contaminating ATP-containing structures such as mitochondria, which release adenosine through the action of ATPases and nucleotidases. For this reason it is advisable to conduct the binding assay in the presence of low concentrations of adenosine deaminase.

Binding of adenosine radioligands has also been performed with solubilized membrane preparations without loss of important regulatory functions of the receptors (Gavish *et al.*, 1982). Similarly to other receptor systems, solubilized membrane preparations may be a useful starting material for the purification and molecular characterization of adenosine receptors.

If functional data cannot be obtained in a broken cell preparation, it may be necessary to determine radioligand binding in intact cells. However, preliminary attempts to measure [^{3}H]-PIA binding in intact isolated fat cells have not yet revealed satisfactory results (Ukena, 1982). This was mainly due to the problem of nonspecific uptake of the radioligand into the cells.

An alternative method of studying adenosine receptors in intact tissues is the autoradiographic localization of radioligand binding. A remarkably heterogenous distribution of adenosine receptors was detected in rat brain by [^{3}H]-CHA (Lewis *et al.*, 1981; Goodman and Snyder, 1982) and in guinea pig intestine by [^{3}H]-NECA (Buckley and Burnstock, 1983). This approach will be especially useful for detecting adenosine receptors in small tissue compartments not readily accessible for the usual biochemical analysis of binding. A general introduction into the basic techniques of this method has been described elsewhere (Young and Kuhar, 1979).

C. Incubation Conditions

The incubation conditions for radioligand binding are usually designed to permit the comparison of binding data with functional parameters. Therefore, incubation should be carried out under physiological conditions with respect to temperature, pH, and ionic concentrations. Further variables are incubation volume and concentration of radioligand and membrane protein.

1. Temperature

Of all incubation conditions the temperature is most important, since binding to both R_i and R_a adenosine receptors is strongly dependent on temperature. R_i adenosine receptors show a relatively narrow temperature optimum at 37°C with more than 50% reduction of specific binding at 25°C (Trost and Schwabe, 1981). Furthermore, the affinity of agonists and antagonists is inversely affected by temperature. Adenosine agonists have higher affinities at 30°C than at 0°C, whereas the reverse order is observed for antagonists (Murphy and Snyder, 1982). Sometimes it is necessary to select the incubation temperature according to the properties of the radioligand, especially its binding affinity. High affinity agonist ligands with K_D values of approximately 1 n*M* such as [^{3}H]-PIA and [^{3}H]-CHA can be studied without difficulties at high incubation temperatures (37°C), since dissociation of binding proceeds slowly with a $t_{1/2}$ of about 20 min for these two ligands (Trost and Schwabe, 1981; Murphy and Snyder, 1982). Radioligands with lower affinities with K_D values above 10 n*M* may show a considerable loss of binding because of dissociation of the receptor–ligand complex during separation (Bennett, 1978). This problem is usually circumvented by diluting the samples with cold buffer, since dissociation of some radioligands is slower at low temperatures. However, some radioligands may dissociate rapidly even at 0°C and binding will be further lowered by an additional dilution step. Under these conditions, it is advisable to conduct the binding assay at lower incubation temperatures followed by immediate filtration without previous dilution. An example for this procedure is the measurement of [^{3}H]-DPX binding in guinea pig brain membranes at 0°C, since at higher temperatures no specific binding could be detected, because of the low K_D (Bruns *et al.*, 1980). In other tissues with higher K_D values for [^{3}H]-DPX, the binding can be measured at higher temperatures (Murphy and Snyder, 1982; Goodman *et al.*, 1982). A low incubation temperature is also recommended for the measurement of [^{3}H]-NECA binding to R_a adenosine receptors, because this radioligand has also relatively low affinities with K_D values between 50 and 200 n*M* (Schütz *et al.*, 1982a; Hüttemann *et al.*, 1984).

2. *Buffer and pH*

Nearly all radioligand binding studies of adenosine receptors have been conducted in 50 m*M* Tris-HCl buffer at pH from 7.4 to 7.7. Two other buffer systems, glycylglycin and Hepes, have also been used in order to adapt buffer conditions to accompanying cyclase experiments (Schütz *et al.*, 1982a; Yeung and Green, 1983). Specific binding of [^{3}H]-PIA is dependent on pH, showing a broad optimum over the pH range from 5.0 to 7.4 and a marked decline at pH 4.5 and 8.0.

3. *Ions*

Several different protocols for the ionic composition of radioligand binding assay for adenosine receptors have been used. Binding studies have been conducted without addition of ions (Bruns *et al.*, 1980; Williams and Risley, 1980b; Goodman *et al.*, 1982) or in the presence of 1–5 mM Mg^{2+} (Schwabe and Trost, 1980; Trost and Schwabe, 1981; Schütz *et al.*, 1982a; Yeung and Green, 1983). Magnesium was always added to adapt the ionic composition to previous or concomitant adenylate cyclase experiments. Magnesium ions enhance binding of [^{3}H]-CHA and [^{125}I]-HPIA in brain membranes, but this effect can only be demonstrated in EDTA-pretreated membranes (Goodman *et al.*, 1982; Schwabe *et al.*, 1982). Sodium ions inhibit the binding of [^{3}H]-CHA in brain membranes (Goodman *et al.*, 1982), whereas in other tissues the effect of these cations has not been systematically studied.

4. *Concentration of Radioligand and Membrane Protein*

The use of low concentrations of the radioligand is always advantageous, since nonspecific binding increases linearly with the concentration of the radioligand. The optimal concentration depends on the affinity and the specific radioactivity of the radioligand. The two agonist ligands for R_i adenosine receptors [^{3}H]-CHA and [^{3}H]-PIA are available with specific radioactivities of 20–50 Ci/mmole and yield best results at concentrations of 1 n*M*. The antagonist ligand [^{3}H]-DPX can be used at 1 n*M* concentration for radioligand-binding studies with bovine brain membranes, but higher concentrations (5–25 n*M*) are necessary for most of the other tissues in which the K_D values are in the range between 30 and 500 n*M* (Bruns *et al.*, 1980; Goodman *et al.*, 1982; Yeung and Green, 1983; Ukena *et al.*, 1984b; Lohse *et al.*, 1984). [^{3}H]-NECA has been used at higher concentrations (10–25 n*M*) for the study of R_a adenosine receptors because of the lower affinity of this receptor subtype compared with R_i adenosine receptors (Schütz *et al.*, 1982a; Hüttemann *et al.*, 1984). The iodinated ligand [^{125}I]-HPIA has the principal advantage of a very high specific radioactivity (2175 Ci/mmole) and can therefore be used at concentrations of 0.03–0.06 n*M* (Schwabe *et al.*, 1982). This ligand may be superior if the amount of biological material is very limited or the receptor density is very low.

The concentration of membrane protein in radioligand binding assays is usually kept as low as possible merely to save membrane protein of highly purified preparations. For ligands with low affinity or low specific radioactivity, it may be desirable to use higher concentrations of protein in order to increase the amount of bound radioactivity. Under these conditions, it is particularly important to take care that the receptor concentration is less (<5%) than the concentration of the free radioligand (Williams *et al.*, 1976). The large excess of the free ligand is a necessary requirement for kinetic and saturation experiments in which quantitative calculations are based on the free ligand concentration. In addition, protein linearity should always be examined in order to exclude artifacts. If the protein concentration exceeds the permissible upper limit, the incubation volume may be increased. We have usually worked with total volumes of 250–500 μl, but volumes up to 2 ml have also been employed. The latter incubation condition may be particularly helpful in systems with a high level of nonspecific binding. This will be reduced if low concentrations of the radioligand and membrane protein are incubated in large volumes.

D. Assay of Radioligand Binding

The methods for measurement of radioligand binding to adenosine receptors are based on the same principle as those used in the study of other receptors for hormones and neurotransmitters. In general, the receptor preparation is incubated with the radioligand until equilibrium is attained. Subsequently, bound and free ligand are rapidly separated in order to enable determination of the receptor-bound radioligand. The methods for separation include filtration, centrifugation, equilibrium dialysis, gel filtration chromatography, precipitation of the receptor–ligand complex, and adsorption of the free radioligand. The choice of these separation techniques depends on the properties of the receptor preparation. Filtration and centrifugation are most suitable for receptor preparations in particulate form, whereas soluble receptor preparations are usually separated by other methods. The general aspects of these procedures including many experimental details are extensively discussed in the methodological literature dealing with this subject (Kahn, 1974; Williams and Lefkowitz, 1978; Bennett, 1978).

1. Filtration

For adenosine receptor studies, filtration has been most widely used as method of separation (Bruns *et al.*, 1980; Schwabe and Trost, 1980; Williams and Risley, 1980b). Bound and free radioligand are separated by rapid filtration through glass fiber filters. Usually an aliquot of 0.2 to 0.9 ml of the incubation mixture is filtered, followed immediately by two washes with 5 ml of cold buffer to remove free ligand nonspecifically trapped in the filter and to the membrane preparation. These wash volumes have been found to be optimal, but they should be reexamined if a maximal reduction of nonspecific binding is not achieved or specific binding is already diminished by this procedure. For binding assays with very small incubation volumes, it may be convenient to rapidly dilute the sample with several milliliters of cold buffer and to pour the diluted sample on the filter, again followed by appropriate washing.

A potential source of error in the filtration procedure is the adsorption of radioligands to the filter material. Some glass fiber filters showed even stereospecific binding of radiolabeled opiates (Snyder *et al.*, 1975). Therefore, filter blanks obtained in the absence of the membrane preparation should always be included. One possible way to reduce this artifact is to dilute the incubation aliquot before filtration. When assaying [^{3}H]-PIA, [^{3}H]-DPX, [^{3}H]-NECA, and [^{125}I]-HPIA, nonspecific adsorption to Whatman GF/B or GF/C filters did not exceed 0.05 to 0.2% of the total filtered radioactivity.

A major disadvantage of the filtration method is the inevitable disturbance of the binding equilibrium by the washing step. By this procedure, the free ligand is infinitely diluted and dissociation of the receptor–ligand complex is initiated. Depending on the dissociation rate, a certain loss of receptor–ligand binding will occur. Therefore, rapidly dissociating receptor–ligand complexes will require separation techniques that are of sufficient velocity to minimize the amount dissociated. Under optimal conditions a total separation time including filtration and washing may be achieved in 5–10 sec (Schütz *et al.*, 1982a; Hüttemann *et al.*, 1984). From this time interval, the lower limit of the dissociation half life of the receptor–ligand complex can be calculated. It should be no less than 25–50 sec to avoid a loss of more than 10% of bound ligand. This limit can also be expressed in terms of the dissociation constant from the equilibrium relationship $K_D = k_2/k_1$. The association rate constant for the low affinity R_a adenosine receptors has been determined to be $k_1 = 1.2 \cdot 10^6\ M^{-1} \cdot \text{sec}^{-1}$ (Fox and Kurpis, 1983) and is similar to the values for most neurotransmitter receptors. Since the dissociation rate constant is defined by $k_2 = (\ln 2)/t_{1/2}$, the dissociation constant can be calculated from $t_{1/2}$ from the following equation: $K_D = (ln\ 2/1.2) \cdot 10^{-6}\ M \cdot \text{sec}/t_{1/2}$. Thus, under the conditions defined above a $t_{1/2}$ for dissociation of 25–50 sec is equivalent to a K_D of 12–24 n*M*. From these relationships it can easily be deducted that the two high affinity ligands [^{3}H]-PIA and [^{3}H]-CHA may be safely used as radioligands in filtration assays, since their K_D values are in the range of 0.3 to 6 n*M* and the $t_{1/2}$ of dissociation is at least several minutes (Trost and Schwabe, 1981; Goodman et al., 1982).

On the other hand, low-affinity ligands for R_a adenosine receptors have K_D values between 20 and 160 n*M* and dissociate rapidly from the binding sites. [^{3}H]-NECA binding in human platelets shows a dissociation half life of approximately 20 sec, a value which is very close to the lower limit for the applicability of the filtration procedure (Schwabe, 1983; Hüttemann *et al.*, 1984). Similar kinetic properties have been described for 2-chloro[^{3}H]adenosine binding to R_a adenosine receptors in human placenta (Fox and Kurpis, 1983). R_a adenosine receptors in other tissues with a higher affinity for [^{3}H]NECA, such as brain microvessels, may be studied at higher incubation temperatures (Schütz *et al.*, 1982b).

2. *Centrifugation*

An alternative method for rapid separation of bound and free ligand is centrifugation. This technique is preferable for binding studies with rapidly dissociating ligands or in case of high nonspecific adsorption of the radioligand to the filter material. Usually a microcentrifugation assay is used, which has been described by Rodbell *et al.* (1971). The necessary speed of separation is achieved by use of microcentrifuges with high *g* values (12,000*g*) which enable rapid pelleting of 100- to 300-μl samples within 1–2 min. An even more rapid separation (30 sec) can be obtained by application of a miniature ultracentrifuge (Beckman Airfuge) with 170,000*g* (Albers and Krishnan, 1979). The amount of bound radioactivity is measured in the pellet, which is carefully rinsed without disturbing the pellet surface. The major advantage of centrifugation is that equilibrium conditions are maintained during the separation procedure. A limitation of this methodology is the time needed for centrifugation, since short time intervals of less than 1 min cannot be followed if rapid kinetics of association and dissociation have to be determined.

The major disadvantage of centrifugation as method of separation is the less efficient washing of the particulate pellet compared to the filtration technique. Consequently, higher amounts of unbound ligand are trapped in the water space of the pellet resulting in higher levels of nonspecific binding. [^{14}C]Sucrose has been used to correct total binding for the residual amounts of the free ligand at the walls of the centrifuge tube and in the water space of the protein pellet (Rodbell *et al.*, 1971; Schwabe *et al.*, 1979). An additional modification of the centrifugation procedure employs centrifugation through silicone oil or other oil mixtures placed at the bottom of the centrifuge tube (Klingenberg and Pfaff, 1967; Mackin *et al.*, 1983). These oil mixtures have a higher density than hypotonic aqueous incubation buffers but a lower density than particulate membrane preparations. The samples are incubated on top of the oil phase and the membrane-bound radioligand is centrifuged into the oil phase, resulting in a complete and rapid separation of the bound radioactivity from the free ligand in the incubation buffer. The centrifuge tube may be rinsed or the tip of the tube may be cut off without risk of disturbing the pellet surface. Oil-phase centrifugation may not be suitable for very lipophilic radioligands, which potentially can diffuse into the oil layer, producing inconsistent increases in blank values. For [^{3}H]-PIA no significant accumulation of the ligand into the oil phase has been observed during centrifugation (Ukena, 1982).

The centrifugation technique has not been widely used for adenosine receptor binding studies. The initial attempts to measure [^{3}H]adenosine binding were carried out with this procedure (Schwabe *et al.*, 1979; Schütz and Brugger, 1982; Schütz *et al.*, 1982a), but, as already mentioned, [^{3}H]adenosine cannot be used as a suitable radioligand, since it failed to label physiologically important adenosine receptors for several other reasons. Furthermore, the binding of [^{3}H]-CHA and [^{3}H]-NECA has been determined by the centrifugation assay in a liver membrane preparation. Again, an appropriate structure–activity profile for R_a adenosine receptors was not obtained, possibly because of the interference by a large number of low-affinity, high-capacity binding sites and a high background of nonspecific binding (Schütz *et al.*, 1982a).

3. *Nonspecific Binding*

Nonspecific binding is generally defined as the portion of total radioligand binding that is not displaceable by an excess concentration of unlabeled ligand. The amount of specific binding is then obtained by subtracting nonspecific binding from total binding. Several components contribute to nonspecific binding, such as adsorption to filters and test tubes, free radioligand trapped in the separated material, and the true nonspecific binding to nonreceptor sites in the membrane preparation under study. The concentration of unlabeled ligand used for determination of nonspecific binding is usually 1000 times K_D concentration. If additional amounts of bound radioligand are displaced by higher concentrations, careful examination should be undertaken to determine whether this component represents true specific binding to adenosine receptors. Under such conditions, it is always advisable to use another displacing ligand that is chemically different from the radioligand and improves the specificity of radioligand binding. The amount of nonspecific binding depends linearly on the concentration of the radioligand, which therefore is always kept as low as possible. Values for the percent nonspecific binding usually refer to the K_D concentration of the radioligand. Details on the validity of the determination of nonspecific binding are described in reviews of the general methodology of receptor ligand binding (Bennett, 1978; Williams and Lefkowitz, 1978).

The levels of nonspecific binding of most radioligands used for the study of adenosine receptors are less than 10% of total binding (Bruns *et al.*, 1980; Williams and Risley, 1980b; Trost and Schwabe, 1981; Murphy and Snyder, 1982; Hüttemann *et al.*, 1984). Higher levels of nonspecific binding have been observed with the antagonist ligand [^{3}H]-DPX in some membrane preparations. Assays of brain membrane preparations from calf, rat, and rabbit gave levels of nonspecific binding in the range of 10–30%, but 50–90% for guinea pig and human brain (Bruns *et al.*, 1980; Murphy and Snyder, 1982). In rat fat cells only 10–15% of [^{3}H]-DPX was nonspecifically bound (Ukena *et al.*, 1984b). These data confirm observations obtained with other receptor systems that marked variations of nonspecific binding depending on tissue and species may be obtained.

III. IDENTIFICATION OF R_i ADENOSINE RECEPTORS BY RADIOACTIVELY LABELED AGONISTS

Several radioactively labeled adenosine agonists have been used in binding studies of R_i adenosine receptors. These include the tritiated adenosine analogs [^{3}H]-CHA, [^{3}H]-PIA, and 2-chloro[^{3}H]adenosine, as well as the iodinated radioligand [^{125}I]-HPIA. All agonist ligands are characterized by a high affinity for R_i adenosine receptors, often more than 100-fold higher than that of potent antagonists such as DPX. The first successful binding studies were performed with particulate preparations from brain tissue (Bruns *et al.*, 1980; Schwabe and Trost, 1980; Williams and Risley, 1980b). The data obtained with various radioligands were in reasonably good agreement. Subsequently, several other tissues have been studied (Table I).

Table I. Characterization of R_i Adenosine Receptors in Various Tissues by Radioligand Binding

Tissue	Radioligand	*KD* (n*M*)	B_{max} (fmoles/mg)	Reference
Rat brain	[^{3}H]-ClA[a]	1.3/16	590	Williams and Risley (1980b)
	[^{3}H]-CHA	0.7/2.4	350	Patel *et al.* (1982)
	[^{3}H]-PIA	1.4/139	740	Lohse *et al.* (1984)
	[^{3}H]-DPX	68	1220	Lohse *et al.* (1984)
	[^{125}I]-HPIA	0.5	230	Schwabe *et al.* (1982)
Bovine brain	[^{3}H]-CHA	0.3/1.8	540	Bruns *et al.* (1980)
	[^{3}H]-DPX	5	1000	Bruns *et al.* (1980)
Guinea pig brain	[^{3}H]-CHA	6	370	Bruns *et al.* (1980)
	[^{3}H]-DPX	70	500	Bruns *et al.* (1980)
Rat fat cell	[^{3}H]-PIA	6	1900	Trost and Schwabe (1981)
	[^{3}H]-PIA	0.3/11	1400	Ukena *et al.* (1984b)
	[^{3}H]-DPX	63	1990	Ukena *et al.* (1984b)
	[^{125}I]-HPA	0.7/7.6	1900	Ukena *et al.* (1984a)
Rat testes	[^{3}H]-CHA	2.0	200	Murphy and Snyder (1982)

[a] 2-Chloro[^{3}H]adenosine.

A. Radioligands

Each of these radioligands has specific advantages for the characterization and identification of R_i adenosine receptors. Most studies have been conducted with the radiolabeled N^6-substituted adenosine derivatives, [^{3}H]-CHA and [^{3}H]-PIA. (−)PIA, originally developed as a coronary vasodilator, was first described as an antilipolytic agent in adipose tissue (Westermann and Stock, 1970). Subsequently, it was identified as a potent agonist in many adenosine-sensitive systems, such as platelets (Dietmann *et al.*, 1970), coronary vessels (Vapaatalo *et al.*, 1975), Leydig cell tumors (Londos and Wolff, 1977), cultured brain cells (Van Calker *et al.*, 1979), and brain slices (Smellie et al., 1979). The most potent effects of (−)PIA were observed for the inhibition of adenylate cyclase and lipolysis of isolated fat cells with an IC_{50} of 0.2 n*M* (Londos *et al.*, 1980). Similarly, (−)PIA was the most potent adenosine analog to inhibit hormone-induced cyclic AMP formation in mouse brain cell cultures (Van Calker *et al.*, 1979). In adenosine-responsive tissues that mediate stimulation of adenylate cyclase (−)PIA was less potent than adenosine and NECA (Van Calker *et al.*, 1979; Londos *et al.*, 1980). These results were the basis for the present concept of inhibitory R_i (A_1) and stimulatory R_a (A_2) adenosine receptors linked to adenylate cyclase. For all these reasons, [^{3}H]-PIA appears particularly appropriate as radioligand for R_i adenosine receptor studies. The same holds true for [^{3}H]-CHA, with the only limitation being that the pharmacological properties of CHA have been less extensively investigated than that of (−)PIA.

2-Chloro[^{3}H]adenosine is another tritiated ligand that has been used in radioligand-binding studies of R_i adenosine receptors (Williams and Risley, 1980b; Wu and Phillis, 1982). However, previous adenylate cyclase studies have shown that 2-chloroadenosine acts on both R_a and R_i adenosine receptors (Londos *et al.*, 1980). Actually, binding of 2-chloro[^{3}H]adenosine to R_a adenosine receptors has recently been identified in human placenta (Fox and Kurpis, 1983). Therefore, precautions are necessary if 2-chloro[^{3}H]adenosine is used for binding studies in tissues containing both adenosine receptor subtypes. Further disadvantages of this compound are the relatively low specific radioactivity of 12 Ci/mmole and problems of its chemical stability (Williams and Risley, 1982).

[^{125}I]-HPIA has a high affinity for R_i adenosine receptors and the same structure–activity profile as [^{3}H]-PIA (Schwabe *et al.*, 1982; Ukena *et al.*, 1984a). The incorporation of one [^{125}I]atom per molecule of ligand results in a compound with a specific radioactivity of 2175 Ci/mmole which exceeds that of tritiated ligands 50- to 100-fold. This high specific radioactivity permits the study of R_i adenosine receptors in very small tissue samples or in tissues with low density of adenosine receptors. Another advantage appears likely for autoradiographic studies in which the exposure time might be shortened from several weeks to a few days by using this radioiodinated ligand.

Measurement of radioligand binding to R_i adenosine receptors is generally performed in membrane preparations. Binding has been studied in membrane fractions derived from brain (Bruns *et al.*, 1980; Schwabe and Trost, 1980; Williams and Risley, 1980b; Goodman *et al.*, 1982; Murphy and Snyder, 1982), isolated fat cells (Trost and Schwabe, 1981), and testes (Williams and Risley, 1980b; Murphy and Snyder, 1981). Fat cells offer the advantage of studying R_i adenosine receptors in a single cell type without interference by R_a receptors, whereas in brain both receptor subtypes may contribute to overall radioligand binding. Therefore, the fat cell system has been selected for the detailed description of the binding assay for R_i adenosine receptors. This binding assay can also be used for membrane preparations of other tissues and for other R_i selective radioligands such as [^{3}H]-CHA.

B. Description of the Binding Assay

1. Materials

[^{3}H]-PIA with a specific radioactivity of 49.9 Ci/mmole (New England Nuclear Corporation, Boston, Mass., USA).

Adenosine deaminase from calf intestine (200 U/mg) (Boehringer Mannheim, Mannheim, Federal Republic of Germany).

(−)PIA (Boehringer Mannheim, Mannheim, Federal Republic of Germany)

50 m*M* Tris-HCl buffer, pH 7.4.

Whatman GF/B glass fiber filter (25 mm diameter).

Vacuum filtration apparatus (Millipore).

Triton-based scintillation cocktail, Quickszint 402 (Zinsser Analytic GmbH, Frankfurt, Federal Republic of Germany).

Rat fat cell plasma membranes, prepared according to the method of McKeel and Jarett (1970) and stored in 50 m*M* Tris-HCl, pH 7.4, in liquid nitrogen after the last centrifugation step.

2. *Preparation of [^{125}I]-HPIA*

The preparation is performed as described by Schwabe *et al.* (1982). [^{125}I]-HPIA is iodinated by the method of Hunter and Greenwood (1962). 10 μl of 2.5 m*M* (−)HPIA (in 50% ethanol) are mixed with 20 μl 0.3 *M* sodium phosphate buffer, pH 7.55, in an Eppendorf test tube (1.5 ml), followed by addition of 1 mCi Na[^{125}I] as carrier-free Na[^{125}I] and 20 μl of chloramine T (0.3 mg/ml of 0.3 *M* sodium phosphate buffer, pH 7.55). After 4.5 min the reaction is stopped by addition of 300 μl aqueous solution of sodium metabisulfite (1 mg/ml). The iodinated product is extracted three times with ethylacetate containing 0.01% phenol. Phases are separated by a 1-min spin at 12,000*g*. The three ethylacetate washes are combined and concentrated to 20–50 μl by a stream of nitrogen. The ethylacetate extract is spotted on Whatman 3MM paper under constant flow of nitrogen and chromatographed in a descending manner at 4°C for 6 hr with 50 m*M* ammonium formate, pH 8.5. The wet chromatogram is cut into 1-cm strips, which are immediately placed in 2 ml methanol containing 0.01% phenol and stored at −25°C.

Purification of [^{125}I]-HPIA is also achieved by high-pressure liquid chromatography (Spectra Physics 8100 liquid chromatograph) on a Waters C18 μBondapak steel column (30 × 0.4 cm) with 0.02 *M* KH_2PO_4 (pH 5.6)/acetonitrile in a linear gradient from 70/30 (v/v) to 20/80 (v/v) at 40°C and a flow rate of 1 ml/min for 15 min. The elution profile is monitored at 254 nm. Uniodinated (−)HPIA elutes as a single sharp peak with a retention time of 4.3 min and (−)IHPIA follows with a retention time of 7.1 min. A tracer amount of [^{125}I]-HPIA (100,000 cpm) gives essentially the same elution profile (Ukena *et al.*, 1984a).

[^{125}I]-HPIA can further be characterized by thin-layer chromatography with three solvent systems. Solvent system I for thin-layer cellulose (Merck, Darmstadt, Federal Republic of Germany) contains 50 m*M* ammonium formate, pH 8.4; solvent system II for cellulose thin layer plates, 250 m*M* lithium chloride; solvent system III for silica gel plates, *n*-butanol/methanol/25% NH_4OH (80:20:20, v/v). The R_f values in system I are [^{125}I]-HPIA 0.39 and HPIA 0.61; in system II, [^{125}I]-HPIA 0.35 and HPIA 0.59; and in system III; [^{125}I]-HPIA 0.40 and HPIA 0.44. The radiochemical purity of [^{125}I]-HPIA as analyzed by thin-layer chromatography is more than 95%. The ligand is stable for at least 4 weeks under the storage conditions mentioned above. After prolonged storage for 4 months, uncharacterized radioactive impurities of up to 15% of the total radioactivity may occur.

3. *Binding Assay for [^{3}H]-PIA*

[^{3}H]-PIA binding to rat fat cell membranes is determined by a vacuum filtration technique. The following steps are performed in 1.5-ml polypropylene microtubes (Eppendorf) at 37°C in an Eppendorf thermostat 5320. The final assay volume is 500 μl and all samples should be assayed in duplicates.

a. Incubation. Add 50 μl of the displacing agent; add 50 μl of 10 n*M* [^{3}H]-PIA (approximately 24,000 cpm per assay tube), resulting in a final radioligand concentration of 1 n*M*; add 300 μl of water or additional compounds dissolved in water; add 50 μl 500 m*M* Tris-HCl buffer, pH 7.4, resulting in a final concentration of 50 m*M*; preincubate for 5 min at 37°C for temperature equilibration. Start binding reaction by addition of 50 μl freshly thawed fat cell membrane suspension containing 10–20 μg protein and 0.5 μg (0.1 U) adenosine deaminase. Mix by vortexing and incubate in 37°C for 60 min.

b. Filtration. Stop reaction by removal of 400 μl-aliquot and rapid filtration through Whatman GF/B glass fiber filters. Wash the filters immediately with two 5-ml portions of ice-cold incubation buffer and transfer the filter quickly from the filter holder into a counting vial. The whole filtration from application of the aliquot to the filter until removal of the filter should not exceed 10 sec.

c. Preparation of Standards and Blanks. Total binding: Add 50 μl 10 n*M* [^{3}H]-PIA, 350 μl H_2O, 50 μl 500 m*M* Tris-HCl buffer, pH 7.4, and start by addition of 50-μl membrane suspension together with the other samples as described above. Prepare four samples and place two samples at the first and two samples at the last places of the complete binding assay.

Nonspecific binding: Add 50 μl 100 μ*M* (−)PIA as displacing agent (final concentration in the assay 10 μ*M*) and add all other compounds as described above in step a. Prepare four samples and place two samples at the first and two samples at the last places of the complete binding assay.

Counting standard: Add 50 μl of 10 n*M* [^{3}H]-PIA standard solution directly on a glass fiber filter placed in a counting vial and previously washed with two 5-ml portions of the incubation buffer.

Filter blank: Add 50 μl 10 n*M* [^{3}H]-PIA, 400 μl H_2O, and 50 μl 500 m*M* Tris-HCl buffer, pH 7.4; mix, incubate, and filtrate as described above.

Add 10-ml scintillation solution, cap scintillation vials, vortex vigorously two times for at least 10 sec and count in a liquid scintillation counter after 6-hr storage of the samples to allow for complete solution of the filter-trapped radioactivity.

d. Calculations. The amount of [^{3}H]-PIA specifically bound to fat cell membranes expressed in fmoles [^{3}H]-PIA per milligram protein is calculated as follows:

$$\text{Specific binding} = (\text{T} - \text{N}) \frac{\text{I} \times \text{R}}{\text{F} \times \text{S} \times \text{P}}$$

where T = mean cpm of total (or displaced) binding,
N = mean cpm of nonspecific binding,
S = mean cpm of counting standard,
I = incubation volume (μl),
F = filtrated volume (μl),
R = amount of radioligand per sample (fmoles[^{3}H]PIA), and
P = amount of membrane protein per sample (mg).

Under these assay conditions, total [^{3}H]-PIA binding is 1200 cpm and nonspecific binding is 50 cpm (3–5%) in typical experiments. The filter blank is less than 0.1% of total radioactivity per sample and thus in the range of the counter background. By use of suitable protein concentrations, it should always be assured that less than 5% of the added radioligand is bound to the membrane preparation. This is an important requirement, since the free radioligand concentration must be kept constant in order to enable the calculation of binding constants from association and displacement experiments. If the amount of bound radioligand is greater than 5% of total radioligand added, binding constants will be underestimated unless appropriate corrections of the actual free ligand concentration are made.

The samples for total and nonspecific binding at the beginning and the end of the assay are used as internal quality control and should not differ more than 5%. Higher deviations may be due to incomplete stability of the membrane preparation and of the radioligand, insufficient activity of the added adenosine deaminase, or differences in filtration conditions. The last point may occur with the use of manifold filtration machines, which do not allow the immediate removal of the filter from its support after the washing procedure.

4. *Binding Assay for [^{125}I]-HPIA*

The assay for [^{125}I]-HPIA binding to rat fat cell membranes is carried out in a total volume of 500 μl under the same conditions as those described for [^{3}H]-PIA binding, except the following changes in the concentration of radioligand and membrane protein.

a. Specific Binding. Add 50 μl of 1 n*M* [^{125}I]-HPIA (approximately 100,000 cpm per assay tube) resulting in a final concentration of 0.1 n*M*; add 50 μl of displacing agent (or H_2O for determination of total binding); add 300 μl H_2O or additional compounds dissolved in H_2O; add 50 μl 500 μ*M* Tris-HCl buffer, pH 7.4; and start binding reaction by addition of 50-μl membrane suspension containing 5–10 μg protein and 0.5 μg (0.1 U) adenosine deaminase. Mix by vortexing, incubate at 37°C for 60 min, and stop reaction by filtration as described for [^{3}H]-PIA binding (see Section 3b).

b. Nonspecific Binding. Add 50 μl of 10 μ*M* (−)PIA as displacing agent and all other compounds as listed above for specific binding. Other blanks and standards are prepared as described for [^{3}H]-PIA binding (see Section 3c).

c. Calculations. Count the filters directly in a gamma counter and calculate [^{125}I]-HPIA binding as described for [^{3}H]-PIA (see Section 3d).

The advantage of [^{125}I]-HPIA compared to [^{3}H]-PIA is the use of lower concentrations of the radioligand and of membrane protein. If it is desirable to use even less radioligand and protein, the incubation volume may be reduced to 200 μl. In this case, it is convenient to dilute the incubated sample with 1 ml of cold incubation buffer immediately before filtration and to filtrate an appropriate aliquot.

C. Analysis of Binding Data

The characterization of physiologically relevant adenosine receptors always requires that several criteria be satisfied. The binding of the radioligand to its receptor should be saturable, rapid, reversible, and specific as demonstrated by appropriate structure–activity profiles in displacement experiments with agonists

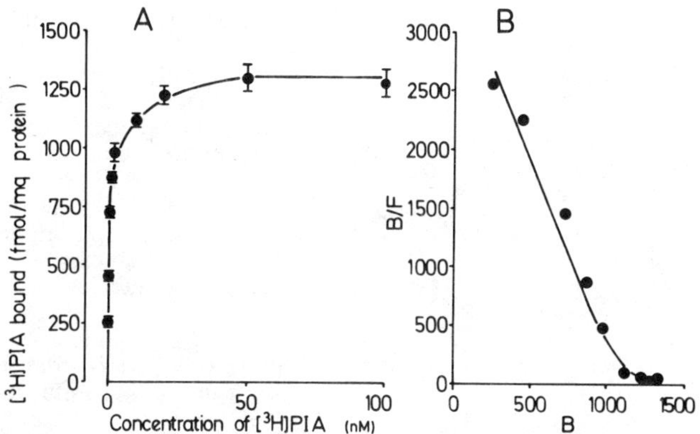

Figure 2. (A) Saturation of [^{3}H]-PIA binding to rat fat cell membranes. Binding was determined after 60 min incubation at 37°C. Each value is the mean of four experiments ± S.E.M.(B) Scatchard plot of the same data. B = fmoles [^{3}H]-PIA bound per milligram protein; F = free concentration of [^{3}H]-PIA (n*M*). K_D and B_{max} values of the high- and low-affinity binding were obtained by a curve-fitting program (SCTFIT) according to De Lean *et al.* (1982). The high-affinity site has a K_D of 0.26 n*M* and a B_{max} of 1.1 pmoles/mg protein, the low-affinity site a K_D of 10.5 n*M* and a B_{max} of 0.29 pmoles/mg protein. Data from Ukena *et al.* (1984b).

and antagonists. In addition, the data obtained in binding experiments should be reflected in corresponding data on the biological response.

1. Saturation Experiments

Saturation experiments are performed in order to determine the affinity expressed as dissociation constant K_D and the maximal number of [^{3}H]-PIA binding sites expressed as B_{max}. Increasing concentrations of the radioligand are incubated with a constant amount of the membrane preparation and the data for specific binding are analyzed according to the Scatchard equation (Scatchard, 1949). A typical saturation experiment for [^{3}H]-PIA binding to rat fat cell membranes is shown in Figure 2. The specific binding appears to be a saturable process, whereas nonspecific binding increases linearly with the [^{3}H]-PIA concentration. Scatchard analysis of these binding data reveals a curvilinear plot. Quantitative analysis of the data by a computer-assisted curve-fitting program (SCTFIT) according to De Lean *et al.* (1982) indicates a two-site model with different affinities. For the high affinity site, a K_D of 0.26 n*M* and a maximal number of binding sites of 1.1 pmoles/mg protein were calculated. For the low affinity site, the corresponding data were 10.5 n*M* for K_D and 0.29 pmoles/mg protein for B_{max}. Thus, 79% of the total [^{3}H]-PIA binding sites are of high affinity and 21% are of low affinity. These two portions of total binding reflect different affinity states of a single receptor type and not the existence of two separate adenosine receptors, as demonstrated by the interconversion in response to endogenous modulators. By addition of GTP, 90% of the high-affinity binding sites can be converted into the low-affinity state (Ukena *et al.*, 1984c).

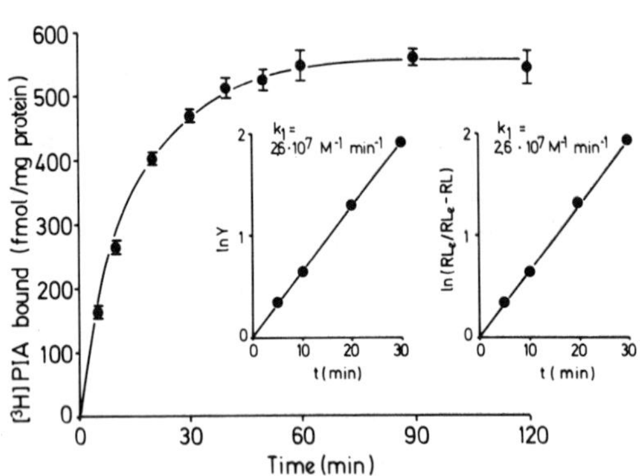

Figure 3. Association of [^{3}H]-PIA to rat fat cell membranes. [^{3}H]-PIA binding was determined at 37°C. Each value is the mean of 4 experiments. Left inset: [^{3}H]-PIA binding is plotted according to the integrated form of the second order rate equation, y $= RL_e\,(L_T - RL \cdot RL_e/R_T)/L_T(RL_e - RL)$. Right inset: [^{3}H]-PIA binding is plotted according to the pseudo-first-order equation. RL_e = concentration of bound radioligand at equilibrium; RL = concentration of bound radioligand at time t; L_T = total concentration of radioligand; R_T = total concentration of binding sites (B_{max}). Data from Ukena *et al.* (1984b).

The K_D value for the high-affinity site is in close agreement with the apparent IC_{50} of (−)PIA for the inhibition of hormone-induced cyclic AMP accumulation and of lipolysis in isolated fat cells (Londos *et al.*, 1980). The low-affinity component of [^{3}H]-PIA binding has not been found in previous studies of [^{3}H]-PIA binding (Trost and Schwabe, 1981). This is probably due to the fact that the radioligand concentration was varied over a smaller concentration range and that the saturation isotherm was not evaluated by means of computer-assisted curve fitting. Usually it is sufficient to extend saturation curves to the 10-fold K_D value. However, if a receptor is assumed to exist in two different affinity states, the saturation curve should extend to 10-fold the higher K_D value. Otherwise, the total number of binding sites may be underestimated and differences in agonist and antagonist radioligand binding data may occur, since antagonist radioligands do not distinguish between the high- and low-affinity states of adenosine receptors, as outlined below.

2. *Rate Constants: Association*

A second important criterion of receptor analysis is the rapid and reversible interaction between radioligand and receptor. In order to characterize these properties, time courses for association and dissociation of [^{3}H]-PIA binding are measured. Experimentally, it is convenient to perform the time course experiments in a batch procedure with a larger incubation volume that allows the removal of at least 15 aliquots. Thus, the total incubation volume is increased to 7 ml. The association reaction is started by addition of the fat cell membrane suspension and 400-μl aliquots (10–20 μg protein) are removed at appropriate time intervals for filtration. In order to ensure homogeneity of the samples, the incubation should be performed in a shaking water bath. As shown in Figure 3, specific binding of [^{3}H]-PIA to fat cell membranes is relatively slow at the radioligand concentration of 1 n*M*, reaching equilibrium within 60 min at 37°C. At higher radioligand concentrations (10 n*M*) steady-state binding is already achieved at 10 min (Trost and Schwabe, 1981).

The data of the time course are used for the calculation of the association rate constant k_1 for the reaction $R + L \rightarrow RL$ in which R is the free receptor, L the free ligand, and RL the receptor–ligand complex. This bimolecular process is described by a second-order reaction, but can be considered as a pseudomonomolecular first-order reaction if the concentration of the free ligand is much higher than that of the receptor sites. Under this condition a pseudo-first-order rate constant $k_i = k_1 [L]$ can be defined. In the association experiment shown in Figure 3, the receptor concentration was 15 μg protein/0.5 ml incubation volume and, with regard to the total B_{max} value (1.4 pmoles/mg protein) obtained in the saturation experiment, equivalent to 0.042 nM, which is less than 5% of the free concentration of [^{3}H]-PIA (1 nM). The observed forward rate constant ($k_{ob} = k_1 \cdot L + k_2$) can be calculated from the slope of a plot of the term $ln[(RL_e)/(RL_e - RL)]$ versus time (Williams *et al.*, 1976; Williams and Lefkowitz, 1978). In this equation RL_e represents the concentration of bound radioligand at equilibrium and RL the concentration of bound radioligand at each time. The second order rate constant, k_1, can be calculated from the equation $k_1 = (k_{ob} - k_2)/L$, in which k_2 is the independently determined rate constant for the dissociation reaction (see below). In the experiment shown in Figure 3 the association constant is $k_1 = 2.6 \times 10^7\ M^{-1} \cdot min^{-1}$.

An alternative method for determination of the kinetic association constant, k_1, from the time course of association is to use the integrated second order rate equation (Weiland and Molinoff, 1981):

$$ln \left[\frac{RL_e\,(L_T - RL \times RL_e/R_T)}{L_T(RL_e - RL)} \right] = k_1 \left[\frac{L_T \times R_T}{RL_e} - RL_e \right] t$$

In this equation L_T is the total concentration of ligand, R_T the total concentration of binding sites (B_{max}), RL_e the concentration of radioligand bound at equilibrium, and RL the concentration of receptor–ligand complex at time t. The association constant k_1 is determined from the slope of a plot of the left side of the equation versus time (see Figure 3). The use of the full second-order equation has the advantage of making no assumptions concerning the relative concentrations of the radioligand and the receptor sites, but it requires an independent estimate of the total number of binding sites as obtained from saturation experiments. The association constant according to the second-order rate equation for the experiment shown in Figure 3 is $k_1 = 2.6 \times 10^7\ M^{-1} \cdot min^{-1}$ and thus identical with the value derived from the first-order equation.

Furthermore, both methods for the determination of the rate constants yield linear plots, as shown in Figure 3, thereby confirming that the binding reaction is a simple second-order process. Biphasic plots may occur that indicate heterogeneity of binding sites, a ligand-induced site–site interaction, a two-step ligand–receptor interaction, or a ligand-induced conformational change of the receptor. Analysis of these more complex reactions may require detailed kinetic and equilibrium experiments.

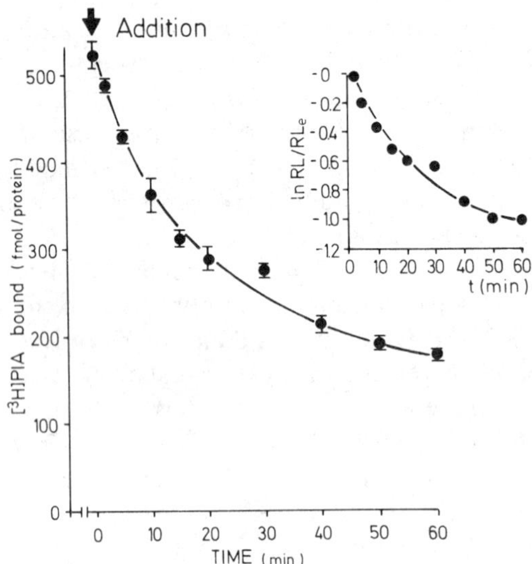

Figure 4. Dissociation of $[^3H]$-PIA binding from rat fat cell membranes. Dissociation of $[^3H]$-PIA (1 n*M*) was measured at 37°C after 60 min of equilibration and was induced by rapid addition of 10 μM (−)PIA (arrow). Values are the mean of four experiments ±S.E.M. Inset: Dissociation is plotted as a first order reaction: $\ln(RL/RL_e) = -k_2 t$; RL = concentration of bound radioligand at time t, RL_e = concentration of bound radioligand at equilibrium. Data from Ukena *et al.* (1984b).

3. *Rate Constants: Dissociation*

The dissociation is a monomolecular process that follows first-order kinetics. Therefore, the dissociation rate constant k_2 can be calculated more easily than the association constant. The rate equation for dissociation is described by $ln(RL/RL_e) = -k_2t$, in which RL_e is the concentration of the equilibrated ligand–receptor complex just prior to the "infinite" dilution of the radioligand and RL the concentration of bound radioligand at time t after initiation of the dissociation. The dissociation constant k_2 can be estimated from the negative slope of a plot of $ln(RL/RL_e)$ versus t. Alternatively, the half-life ($t_{1/2}$) for the loss of specific radioligand binding can be calculated from the equation $t_{1/2} = ln\ 2/k_2$. Nonlinear first-order dissociation plots may reflect heterogeneity of binding sites, cooperative site–site interactions, or conformational changes of the binding sites.

Experimentally, the dissociation rate constant is determined at equilibrium by elimination of the association reaction. This can be achieved either by an "infinite" dilution of a concentrated solution of the binding assay with at least a 100-fold volume excess of incubation buffer at the desired temperature or by addition of a 1000-fold excess of the unlabeled ligand. Aliquots of the receptor–ligand mixture are assayed for specific binding at various time intervals after the dilution step. In practice, the second method of dissociation can be performed more easily than the true dilution method by volume addition. Figure 4 shows the data demonstrating the dissociation of $[^3H]$-PIA from rat fat cell membranes as determined by adding an excess of unlabeled (−)PIA to an equilibrated mixture of the radioligand and the membranes. The dissociation was relatively slow and showed a biphasic curve with a $t_{1/2}$ of about 13 min for the initial phase and about 165 min for the second phase. The rate constants of dissociation, k_{2H} and k_{2L}, as calculated by the method described by Lohse *et al.* (1984) were 0.0042 min^{-1} and 0.053 min^{-1}, respectively.

The ratio k_{2H}/k_1 and k_{2L}/k_1 of the rate constants was 0.16 nM and 2 nM, respectively, and provides an independent estimate of the dissociation constants K_H and K_L for the interaction of the radioligand with its binding sites in fat cell plasma membranes. This value is in reasonable agreement with the high and low affinity K_D values calculated from the saturation experiment illustrated in Figure 2.

4. *Specificity of Binding Sites*

The structural specificity of radioligand binding to adenosine receptors is determined by the ability of a series of unlabeled agents to compete for the binding sites. Adenosine receptor agonists and antagonists, as well as compounds devoid of biological activity, are included in the competition experiments. The order of potency of these compounds in inhibiting radioligand binding should correlate with the potencies determined for the physiological response mediated by R_i adenosine receptors. If stereoselectivity can be demonstrated by measurement of functional parameters, it should always be detectable in binding experiments.

The potency of the displacing drugs can be estimated from the concentration of the compound that inhibits specific binding by 50% (IC_{50}) at equilibrium. The IC_{50} value is determined from displacement curves or more accurately after transformation of the data to indirect Hill plots (also called logit-log plots) according to the following equation:

$$\log \frac{RL_I}{RL - RL_I} = -n \log I + n \log IC_{50}$$

In this equation RL is the amount of radioligand specifically bound in the absence of the inhibitor, RL_I the amount specifically bound in the presence of the inhibitor, I the concentration of the inhibiting drug and n the indirect Hill coefficient, which expresses the theoretical number of ligand binding sites per receptor molecule. A plot of log ($RL_I/RL - RL_I$) versus log I has an intercept on the abscissa equal to the IC_{50} and a slope of $-n$.

Steep competition curves as characterized by a Hill coefficient of approximately 1.0 are indicative of the interaction of the displacing compound with one population of binding sites and can be used to indirectly estimate the dissociation constant (K_D) of the displacing compound. The relationship between IC_{50} and K_D is described by the equation of Cheng and Prusoff (1973) $K_i = IC_{50}/(1 + L/K_{DL})$, in which L is the concentration of free labeled ligand and K_{DL} is the dissociation constant of the labeled ligand usually determined by saturation experiments. This equation can only be applied if the interaction between radioligand and unlabeled drug is competitive, if the Hill coefficient is 1, and if less than 10% of the total radioligand is bound and the K_D of the radioligand is much greater than the concentration of binding sites. Otherwise, more complex corrections have to be introduced (Jacobs *et al.*, 1975). Furthermore, it should be considered that the competing drug affects the time required to reach equilibrium and appropriate adjustments of the incubation time have to be made. It has been calculated that

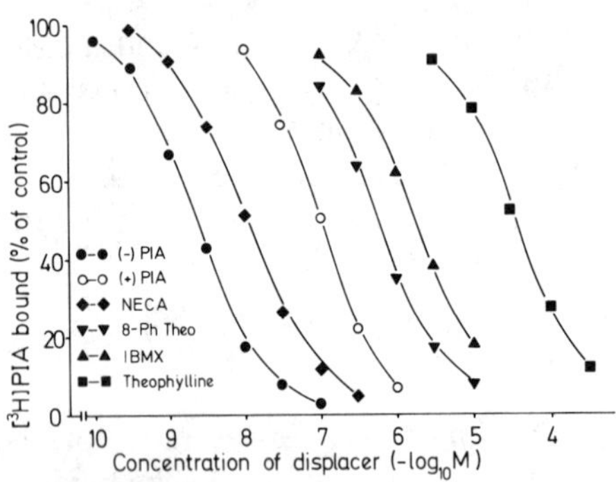

Figure 5. Inhibition of [^{3}H]-PIA binding to rat fat cell membranes by adenosine agonists and antagonists. Binding was measured at a radioligand concentration of 1 n*M* at 37°C for 60 min; 8-Ph Theo = 8-phenyltheophylline. Mean values of triplicate experiments are shown. Data from Ukena *et al.* (1984c).

the $t_{1/2}$ of association can be increased by a factor of $1 + L/K_{DL}$ in presence of the inhibitor (Weiland and Molinoff, 1981).

Shallow displacement curves as characterized by Hill coefficients of less than 1.0 and curvilinear Hofstee plots may indicate a complex interaction between ligand and receptor. Low indirect Hill coefficients of competition curves are most commonly due to heterogeneity of binding sites. Several analytical methods have been proposed to quantitate the relative proportions of receptor subtypes. Rugg *et al.* (1978) have transformed their data into Hofstee plots and analyzed it graphically. Minneman *et al.* (1979) used the same transformation with a subsequent computer-aided iterative analysis. A procedure using untransformed binding data was proposed by Hancock *et al.* (1979) who analyzed displacement curves directly by a computer-assisted nonlinear least-square curve fitting. This technique results in increased accuracy, since the transformation into percentage data and the approximate correction according to Cheng and Prusoff (1973) is not required. Furthermore, it permits the comparison of different models and the simultaneous analysis of several curves. The same methodology has also been used to characterize agonist-induced changes of affinity states in systems regulated by guanine nucleotides (Kent *et al.*, 1980). These curve-fitting procedures will provide reliable data only if the mass action principles are fully satisfied for all ligands at all sites. Furthermore competition curves should be designed to contain 12 to 18 concentrations of the displacing ligand in order to obtain enough data for a precise definition of two subtypes (Minneman *et al.*, 1979).

Typical competition curves of [^{3}H]-PIA binding by agonists and antagonists in rat fat cell membranes are shown in Figure 5. The binding sites for [^{3}H]-PIA are highly stereospecific, as is demonstrated by a 40-fold higher K_i value for (+)PIA (18 n*M*) as compared to (−)PIA (0.47 n*M*). The adenosine antagonists IBMX and theophylline are more than 1000-fold less potent in competing with [^{3}H]-PIA. Transformation of the competition data to indirect Hill plots reveals that the slope factors for all compounds are close to unity (Table II),, consistent with an interaction at a single type of high-affinity adenosine receptors, whereas the portion of low affinity receptors (21%) does not significantly contribute to total specific binding at a radioligand concentration of 1 n*M* (Ukena *et al.*, 1984a).

Table II. Inhibition of Radioligand Binding to R_i Adenosine Receptors of Rat Fat Cell Membranes[a]

Compound	[^{3}H]-PIA binding K_H (nM)	[^{3}H]-PIA binding n_H	[^{125}I]-HPIA binding KH (nM)	[^{125}I]-HPIA binding K_L (nM)	[^{125}I]-HPIA binding n_H
(−)PIA	0.5	0.98	0.6	1.5	0.81
CHA	0.7	1.01	0.3	2.4	0.78
(−)IHPIA	0.7	0.92	0.6	7.6	0.60
(−)HPIA	0.9	1.01	0.8	21.7	0.60
NECA	1.9	0.93	2.3	16.6	0.70
2-Chloroadenosine	2.7	0.97	2.2	44.3	0.76
(+)PIA	18.1	0.98	11.1	86.2	0.76
DPX	72	0.95	67[b]		0.95
8-Phenyltheophylline	103	0.95	83[b]		0.98
IBMX	3,600	0.90	960[b]		0.86
Theophylline	7,400	0.99	2,000[b]		0.85
2′,5′-Dideoxyadenosine	11,600	0.89	6,000[b]		0.89
Caffeine	36,000	0.93	21,000[b]		0.89
Dipyridamole	>100,000 (43%)		>100,000 (36%)		
Adenine	>100,000 (34%)		>100,000 (41%)		
Inosine	>100,000 (31%)		>100,000 (38%)		

[a] Competition experiments were performed with 1 nM [^{3}H]-PIA or 0.1 nM [^{125}I]-HPIA at 37°C for 60 min. For [^{3}H]-PIA binding IC_{50} values are calculated from the competition curves after logit-log transformation by last-square linear regression and transformed into K_H values according to Cheng and Prusoff (1973) using the high affinity K_D value of [^{3}H]-PIA (0.26 nM) from the saturation curve (Figure 2). For the [^{125}I]-HPIA competition curves, the relative proportions of high- and low-affinity sites have been calculated by curve-fitting analysis according to De Lean *et al.* (1982) and the inhibition constants for the high (K_H) and low (K_L) affinity sites are shown. In addition, the indirect Hill coefficients (n_H) and low (K_L) affinity sites are shown. In addition, the indirect Hill coefficients (n_H) are shown. Each value is the geometric mean of four experiments. If inhibition is less than 50% at 100 μM, the percentage of inhibition is given in parenthesis. Data from Ukena *et al.* (1984a).
[b] Models to one state of homogeneous affinity (K_H = K_L), values given under K_H.

In addition to these compounds, a great number of adenosine analogs, methylxanthines, and other compounds have been analyzed for competition with [^{3}H]-PIA and [^{125}I]-HPIA binding. In contrast to [^{3}H]-PIA binding, the competition curves obtained with [^{125}I]-HPIA showed low Hill coefficients for all agonists (0.6–0.81). Therefore, the relative proportion of high- and low-affinity sites have been calculated by curve-fitting analysis and the values for both, K_H and K_L are given in Table II. In both radioligand binding systems, (−)PIA, CHA, (−)IHPIA, and (−)HPIA are the most potent adenosine agonists, as shown by K_i values of approximately 0.3–0.9 nM, followed by NECA and 2-chloroadenosine. These results demonstrate that the iodinated adenosine derivative IHPIA has nearly the same potency as (−)PIA, confirming data obtained in adenylate cyclase studies (Ukena *et al.*, 1984a). NECA, which has been classified as an R_a receptor agonist is approximately 4-fold less potent than (−)PIA. 2′,5′-Dideoxyadenosine, the most potent adenosine derivative at the P site, is 4 orders of magnitude less effective than (−)PIA. The adenosine antagonists, such as DPX, IBMX, and theophylline, have K_i values between 0.1 and 10 μM, which are comparable to those obtained in adenylate cyclase studies (Londos *et al.*, 1978). As would be expected, the adenosine uptake blocker dipyridamole does not compete with [^{3}H]-PIA binding, indicating that adenosine uptake sites are not labeled. Agents devoid of adenosinelike activity, such as inosine and adenine, do not compete for the binding sites. All these data emphasize that the pharmacological profile of radioligand binding sites is in excellent agreement with that of R_i adenosine receptors mediating the inhibitory effects on adenylate cyclase. Adenosine itself is not listed in this table, since it cannot be examined in adenosine deaminase-treated membranes. When adenosine was studied in the absence of adenosine deaminase, half-maximal inhibition of [^{3}H]-PIA binding was obtained at 180 nM (Trost and Schwabe, 1981). Although relatively high, this K_i value for adenosine demonstrates that the endogenous ligand of the R_i receptor is able to inhibit radioligand binding.

IV. IDENTIFICATION OF R_i ADENOSINE RECEPTORS BY RADIOACTIVELY LABELED ANTAGONISTS

A. Radioligand

Radioligand binding of adenosine antagonists to adenosine receptors has been less intensively investigated than that of agonists. The first, and so far only, antagonist ligand is tritiated 1,3-diethyl-8-phenylxanthine ([^{3}H]-DPX). This compound belongs to the class of xanthine derivatives that includes the well-known methylxanthines theophylline and caffeine. The alkylxanthines are equally effective as adenosine antagonists at R_i and R_a adenosine receptors and selective antagonists have not yet been developed. DPX is a suitable candidate for radioligand binding studies, since it has the highest potency as antagonist of adenosine receptor-mediated cyclic AMP responses (Fredholm and Persson, 1982). Radioligand binding of [^{3}H]-DPX has first been investigated in brain tissue (Bruns *et al.*, 1980). The compound proved to be a suitable ligand for R_i adenosine receptors in bovine brain but exhibited 50- to 1000-fold lower affinities in brain membranes of other species (Murphy and Snyder, 1982). Other disadvantages are a relatively low specific radioactivity of about 13 Ci/mmole and high levels of nonspecific binding in some tissue preparations. However, in several tissues, such as bovine brain, rat brain, and rat fat cells, [^{3}H]-DPX binding may be studied with sufficient accuracy under the conditions outlined below.

B. Assay Description for [^{3}H]-DPX Binding

1. Materials

1,3-Diethyl-8-[^{3}H]phenylxanthine ([^{3}H]-DPX) with a specific radioactivity of 13.4 Ci/mmole (New England Nuclear Corporation, Boston, Mass., USA).

Adenosine deaminase from calf intestine (200 U/mg) (Boehringer Mannheim, Mannheim, Federal Republic of Germany).

(–)N^6-Phenylisopropyladenosine (Boehringer Mannheim, Mannheim, Federal Republic of Germany).

250 mM Tris-HCl buffer, pH 7.4.

Whatman GF/B glass fiber filter (25 cm diameter).

Vacuum filtration apparatus (Millipore).

Triton-based scintillation cocktail, Quickszint 402 (Zinsser Analytic GmbH, Frankfurt, Federal Republic of Germany).

Rat brain membranes, P_2 fraction prepared according to Whittaker (1969).

2. *Binding Assay*

[^{3}H]-DPX binding to rat brain membranes is determined by a vacuum filtration technique. The following steps are performed in 1.5-ml polypropylene microtubes (Eppendorf) at 37°C in an Eppendorf thermostat 5320. The final assay volume is 250 μl and all samples should be assayed in duplicate.

a. Incubation. Add 50 μl of the displacing agent; add 50 μl of 50 n*M* [^{3}H]-DPX (approximately 30,000 cpm per assay tube), resulting in a final radioligand concentration of 10 n*M*; add 50 μl H_2O or additional compounds dissolved in H_2O; add 50 μl 250 m*M* Tris-HCl buffer, pH 7.4, resulting in a final concentration of 50 m*M*; preincubate for 5 min at 37°C for temperature equilibrium, and start the binding reaction by addition of 50-μl freshly thawed brain membrane suspension containing 200 μg protein and 0.5 μg (0.1 U) adenosine deaminase. Mix by vortexing and incubate at 37°C for 15 min.

b. Filtration. Stop reaction by removal of a 200-μl aliquot and rapid filtration through Whatman GF/B glass fiber filters; wash the filters immediately with two 3-ml portions of ice-cold incubation buffer and remove filters quickly from the filter holder. The whole filtration from application of the aliquot to the filter until removal of the filter should not exceed 10 sec. This time limitation is essential, since [^{3}H]-DPX is a fast-dissociating ligand.

c. Preparation of Standards and Blanks.

Total binding: Add 50 μl 50 n*M* [^{3}H]-DPX, 100 μl H_2O, 50 μl 250 m*M* Tris-HCl buffer, pH 7.4, and start by addition of 50-μl membrane suspension. Prepare four samples and place two samples as the first and two samples as the last of the complete binding assay.

Nonspecific binding: Add 50 μl 50 μ*M* (–)PIA as displacing agent (final concentration 10 μ*M*) and all other compounds as described above for incubation.

Counting standard: Add 50 μl 50 n*M* [^{3}H]-DPX standard solution directly to a glass fiber filter placed in a scintillation vial that was previously washed with two 3-ml portions of the incubation buffer.

Filter blank: Add 50 μl 50 n*M* [^{3}H]-DPX, 150 μl H_2O, and 50 μl 250 m*M* Tris-HCl buffer, pH 74; mix, incubate, and filtrate as described above.

d. Counting. Add 10 ml scintillation solution, cap vials, vortex vigorously two times for at least 10 sec, and count in a liquid scintillation counter after 6-hr storage of the samples to allow for complete solution of the filter-trapped radioactivity.

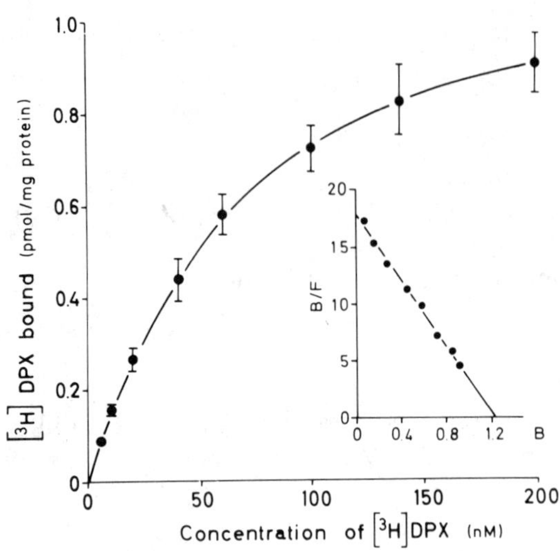

Figure 6. Saturation of [^{3}H]-DPX binding to rat brain membranes. Binding was determined after 15 min incubation at 37°C. Each value is the mean of four experiments ±S.E.M. Inset: Scatchard plot of the same data; B = pmoles [^{3}H]-DPX bound per milligram protein; F = free concentration of [^{3}H]-DPX (n*M*). The K_D is 68 n*M* and B_{max} is 1250 fmoles/mg protein. Data from Lohse *et al.* (1984).

e. Calculations. The amount of [^{3}H]-DPX specifically bound to brain membranes, expressed as fmoles [^{3}H]-DPX/mg protein, is calculated as described for [^{3}H]-PIA binding (see Section IIIB3).

Under these assay conditions, total [^{3}H]-DPX binding to rat brain membranes is approximately 600 cpm and nonspecific binding 150 cpm (25%) in typical experiments. The filter blank is less than 0.1% of total radioactivity per sample. At lower incubation temperatures (0°C), specific [^{3}H]-DPX binding is approximately 100% higher compared to the values obtained at 37°C. However, affinity of adenosine agonists and effects of GTP cannot be adequately analyzed at low temperatures. Furthermore, correlation of binding data with those of adenylate cyclase assays is only possible if [^{3}H]-DPX binding is done at higher temperatures.

C. Binding Studies with [^{3}H]-DPX

1. General Properties of [^{3}H]-DPX Binding

The characterization of R_i adenosine receptors by an antagonist radioligand follows the same procedures as outlined for the agonist ligand [^{3}H]-PIA. All essential criteria for R_i adenosine receptors are satisfied by [^{3}H]-DPX binding studies.

The kinetic properties of [^{3}H]-DPX binding to rat brain membranes are markedly different from those of [^{3}H]-PIA binding. At 37°C, specific binding occurs rapidly and achieves equilibrium after 1 min of incubation. The dissociation of [^{3}H]-DPX is also very fast and nearly complete after 15 sec.

The saturation of [^{3}H]-DPX binding to rat brain membranes is shown in Figure 6. The binding is saturable with a K_D of 68 n*M* and a maximal number of binding sites of 1250 fmoles/mg protein. The Scatchard plot of these data is linear, indicating a single class of binding sites.

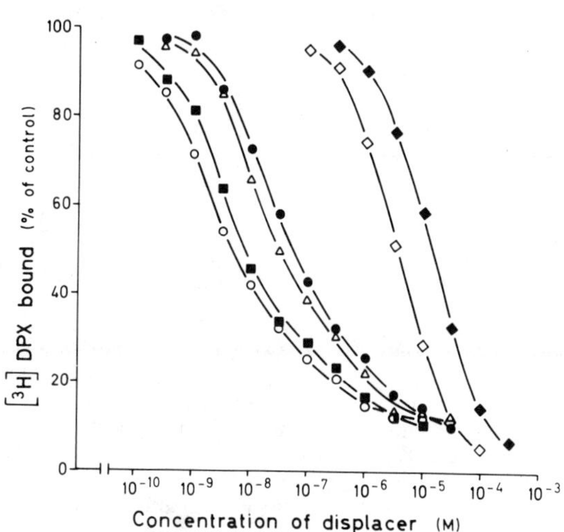

Figure 7. Inhibition of [^{3}H]-DPX binding to rat brain membranes by adenosine agonists and antagonists. Binding was measured at a radioligand concentration of 10 n*M* at 37°C for 15 min. Mean values of five experiments are shown. (○—○) (−)PIA; (■—■)CHA; (△—△)NECA; (●—●)2-chloroadenosine; (◇—◇)IBMX; (◆—◆) theophylline. Data from Lohse *et al.* (1984).

The structural specificity of [^{3}H]-DPX binding is determined by competition experiments with several adenosine analogs and xanthine derivatives. Figure 7 shows a remarkable difference between the displacement curves of agonists and antagonists. The curves of the agonists are biphasic with Hill coefficients between 0.49 and 0.51. The analysis by computer-assisted curve fitting according to De Lean *et al.* (1982) revealed a better fit with a two-site model indicating two affinity states of the receptor, a result that was also confirmed by the data obtained in presence of GTP, as outlined below. The competition curve for (−)PIA is resolved to contain 72% of the binding sites in the high-affinity state with a dissociation constant K_H = 1.3 n*M* and 28% of the binding sites in the low-affinity state with a dissociation constant K_L = 194 n*M*. Similar proportions of the two affinity states were obtained for the other adenosine agonists. The displacement of [^{3}H]-DPX by the antagonists IBMX and theophylline is monophasic with a Hill coefficient of 0.95, indicating a single class of binding sites. The dissociation constants of the antagonists and for each state of the agonists are listed in Table III. These values are in close agreement with those obtained in competition experiments with [^{3}H]-PIA binding shown in Table II.

2. *Use of Guanine Nucleotides to Distinguish Adenosine Agonists and Antagonists*

Radioligand binding of several hormone and neurotransmitter receptors that are linked to adenylate cyclase is regulated by guanine nucleotides (Rodbell, 1980). Similar properties have recently been described for the R_i adenosine receptor. The affinity of agonists for adenosine receptors is selectively decreased by guanine nucleotides, whereas the affinity of antagonists is not affected (Goodman *et al.*, 1982; Lohse *et al.*, 1984). Therefore, guanine nucleotides can be used as an experimental tool to distinguish between adenosine agonists and antagonists if newly

Table III. Inhibition of [^{3}H]-DPX Binding by Adenosine Agonists and Antagonists in Rat Brain Membranes[a]

Compound	B_{max} (fmoles/mg)	R_H (%)	K_H (nM)	K_L (nM)	n_H
(−)PIA	950	72	1.3	194	0.51
CHA	930	78	2.6	224	0.49
NECA	960	72	8.2	503	0.50
2-Chloroadenosine	1,040	74	14.4	1,205	0.49
IBMX	1,030		3,170[b]		0.92
Theophylline	1,120		11,000[b]		0.88

[a] Competition experiments were performed with 10 nM [^{3}H]-DPX at 37°C for 15 min. For each experiment with the various compounds, estimates of the high (K_H) and low (K_L) affinity dissociation constants, the maximal number of binding sites (B_{max}), the percentage of total receptors in the high-affinity states (% R_H), and the slope factor as indirect Hill coefficient (n_H) are calculated. Each value is the mean of five experiments. Data from Lohse *et al.* (1984).

[b] Models to one state of homogeneous affinity ($K_H = K_L$), values given under K_H.

developed derivatives of adenosine and xanthine have to be classified in radioligand binding experiments.

In principle, two different procedures can be employed to evaluate the effect of guanine nucleotides on agonist affinity. First, a radiolabeled agonist, such as [^{3}H]-PIA, can be used to conduct competition experiments with unlabeled compounds in the absence and the presence of GTP. However, in several tissues, [^{3}H]-PIA binding is reduced to very low values (10–20% of control values) that are difficult to analyze by additional displacement curves. In addition, GTP changes the affinity of the radioligand, and competition curves are also biphasic in the presence of GTP. The alternative procedure is to investigate antagonist radioligand binding, which is not changed by GTP. This approach offers the advantage that competition curves start from the same level of radioligand binding. A possible disadvantage is the lower affinity of [^{3}H]-DPX compared to that of agonist ligands such as [^{3}H]-PIA and [^{3}H]-CHA.

Figure 8 shows the competition curves of (−)PIA and IBMX displacing [^{3}H]-DPX binding to rat brain membranes in the presence and absence of GTP. It is clearly demonstrated that the competition curve of (−)PIA is shifted to the right and is steeper in the presence of the nucleotide. The competition curve of the antagonist IBMX is not changed by GTP. As already mentioned above, the shallow competition curve of (−)PIA in absence of GTP can be resolved into a portion with high affinity (K_H 1.3 nM) and a second portion with low affinity (K_L 194 nM). The addition of GTP results in a monophasic competition curve with 100% low affinity sites (K_L 200 nM). From these data it can be concluded that GTP converts the heterogeneous two-affinity state into a basically homogeneous state of low affinity. The ratio of the dissociation constants K_L/K_H indicates a 150-fold loss of affinity for (−)PIA in the presence of the nucleotide. In bovine membrane, the GTP-induced loss of agonist affinity is only 3- to 10-fold (Goodman *et al.*, 1982; Lohse *et al.*, 1984). Therefore, rat brain membranes presently offer the most

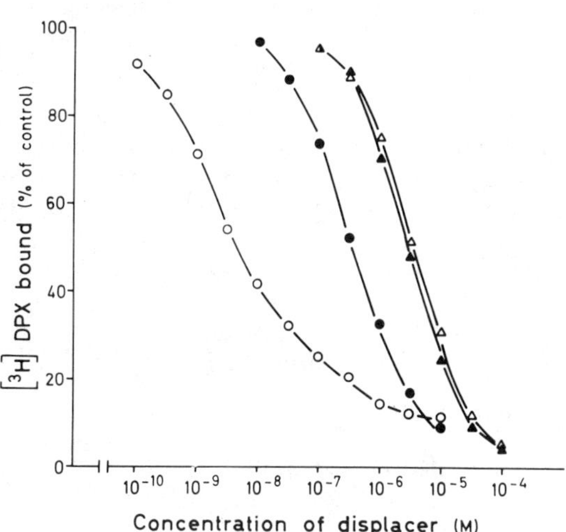

Figure 8. Effect of GTP on displacement of [^{3}H]-DPX binding by (−)PIA and theophylline. [^{3}H]-DPX binding to rat brain membranes was measured at a radioligand concentration of 10 n*M* at 37°C for 15 min. Mean values of triplicate experiments are shown. (○—○) (−)PIA; (●—●) (−)PIA + 100 μ*M* GTP; (△—△) theophylline; (▲—▲) theophylline + 100 μ*M* GTP. Computer analysis of the (−)PIA displacement curve indicates two affinity states with 72% of the binding sites in the high-affinity state (K_H 1.3 n*M*) and 28% in the low-affinity state (K_L 194 n*M*); in the presence of GTP, all sites have a low affinity (K_L 200 n*M*). The displacement curve for theophylline (K_i 3.1 n*M*) was not substantially changed by GTP (K_i 2.4 μ*M*). Data from Lohse *et al.* (1984).

convenient model to evaluate agonist/antagonist properties of newly developed compounds for adenosine receptors.

V. IDENTIFICATION OF R_a ADENOSINE RECEPTORS BY RADIOLIGAND BINDING

The pharmacological definition of R_a adenosine receptors is based on the ability of adenosine analogs to stimulate adenylate cyclase in a specific order of potency. R_a adenosine receptors have a higher affinity for NECA than for adenosine and (−)PIA (Van Calker *et al.*, 1979; Londos *et al.*, 1980). In addition, the affinity of R_a receptors for adenosine is in the micromolar range, whereas that of R_i receptors is in the nanomolar range.

A. Radioligands

A number of radioligands has been used for the study of R_a adenosine receptors. These include cyclopropylcarboxamido[^{3}H]adenosine([^{3}H]-CPCA), [^{3}H]DPX, [^{3}H]NECA, and 2-chloro[^{3}H]adenosine. Initial binding studies in brain and liver tissue did not succeed in labeling physiologically relevant R_a adenosine receptors (Daly *et al.*, 1979; Bruns *et al.*, 1980; Schütz *et al.*, 1982a). Although partial labeling of R_a adenosine receptors was achieved, several discrepancies in the structure–activity profile were observed. Some of the difficulties may arise from the relatively low affinity of these sites and from the common occurrence of both receptor subtypes in these tissues.

Recently, progress has been made in radiolabeling R_a adenosine receptors by selecting tissues that contain only this receptor subtype. Human platelets proved to be a suitable candidate for this kind of approach. This cell type has previously been classified as possessing only R_a adenosine receptors, which mediate inhibition of platelet aggregation via an activation of adenylate cyclase (Haslam and Cusack, 1981). The binding of [^{3}H]-NECA to human platelet membranes satisfies essential criteria for R_a adenosine receptors and, with some limitations mentioned below, may be used for the characterization and study of adenosine receptors in subtype-selective cells (Hüttemann *et al.*, 1984). Similar properties have been reported for [^{3}H]-NECA binding to calf thymocytes (Ukena *et al.*, 1982) and for the binding of 2-chloro[^{3}H]adenosine to R_a adenosine receptors of human placenta (Fox and Kurpis, 1983).

B. Assay Description for [^{3}H]-NECA Binding

1. Materials

5′-*N*-Ethylcarboxamido[^{3}H]adenosine ([^{3}H]-NECA) with a specific radioactivity of 27 Ci/mmole (Amersham Buchler, 3500 Braunschweig, Federal Republic of Germany).

5′-*N*′-Ethylcarboxamidoadenosine (NECA) (donated by Prof. Klemm [Byk Gulden Lomberg Chemische Fabrik, 7750 Konstanz, Federal Republic of Germany]).

250 m*M* Tris-HC1 buffer, pH 7.4.

Whatman GF/B glass fiber filter (25 mm diameter).

Vacuum filtration apparatus (Millipore).

Triton-based scintillation cocktail, Quickszint 402 (Zinsser Analytic GmbH, Frankfurt, Federal Republic of Germany).

Human platelet membranes, prepared as described by Tsai and Lefkowitz (1979).

2. Binding Assay

[^{3}H]-NECA binding to human platelet membranes is determined by a vacuum filtration technique. The following steps are performed in 1.5-ml polypropylene microtubes (Eppendorf) at 0°C in an ice-cold aluminum block with appropriate boreholes. The final assay volume is 250 μl and all samples should be assayed in duplicates.

a. Incubation. Add 50 μl of the displacing agent; add 50 μl of 50 n*M* [^{3}H]-NECA (approximately 60,000 cpm per assay tube), resulting in a final concentration of 10 n*M*; add 50 μl H_2O or additional compounds dissolved in H_2O; add 50 μl 250 m*M* Tris-HCl buffer, pH 7.4, resulting in a final concentration of 50 m*M*; preincubate for at least 5 min at 0°C for temperature equilibration, and start the binding reaction by addition of 50 μl freshly thawed platelet membrane suspension containing approximatley 100 μg protein. Mix by vortexing and incubate at 0°C for 30 min.

b. Filtration. Stop reaction by removal of a 200-μl aliquot and rapid filtration through Whatman GF/B glass fiber filters. Wash the filters immediately with two 5-ml portions of ice-cold incubation buffer and remove filters quickly from the filter holder. The whole filtration from application of the aliquot to the filter until removal of the filter should not exceed 10 sec. This time limitation is essential, since [^{3}H]-NECA is a fast-dissociating ligand.

c. Preparation of standards and blanks.

Total binding: Add 50 μl 50 n*M* [^{3}H]-NECA, 100 μl H_2O, 50 μl 250 m*M* Tris-HCl buffer, pH 7.4, and start reaction by addition of 50 μl membrane suspension. Prepare four samples and place two samples as the first and two as the last samples of the complete binding assay.

Nonspecific binding: Add 50 μl 5 m*M* NECA as displacing agent (final concentration 1 m*M*) and all other compounds as described above for incubation.

Counting standard: Add 50 μl 50 n*M* [^{3}H]-NECA standard solution directly on a filter placed into a scintillation vial and previously washed with two 5-ml portions of the incubation buffer.

Filter blank: Add 50 μl 50 n*M* [^{3}H]-NECA, 150 μl H_2O, and 50 μl 250 m*M* Tris-HCl buffer, pH 7.4; mix, incubate, and filtrate as described above.

d. Counting. Add 10-ml scintillation solution, cap vials, vortex vigorously two times for at least 10 sec, and count in a liquid scintillation counter for radioactivity after 6-hr storage of the samples to allow for complete solution of the filter-trapped radioactivity.

e. Calculations. The amount of [^{3}H]-NECA specifically bound to platelet membranes, expressed as fmoles [^{3}H]-NECA/mg protein, is calculated as described for [^{3}H]-PIA binding (see Section IIIB3).

Under these assay conditions, total [^{3}H]-NECA binding to human platelet membranes is approximately 800 cpm and nonspecific binding 40 cpm (5%) in typical experiments. The filter blank is less than 0.05% of total radioactivity per sample. In contrast to [^{3}H]-PIA binding to rat fat cell membranes, [^{3}H]-NECA binding is not changed by pretreatment with adenosine deaminase for 30 min at 37°C (Hüttemann *et al.*, 1984). Therefore, adenosine deaminase is not included in the [^{3}H]-NECA binding assay. For further general comments to the assay procedure, see Section IIIB3.

C. Binding Studies with [^{3}H]-NECA

[^{3}H]-NECA binding sites in human platelet membranes fulfill essential criteria for R_a adenosine receptors. The binding is rapid, reversible, saturable, and specific, as demonstrated by appropriate structure–activity relationships for R_a adenosine agonists. There are some considerations to keep in mind concerning the properties of [^{3}H]-NECA binding. At high concentrations, [^{3}H]-NECA binds to low-affinity sites of high capacity, and therefore binding should always be performed at sufficiently low radioligand concentrations. Furthermore, [^{3}H]-NECA binding is considerably reduced at incubation temperatures above 0°C, rendering correlation of binding data with adenylate cyclase activity more difficult. Binding studies in rat fat cell membranes have shown that [^{3}H]-NECA also binds to R_i receptors, indicating that [^{3}H]-NECA is not a subtype selective ligand for R_a receptors. However, in several tissues containing only R_a adenosine receptors, such as human platelets, [^{3}H]-NECA may be used as a suitable ligand for this adenosine receptor subtype.

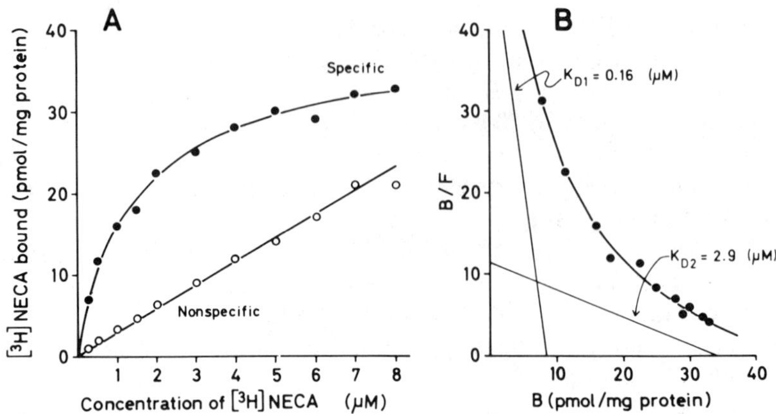

Figure 9. (A) Saturation of [^{3}H]-NECA binding to human platelet membranes. Binding was determined after 30 min of incubation at 0°C. Each value is the mean of four experiments. (B) Scatchard plot of the same data. K_D and B_{max} values of the high- and low-affinity binding were obtained by computer-assisted curve fitting. Data from Hüttemann *et al.* (1984).

1. Saturability of [^{3}H]-NECA Binding

The specific binding of [^{3}H]-NECA to human platelet membranes appears to be saturable at ligand concentrations between 0.25 and 8 μM (Figure 9). Scatchard analysis of the binding data reveals a curvilinear plot suggesting the presence of two classes of binding sites. With the use of computer-assisted curve fitting, the saturation curve is resolved to indicate the presence of a high-affinity site with a K_D of 0.16 μ*M* and a B_{max} of 8.4 pmoles/mg protein and a low-affinity site with a K_D of 2.9 μ*M* and a B_{max} of 33.7 pmoles/mg protein. As would be expected for R_a adenosine receptors, the affinity of the high-affinity site is about 100-fold lower than that of R_i adenosine receptors.

2. Kinetic Characteristics of [^{3}H]-NECA Binding

Figure 10 shows the time course of [^{3}H]-NECA binding to membranes at 0°C. The specific binding occurs very rapidly, being 50% complete after approximately 20 sec. Equilibrium is reached after 30 min and binding remains constant for up to 60 min.

[^{3}H]-NECA binding is reversible, as determined by adding an excess of the unlabeled compound (1 m*M* NECA) to an equilibrated mixture of the radioligand and platelet membranes (Figure 10). The dissociation at 0°C is extremely rapid, since more than 50% of the radioligand specifically bound to the membranes is dissociated from its binding sites within 20 sec after addition of the unlabeled ligand. As reported by Fox and Kurpis (1983), the binding of 2-chloro[^{3}H]adenosine to human placenta microsomes follows a similar time course. Both examples show that binding kinetics of agonists to R_a adenosine receptors are much faster than that to R_i receptors.

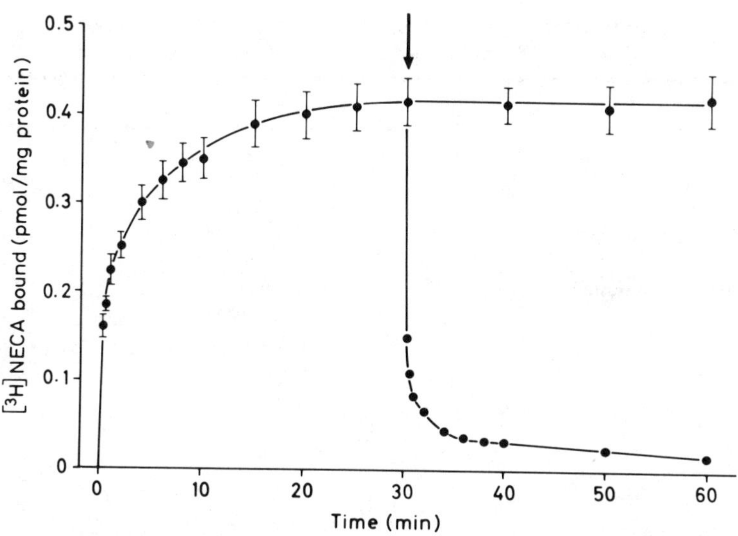

Figure 10. Time course of [^{3}H]-NECA binding to human platelet membranes. Association and dissociation of [^{3}H]-NECA (10 n*M*) were measured at 0°C. Dissociation was induced by rapid addition of 1 m*M* NECA after 30 min of equilibration (arrow). Values are the mean ±S.E.M. of five experiments. Data from Hüttemann *et al.* (1984).

3. *Specificity of [^{3}H]-NECA Binding Sites*

The ability of adenosine analogs and methylxanthines to compete for [^{3}H]-NECA binding sites of human platelet membranes is shown in Table IV. The competition curves for NECA, adenosine, and caffeine are monophasic with Hill coefficients between 0.82 and 1.03, whereas competition curves for 2-chloroadenosine, IBMX, and theophylline are biphasic, as indicated by Hill coefficients between 0.51 and 0.76. NECA is the most potent adenosine agonist, with an IC_{50} value of 0.5 μM, followed by 2-chloroadenosine and adenosine. By contrast, selective R_i receptor agonists, such as (−)PIA and CHA cause only 30% inhibition of binding at concentrations of 1000 μM. This order of potencies is typical for R_a adenosine receptors, as defined by Londos *et al.* (1980). However, it is important to mention that both N^6-substituted adenosine agonists are more potent to stimulate adenylate cyclase than to compete for [^{3}H]-NECA binding. This comparison shows that the R_a activity of potent R_i-selective adenosine analogues is not sufficiently recognized by [^{3}H]-NECA binding.

Among the adenosine antagonists studied, IBMX is the most potent agent with an IC_{50} value of 98 μM. Theophylline is approximately 7 times as potent as caffeine. The IC_{50} values are approximately 10-fold higher than those determined at R_i adenosine receptors and in adenylate cyclase studies of R_a receptors. A relatively low IC_{50} value is observed for 2′,5′-dideoxyadenosine, a P-site adenosine agonist that is expected to be inactive at R_a adenosine receptors. However, 2′,5′-dideoxyadenosine has been shown to antagonize adenosine-mediated increases of cyclic AMP in human fibroblasts, and therefore has been classified as an R_a receptor antagonist (Bruns, 1981). Compounds that are inactive as stimu-

Table IV. Inhibition of [^{3}H]-NECA Binding to Human Platelet Membranes by Adenosine Analogues and Related Compounds[a]

Compound	IC_{50} μM	Hill coefficient
NECA	0.5 (0.4–0.7)	0.97
2-Chloroadenosine	6.3 (3.4–11.7)	0.51
Adenosine	11.9 (7.2–19.4)	0.82
2′,5′-Dideoxyadenosine	14.8 (12.5–17.4)	0.92
Adenine	91 (64–131)	0.62
3-Isobutyl-1-methylxanthine	98 (79–121)	0.57
Theophylline	827 (678–1008)	0.76
Caffeine	5,600 (4650–6750)	1.03
Eritadenine	>100 (17%)	
(−)Adrenaline	>100 (8%)	
ADP	>100 (7%)	
Dipyridamole	>100 (3%)	
(+)PIA	>1000 (38%)	
(−)PIA	>1000 (29%)	
CHA	>1000 (25%)	
ATP	>1000 (21%)	
GTP	>1000 (7%)	
Inosine	>1000 (9%)	

[a] Competition experiments were performed with 10 nM [^{3}H]-NECA at 0°C for 30 min. IC_{50} values were calculated from the displacement data after logit-log transformation by least-square linear regression. Each IC_{50} value is the geometric mean of four to five separate experiments with 95% confidence limits in parentheses. If inhibition was less than 50%, the percentage of inhibition is given in parentheses. Data from Hüttemann *et al.* (1984).

lators of platelet adenylate cyclase (e.g., ADP, dipyridamole, and inosine) do not displace [^{3}H]-NECA binding. Of particular significance is ADP, an inhibitor of platelet adenylate cyclase. This adenine nucleotide does not affect [^{3}H]-NECA binding in concentrations up to 100 μM whereas half-maximal inhibition of platelet aggregation is observed at 1 μM. This finding confirms previous results obtained in cyclase studies that platelet receptors for ADP and adenosine are independent entities (Haslam and Rosson, 1975).

The use of [^{3}H]-NECA offers a considerable advantage over other radioligands that have been tested for the study of R_a adenosine receptors. [^{3}H]-DPX, for example, binds with moderate affinity to sites in guinea pig brain that seem to resemble R_a adenosine receptors (Bruns *et al.*, 1980). But several findings were not consonant with this suggestion, because [^{3}H]-DPX binding was displaced by biologically inactive compounds such as 8-bromoadenosine, whereas the potent R_a agonist, 5′-*N*-cyclopropylcarboxamidoadenosine (CPCA), was only marginally effective (IC_{60} = 100 μM). Another example is the binding of [^{3}H]-CHA in rat liver membranes. The structure–activity profile of this ligand differs markedly from the findings obtained in adenylate cyclase studies, and the radioligand binding contains a large component of low-affinity binding to apparently nonreceptor sites (Schütz *et al.*, 1982a). In the same report, [^{3}H]-NECA was first used as a radioligand for R_a adenosine receptors, but for unknown reasons [^{3}H]-NECA binding to liver membranes was even less sensitive to displacement by adenosine agonists than that of [^{3}H]-CHA (Schütz *et al.*, 1982a). Similar equivocal specificity was obtained for the binding of [^{3}H]-NECA to rat brain microvessels (Schütz *et al.*, 1982b).

On the other hand, [^{3}H]-NECA cannot be regarded as a highly selective radioligand for R_a adenosine receptors. [^{3}H]-NECA binds to a large component of low affinity that has not yet been evaluated with respect to its binding specificity. Due to the rapid dissociation, [^{3}H]-NECA binding can be assessed accurately only at low incubation temperatures. Finally, the potencies of N^6-substituted adenosine analogs, such as (−)PIA and CHA, and of several methylxanthines are underestimated if the binding data are compared to that of adenylate cyclase studies. However, if these limitations are properly taken into account, [^{3}H]-NECA should be of value in the characterization of adenosine receptors in R_a subtype selective cells.

VI. CONCLUSIONS

This review has attempted to give detailed information about the methods developed for radioligand binding assays of adenosine receptors. Examples of binding data have been presented for several tissues in which adenosine receptors have been defined on the basis of adenylate cyclase studies. Subtype-selective radioligands for R_i adenosine receptors are available. In contrast to other receptor systems, agonist radioligands have been predominantly employed.

The most suitable agonist radioligands for labeling R_i receptors are N^6-substituted analogues of adenosine. These ligands exhibit high subtype selectivity. The iodinated ligand [^{125}I]-HPIA, which has nearly the same biological activity as (−)PIA provides a very high specific radioactivity and offers the possibility of identifying R_i adenosine receptors in tissues with low receptor densities. R_i receptors can also be labeled by the antagonist ligand [^{3}H]-DPX, which with the aid of GTP offers the most convenient model to evaluate the agonist/antagonist properties of newly developed adenosine and xanthine derivatives.

The identification of R_a adenosine receptors by radioligand binding has been improved but still lags behind that of R_i adenosine receptors. With the limitations mentioned, [^{3}H]-NECA appears to be a useful radioligand for R_a receptors. Possible disadvantages such as a large low-affinity component and a relative underestimation of the potency of R_i-selective ligands should be considered. Another ligand used in binding studies of this receptor subtype is 2-chloro[^{3}H]adenosine. This compound may turn out as a possible alternative to [^{3}H]-NECA, since interference by low-affinity binding was not observed. However, comparative data from the same tissues are not yet available and stability problems may occur. Attempts to use the antagonist ligand [^{3}H]-DPX for labeling R_a receptors have not been satisfactory. In analogy to other receptor systems, subtype-selective antagonists could provide an important tool for this approach.

The two important differences of the adenosine receptor subtypes refer to the affinity range for adenosine and the relative potency of subtype-selective agonists. These properties have been defined from adenylate cylcase studies and were confirmed by radioligand binding data. Additional criteria can now be checked to distinguish R_i and R_a adenosine receptors. Radioligand binding to R_i receptors is increased several-fold by adenosine deaminase treatment, but [^{3}H]-NECA binding to R_a receptors is not (Hüttemann *et al.*, 1984). A second property that may be used for discrimination of both receptor subtypes is the response to guanine nucleotides. Radioligand binding to R_i receptors is decreased by GTP (Goodman *et al.*, 1982; Lohse *et al.*, 1984; Ukena *et al.*, 1984c), whereas [^{3}H]-NECA binding to platelets is not changed by GTP alone (Hüttemann *et al.*, 1984). Similarly to GTP, *N*-ethylmaleimide reduces radioligand binding to R_i, but not to R_a, adenosine receptors (Yeung and Green, 1983; Ukena *et al.*, 1984b).

The methods that are now available to characterize receptor subtypes provide an additional approach for the investigation of the occurrence, nature, and regulation of adenosine receptors. The extension of these studies to other cellular systems will provide further insight into the physiological functions modulated by adenosine.

ACKNOWLEDGMENTS

The author's research cited herein has been supported by the Deutsche Forschungsgemeinschaft (Schw 83/13-1). I would like to acknowledge the useful comments of Drs. M. J. Lohse and D. Ukena on this manuscript. I would also like to thank Mrs. Carola Maier-Reimer for her expert secretarial assistance.

REFERENCES

Albers, R. W., and Krishnan, N. 1979. Application of the miniature ultracentrifuge in receptor-binding assays. *Anal. Biochem.*, *96*:395–402.

Bennett, J. P. 1978. Methods in binding studies. In: *Neurotransmitter Receptor Binding*, pp. 57–90. Ed. by Yamamura, H. I., Enna, S. J., and Kuhar, M. J. Raven Press, New York.

Bruns, R. F. 1981. Adenosine antagonism by purines, pteridines and benzopteridines in human fibroblasts. *Biochem. Pharmacol.*, *30*:325–333.

Bruns, R. F., Daly, J. W., and Snyder, S. H. 1980. Adenosine receptors in brain membranes: Binding of N^6-cyclohexyl[^{3}H]adenosine and 1,3-diethyl-8-[^{3}H]phenylxanthine. *Proc. Natl Acad. Sci. USA*, *77*:5547–5551.

Bruns, R. F., Daly, J. W., and Snyder, S. H. 1983. Adenosine receptor binding: Structure-activity analysis generates extremely potent xanthine antagonists. *Proc. Natl Acad. Sci. USA*, *80*:2077–2080.

Buckley, N., and Burnstock, G. 1983. Autoradiographic demonstration of peripheral adenosine binding sites using [^{3}H]-NECA. *Brain Res.*, *269*:374–377.

Cheng, Y., and Prusoff, W. H. 1973. Relationship between the inhibition constant (K_I) and the concentration of inhibitor which causes 50% inhibition (I_{50}) of an enzymatic reaction. *Biochem. Pharmacol.*, *22*:3099–3108.

Cuatrecasas, P. 1971. Insulin-receptor interactions in adipose tissue cells: Direct measurement and properties. *Proc. Natl Acad. Sci. USA*, *68*:1264–1268.

Daly, J. W., Nimitkitpaisan, Y., Pons, F., Bruns, R. F., Smellie, F., and Skolnick, P. 1979. Binding sites for adenosine analogs: Possible relationship to cyclic AMP-generating systems in brain tissue. *Pharmacologist*, *21*:253.

De Lean, A., Hancock, A. A., and Lefkowitz, R. J. 1982. Validation and statistical analysis of a computer modeling method for quantitative analysis of radioligand binding data for mixtures of pharmacological receptor subtypes. *Mol. Pharmacol., 21:*5–16.

Dietmann, K., Birkenheier, H., and Schaumann, W. 1970. Hemmung der induzierten Thrombozyten-Aggregation durch Adenosin und Adenosin-Derivative. II: Korrelation zwischen Hemmung der Aggregation und peripherer Vasodilatation. *Arzneimittelforsch., 20:*1749–1751.

Fox, I.H., and Kurpis, L. 1983. Binding characteristics of an adenosine receptor in human placenta. *J. Biol. Chem., 258:*6952–6955.

Fredholm, B. B. 1980. Are methylxanthine effects due to antagonism of endogenous adenosine? *Trends Pharmacol. Sci., 1:*129–132.

Fredholm, B. B., and Persson, C. G. A. 1982. Xanthine derivatives as adenosine receptor antagonists. *Eur. J. Pharmacol., 81:*673–676.

Freychet, P., Roth, J., and Neville, D. M. 1971. Insulin receptors in the liver: Specific binding of [^{125}I]insulin to the plasma membrane and its relation to insulin bioactivity. *Proc. Natl Acad. Sci. USA, 68:*1833–1837.

Gavish, M., Goodman, R. R., and Snyder, S. H. 1982. Solubilized adenosine receptors in the brain: Regulation by guanine nucleotides. *Science, 215:*1633–1635.

Goodman, R. R., and Snyder, S. H. 1982. Autoradiographic localization of adenosine receptors in rat brain using [^{3}H]cyclohexyladenosine. *J. Neurosci., 2:*1230–1241.

Goodman, R. R., and Cooper, M. J., Gavish, M., and Snyder, S. H. 1982. Guanine nucleotide and cation regulation of the binding of [^{3}H]cyclohexyladenosine and [^{3}H]diethylphenylxanthine to adenosine A_1 receptors in brain membranes. *Mol. Pharmacol., 21:*329–335.

Hancock, A. A., DeLean, A. L., and Lefkowitz, R. J. 1979. Quantitative resolution of beta-adrenergic receptor subtypes by selective ligand binding: Application of a computerized model fitting technique. *Mol. Pharmacol., 16:*1–9.

Haslam, R. J., and Cusack, N J. 1981. Blood platelet receptors for ADP and for adenosine. In: *Purinergic receptors.*, pp. 223–285. Ed. by Burnstock, G. Chapman and Hall, London.

Haslam, R. J., and Lynham, J. A. 1972. Activation and inhibition of blood platelet adenylate cyclase by adenosine or by 2-chloroadenosine. *Life Sci., 11:*1143–1154.

Haslam, R. J., and Rosson, G. M. 1975. Effects of adenosine on levels of adenosine cyclic 3′,5′-monophosphate in human blood platelets in relation to adenosine incorporation and platelet aggregation. *Mol. Pharmacol., 11:*528–544.

Hunter, W. M., and Greenwood, H. 1962. Preparation of ^{131}iodine labelled human growth hormone of high specific activity. *Nature, 194:*495–496.

Hüttemann, E., Ukena, D., Lenschow, V., and Schwabe, U. 1984. R_a Adenosine receptors in human platelets: Characterization by 5′-N-ethylcarboxamido[^{3}H]adenosine binding in relation to adenylate cyclase activity. *Naunyn-Schmiedebergs Arch. Pharmacol., 325:*226–233.

Jacobs, S., Chang, K.-J., and Cuatrecasas, P. 1975. Estimation of hormone receptor affinity by competitive displacement of labeled ligand: Effect of concentration of receptor and of labeled ligand. *Biochem. Biophys. Res. Comm., 66:*687–692.

Kahn, C. R. 1974. Membrane receptors for polypeptide hormones. In: *Methods in Membrane Biology*, Vol. 3, pp. 81–128. Ed. by E.D. Korn, Plenum Press, New York.

Kent, R. S., De Lean, A., and Lefkowitz, R. J. 1980. A quantitative analysis of beta-adrenergic receptor interactions: Resolution of high and low affinity states of the receptor by computer modeling of ligand binding data. *Mol. Pharmacol., 17:*14–23.

Klingenberg, M., and Pfaff, E. 1967. Means of terminating reactions, in: *Methods in Enzymology*, Vol. 10, pp. 680–684. Ed. by Eastabrook, R. W., and Pullman, M. E. Academic Press, New York.

Lefkowitz, R. J., Roth, J., Pricer, W., and Pastan, I. 1970. ACTH receptors in the adrenal: Specific binding of ACTH-[^{125}I] and its relation to adenyl cyclase. *Proc. Natl Acad. Sci. USA, 65:*745–752.

Lewis, M. E., Patel, J., Edley, S. M., and Marangos, P. J. 1981. Autoradiographic visualization of rat brain adenosine receptors using N^6-cyclohexyl[^{3}H]adenosine. *Eur. J. Pharmacol., 73:*109–110.

Lohse, M. J., Lenschow, V., and Schwabe, U. 1984. Two affinity states of R_i adenosine receptors in brain membranes: Analysis of guanine nucleotide and temperature effects on radioligand binding. *Mol. Pharmacol., 26:*1–9.

Londos, C., and Wolff, J. 1977. Two distinct adenosine-sensitive sites on adenylate cyclase. *Proc. Natl Acad. Sci. USA, 74:*5482–5486.

Londos, C., Cooper, D. M. F., Schlegel, W., and Rodbell, M. 1978. Adenosine analogs inhibit adipocyte adenylate cyclase by a GTP-dependent process: Basis for actions of adenosine and methylxanthines on cyclic AMP production and lipolysis. *Proc. Natl Acad. Sci. USA, 75:*5362–5366.

Londos, C., Cooper, D. M. F., and Wolff, J. 1980. Subclasses of external adenosine receptors. *Proc. Natl Acad. Sci. USA, 77:*2551–2554.

Londos, C., Wolff, J., and Cooper, D. M. F. 1981. Adenosine as a regulator of adenylate cyclase. In: *Purinergic receptors,* pp. 289–323. Ed. by Burnstock, G. Chapman and Hall, London.

Mackin, W. M., Huang, C.-K., Bormann, B.-J., and Becker, E. L. 1983. A simple and rapid assay for measuring radiolabeled ligand binding to purified plasma membranes. *Anal. Biochem., 131:*430–437.

Malbon, C. C., Hert, R. C., and Fain, J. N. 1978. Characterization of [^{3}H]adenosine binding to fat cell membranes. *J. Biol. Chem., 253:*3114–3122.

McKeel, D. M., and Jarett, L. 1970. Preparation and characterization of a plasma membrane fraction from isolated fat cells. *J. Cell. Biol., 44:*417–432.

Minneman, K. P., Hegstrand, L. R., and Molinoff, P. B. 1979. Simultaneous determination of beta-1 and beta-2-adrenergic receptors in tissues containing both receptor subtypes. *Mol. Pharmacol., 16:*34–46.

Munshi, R., and Baer, H. P. 1982. Radioiodination of p-hydroxyphenylisopropyladenosine: development of a new ligand for adenosine receptors. *Can. J. Physiol. Pharmacol., 60:*1320–1322.

Murphy, K. M. M., and Snyder, S. H. 1981. Adenosine receptors in rat testes: Labelling with ^{3}H-cyclohexyladenosine. *Life Sci., 28:*917–920.

Murphy, K. M. M., and Snyder, S. H. 1982. Heterogeneity of adenosine A_1 receptor binding in brain tissue. *Mol. Pharmacol., 22:*250–257.

Newman, M. E., Patel, J., and McIlwain, H. 1981. The binding of [^{3}H]adenosine to synaptosomal and other preparations from the mammalian brain. *Biochem. J. 194:*611–620.

Nimit, Y., Law, J., and Daly, J. W. 1982. Binding of 2′,5′-dideoxyadenosine to brain membranes. *Biochem. Pharmacol., 31:*3279–3287.

Patel, J., Marangos, P. J., Stivers, J., and Goodwin, F. K. 1982. Characterization of adenosine receptors in brain using N^6-cyclohexyl[^{3}H]adenosine. *Brain Res., 237:*203–214.

Rodbell, M. 1980. The role of hormone receptors and GTP-regulatory proteins in membrane transduction. *Nature, 284:*17–22.

Rodbell, J., Krans, H. M. J., Poh. S. L., and Birnbaumer, L. 1971. The glucagon-sensitive adenyl cyclase system in plasma membranes of rat liver. III. Binding of glucagon: method of assay and specificity. *J. Biol. Chem., 246:*1861–1871.

Rugg, E. L., Barnett, D. B., and Nahorski, S. R. 1978. Coexistence of $beta_1$ and $beta_2$ adrenoceptors in mammalian lung: Evidence from direct binding studies. *Mol. Pharmacol., 14:*996–1005.

Sattin, A., and Rall, T. W. 1970. The effect of adenosine and adenine nucleotides on the cyclic adenosine 3′,5′-phosphate content of guinea pig cerebral cortex slices. *Mol. Pharmacol., 6:*13–23.

Scatchard, G. 1949. The attractions of proteins for small molecules and ions. *Ann. N.Y. Acad. Sci., 51:*660–672.

Schütz, W., and Brugger, G. 1982. Characterization of [^{3}H]-adenosine binding to media membranes of hog carotid arteries. *Pharmacology, 24:*26–34.

Schütz, W., and Tuisl, E. 1981. Evidence against adenylate cyclase-coupled adenosine receptors in the guinea pig heart. *Eur. J. Pharmacol., 76:*285–288.

Schütz, W., Tuisl, E., and Kraupp, O. 1982a. Adenosine receptor agonists: Binding and adenylate cyclase stimulation in rat liver plasma membranes. *Naunyn-Schmiedebergs Arch. Pharmacol., 319:*34–39.

Schütz, W., Steurer, G., and Tuisl, E. 1982b. Functional identification of adenylate cyclase-coupled adenosine receptors in rat brain microvessels. *Eur. J. Pharmacol., 85:*177–184.

Schwabe, U. 1983. General aspects of binding of ligands to adenosine receptors. In: *Regulatory Function of Adenosine*, pp. 77–96. Ed. by Berne, R. M., Rall, T. W., and Rubio R. Martinus Nijhoff, The Hague.

Schwabe, U., and Trost, T. 1980. Characterization of adenosine receptors in rat brain by (−) [^{3}H]N^6-phenylisopropyladenosine. *Naunyn-Schmiedebergs Arch. Pharmacol., 313:*179–187.

Schwabe, U., Kiffe, H., Puchstein, C., and Trost, T. 1979. Specific binding of ^{3}H-adenosine to rat brain membranes. *Naunyn-Schmiedebergs Arch. Pharmacol., 310:*59–67.

Schwabe, U., Lenschow, V., Ukena, D., Ferry, D. R., and Glossmann, H. 1982. [^{125}I]N^6-p-Hydroxyphenylisopropyladenosine, a new ligand for R_i adenosine receptors. *Naunyn-Schmiedebergs Arch. Pharmacol., 321:*84–87.

Smellie, F. W., Daly, J. W., Dunwiddie, T. V., and Hoffer, B. J. 1979. The dextro and levorotatory isomers of N-phenylisopropyladenosine: Stereospecific effects on cyclic AMP-formation and evoked synaptic responses in brain slices. *Life Sci., 25:*1739–1748.

Snyder, S. H., Pasternak, G. W., and Pert, C. B. 1975. Opiate receptor mechanisms. In: *Handbook of Psychopharmacology* pp. 329–360. Ed. by Iversen, L. L., Iversen, S. D., and Snyder, S. H. Plenum Press, New York.

Trost, T., and Schwabe, U. 1981. Adenosine receptors in fat cells. Identification by (−)-N^6-[^{3}H]phenylisoproyladenosine binding. *Mol Pharmacol., 19:*228–235.

Tsai, B. S., and Lefkowitz, R. J. 1979. Agonist-specific effects of guanine nucleotides on alpha-adrenergic receptors in human platelets. *Mol. Pharmacol., 16:*61–68.

Ukena, D. 1982. Identification of adenosine receptors on intact fat cells. *Naunyn-Schmiedebergs Arch. Pharmacol., Suppl. 319:*R6.

Ukena, D., Martens, D., and Schwabe, U. 1982. Specific binding of 5′-N-ethylcarboxamido [^{3}H]adenosine to calf thymocyte membranes. *Naunyn-Schmiedebergs Arch. Pharmacol., Suppl. 321:*R39.

Ukena, D., Furler, R., Lohse, M. J., Engel, G., and Schwabe, U. 1984a. Labelling of R_i adenosine receptors in rat fat cell membranes with (−)[^{125}Iodo]N^6-hydroxyphenylisopropyladenosine receptors. *Naunyn-Schmiedebergs Arch. Pharmacol., 326:*233–240.

Ukena, D., Poeschla, E., Hüttemann, E., and Schwabe, U. 1984b. Effects of N-ethylmaleimide on adenosine receptors of rat cells and human platelets. *Naunyn-Schmiedebergs Arch. Pharmacol., 327:*247–253.

Ukena, D., Poeschla, E., and Schwabe, U. 1984c. Guanine nucleotide and cation regulation of radioligand binding to R_i adenosine receptors of rat fat cells. *Naunyn-Schmiedeberg's Arch. Pharmacol., 326:*241–247.

Van Calker, D., Müller, M., and Hamprecht, B. 1979. Adenosine regulates via two different types of receptors, the accumulation of cyclic AMP in cultured brain cells. *J. Neurochem., 33:*999–1005.

Vapaatalo, H., Onken, D., Neuvonen, P. J., and Westermann, E. 1975. Stereospecificity in some central and circulatory effects of phenylisopropyladenosine (PIA). *Arzneim.-Forsch., 25:*407–410.

Weiland, G. A. and Molinoff, P. B. 1981. Quantitative analysis of drug-receptor interactions: I. Determination of kinetic and equilibrium properties. *Life Sci., 29:*313–330.

Westermann, E., and Stock, K. 1970. Inhibitors of lipolysis: Potency and mode of action of α- and β-adrenolytics, methoxamine derivatives, prostaglandin E_1 and phenylisopropyl adenosine. In: *Adipose Tissue, Regulation and Metabolic Functions* pp. 47–54. Ed. by Jeanrenaud, B. and Hepp, D. Georg Thieme Verlag, Stuttgart, Academic Press, New York.

Whittaker, V. P. 1969. The synaptosome. In: *Handbook of Neurochemistry*, Vol. 2, pp. 327–364. Ed. by Lajtha, A. Plenum Press, New York.

Williams, L. T., and Lefkowitz, R. J. 1978. *Receptor Binding Studies in Adrenergic Pharmacology.* Raven Press, New York.

Williams, L. T., Jarett, L., and Lefkowitz, R. J. 1976. Adipocyte β-adrenergic receptors. Identification and subcellular localization by (−)-[^{3}H]dihydroalprenolol binding. *J. Biol. Chem., 251:*3096–3104.

Williams, M., and Risley, E. A. 1980a. High affinity binding of 2-chloroadenosine to rat brain synaptic membranes. *Eur. J. Pharmacol., 64:*369–370.

Williams, M., and Risley, E. A., 1980b. Biochemical characterization of putative central purinergic receptors by using 2-chloro[^{3}H]adenosine, a stable analog of adenosine. *Proc. Natl Acad. Sci. USA, 77:*6892–6896.

Williams. M., and Risley, E. A. 1982. Interaction of the benzodiazepine antagonists, CGS 8216 and Ro 15-1788, with central adenosine A-1 receptors. *Arch. Int. Pharmacodyn. Ther., 260:*50–53.

Wu, P. H., and Phillis, J. W. 1982. Adenosine receptors in rat brain membranes: characterization of high affinity binding of [^{3}H]-2-chloroadenosine. *Int. J. Biochem., 14:*399–404.

Wu, P. H., Phillis, J. W., Balls, K., and Rinaldi, B. 1980. Specific binding of 2-[^{3}H]chloroadenosine to rat brain cortical membranes. *Can. J. Physiol. Pharmacol., 58:*576–579.

Yeung, S.-M. and Green, D. 1983. Agonist and antagonist affinities for inhibitory adenosine receptors are reciprocally affected by 5′-guanylyl-imidodiphosphate or N-ethylmaleimide. *J. Biol. Chem., 258:*2334–2339.

Young, W. C., and Kuhar, M. J. 1979. A new method for receptor autoradiography: [^{3}H]opioid receptors in rat brain. *Brain Res., 179:*255–270.

Chapter **14**

Use of Photoaffinity Labels as P_2-Purinoceptor Antagonists

Jeffrey S. Fedan,*,† G. Kurt Hogaboom,† John P. O'Donnell,‡ and David P. Westfall**

Physiology Section*,†
National Institute for Occupational Safety and Health
Department of Pharmacology and Toxicology,†
School of Pharmacy,‡ West Virginia University Medical Center,
Morgantown, West Virginia, and Department of Pharmacology,
University of Nevada School of Medicine,**
Reno, Nevada

I. INTRODUCTION

In recent years there has been considerable interest in the possible role of adenine nucleotides, such as ATP, as neuromodulators (Su, 1977; De Mey *et al.*, 1979; Katsuragi and Su, 1982), neurotransmitters (Burnstock *et al.*, 1970; Burnstock, 1979), or cotransmitters (Westfall *et al.*, 1978; Fedan *et al.*, 1981; Sneddon *et al.*, 1982a). The chief impediment to accepting the notion that adenine nucleotides act as neuromodulators or neurotransmitters has been the unavailability of a specific pharmacological antagonist of responses to ATP (see, for example, Campbell and Gibbons, 1979). Although a number of compounds have been investigated in this regard, including 2-2′-pyridylisatogen, 2-2′-methoxyphenylisatogen, quinidine, apamin, and 2-substituted imidazolines, the antagonism afforded by these drugs in several autonomic nerve-smooth muscle preparations is nonspecific; i.e., in concentrations sufficient to antagonize responses to ATP, the responses to other agonists are also reduced (Weetman and Turner, 1977; Burnstock, 1979, 1983).

In 1980, it was reported that 3′-*O*-{3[*N*-(4-azido-2-nitro-phenyl)amino] propionyl}adenosine 5′-triphosphate ($ANAPP_3$), a photoaffinity analog of ATP,

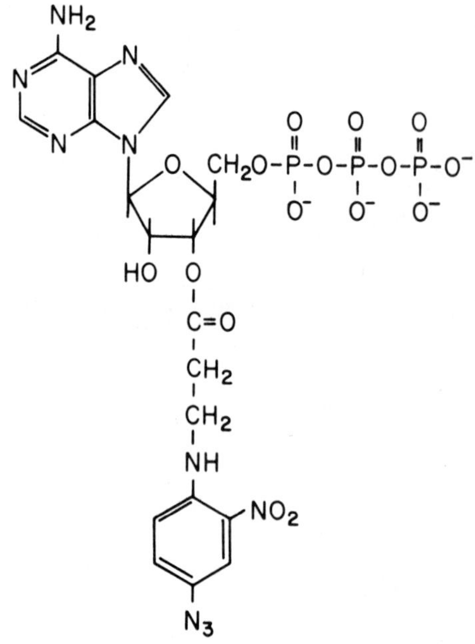

Figure 1. Structure of 3′-O-{3[*N*-(4-azido-2-nitrophenyl)amino]propionyl} adenosine 5′-triphosphate or $ANAPP_3$.

antagonized contractile responses of the guinea-pig vas deferens to adenine nucleotides, but not to a number of other agonists, including norepinephrine, acetylcholine, histamine, or KCl (Hogaboom *et al.*, 1980). Subsequent studies with a number of smooth muscle preparations have confirmed the specificity of antagonism by $ANAPP_3$, and, further, have demonstrated the utility of this substance as an antagonist of P_2 purinoceptors. The goal of this chapter is to provide a guide for the use of this photoaffinity label to produce a blockade of P_2 purinoceptors in isolated, intact tissue preparations.

II. THEORETICAL ASPECTS OF PHOTOAFFINITY LABELING

A thorough discussion of the theory of photoaffinity labeling is beyond the scope of this chapter. However, there are a number of general reviews that discuss in considerable detail the theoretical basis of this technique. Included among these are the following: Cooperman (1976); Bayley and Knowles (1977); Chowdry and Westheimer (1979); Fedan *et al.* (1983a,b); Guillory and Jeng (1983).

Photoaffinity labels are analogs of parent compounds that have an inherent affinity for a binding site and that also contain a light-sensitive grouping that, when irradiated with light, are capable of forming a covalent bond at or near the binding site. The light-sensitive moiety of $ANAPP_3$ (Figure 1) is an arylazide that is connected to the 3′-hydroxyl grouping of the parent ATP molecule through a β-alanine bridge. The rationale for the use of this compound to study P_2 purinoceptors is that the ATP portion of the molecule directs the binding of the compound to the receptors, and photolysis of the compound that is bound to the receptor results in the formation of a reactive nitrene intermediate that is capable of forming covalent bonds at or near the receptor. The result is a specific pharmacological antagonism of responses mediated via the receptors for ATP. Furthermore, the covalent attachment of $ANAPP_3$ to the receptors provides a means for biochemical characterization (Fedan *et al.*, 1983b) and isolation of the receptors.

III. SYNTHESIS OF $ANAPP_3$

At the present time, $ANAPP_3$ is not commercially available, thus, synthesizing the compound is necessary. The original synthesis of $ANAPP_3$ was described by Jeng and Guillory (1975). In the Appendix to this chapter, an expanded working protocol for the preparation of $ANAPP_3$ is provided.

IV. PHOTOLABELING AND BLOCKADE OF P_2 RECEPTORS

In this section, we summarize the procedures that have been used to establish a blockade of P_2 receptors in isolated smooth muscles. Among the preparations in which this has been accomplished are the vas deferens, urinary bladder, and taenia coli of several species (Hogaboom *et al.*, 1980; Westfall *et al.*, 1982; Westfall *et al.*, 1983). The approaches we have used should be applicable, with some modification, to other muscle and nonmuscle preparations. This discussion begins with general concepts and then amplifies certain details.

When possible, we treat preparations with $ANAPP_3$ under conditions in which the function of the tissue can be monitored; i.e., for smooth muscle preparations this would be in an organ bath so that tension can be recorded. (The reason for this is that $ANAPP_3$ is a P_2-receptor agonist and may therefore evoke responses when initially added.) After an appropriate equilibration period, $ANAPP_3$ is added to the bath, in *near darkness*, and allowed to incubate with the tissue for as long a period as is required for the compound to reach binding equilibrium with the receptor. This is taken as the time required for the response to $ANAPP_3$ to stabilize. At this point, the organ chamber, containing the tissue bathed in $ANAPP_3$-containing solution, is irradiated with high-intensity visible light for a predetermined period of time to induce photoactivation or photolysis of receptor-bound $ANAPP_3$ and the formation of covalent bonds. At the end of the photolysis period, $ANAPP_3$ is washed from the bath and the analysis of the effect of P_2-receptor antagonism is begun.

A. Light Sensitivity of $ANAPP_3$: Storage; Stability

Because $ANAPP_3$ is light sensitive, all preparative procedures, i.e., weighing, preparing solutions, and so on, and the organ bath procedures, until photolysis is begun, should be done in near darkness. The compound is extremely soluble in water. It should be stored dessicated at −20°C when in powder form and solutions should be frozen. When it is stored in this fashion, we have observed no appreciable degradation of the compound over periods of several months.

B. Photolysis

$ANAPP_3$ can be photolyzed by visible or UV light. Glass quenches UV frequencies and therefore photolysis is more easily achieved with glass organ chambers using visible light. As a light source, DYH and DVY projector lamps, available at most photography suppliers, are quite satisfactory. It is likely that other bulbs can be used also, but the kinetics of photoactivation need to be established (see below). Visible lamps such as the DYH and DVY generate a great deal of heat so that one must insure that during photolysis the temperature in the organ bath is not elevated. Water-jacketed organ chambers or the immersion of chambers near the wall of a glass, water-filled aquarium can be used to maintain temperature at levels that will not disrupt the tissue. Chilling the preparation is less desirable than maintaining temperature at near-physiological levels, because active transport processes and the affinity of receptors for ligands may be compromised at low temperature. If the organ chamber assembly has rubber or plastic tubing, these should be covered with aluminum foil to protect them from the heat of the lamp. A fan to help dissipate heat is also quite useful.

UV light (254 nm) will cause the photolysis of $ANAPP_3$, so that a UV light source (Mineral Lite) could be used rather than the high-intensity projector bulbs. However, a quartz organ chamber would need to be used.

The intensity of light contacting the tissue and the time course of photolysis of $ANAPP_3$ will be a function of several factors:

1. Wattage and spectral characteristics of the lamp. Light intensity and wattage are directly related. The visible light bulb must emit blue wavelengths, since $ANAPP_3$ has an absorption peak at 460–480 nm, that is, in the blue range.
2. Composition and geometry of the lamp housing. A home-made apparatus for irradiating tissues, such as a desk lamp fitted with a projector bulb, can work quite satisfactorily. The amount of light reaching the tissue will be increased if, rather than a desk lamp, an apparatus is used that has a metallic parabolic reflector such as a Dyna Lume Heat Projector (Cole Parmer, Chicago).
3. Glass and water-jacket thickness, chamber diameter, and degree of gassing of the physiological solution. These factors will vary in different laboratories but should be standardized for a given apparatus.
4. Distance of the bulb *filament* from the tissue. Light intensity declines with the inverse square of distance. Therefore, the bulb alignment must be made carefully and consistently. A balance must be struck so as to maximize light intensity and to minimize heat delivery.

As demonstrated for $ANAPP_3$ (Hogaboom *et al.*, 1980), photoaffinity labels bind in an equilibrium fashion prior to photolysis and, because of the formation of covalent bonds, irreversibly after photolysis. The latter is a time-dependent process (see below). It is important that the binding of $ANAPP_3$ to the P_2 receptor be at equilibrium prior to photolysis. If not, then three time-dependent processes will be occurring during photolysis, i.e. establishment of equilibrium binding of native $ANAPP_3$, time course of photolysis, and time course of covalent bond formation.

Experiments should be done in which tissues are irradiated in the absence of $ANAPP_3$. This must be done to control for the possible effect of irradiation *per se*. Although the DVY and DYH lamps used in our studies have not produced an effect by themselves, irradiation with light of other wavelengths is known to affect smooth muscle function (Somylo and Somylo, 1970; Burnstock and Wong, 1978; Hogaboom *et al.*, 1980; Galardy and LaVorgna, 1981).

In order to produce a consistent antagonism in each experiment, the same fraction of P_2 receptors should be blocked. For a given concentration of $ANAPP_3$, the extent of receptor blockade is a function of two processes: the time course of photolysis (nitrene intermediate formation) and the time course of covalent insertion. While the time courses of these events are somewhat different, they are related in that the second is obviously dependent on the first. It should be recognized that after a certain point, however, further photolysis will not increase appreciably the extent of antagonism, because the photoaffinity label that is in solution will have been consumed during the process. This is unlike the case with conventional irreversible antagonists, such as phenoxybenzamine, in which the extent of antagonism increases the longer the preparation is exposed to the antagonist.

It is necessary to assess the time course of photoactivation in order to know the extent to which $ANAPP_3$ is photolyzed during irradiation. Such information can be obtained using spectrophotometric methods to assess changes in absorption of samples removed at various times during irradiation. An example is shown in Figure 2 in which is depicted the native spectrum of $ANAPP_3$ prior to photolysis and after extensive photolysis of the compound to cause completion of the photolysis reaction. The spectrum is altered in a characteristic fashion. Figure 2 also illustrates the absorbance changes at 260 nm obtained from spectra of samples removed at various intervals during photolysis. The curve provides an indication of the extent of photolysis of $ANAPP_3$. Thus, photolysis of $ANAPP_3$ in our 3-ml organ chambers for 15 min with a DYH bulb, the filament of which was 15 cm from the center of the chamber, results in photolysis of 80% of the compound. This degree of photolysis would not necessarily occur if different conditions were used, e.g., a bulb of different wattage, a different distance of the filament from the chamber, and so on. Since 80% of the $ANAPP_3$ is photolyzed in 15 min under the conditions stated above, little more is gained by irradiating for longer time periods. If a more substantial P_2-receptor blockade is desired than that produced by a 15 min photolysis period, an approach would be to add additional fresh $ANAPP_3$ and photolyze again.

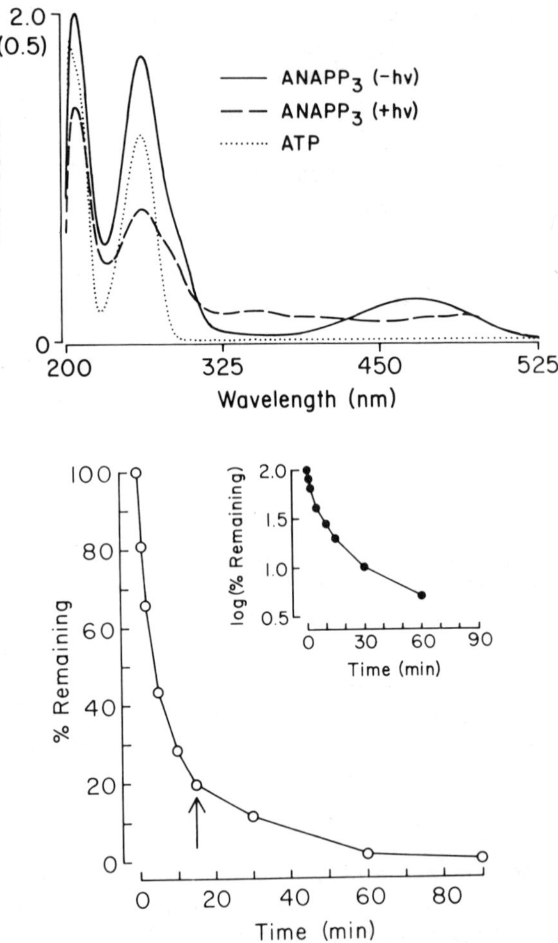

Figure 2. Upper panel: Spectra of $ANAPP_3$ ($10^{-4}M$) before ($-h\nu$) and 30 min after ($+h\nu$) photolysis of the compound in 20-ml organ chambers. A DVY bulb was used for irradiation and the $ANAPP_3$ was dissolved in modified Krebs–Henseleit solution. The reference cuvette contained modified Krebs–Henseleit solution. For comparison, the spectrum of ATP (2×10^{-5} *M*) is also shown (0.5 full-scale absorbance). Photolysis of $ANAPP_3$ produced a characteristic alteration in its spectrum, as shown, from which information on the time course of photolysis may be obtained, i.e., from the reduction in A_{260}. From Hogaboom *et al.* (1980). Copyright 1980 by the American Association for the Advancement of Science. Lower panel: Time course of reduction in A_{260} for 10^{-4} *M* $ANAPP_3$ (dissolved in modified Krebs–Henseleit solution) during photolysis with DYH bulb of the compound in 3-ml organ chambers. The reference cuvette contained modified Krebs–Henseleit solution. The bulb filament was 15 cm from the center of the organ chamber. Percent remaining was determined from the ΔA_{260} obtained at sampling intervals compared to the total ΔA_{260} between $t = 0$ and when the reaction reached completion (90 min), i.e., $100\% - [(A_{t=0} - A_{t=i})/A_{\text{total}} \times 100]$ where i = time of sample. The arrow indicates that 15 min was required to produce 80% of the maximum ΔA_{260}. This period (15 min) is used routinely in our experiments as the standard photolysis period. Inset: Logarithmic transform of the data. The plot yields a curve instead of a straight line. Photolysis of $ANAPP_3$ thus is not a simple exponential or first-order process, but proceeds with order 1.5. From O'Donnell *et al.* (1983), with permission.

C. Specificity of Antagonism

When $ANAPP_3$ is used as a tool to investigate P_2 receptors, the specificity of its antagonism needs to be evaluated. Although the evidence to date indicates a high degree of specificity, it remains possible that the reactive nitrene intermediate that is generated by photolysis of $ANAPP_3$ could react with sites in the preparation other than P_2 receptors. In our studies, the effects of $ANAPP_3$ treatment on responses to agonists that act via receptors other than purinoceptors has been investigated. For example, in several different smooth muscle preparations, photolysis of $ANAPP_3$ results in antagonism of ATP-induced responses, but not those to norepinephrine, acetylcholine, isoproterenol, or KCl (Hogaboom *et al.*, 1980; Westfall *et al.*, 1982, 1983). Thus it appears that $ANAPP_3$ does not antagonize responses mediated by α- or β-adrenergic receptors or muscarinic receptors. Additionally, $ANAPP_3$ does not antagonize responses induced by KCl-induced membrane depolarization.

A question that has not been completely answered is whether $ANAPP_3$ antagonizes responses mediated by P_1 purinoceptors, although the evidence to date indicates that it does not. Part of the difficulty in answering this question resides in the fact that in a number of preparations in which the effects of $ANAPP_3$ have been investigated, ATP, the prototype P_2 agonist, and adenosine, the prototype P_1 agonist, produce qualitatively dissimilar effects. For example, in the guinea pig vas deferens, ATP, ADP, and a number of nucleotide analogs, produce contraction. Adenosine, however, does not produce contraction, so that the potential antagonism by $ANAPP_3$ cannot be assessed. In a preparation in which ATP and adenosine produce similar effects, the results are equivocal. Experiments conducted with the guinea-pig taenia coli show that $ANAPP_3$ produces an approximate 6-fold antagonism of relaxation responses to ATP, but only a 2-fold antagonism of relaxation responses to adenosine (Westfall *et al.*, 1982). One interpretation of this finding is that $ANAPP_3$ antagonizes responses mediated by P_1 receptors, although somewhat less effectively than those mediated by P_2 receptors. However, it is also possible that a component of the response to adenosine is mediated by its interaction with P_2 receptors, thereby accounting for the antagonism by $ANAPP_3$.

In some preparations, responses to ATP are not antagonized by $ANAPP_3$. For example, Sneddon *et al.* (1982b) have found that relaxations of the rabbit anococcygeus muscle produced by ATP and adenosine were not blocked by $ANAPP_3$. ATP and adenosine were nearly equipotent, and, on the basis of other experiments, it was determined that $ANAPP_3$ was ineffective against ATP because responses to the nucleotide followed its conversion to adenosine, which actually mediated the response. Similarly, Frew and Lundy (1982a) reported that $ANAPP_3$ was unable to antagonize ATP-induced relaxation of the fundus of the guinea-pig stomach. Additional studies indicated that these responses are mediated by P_1 receptors because they are antagonized by 8-phenyltheophylline (Frew and Lundy, 1982b); this implies that a conversion of ATP to adenosine occurs. The cumulative evidence obtained by us and others therefore indicates that the antagonism by $ANAPP_3$ is selective for the P_2-receptor.

D. Effects of Nonphotolyzed $ANAPP_3$

Nonphotolyzed $ANAPP_3$ is an agonist and, upon initial application, produces responses that resemble those produced by ATP. If $ANAPP_3$ is allowed to remain in the organ bath during subsequent exposure to ATP, the responses to ATP are reduced, whereas those to chemically unrelated agonists are not (Hogaboom *et al.*, 1980; Fedan *et al.*, 1981; Westfall *et al.*, 1983).

The effects of nonphotolyzed $ANAPP_3$ on responses of the guinea-pig vas deferens to ATP are illustrated in Figure 3. (Also shown in Figure 3 are the effects

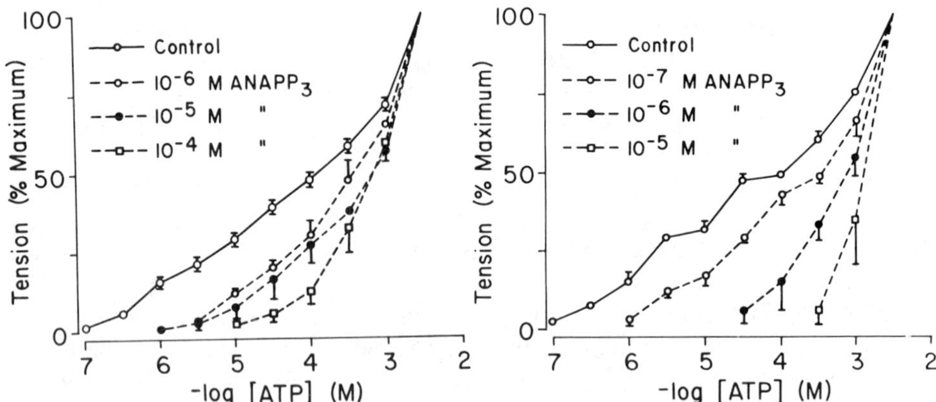

Figure 3. Left panel: Effect of several concentrations of $ANAPP_3$, following its photolysis (DVY bulb, 30-min irradiation period) in organ chamber containing the guinea-pig vas deferens, on contractile responses of the tissue to ATP. The $ANAPP_3$ was no longer present during the ATP concentration–response determinations. Right panel: Effect of nonphotolyzed $ANAPP_3$ on ATP concentration–response curves of isolated guinea-pig vas deferens. In these experiments, which were performed in the dark, the $ANAPP_3$ was continually present during the additions of ATP. From Hogaboom et al. (1980). Copyright 1980 by the American Association for the Advancement of Science.

of photolyzed $ANAPP_3$ on responses to ATP.) This ATP-specific antagonism by nonphotolyzed $ANAPP_3$ is reversed readily by washing out the $ANAPP_3$; i.e., covalent bonds are not formed if the compound is not photolyzed. A similar phenomenon occurs *in situ*. Nonphotolyzed $ANAPP_3$ administered intraarterially to the cat urinary bladder produces a contraction followed by an antagonism of intraarterially administered adenine nucleotides (Theobald, 1982, 1983).

The reversible antagonistic effects of nonphotolyzed $ANAPP_3$ could result from a conventional equilibrium-competitive antagonism of P_2 receptors. Alternatively, because a similar antagonistic effect occurs after administration of ATP itself, the antagonism by nonphotolyzed $ANAPP_3$ may be a manifestation of an autoinhibition phenomenon known to be induced by adenine nucleotides in smooth muscle (Ambache and Zar, 1970; Dean and Downie, 1978; Baer and Frew, 1979; Meldrum and Burnstock, 1983). Definitive evidence to support either possibility is not available. However, because the agonistic potency of nonphotolyzed $ANAPP_3$ and ATP are virtually identical (O'Donnell *et al.*, 1983), whereas nonphotolyzed $ANAPP_3$ is more effective than ATP in reducing ATP-induced responses (Hogaboom *et al.*, 1980), it would seem that part of the antagonism produced by nonphotolyzed $ANAPP_3$ results from a true competitive antagonism.

E. Structural Considerations in the Design of P_2-Receptor Photoaffinity Labels.

The potency of photoaffinity labels under equilibrium binding conditions (i.e., before photolysis) and the extent of photolabeling upon photolysis will be influenced by the location of the photolabile moiety on the ATP molecule. Information on where the photosensitive grouping can be added to ATP without reducing potency at the P_2 receptor can be obtained *a priori* from the ability of ATP analogs to induce responses. This information also provides a useful comparison to the structural requirements of ligands for the P_1 receptor.

In general, additions of varying size to the adenine ring at N^1, N^6, and C^8 all reduce agonist activity. The replacement of the N^6 amino group of ATP with a hydroxyl (e.g., inosine triphosphate) reduces agonist activity substantially. It seems clear that the adenine ring is involved in receptor recognition and even slight modifications reduce activity (Fedan *et al.*, 1982). An ATP photoaffinity label used widely in biochemical studies is 8-azido ATP (Haley, 1975; Pomerantz *et al.*, 1975; Owens and Haley, 1978). While we have had no direct experience with this compound, it would be predicated that 8-azido ATP would be less useful than $ANAPP_3$ as a P_2 antagonist, based on the finding that other 8-substituted compounds, such as 8-bromo ATP and 8-(6-aminohexyl) amino ATP, are less potent than ATP in the guinea-pig vas deferens.

Modification of ribose are better tolerated than modifications of the adenine moiety. While there is some loss of potency with 2′-deoxy ATP, two other modifications, e.g., 3′-deoxy-ATP and 9-β-D-ribofuranosyl ATP yield compounds that are nearly equivalent to ATP. $ANAPP_3$ is a 3′ derivative of ATP, as is arylazido aminobutyryl ATP ($ANABP_3$), another photoaffinity analog; these compounds have agonist potency similar to ATP (O'Donnell *et al.*, 1983).

The replacement of 5′-phosphates with sulfate, amidate, morpholidate, or other groups results in compounds with little agonist activity. In terms of structure–activity relationships, therefore, an intact adenine and the presence of 5′-phosphates are critical for receptor recognition, whereas modifications of the ribose are better tolerated. These structural features are quite different from those for P_1 receptors, where N^6 and 5′ hydroxyl additions confer receptor specificity without loss of potency. From this analysis, it seems that for P_2 receptor interaction the best location for a photolabile moiety is on the 3′ hydroxyl of ribose, which is where ATP is derivitized in the case of $ANAPP_3$.

V. CONCLUDING COMMENTS

There are both disadvantages and advantages to the use of the photoaffinity label $ANAPP_3$ in the study of P_2 receptors. The most obvious disadvantage is that $ANAPP_3$ cannot be used as an irreversible antagonist *in vivo*, because there is no mechanism, at present, to irradiate the compound under these conditions. Related to this is the potential difficulty of photolyzing $ANAPP_3$ *in vitro* if relatively thick tissue preparations are being investigated. The novelty of dealing with photoaffinity compounds, as well as the unusual apparatus, such as the lamps that are required, may seem to be a disadvantage as well. In spite of these difficulties, however, $ANAPP_3$ is an important tool for investigators interested in the pharmacology and physiology of adenine nucleotides and nucleosides. $ANAPP_3$ has the advantage of being the only specific antagonist of responses mediated through P_2 receptors. Thus, the compound is of considerable value in probing the potential physiological role of ATP and in helping to distinguish between responses mediated by ATP and by adenosine.

APPENDIX: PROCEDURE FOR PREPARATION OF ANAPP$_3$ (based on Jeng and Guillory, 1975)

Step I. Preparation of 4-fluoro-3-nitrophenyl azide

Supplies

Acetone, sodium nitrite, dry ice, sodium azide, hydrochloric acid, petroleum ether, 4-fluoro-3-nitroaniline.

Equipment

Filter flask and funnel (3) two 250 ml, one 1000 ml; 50–100 ml beaker; Pasteur pipettes and bulbs; stir bars and stir rods (glass); 100-ml 3-neck round bottom flask (2); stir/heat plate; ice bucket; 2-liter Erlenmeyer flask; two acetone-dry Ice Baths (any small cold-proof bowl will suffice); filter paper.

Procedure

Heat gently 30-ml conc. HCl/5 ml H_2O on a stir/heat plate in a hood. Place 4.4 g of 4-fluoro-3-nitroaniline in the 100-ml beaker and stir well for 10 min at 40–50°C. While heating, cool a 100-ml 3-neck round bottom flask to −20° to −30°C in an acetone/dry ice bath. After heating/stirring the 4-floro-3-nitroaniline, filter through a filter flask/funnel and discard the black residue on the filter paper. Place the light brown filtrate in the 100-ml round bottom (RB) flask and maintain the slush bath at −20 to −30°C while stirring. At this time dissolve 2.4 g of sodium nitrite in 5 ml of water and 2.2 g of sodium azide in 8 ml of water. Also cool the 250-ml filter flask in a second acetone/dry ice bath to −20° to −30°C. Set up this apparatus for filtering. With a pasteur pipette, add slowly (about a drop a second) the sodium nitrite to the cold (−20°C) well-stirred 4-floro-3-nitroanline/acid medium. Stir for 10 min and keep at −20°. Filter the mixture into the −20°C filter flask and cool another 100-ml RB flask (3 neck) to −20°C in a slush bath. Discard the residue and place the light brown filtrate into the −20°C RB flask. Cool the mixture to −20°C and add the sodium azide slowly (about a drop every 5 sec). Stir well with a medium-sized stir bar. After about a minute, stir the mixture with a glass rod as an insoluble layer forms over the top of the reaction mixture. This layer must be dispersed to insure even mixing. Repeat this until the azide has been added. Keep the dry ice/acetone bath at −20°C to −30°C at all times. Filter the light brown mixture. Rinse the residue in the RB flask with ice-cold distilled water. Wash the solid with about 2 liters of cold distilled H_2O. Take the light brown solid on the filter paper and dry by vacuum dessication. When absolutely dry, recrystallize with hot petroleum ether. Allow the crystals to form in a cool dark dry area over night. (*The reactions were carried out in a lab room with no outside lighting. The lights were dimmed in the room. These were the only precautions taken. However, there is a constant danger of the azides exploding.)*

Step II: Preparation of *N*-4-Azide-2-nitrophenyl-β-alanine

Supplies

β-Alanine, ether, sodium carbonate, pH paper, ethanol (95%), sodium chloride, hydrochloric acid, magnesium sulfate, 4-fluoro-3-nitrophenyl azide.

Equipment

Oil bath with heating device and rheostat, small beakers, 100-ml round-bottom flask, cooling condenser, rotating evaporator (roto-vap), separatory funnel (500 ml), 500-ml round-bottom flask (2), filter funnel and paper.

Procedure

All of the following steps take place in a hood. Dissolve 0.534 g of β-alanine and 1.08 g of sodium carbonate in 5.4 ml of water using a 100-ml round-bottom flask. Add 0.9000 g of 4-fluoro-3-nitrophenyl azide and stir well. Add 6.75 ml of ethanol, 5.4 ml of water, and then 13.5 ml of ethanol. Cover with foil, place in a hood, and stir at 52–55°C overnight (12–18 hr). Reduce the volume to about 10 ml using a roto-vap apparatus. Extract with 45 ml of ether (twice) to remove the starting azide. Save the red aqueous layer and add 3 *N* HCl until the solution is a pH of 2 or less. The solution becomes somewhat opaque. Extract with 90 ml of ether (three times) and save the ether layer (clear orange-red). Wash the ether layer three times with 50 ml of saturated NaCl. Place the ether layer in a 500-ml round-bottom flask and add in magnesium sulfate (2–3 g) and allow to stand for 15–30 min. Filter the ether into a 500-ml round-bottom flask and evaporate to dryness using a roto-vap. Add in 20–40 ml of hot ethanol and heat until the residue is dissolved. Place the hot ethanol in a 100-ml beaker and set in the hood covered with foil until dry. The resulting dark red solid is used in the next step.

Step III: Preparation of 3′-*O*-{3[*N*-(4-Azido-2-nitrophenyl)amino-propionyl} adenosine 5′-triphosphate (ANAPP$_3$)

Supplies

Carbonyldiimidazole, acetone, N,N-dimethylformamide, n-butanol, Whatman 3MM Chromatography Sheets, Glacial Acetic acid.

Equipment

50-ml round-bottom flask (2) (*dry*), rotating evaporator, small beakers, 16 × 100 test tubes, table top centrifuge, vacuum dessicator, chromatography tank, Pasteur pipette and bulb, vortex.

Procedure

Dissolve carbodiimidazole (1.35 g) in 2.5 ml of dimethylformamide (dried over molecular sieves) in a 50-ml RB flask. Add and dissolve by stirring well 0.630 g of *N*-4-azide-2-nitrophenyl-β-alanine. The dark-red solution will turn into thick orange-red viscous material after about 5 min. Pour in 0.325 g of Na_2ATP dissolved in 12.5 ml of water. (A ratio of 5:1 water to dimethylformamide is essential). The solution will immediately become an orange foamy solution. Cover with foil, set in the hood, and stir well overnight (18–24 hr). Using a roto-vap, dry the solution to a dark-red residue. Add acetone (20 ml) to the 50-ml round-bottom flask. An orange precipitate will form in the red acetone solution. Pipette the solution and precipitate into 16 × 100 mm test tubes. Use as much acetone as needed to get the precipitated material out of the flask (usually 50 ml). Centrifuge the tubes 10 min at 2000 rpm. Aspirate out the clear red supernatant and discard. Add 2 ml of acetone to each tube and disperse the precipitate using a vortex and a small spatula. Combine the acetone mixture into two tubes. Disperse the precipitate very well in the acetone. Centrifuge again 2000 rpm for 10 min. Aspirate off the acetone. Add fresh acetone, disperse, centrifuge. Repeat this step 3–5 times until the acetone supernatant becomes a faint clear orange. Combine the dispersed precipitate–acetone mixture into one tube, centrifuge, aspirate the acetone, place a foil cap over the test tubes, and punch small holes in the foil. Tape the foil on the sides of the tube to keep the foil on and vaccuum dessicate overnight. *Once the dried solid is obtained, make attempts to keep the orange solid away from light.* Add 1 ml of distilled water to make a dark-red solution. Apply to Whatman 3MM chromatography sheets and chromatograph using *n*-butanol, water, and acetic acid (5:3:2) *in the dark.* Let the solvent front run to about an inch from the bottom and then *dry in the dark.* Cut out the orange band eluting at R_f = 0.30–0.50, cut the paper into fine strips (0.5 cm × 2 cm), and place in distilled water overnight *in the dark* at room temperature (50–100 ml water). Pour off the orange solution and filter twice through glass wool. Add 50 ml of water to the remaining strips and repeat as above. Lyophilize the solution *in the dark* to a resulting fluffy orange powder. *Store in the dark, dessicated at −20°C.*

REFERENCES

Ambache, N., and Zar, M. S. 1970. Non-cholinergic transmission by post-ganglionic motor neurones in the mammalian bladder. *J. Physiol.* (*London*), *210:*761–783.

Baer, H. P., and Frew, R. 1979. Relaxation of guinea-pig fundic strip by adenosine, adenosine triphosphate and electrical stimulation: Lack of antagonism by theophylline or ATP treatment. *Br. J. Pharmacol.*, *67:*293–299.

Bayley, H., and Knowles, J. R. 1977. Photoaffinity labeling. *Methods Enzymol. 46:*69–114.

Burnstock, G. 1979. Past and current evidence for the purinergic nerve hypothesis. In: *Physiological and Regulatory Functions of Adenosine and Adenine Nucleotides*, pp. 3–32. Ed. by Baer, H. P. and Drummond, G. I. Raven Press, New York.

Burnstock, G. 1983. A comparison of receptors for adenosine and adenine nucleotides. In *Regulatory Function of Adenosine*, pp. 49–59. Ed. by Berne, R. M., Rall, T. W., and Rubio, R. Martinus Nijhoff, Boston.

Burnstock, G., and Wong, H. 1978. Comparison of the effects of ultraviolet light and purinergic nerve stimulation on the guinea-pig taenia coli. *Br. J. Pharmacol., 62*:293–302.

Burnstock, G., Campbell, G., Satchell, D., and Smythe, A. 1970. Evidence that adenosine triphosphate or a related nucleotide is the transmitter substance released by non-adrenergic inhibitory nerves in the gut. *Br. J. Pharmacol.*, 40:668–688.

Campbell, G., and Gibbons, I. L. 1979. Non-adrenergic, non-cholinergic transmission in the autonomic nervous system: purinergic nerves. In: *Trends in Automatic Pharmacology*, Volume 1, pp. 103–144. Ed. by Kalsner, S. Urban and Schwarzenberg, Baltimore.

Chowdry, V., and Westheimer, F. H. 1979. Photoaffinity labeling of biological systems. *Ann. Rev. Biochem., 48*:293–325.

Cooperman, B. S. 1976. Photoaffinity labeling of proteins and more complex receptors. In: *Ageing, Carcinogenicity and Radiation Biology*, pp. 315–339. Ed. by Kendric, C. Plenum, New York.

Dean, D. M., and Downie, J. W. 1978. Contribution of adrenergic and 'purinergic' neurotransmission to contraction in rabbit detrusor. *J. Pharmacol. Exp. Ther., 207*:431–445.

De Mey, J., Burnstock, G., and Vanhoutte, P. M. 1979. Modulation of the evoked release of noradrenaline in canine saphenous vein via presynaptic receptors for adenosine but not ATP. *Eur. J. Pharmacol., 55*:401–405.

Fedan, J. S., Hogaboom, G. K., O'Donnell, J. P., Colby, J., and Westfall, D. P. 1981. Contribution by purines to the neurogenic response of the vas deferens of the guinea pig, *Eur. J. Pharmacol., 69*:41–53.

Fedan, J. S., Hogaboom, G. K., Westfall, D. P., and O'Donnell, J. P. 1982. Comparison of contractions of the smooth muscle of the guinea-pig vas deferens induced by ATP and related nucleotides. *Eur. J. Pharmacol., 81*:193–204.

Fedan, J. S., Hogaboom, G. K., Westfall, D. P., and O'Donnell, J. P. 1983a. Photoafinity labeling of P_2-purinergic and H_1-histamine receptors in intact smooth muscle. *Fed. Proc., 42*:2846–2850.

Fedan, J.S., Hogaboom, G. K., and O'Donnell, J. P. 1983b. Photoaffinity labels as pharmacological tools. *Biochem. Pharmacol.*, in press.

Frew, R., and Lundy, P. M. 1982a. Effect of arylazido aminopropionyl ATP ($ANAPP_3$), a putative ATP antagonist, on ATP responses of isolated guinea pig smooth muscle. *Life Sci., 30*:259–267.

Frew, R., and Lundy, P. M. 1982b. Evidence against ATP being the nonadrenergic, noncholinergic inhibitory transmitter in guinea pig stomach, *Eur. J. Pharmacol., 81*:333–336.

Galardy, R. E., and LaVorgna, K. A. 1981. Photochemical inactivation of the angiotensin receptor of rabbit aorta by *N* (2-nitro-5-azidobenzoyl)-[1-aspartic, 5-isoleucine] angiotensin II. *J. Med. Chem., 24*:362–366.

Guillory, R. J., and Jeng, S. J. 1983. Photoaffinity labeling: Theory and practice. *Fed. Proc., 42*:2826–2830.

Haley, B. E. 1975. Photoaffinity labeling of cAMP binding sites of human red blood cell membranes. *Biochemistry, 14*:3852–3857.

Hogaboom, G. K., O'Donnell, J. P., and Fedan, J. S. 1980. Purinergic receptors; Photoaffinity analog of adenosine triphosphate is a specific adenosine triphosphate antagonist. *Science, 208*:1273–1276.

Jeng, S. J., and Guillory, R. J. 1975. The use of arylazido ATP analogs as photoaffinity labels for myosin ATPase. *J. Supramolec. Struct., 3*:448–468.

Katsuragi, R., and Su, C. 1982. Augmentation by theophylline of [^{3}H]purine release from vascular adrenergic nerves: Evidence for presynaptic autoinhibition. *J. Pharmacol. Exp. Ther., 220*:152–156.

Meldrum, L. A., and Burnstock, G., 1983. Evidence that ATP acts as a co-transmitter with noradrenaline in sympathetic nerves supplying the guinea-pig vas deferens. *Eur. J. Pharmacol., 92*:161–163.

O'Donnell, J. P., Hogaboom, G. K., and Fedan, J. S. 1983. Comparison of photoaffinity labeling of P_2-purinergic receptors of isolated guinea-pig vas deferens by arylazido aminopropionyl ATP and by arylazido aminobutyryl ATP. *Eur. J. Pharmacol., 86*:435–440.

Owens, J. R., and Haley, B. E. 1978. Use of photoaffinity nucleotide analogs to determine the mechanism of ATP regulation of a membrane bound, cAMP activated protein kinase. *J. Supramolec. Struct., 9*:57–68.

Pomerantz, A. H., Rudolf, S. A., Haley, B. E., and Greengard, P. 1975. Photoaffinity labeling of a protein kinase from bovine brain with 8-azido adenosine 3′, 5′-monophosphate. *Biochemistry 14:*3858–3862.

Sneddon, P., Westfall, D. P., and Fedan, J. S. 1982a. Cotransmitters in motor nerves of the guinea pig vas deferens: Electrophysiological evidence. *Science, 218:*693–695.

Sneddon, P., Westfall, D. P., and Fedan, J. S. 1982b. Investigation of relaxations of the rabbit anococcygeus muscle by nerve stimulation and ATP using the ATP antagonist $ANAPP_3$. *Eur. J. Pharmacol., 80:*93–98.

Somylo, A. P., and Somylo, A. V. 1970. Vascular smooth muscle. II. Pharmacology of normal and hypertensive vessels, *Pharm. Rev. 22:*249–353.

Su, C. 1977. Purinergic inhibition of adenergic transmission in rabbit blood vessels. *J. Pharmacol. Exp. Ther., 204:*351–361.

Theobald, R. J., Jr., 1982. Arylazido aminopropionyl ATP ($ANAPP_3$) antagonism of cat urinary bladder contractions. *J. Autonom. Pharmacol., 3:*175–179.

Theobald, R. J., Jr., 1983. The effect of arylazido aminopropionyl ATP on atropine resistant contractions of the cat urinary bladder. *Life Sci., 32:*2479–2484.

Weetman, D. F., and Turner, N. 1977. The effects of ATP-receptor blocking agents on the response of the guinea-pig isolated bladder preparation to hyoscine-resistant nerve stimulation. *Arch. Int. Pharmacodyn, 228:*10–14.

Westfall, D. P., Stitzel, R. E., and Rowe, J. N. 1978. The postjunctional effects and neuronal release of purine compounds in the guinea pig vas deferns, *Eur. J. Pharmacol., 50:*27–38.

Westfall, D. P., Hogaboom, G. K., Colby, J., O'Donnell, J. P., and Fedan, J. S. 1982. Direct evidence against a role of ATP as the nonadrenergic, noncholinergic inhibitory neurotransmitter in guinea pig tenia coli. *Proc. Natl. Acad. Sci. USA, 49*: 7041–7045.

Westfall, D. P., Fedan, J. S., Colby, J., Hogaboom, G. K., and O'Donnell, J. P. 1983. Evidence for a contribution by purines to the neurogenic response of the guinea-pig urinary bladder. *Eur. J. Pharmacol., 87:*415–422.

Chapter **15**

Use of Structure–Activity Relationships in the Study of Adenosine Receptors

R. A. Olsson*, R. D. Thompson, and S. Kusachi

Suncoast AHA Chapter Cardiovascular Research Laboratory
Department of Internal Medicine, and Departments of Internal Medicine and Biochemistry*
University of South Flordia
College of Medicine
Tampa, Florida

I. INTRODUCTION

The study of structure–activity correlations uses information about the chemical attributes and biological activities of ligands to draw indirect inferences about the structure of a receptor and the physical forces that govern the receptor–ligand interaction. Knowledge of this kind can guide the design of artifical ligands, drugs that preserve the essential features of a natural ligand for receptor recognition and activation (or inhibition) at some advantage over the natural ligand, such as lower cost, greater selectivity, or better stability.

This chapter describes and illustrates with examples the conceptual approach that we have used to characterize the dog coronary artery adenosine receptor. The fundamental principles that underlie our approach are generally applicable to the study of adenosine receptors in other preparations, such as isolated cell membranes or intact organs.

In common with other quantitative structure–activity relationship (QSAR) approaches, our studies of the coronary adenosine receptor are based on the chemical dynamics of receptor activation, particularly the extrathermodynamic linear free energy theorem, and on the types of forces that govern the binding of a ligand to its receptor (Osman *et al.*, 1979; Weinstein *et al.*, 1979; Israelachvili, 1974). A formal mathematical analysis of our results by one of the QSAR techniques is certainly feasible. However, we have followed a largely nonmathematical approach, interpreting experimental results in terms of probable chemical mechanisms and placing great reliance on the predictive power of such inferences as tested by further experiment. That it was possible to take this course owes to the wealth of structure–activity data on the coronary vasoactivity of adenosine analogs already available to us at the outset (Gough and Maguire, 1965; Jahn, 1965; Jahn, 1969; Angus *et al.*, 1971; Shimizu *et al.*, 1971; Scholtholt *et al.*, 1972; Cobbin *et al.*, 1974; Marumoto *et al.*, 1975; Vapaatalo *et al.*, 1975; Prasad *et al.*, 1976; Raberger *et al.*, 1977; Olsson *et al.*, 1979; Prasad *et al.*, 1980). Additionally, we exploited the chemical complexity of the adenosine molecule and the principle that a ligand contains information about its receptor in proportion, at least roughly, to its complexity. Further, the availability of an adenosine antagonist, theophylline, provided evidence complementary to that yielded by agonists. Finally, the parallel activity of adenosine analogs as coronary vasodilators and inhibitors of platelet aggregation (Dietmann *et al.*, 1970) opened to us the extensive literature on this subject (Kikugawa *et al.*, 1972; 1973; Mills *et al.*, 1983). Information from such varied sources was an important base for the "thought experiments" that led to models for experimental test.

The results described below come from studies of appropriately instrumented conscious or anesthetized, open-thorax dog preparations (Olsson *et al.*, 1979; Kusachi *et al.*, 1983). Measurements of coronary blood flow rate and perfusion pressure during the steady-state responses to the direct intracoronary infusion of adenosine analogs served for the construction of cumulative dose–response curves from which we estimated EC_{50}, the agonist concentration that produced a half-maximum change in coronary conductance (reciprocal resistance). In order to account for between-dog differences in coronary reactivity and to compare our observations with those from other laboratories (Angus *et al.*, 1971; Cobbin *et al.*, 1974; Marumoto *et al.*, 1975), we normalize the potency of an analog by referring its potency to that of adenosine in the same dog, a molar potency ratio (MPR).

The coronary vasoactivity of adenosine depends absolutely on both the adenine and ribose moieties; accordingly, we model the coronary receptor as discrete purine and ribose domains. The illustrative examples given below concern only the fine structure of the purine domain.

II. ADENOSINE RECEPTORS

A. General

The demonstration in 1970 (Sattin and Rall, 1970) that adenosine stimulates the adenylate cyclase of brain and that theophylline specifically antagonizes this effect established the existence of adenosine receptors. Within a decade of their discovery, additional work showed that there are at least two kinds of adenosine receptors associated with adenylate cyclase, those which stimulate (R_a or Ai2) and those which inhibit (R_i or A_i) the enzyme (Van Calker *et al.*, 1979; Londos *et al.*, 1980). Like many other hormone receptors, R_a and R_i receptors require the intermediacy of the GTP-binding G/N proteins. A distinct inhibitory "P site" neither requires GTP nor is sensitive to inhibition by dialkylxanthines and thus seems to operate distal to the G/N proteins, perhaps directly on the catalytic site (Wolff *et al.*, 1981). Available evidence neither strongly supports nor excludes the possibility that there are additional kinds of adenosine receptors that do not act through adenylate cyclase, e.g., receptors coupled directly to receptor-operated ion channels.

Two receptor-selective adenosine analogs, ethyl adenosine-5′-uronamide, "NECA", and N^6-(*R*-1-phenyl-2-propyl)adenosine, "*R*-PIA", are important reagents for identifying R_a and R_i receptors. R_a receptors exhibit a potency order NECA > *R*-PIA, whereas R_i receptors exhibit a reverse order and also a high degree of stereoselectivity, such that *R*-PIA is 50–100 times more potent than its *S* diastereomer (Bruns *et al.*, 1980).

B. The Coronary Adenosine Receptor

Several lines of evidence suggest that R_a receptors mediate the coronary vasoactivity of adenosine. Adenosine elicits cyclic AMP accumulation in parallel with the relaxation of bovine coronary rings and stimulates adenylate cyclase activity in coronary homogenates (Kukovetz *et al.*, 1979). In rabbit coronary microvessels, NECA stimulates adenylate cyclase more potently than either adenosine or *R*-PIA (Mistry and Drummond, 1983). Because blood vessels contain several types of cells besides myocytes, inferences drawn from studies of whole arteries must await confirmation through studies of purified coronary myocyte plasma membranes. In the open-chest dog, the coronary vasoactivity of adenosine is two orders of magnitude greater than that of *R*-PIA (Kusachi *et al.*, 1983). However, *R*-PIA stereoselectively activates the coronary receptor (Vapaatalo *et al.*, 1975; Kusachi *et al.*, 1983), albeit to a much lower degree than its action at R_i receptors. Such a result suggests that the coronary receptor may be an R_a receptor that retains the specialized N-6 region characteristic of R_i receptors. Similarly to its effect on R receptors generally, theophylline competitively inhibits the coronary vasoactivity of adenosine (Afonso, 1970; Bünger *et al.*, 1975).

III. STRUCTURE OF THE CORONARY RECEPTOR PURINE DOMAIN

Herein we describe how we proceed from an analysis of the chemical features of a ligand to hypothetical receptor models and, through the results of testing, further refinement of these models. Unfortunately, as the model becomes more detailed, the synthesis of the analogs needed for experimental test becomes more difficult. Consequently, the account that follows is more a progress report drawn from unpublished observations than a definitive description of the receptor.

A. Chemistry of Adenine

Figure 1A diagrams the formal structure and numbering system and Figure 1B the results of a molecular arbital calculation of the atomic charge distribution of adenine.

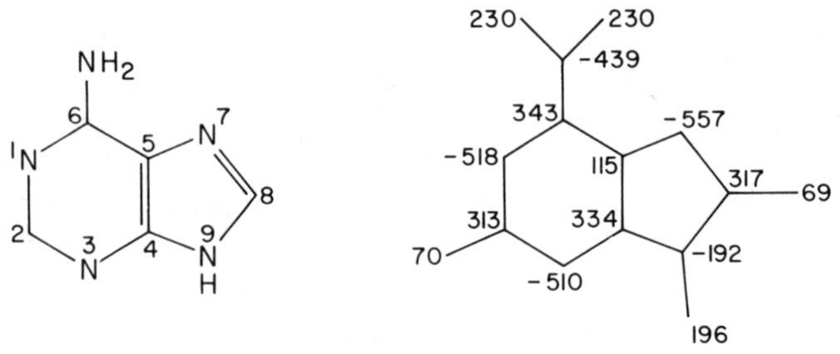

Figure 1. (A) Structure of adenine, showing the IUPAC system for numbering individual atoms as estimated by molecular orbital calculations (Redrawn from Pullman, 1969, Figure 6). Note that the charges on each atom differ. Such as asymmetric charge distribution is the origin of the permanent dipole of adenine.

Purine is a nitrogen heterocycle. The lone pair electrons of nitrogen make these atoms centers of electron density. As a consequence, each nitrogen could act as a local polar center that participates in binding to the receptor electrostatically through a dipole–dipole or induced dipole interaction. Alternatively, the asymmetric spatial disposition of the four nitrogens gives rise to a dipole moment, a global property of a molecule. The dipole moment of purine is rather strong, 4.3 D, and that of adenine only slightly less so, 3.2 D (Bergmann and Weiler-Feilchenfeld, 1972). Any or all of the purine nitrogens can, through their lone pair electrons, act as hydrogen bond acceptors. For example, an intramolecular H bond between purine N-3 and the C-5′ amide N of NECA is thought to stabilize the nucleoside in a *syn* conformation favored for binding; such an explanation has been invoked to account for the vasoactivity of NECA (Prasad et al., 1980). Intermolecular H bonds between a purine nitrogen and the receptor would, of course, contribute to binding affinity. The carbons and nitrogens of purine alike contribute electrons to a π system; however, the degree of delocalization and, consequently, the aromatic character of purine are small. Indeed, convincing evidence that adenines can undergo reactions typical of aromatic compounds, e.g., the formation of diazonium ions, has appeared only recently (Robins and Uznański, 1981; Nair and Richardson, 1982). Nevertheless, these delocalized electrons might contribute to binding through Van der Waals forces. Finally, the dimensions of purine govern susceptibility to steric hindrance, which, on the atomic level, is but another manifestation of Van der Waals forces.

The low coronary vasoactivity of purine riboside, MPR 0.023, shows how strongly the vasoactivity of adenosine depends on the 6-amino group. Either the intrinsic properties of this nitrogen or its influence on the chemistry of the purine base could contribute to activity. N-6 may act as a polar center, as a hydrogen bond acceptor, and also as a hydrogen bond donor. Although this nitrogen is basic and has the potential for protonation, such is not the case. Rather, N-6 contributes electrons to the π deficient purine system, thereby increasing its aromaticity, its stability, and the basicity of N-1, which is the site of protonation and alkylation of adenosine (Jones and Robbins, 1963). The 6-amino group also weakens the purine dipole moment and shifts it counterclockwise.

B. Purine Region

A specific interaction of the adenine base with a base region of the receptor contributes to the coronary vasoactivity of adenosine. The first step in obtaining support for this idea is to decide whether binding owes to the properties of one or more individual atoms or to a global property of the entire purine base. Analogs whose bases are purine isosteres, the aza and deaza adenosines, serve to test the hypothesis that the local interaction of a single atom accounts for binding. This hypothesis predicts that an isosteric C for N or N for C substitution at the key position will abolish activity, whereas such modifications at other positions will have little or no effect. Not all the purine isosteres of adenosine have been tested for coronary vasoactivity; except for 2-aza-adenosine, which has an MPR of 0.15, those which have been tested are essentially inactive. Such a result excludes the "single atom" hypothesis. While it is conceivable that binding of the purine base requires polar interactions of hydrogen bonding at every one of the purine nitrogens, such a possibility seems remote.

An alternative hypothesis, that a dipole–dipole interaction determines the binding of the purine to the base region, is more parsimonious and enjoys experimental support from both agonists and antagonists. The original test of this hypothesis (Olsson, 1983) included all the purine ribosides for which estimates of vasoactivity were available, because at that time we did not appreciate that factors such as tautomerism of the purinones and the interaction of large exocyclic substituents with contiguous receptor regions were overshadowing the dipole moment effects we wished to study. By restricting the analysis to adenosines with small C-2 and C-8 substituents and to certain 2,6-disubstituted purine ribosides, and specifically excluding analogs with sterically hindering C-6 and C-8 substituents such as −SH or Br, one finds that activity varies according to dipole moment about an optimum of ≅ 4 D, 70° (S. Kusachi, R. D. Thompson, and R. A. Olsson, unpublished).

The low activity of the purine isosteres of adenosine is probably the result of the profound change in dipole moment that accompanies an isosteric substitution. The effect on base dipole moment of an isosteric N for C substitution at position 2 will resemble that of a moderately strong electron-withdrawing purine C-2 substituent. Perhaps this is why "2-aza-adenosine" retains a modest degree of vasoactivity.

The dipole moment hypothesis draws important additional support from its ability to account for the antagonistic action of theophylline. This dialkylxanthine has little structural resemblance to adenosine and a dipole moment of μ 4.3 D, oriented at 102° (Bergmann and Weiler-Feilchenfeld, 1972), far outside the optimum range for binding. However, a 180° rotation of this molecule around its long axis such that N-1, N-3, N-7 and N-9 occupy, respectively, the same loci as C-2, C-6, N-9, and N-7 of adenosine, results in a dipole moment equivalent to 180° − 102° or 78°, much closer to the optimum angle identified by studies of agon-

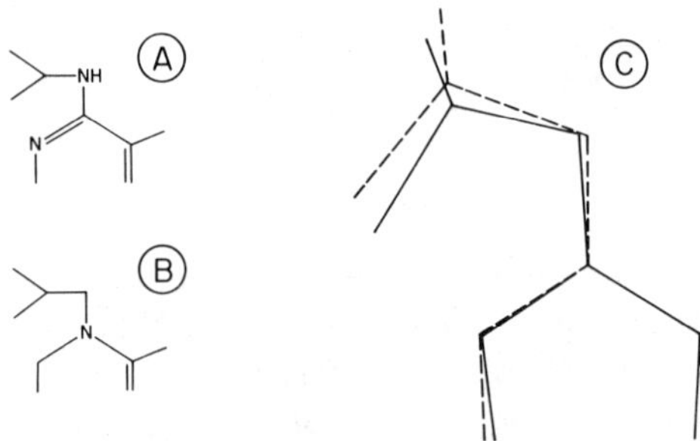

Figure 2. Structural similarity of the C-6 substituent of N^6-2-propylandenosine (A) to the N-3 substituent of 3-*iso*butyl-1-methylxanthine (IBMX) (B). In (C) two molecules are superimposed such that the C-4–C-5 bond of the adenosine (solid lines) lies over the N-3–C-4 bond of the xanthine (dashed lines). Bond lengths and angles are drawn to scale. Note how closely the two exocyclic substituents resemble each other with respect to shape and spatial orientation.

ists. An analysis of this sort would be mere prestidigitation if it did not yield predictions testable by experiment. One such prediction is that theophylline-7-riboside will be an antagonist, whereas theophylline-9-riboside will not. A second prediction derives from studies of the N-6 receptor region (see below), which show that certain N-6 substituents greatly enhance coronary vasoactivity, presumably through interaction with a specialized region distal to the N-6 site. Accordingly, we reasoned that theophylline analogs with sterically similar N-3 substituents might be stronger antagonists than theophylline itself. By way of illustration, the comparison made in Figure 2 shows how closely the shape of the N-3 substituent of 1-*iso*butyl-3-methylxanthine (IBMX) resembles that of the C-6 substituent of N^6-2-propyladenosine. Table I summarizes results from preliminary experiments that show that theophylline-7-riboside does indeed antagonize the coronary vasoactivity of adenosine and that the antagonist potency of N-3-substituted theophyoline analogs parallels the agonist potency of their N-6-substituted adenosine isosteres. We have not yet tested the antagonist potency of theophylline-9-riboside.

Although results such as those shown in Table I are encouraging, there are important obstacles to straightforward interpretation. Theophylline and its analogs

Table I. Dialkylxanthine Inhibition Of Adenosine Coronary Vasoactivity

N-3 substituent of 1-methylxanthine	K_i (μM)	N-3 substituent compared with C-6 substituent of	Adenosine MPR
Methyl (theophylline)	15	Adenosine	1.0
Theophylline-7-riboside	9	Adenosine	1.0
Cyclohexanemethyl	13	N^6-cyclohexyl adenosine	1.5
2-phenethyl	8	N^6-benzyl adenosine	0.5
3-phenylpropyl	3	N^6-2-phenethyl adenosine	2.0
*iso*butyl[a]		N^6-2-propyl adenosine	0.7
2-ethylbutyl		N^6-3-pentyl adenosine	4.0

[a] Vasodilator.

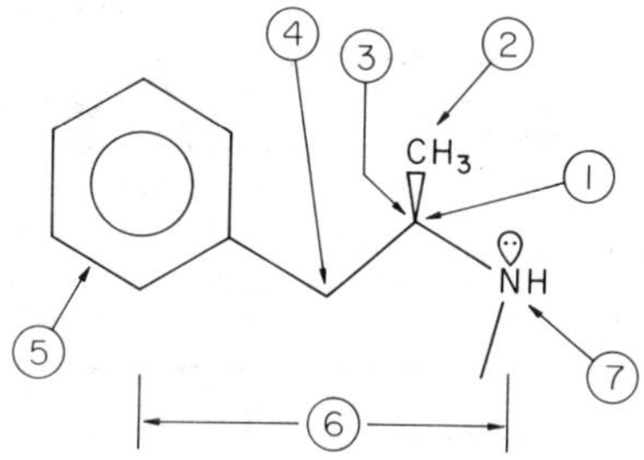

Figure 3. Chemical attributes of the C-6 substituent of *R*-PIA that could contribute to coronary vasoactivity: (1) absolute configuration at the propyl C-2 chiral center; (2) size and hydrophobicity of the propyl C-3; (3) contribution of propyl C-2; (4) chemistry of propyl C-1; (5) chemistry of the phenyl group, e.g., size, aromaticity, and planarity; (6), geometric relationship of phenyl group to the rest of the molecule; and (7) the chemistry of N6.

readily penetrate into cells and there can inhibit cyclic AMP phosphodiesterases and also release Ca^{2+} from intracellular stores. Thus, an effect on coronary vasoactivity is the sum of directionally dissimilar effects at the myocyte surface and in the cell interior. Coupling theophylline to oligosaccharides to prevent penetration into cells is one way to circumvent this problem. However, ligands for coupling to the oligosaccharides are not easy to prepare and batch-to-batch differences in the degree of substitution make between-ligand comparison of potency difficult. Analogs of 8-(*p*-sulfophenyl)theophylline are an attractive solution to these problems. The *p*-sulfophenyl group enhances antagonist activity (Bruns, 1981) and, because the sulfonic acid group is ionized at physiological pH, these purines cannot penetrate to the cell interior.

C. N-6 Region

R-PIA has proved to be a useful lead nucleoside for mapping the N-6 region. Three reasons underlie the choice of *R*-PIA as the lead compound for probing the structure of the N-6 region of the coronary receptor. *R*-PIA exhibits coronary vasoactivity that is both substantial and also rather stereoselective (Vapaatalo *et al.*, 1975; Kusachi *et al.*, 1983). Since activity is substantial, MPR $\cong$ 4, it is possible to use gradations in activity resulting from chemical modifications of the N-6 substituent to assess the relative importance of each attribute being modified. The C-6 substituent is quite complex; in general, a complex ligand will contain more information about a receptor than a simple one. Finally, the C-6 substituent of *R*-PIA is *R*-amphetamine. The extensive chemical literature on analogs of this well-known drug was a valuable guide to the synthesis of *R*-PIA analogs.

The first step in mapping the N-6 receptor region was the analysis of the structure of the C-6 substituent to identify attributes that might contribute to vasoactivity and the kinds of forces which might govern their interaction with the receptor (Figure 3). Next, we designed congeneric series of analogs to define the importance of each attribute. The choice of analogs reflected the complexity of the C-6 substituent and the desire for a certain amount of redundancy as a hedge against spurious correlations. Consonant with these aims, working out the structure of the N-6 region required nearly 100 analogs. However, a rather detailed picture rewarded this effort; the structure–activity correlations shows that: (1)

Table II. Coronary Vasoactivity of *R*-PIA Analogs

Analogs	MPR
N^6-(*R*-1-phenyl-2-butyl)adenosine	9.0
N^6-(*R*-1-phenyl-2-propyl)adenosine	3.7
N^6-(*S*-1-phenyl-3-hydroxyl-2-propyl)adenosine	1.6
N^6-(*S*-1-phenyl-2-butyl)adenosine	0.36

activity depends on the *R* configuration at the propyl C-2 chiral center; (2) propyl C-2 of itself negatively influences activity and can be replaced by a nitrogen atom, but (3) propyl C-1 and C-3 additively promote activity; (4) the propyl C-3 site is large enough to accommodate a two-carbon alkyl fragment; (5) the propyl C-1 site shows only a low degree of stereoselectivity; (6) hydrophobic forces govern binding of propyl C-1 and C-3 to the receptor; (7) the phenyl group promotes activity, but the covariance of attributes such as size, aromaticity, and planarity, precludes precise identification of the factors responsible for this positive effect; and (8) aromatic heterocyles such as pyridine and thiophene promote activity to a greater extent than benzene, an effect that seems related to a dipole moment oriented transversely with respect to the direction to propyl C-1. Although the experimental evidence shows that N-6 is not a hydrogen bond acceptor, it is ambiguous concerning a role for this atom as a hydrogen bond donor. Similarly, it has not been possible to describe the torsional angles around the propyl C-1–C-2 or the propyl C-1–benzene C1 bonds that define the geometric relationship of the phenyl subregion to the rest of the receptor.

Even though our structure–activity approach has not yet yielded a complete description of the N-6 region, the results to date furnish a model that seems to have good predictive power. For example, the deduction that the propyl C-3 site is large enough to hold an ethyl group implies that N^6-(*R*-1-phenyl-2-butyl) adenosine will be a stronger vasodilator than *R*-PIA. Additionally, the inference that hydrophobic forces effect binding to the propyl C-3 site implies that a polar-OH group on propyl C-3, as in N^6-(*S*-1-phenyl-3-hydroxyl-2-propyl)adenosine*, will reduce activity. Unpublished observations (Table II) bear out these predictions.

D. C-8 Region

Most C-8-substituted adenosines lack vasoactivity. The conventional explanation for this fact is that C-8 substituents impinge on ribose C-2′ and thereby hinder rotation around the glycosylic bond. This forces the nucleoside into a *syn* conformation unsuited for binding. Although this explanation is probably correct, steric hindrance may also obscure electronic effects. Comparing the vasoactivity of 8-aminoadenosine with that of 8-chloroadenosine discriminates between steric

* The absolute configuration at the propyl C-2 chiral center of this nucleoside is identical to that of *R*-PIA. However, according to the Cahn–Prelog-Ingold rules of nomenclature, this configuration is designated *S*.

and electronic effects. The two C-8 substituents are approximately the same size and thus exert the same degree of steric hindrance. The electron-donating 8-amino group tends to move the purine dipole moment toward the optimum range, μ = 4.1 D, Θ = 62°. By contrast, the electron-withdrawing 8-chloro group has the opposite effect on purine dipole moment; that of 8-chloroadenosine is μ = 2.3 D, Θ = 27°. The coronary vasoactivity of 8-aminoadenosine is about the same as that of adenosine, MPR = 1.15; 8-chloroadenosine has no coronary vasoactivity.

Intramolecular steric hindrance of this sort precludes using adenosines substituted at C-8 to establish the existence and probe the structure of a specialized C-8 receptor region. However, Bruns (1981) has circumvented this problem through studies of C-8 modifications that enhance the antagonist potency of theophylline. A phenyl group, particularly one having an electron-withdrawing *para* substituent, greatly enhances antagonism at R_a receptors. The best explanation for this observation seems to be that such substituents direct the phenyl dipole moment toward the *para* position. In support of this interpretation, the addition of an amino group *ortho* to a *para* chlorophenyl substituent further augments potency. The electron-donating amino group would be expected to strengthen and slightly rotate the dipole moment of the *para* chlorophenyl group, μ = 1.6 D, Θ = 180°, to a value of μ = 2.3 D, Θ = 157°. By combining this information with the results of other studies showing that 1,3-dipropylxanthine is a stronger antagonist than theophylline, Bruns and his colleagues (1983) have designed an antagonist, 8-(2-amino-4-chlorophenyl)-1,3-dipropylxanthine, which has a K_i of only 12 p*M* at an R_i receptor. The significance of this achievement becomes apparent when one considers that in the same system, the affinity of theophylline for the receptor is five orders of magnitude lower, its K_i being 1.5 μM.

Bruns's work has clearly established that adenosine receptors contain a specialized C-8 region and suggests that a dipole–dipole interaction may be one of the forces governing binding to this region. At this time, it is not known whether the C-8 regions of R_a and R_i receptors are identical. Searching for such structural differences between the two types of receptor is important. Theophylline is an extremely useful drug; modifications that enhance receptor selectivity could only increase its value.

E. C-2 Region

Purine is less tractable to modifications at C-2 than at C-6 or C-8. Probably for this reason, relatively less is known about the structure of the C-2 region of the adenosine receptor. Although the 2-haloadenosines are quite potent coronary vasodilators (Angus *et al.*, 1971; Cobbin *et al.*, 1974), we do not consider this as support for a C-2 receptor region. Rather, small exocyclic substituents such as halogen atoms probably promote activity through their electronic effects on the purine. More persuasive evidence for a specialized C-2 region comes from experiments that show that several adenosines whose C-2 substituents are an alkoxy, alkylamine, or an alkylthio group are more potent coronary vasodilators than adenosine (Cobbin *et al.*, 1974; Marumoto *et al.*, 1975). Our assay of the coronary vasoactivity of 2-phenylaminoadenosine (Kawazoe *et al.*, 1980) estimates an MPR versus adenosine of 90. It is thus one of the most potent adenosines we have ever tested, second only to NECA (MPR 136).

Available evidence does not permit the deduction of a very detailed model of the C-2 region, nor do we have a complex, information-laden ligand like *R*-PIA to guide the mapping of this region. Experience gained in the study of the N-6 region suggests that substituents containing combinations of branched alkyl chains and aromatic residues may be a useful approach to this goal.

ACKNOWLEDGMENTS

This work was supported by Grants-In-Aid from the Suncoast Chapter, Florida AHA Affiliate, by NIH HL 26611, and by a grant from Nelson Research and Development, Irvine, California.

REFERENCES

Afonso, S. 1970. Inhibition of coronary vasodilating action of dipyridamole and adenosine by aminophylline in the dog. *Circ. Res., 26:*743–752.

Angus, J. A., Cobbin, L. B., Einstein, R., and Maguire, M. H. 1971. Cardiovascular actions of substitutes adenosine analogues. *Br. J. Pharmacol., 41:*592–599.

Bergmann, E. D., and Weiler-Feilchenfeld, H. 1972. The dipole moments of purines. In: *The Purines: Theory and Experiment*, pp. 21–28. Ed. by Bergmann, E. D. and Pullman, B., Israel Acad. Sci. Human., Jerusalem.

Bruns, R. F. 1981. Adenosine antagonism by purines, pteridines and beanzopteridines in human fibroblasts. *Biochem. Pharmacol., 30:*325–333.

Bruns, R. F., Daly, J. W., and Snyder, S. H. 1980. Adenosine receptors in brain membranes: Binding of N^6-cyclohexyl [^{3}H]adenosine and 1,3-diethyl-8-[^{3}H]phenyl-xanthine. *Proc. Natl. Acad. Sci. U.S.A., 77:*5547–5551.

Bruns, R. F., Daly, J. W., and Snyder, S. H. 1983. Adenosine receptor binding: Structure-activity analysis generates extremely potent xanthine antagonists. *Proc. Natl. Acad. Sci. U.S.A., 80:* 2077–2080.

Bünger, R., Haddy, F. J., and Gerlach, E. 1975. Coronary responses to dilating substances and competitive inhibition by theophylline in the isolated perfused guinea pig heart. *Pflügers Arch., 358:*213–224.

Cobbin, L. B., Einstein, R., and Maguire, M. H., 1974. Studies on the coronary dilator actions of some adenosine analogues. *Br. J. Pharmacol. 50:*25–33.

Daly, J. W. 1982. Adenosine receptors: Targets for future drugs. *J. Med. Chem., 25:*197–207.

Dietmann, K., Birkenheier, H., and Schaumann, W. 1970. Hemmung der induzierten Thrombocyten-Aggregation durch Adenosin und Adenosine-Derivate. *Arzneim-Forsch., 20:*1749–1751.

Gough, G., and Maguire, M. H. 1965. 2-trifluoromethyladenosine. *J. Med. Chem., 8:*866–867.

Israelachvili, J. N. 1974. Van der Waals forces in biological systems. *Quart. Rev. Biophys., 6:*341–387.

Jahn, W. 1965. Kreislaufwirkungen 5′-substituierter Adensin Derivate. *Naunyn Schmiedebergs Arch. Pharmacol., 251:*95–104.

Jahn, W. 1969. N^6-[Naphthyl-(1)]-methyl-adenosin, ein Adenosin-Derivat mit langer anhaltender Coronarwirkung. *Arzneium-Forsch., 19:*701–704.

Jones, J. W., and Robins, R. K. 1963. Purine nucleosides: III. Methylation studies of certain naturally occurring purine nucleosides. *J. Am. Chem. Soc., 85:*193–201.

Kawazoe, K., Matsumoto, N., Tanabe, M., Fujiwara, S., Yanagimoto, M., Hirata, M., and Kikuchi, K. 1980. Coronary and cardiohemodynamic effects of 2-phenyl-aminoadenosine (CV-1808), *Arzneim-Forsch., 30:*1083–1087.

Kikugawa, K., Iizuka, K., Higuchi, Y., Hirayama, H., and Ichino, M. 1972. Platelet aggregation inhibitors. 2. Inhibition of platelet aggregation by 5′-, 2-, 6-, and 8-substituted adenosines. *J. Med. Chem., 15:*387–390.

Kikugawa, K., Iizuka, K., and Ichino, M. 1973. Platelet aggregation inhibitors. 4. N^6-substituted adenosines. *J. Med. Chem., 16:*358–364.

Kukovetz, W. R., Wurm, A., Holzmann, S., Pöch, G., and Rinner, I. 1979. Evidence for an adenylate cyclase-linked adenosine receptor mediating coronary relaxation. In: *Physiological and Regulatory Functions of Adenosine and Adenine Nucleotides,* pp. 205–213. Ed. by Baer, H. P., and Drummond, G. I., Raven Press, New York.

Kusachi, S., Thompson, R. D., and Olsson, R. A. 1983. Ligand selectivity of dog coronary adenosine receptor resembles that of adenylate cyclase stimulatory (R_a) receptors, *J. Pharmacol. Exp. Ther. 277:*316–321.

Londos, C., Cooper, D. M. F., and Wolff, J. 1980. Subclasses of external adenosine receptors. *Proc. Natl. Acad. Sci. U.S.A., 77:*2551–2554.

Marumoto, R., Yoshioka, Y., Miyashita, O., Shima, S., Imai, K.-I., Kawazoe, K., and Honjo, M. 1975. Synthesis and coronary vasoactivity of 2-substituted adenosines. *Chem. Pharm. Bull., 23:*759–774.

Mills, D. C. B., MacFarlane, D. E., Lemmex, B. W. G., and Haslam, R. J., 1983. In: *Regulatory Functions of Adenosine*, pp. 277–289. Ed. by Berne, R. M., Rall, T. W., and Rubio, R. Martinus Nijhoff, Boston.

Mistry, G., and Drummond, G. I. 1983. Effects of adenosine, its analogs, adrenergic agents and prostaglandins on adenylate cyclase of heart microvessels. In: *Regulatory Function of Adenosine*, pp. 529–530. Ed. by Berne, R. M., Rall, T. W., and Rubio, R. Martinus Nijhoff, Boston.

Nair, V., and Richardson, S. G. 1982. Modification of nucleic acid bases via radical intermediates: Synthesis of dihalogenated purine nucleosides. *Synthesis*, 670–672.

Olsson, R. A. 1983. Adenosine receptors on vascular smooth muscle. In: *Regulatory Function of Adenosine*, pp. 33–47. Ed. by Berne, R. M., Rall, T. W., and Rubio, R. Martinus Nijhoff, Boston.

Olsson, R. A., Khouri, E. M., Bedynek, J. L., Jr., and McLean, J. 1979. Coronary vasoactivity of adenosine in the conscious dog. *Circ. Res., 45:*468–478.

Osman, R., Weinstein, H., and Green, J. P. 1979. Parameters and methods in quantitative structure–activity relationships. In: *ACS Symposium 112, Computer-Assisted Drug Design*, pp. 21–77. Ed. by Olson, E. C., and Christoffersen, R. E. American Chemical Society, Washington, D. C.

Prasad, R. N., Fung, A., Tietje, K., Stein, H. H., and Brondyk, H. D. 1976. Modification of the 5′ position of purine nucleosides. 1. Synthesis and biological properties of alkyl adenosine-5′-carboxylates. *J. Med. Chem., 19:*1180–1186.

Prasad, R. N., Bariana, D. S., Fung, A., Savic, M., Tietje, K., Stein, H. H., Brondyk, H., and Egan, R. 1980. Modification of the 5′ position of purine nucleosides. 2. Synthesis and some cardiovascular properties of adenosine-5′-(*N*-substituted) carboxamides. *J. Med. Chem., 23:*313–319.

Pullman, A. 1969. The electronic structure of purines and pyrimidines. *Ann. N.Y. Acad. Sci., 158:*65–85.

Raberger, G., Schütz, W., and Kraup, O. 1977. Coronary dilatory action of adenosine analogs: A comparative study. *Arch. Int. Pharmacodyn. Ther., 230:*140–149.

Robins, M. J. and Uznański, B. 1981. Nucleic acid related compounds. 34. Nonaqueous diazotization with *tert*-butyl nitrite. Introduction of fluorine, chlorine and bromine at C-2 of purine nucleosides. *Can. J. Chem., 59:*2608–2611.

Sattin, A., and Rall, T. W. 1970. The effects of adenosine and adenine nucleotides on the cyclic 3′,5′-monophosphate content of guinea pig cerebral cortical slices. *Mol. Pharmacol., 6:*13–23.

Scholtholt, J., Nitze, R. E., and Schraven, E. 1972. On the mechanism of the antagonistic action of xanthine derivatives against adenosine and coronary vasodilators. *Arzneim-Forsch., 22:*1255–1259.

Shimizu, G., Kaneko, M., Saito, A., Nishino, H., Mizuno, H., Oshima, I., Nakayama, K., and Koike, H. 1971. An alternate synthesis of N^6 substituted adenosines and their coronary dilator activities. *Ann. Sankyo Res. Lab., 23:*117–123.

Van Calker, D., Müller, M., and Hamprecht, B. 1979. Adenosine regulates via two different types of receptors: The accumulation of cyclic AMP in cultured brain cells. *J. Neurochem., 33*:999–1005.
Vapaatalo, H., Onken, D., Neuvonen, P. J., and Westermann, E. 1975. Stereospecificity of some central and circulatory effects of phenylisopropyl-adenosine (PIA), *Arzneim-Forsch., 25*:407–410.
Weinstein, H., Osman, R., and Green, J. P. 1979. The molecular basis of structure-activity relationships: Quantum chemical recognition mechanisms in drug–receptor interactions. In: *ACS Symposium 112, Computer-Assisted Drug Design*, pp. 161–187. Ed. by Olson, E. C., and Christoffersen, R. E. American Chemical Society, Washington, D.C.
Wolff, J., Londos, C., and Cooper, D. M. F. 1981. Adenosine receptors and the regulation of adenylate cyclase. *Adv. Cyclic Nucleotide Res. 14*:199–214.

Chapter **16**

Classification of Adenosine Receptors in the Central Nervous System

T. W. Stone

Department of Physiology
St. George's Hospital Medical School
University of London
London, United Kingdom

I. INTRODUCTION

It is important to realize that the classifications of adenosine receptors currently in vogue were devised as the result of work on the activity of adenylate cyclase (see Stone, 1981, 1982a). The independent reports from Londos and Wolff (1977), Van Calker *et al.*, (1979), and later Londos *et al.* (1980) established the existence of a receptor accessible from the inside of intact cells, the P site, requiring an intact purine component of the agonist molecule and externally accessible A_1 (or R_i) and A_2 (or R_a) sites with strict structural requirements of the ribose portion of agonists. The P and A_1 sites induce an inhibition of cyclase activity and the A_2 site causes an increase.

The present chapter concentrates on methods to relate these receptor types to functional activity of the central nervous system (CNS), namely, changes of neuronal firing and the modulation of neurotransmitter release.

II. ELECTROPHYSIOLOGICAL STUDIES OF NEURONAL FIRING

In vitro slice preparations can be used for studying the pharmacology of spontaneously active neurons and have many clear advantages, such as the absence of anesthetic, the controllability of ambient conditions, and for receptor classification studies in particular, the fact that drugs can be applied in the bathing medium at known concentrations. However, the differences that exist between *in vitro* slices and *in vivo* systems are still largely unknown and unexplored, and it is still a wise man who confirms his *in vitro* results on an *in vivo* system. The following methodology therefore begins by considering *in vivo* preparations, though the methodology of slices is discussed in the following section and could be easily adapted for the study of single cell activity.

A. Animal Preparation

The animal will be anesthetised and the head secured in a head holder. As long as superficial neurons are to be studied, in the cerebral or cerebellar cortex, for example, no special apparatus other than a means of preventing head movement will be required. If it is intended to examine neurons in subcortical structures, then a precision built unit suitable for use with one of the stereotaxic atlases (for rats: König and Klippel, 1963; De Groot, 1959; Pellegrino *et al.*, 1979) would be needed. Suitable apparatus is available from Kopf, Trent-Wells, Bioscience, and Narashige. Body temperature (usually rectal) must be maintained by a heating blanket or suitable lamp.

After the skull and dura mater have been removed, the exposed brain should be covered with physiological saline solution, warmed liquid paraffin, or agar in order to prevent drying.

B. Electrodes

In order to study single neurons, it is necessary to apply compounds by microiontophoresis or by pressure. Electrode preparation is essentially the same for both methods. "Blanks" are available from Clark Electromedical, Haer, Medical Systems (USA), Wesley Coe (Cambridge, UK), or WP Instruments; they consist of from three to seven glass capillaries fused along their length. These can be pulled into multibarrelled micropipettes using pullers available from Kopf, Bioscience, Narashige, Clark Electromedical, Campden Instruments, and other suppliers. The length of tip and the size of the pipette tip can be modified by adjusting the size of the current supplied to the heating coil and the timing and magnitude of any active pull. It is usual for extracellular work, however, to break the multibarrel tip by bringing it into contact with a smooth surface under microscopic control, such that each barrel has an opening of 1–2 μm. Those multibarrels made using "omega-dot" capillaries, in which a glass fiber is fused along the inside can be filled with the drug solutions of interest immediately before use, as the glass fiber conducts the solution into the electrode tip. Other multibarrels may require centrifugation after solution is placed into the stem of the barrels.

Most workers fill one barrel of the multibarrel assembly with an electrolyte solution for recording neuronal activity, although the signal-to-noise ratio can be greatly increased by fixing a separate single barrel microelectrode alongside the multibarrel (Stone, 1973).

It is also advisable to fill a second barrel with a solution of sodium chloride (165 m*M*) so that the effect of current itself on neuronal firing can be tested (Stone, 1985). The same barrel can be used for "current balancing," in which a current equal in magnitude to the sum of the currents applied to the other barrels, but opposite in sign, is passed continuously through the balance barrel. This is particularly important when ions of different sign are being used (such as adenosine (hemisulphate) and adenosine monophosphate (sodium salt) and when retaining currents are being used. The latter, usually 5 to 15 nA in size, are applied between ejection pulses in order to reduce the diffusional leak of an ion through the barrel tip. Clearly, retaining currents are of little value with compounds existing as zwitterions, though the pH of solutions may be modified to assure the negligible contribution of one or other ionic form.

C. Equipment

Although it is relatively simple to construct current pumps for the application of compounds by microiontophoresis, several manufacturers now market equipment commercially (Medical Systems [USA], Wp Instruments, Dagan) (see Stone, 1985 for details). The first of these has the advantages that ionophoretic and pressure ejection modules can be combined in the same main frame, a continuous check of barrel resistance is available, and the system is compatible with (though not exclusive for) the company's own multibarrels, which can be supplied already pulled if desired.

D. Recording

Standard extracellular unit recording involves connecting the recording barrel to a high-impedance amplifier capable of at least 100-fold amplification and having low noise level. The raw signals may be displayed on oscilloscopes and recorded photographically or stored on magnetic tape. It is usual, however, to process the signals on line in some way, the most common being to pass the action potentials through a window discriminator unit that generates a constant-sized pulse for each action potential over a certain (adjustable) height. The output pulses may then be used to obtain a record of firing rate using a suitable ratemeter, and the ratemeter output may be recorded on a chart recorder.

E. Solutions

Clearly, the solutions used in the multibarrel pipettes will depend on the experiment being undertaken, but a few general points may be useful. For example, many nucleotides are available as sodium salts and should therefore be ejected as anions. It may be advisable in some instances to raise the pH of the solution in order to ensure maximum dissociation, but this is not necessary for most common nucleotides, such as ATP. In general, it is always preferable to use ionized forms of a compound and hence adenosine hemisulphate (which is a sulphate salt, not to be confused with adenosine 5′-monosulphate) is used in preference to the poorly soluble adenosine base. In fact, we have experienced far more difficulties ejecting adenosine as a cation (from its sulphate salt) than occurs when ejecting anionic nucleotides, and, in view of the almost universal similarity of action, the iontophoresis of AMP may be preferred to adenosine, at least in preliminary experiments. S. Grant (personal communication) has noted the formation of a gel by adenosine in aqueous solution, which may explain some of these difficulties.

F. Controls and Precautions

It is essential to perform control experiments for the effects of current and the ejection of ions not of primary interest. As hinted earlier, the effect of current on cell excitability can in theory be minimized by employing "current balancing," the balance current being passed through a NaCl-containing barrel. However, this method is not foolproof (see Stone, 1985), and it is always advisable to pass the same current used for the ejection of a test compound through an unbalanced NaCl barrel. It should always be born in mind that depending on the proximity of electrode and neuron, current of either polarity may cause excitation or inhibition of the cell.

The most important ion controls are for the unwanted ion of a salt pair, as this will be ejected by the current used to retain the active ion, and H^+ or OH^- ions. Most inorganic ions, such as chloride, bicarbonate, sulphate, and so on, have been shown many times not to have significant effects on cell excitability at normal retaining currents. Equally sodium and potassium ions, even at several tens of nanoamperes current ejection have little observable effect. On the other hand, the importance of checking unusual counter-ion effects may be illustrated by aminophylline, a soluble complex of theophylline and ethylenediamine popular in microiontophoresis some years ago as a convenient source of theophylline. The potent inhibitory effects of aminophylline have now been shown to be attributable to ethylenediamine acting on GABA receptors (Perkins *et al.*, 1981).

If a solution is used at a pH below 3, excitation may occur due to the ejection of H^+ (Frederickson *et al.*, 1971; Stone, 1972). Clearly, this becomes more important if the compound of interest is of high molecular weight or present in low concentration, so that a greater proportion of the current will be carried by H^+. The ejection of OH^- from solutions of pH 10 or more can also cause cell activation, and solutions of NaCl adjusted to these pH levels should always be used as controls.

Two other precautions are commonly overlooked by newcomers to microiontophoresis. The first is the need to maintain a constant time cycle of ejection and retention, particularly when testing for potential antagonism of the responses. This is because the retaining current tends to withdraw ions away from the barrel tips, thus making less available for the next ejection pulse (Bradshaw *et al.*, 1973). Ejection pulses separated by variable retention intervals will therefore vary in size, so that control responses 1 min apart followed by a gap of 3 min during which an antagonist is applied may subsequently appear to have been antagonized.

With potent compounds such as some purines, a cycle variation of a few seconds can lead to major changes in response size.

A final neglected precaution is to use a large number of electrodes. Pipette characteristics vary so much that results cannot be trusted from a small selection. Our guiding principle is to use a minimum of five different electrodes yielding the same results. If results are variable, then many more than five may be needed. We tend to use at least three or four electrodes in each animal. The use of several electrodes becomes especially important if the potency of compounds is being studied, since the amount of current being passed does not necessarily reflect the amount of ion ejected (Stone, 1985).

G. Results

A number of studies have reported the effects of purines on neuronal firing, but only two, published almost simultaneously (Stone, 1982b; Phillis, 1982) have specifically addressed the question of which purine receptor might be involved. Stone (1982b) showed that L-N^6-phenylisopropyl-adenosine (L-PIA) and 5′*N*-ethylcarboxamide adenosine (NECA) were both able to mimic adenosine or AMP in causing a depression of spontaneous neuronal firing in the cerebral cortex. The responses to L-PIA tended to outlast by many minutes the ejecting pulse, and this was interpreted to imply the slow metabolism or removal of L-PIA, perhaps giving an exaggerated impression of its potency. As this kind of slow, prolonged action can also be seen on isolated perfused tissues (Stone, 1983), this interpretation may not be correct. However, coupled with the observation that fewer cells responded to L-PIA than to NECA, whether applied by iontophoresis or pressure ejection, Stone (1982b) concluded that the depression of most cells involved an Ra/A_2 receptor (Van Calker *et al.*, 1979; Londos *et al.*, 1980). The blockade of purine responses by methylxanthines (Perkins and Stone, 1980; Stone and Perkins, 1981) is consistent with this conclusion. It is also interesting to note that adenine nucleotides also depress neuronal firing, and these effects can be blocked by methylxanthines (Stone and Perkins, 1981), implying that a P_2 receptor, as proposed by Burnstock (1978), does not contribute greatly to neuronal inhibition by nucleotides.

In the study by Phillis (1982), NECA was shown to be a better depressant of cell firing than PIA and the prolonged time course of the PIA effects was also confirmed. This author thus came to the same conclusion that an A_2 receptor was involved in the neuronal inhibition.

Stone (1982b) made the additional observation that 2′5′-dideoxyadenosine (DDA) applied for several minutes caused a small reduction of firing rate and, in some cases, a reduction of responses to AMP that was not accompanied by any changes of responses to GABA. As DDA is thought to activate an intracellular receptor causing the inhibition of adenylate cyclase, this would be consistent with the activation of an Ra/A_2 receptor by AMP and the involvement of adenylate cyclase in the regulation of cell firing (Bloom, 1975; Stone and Taylor, 1977; Stone *et al.*, 1975).

III. ELECTROPHYSIOLOGICAL STUDIES OF TRANSMITTER RELEASE IN CNS: *IN VITRO* METHODOLOGY

Much of the preceding discussion regarding electrodes, recording, and so on apply also to the use of *in vitro* methods in which microiontophoresis is used to apply compounds to localized parts of neurons in, for example, brain slices. Slice methods have the advantages that drugs can also be applied in the perfusing medium at precisely known concentrations, the ionic environment, as well as other parameters, can be varied and controlled at will, and there is no anxiety about possible influences of anesthetic. A number of different brain areas can be used for the preparation of slices, and the recent volume by Kerkut and Wheal (1981) should be consulted for details. For the present discussion, however, the hippocampal slice is the only preparation that has been used in relevant studies.

The usual procedure is to remove the hippocampus as rapidly as possible after death and transfer it into an artificial physiological medium. Some groups transfer into medium at 0°C in order to reduce cell metabolism (and thus diminish the likelihood of hypoxic damage) and to make the tissue slightly firmer for cutting. Other groups use medium at room temperature. The tissue is now sliced either using a simple chopping action as on the McIlwain apparatus (Mickle, UK) or using a vibratome. The latter method is reputed to produce superior slices for electrophysiology. A third popular alternative is to slice manually using plastic guides. Slices are usually cut between 200 and 400 μm thick in order to permit adequate oxygenation of cells in the center of the slice (McIlwain, 1975).

After transferring a slice to the recording chamber and bathing in solution at 37°C, some time must be allowed for ionic equilibrium to be restored within the tissue. It is generally accepted that no meaningful recordings can be obtained from a slice for at least 1, and probably 2, hr after slicing.

A. Recording Chambers

A variety of more or less complicated baths has been advocated (see Kerkut and Wheal, 1981), but in conversation most workers will recommend that the most simple chambers should be used. Thus simple perspex blocks containing a well for the slice (usually supported on a piece of nylon stocking in order to permit adequate access of solution to both surfaces of the slice), channels for inflow and outflow of medium, and adequate arrangements for oxygenation seem to be widely used.

B. Stimulation and Recording

While the recording of electrical activity and, if desired, the application of compounds by microiontophoresis or pressure ejection involve essentially the same methodology, described above, the hippocampal slice possesses an outstanding advantage over *in vivo* methods with respect to the stimulation of specific pathways. The layers of pyramidal cell bodies and the sites of entry and egress of neuronal pathways are easily identified and can be accessed by stimulating or recording electrodes under direct visual control.

C. Results

In the study by Reddington *et al.* (1982), the effects of several purines were tested on the population postsynaptic potential evoked by stimulation of the fibers traveling in the stratum radiatum and recorded at the CA_1 pyramidal cells. The order of potency cyclohexyladenosine > L-PIA > 2-chloroadenosine>D-PIA suggests a receptor belonging to the A_1 classification of Van Calker *et al.* (1979) and correlated exactly with the order of potency in displacing cyclohexyladenosine binding in the hippocampus. The greater potency of these compounds in reducing the postsynaptic potential rather than the afferent fiber volley or the antidromic CA_1 spike indicated a selective suppression of transmitter release. This action is entirely consistent with the evidence from studies of peripheral neurons in which depression of transmitter has been attributed to activation of an A_1 receptor (Paton, 1981). In a similar study by Smellie *et al.* (1979), L-PIA was shown to be about 100-fold more potent than the D isomer in depressing the CA_1 postsynaptic potential evoked by stimulation of afferent axons in the stratum radiatum of rat hippocampal slices. This is entirely consistent with the mediation of this effect by an A_1 receptor as reported by Reddington *et al.* (1982).

In producing stimulation of adenylate cyclase in guinea pig cerebral cortex, however, L-PIA was only 4 to 5 times more effective than D-PIA, a difference that implied the involvement of an A_2 site. As subsequently pointed out by Fredholm *et al.* (1982), it is not always wise to draw conclusions from a comparison of potencies in different species. In their experiments on the rat hippocampus, it was found that L-PIA was 60 times more potent than D-PIA at elevating cyclic AMP levels. Nevertheless, since NECA was more potent than L-PIA and since these various analogs activated rather than inhibited adenylate cyclase, the authors proposed that an A_2 receptor was involved in the response.

IV. NEUROCHEMICAL STUDIES OF TRANSMITTER RELEASE

Ideally, studies of transmitter release would involve the measurement of endogenous compounds released into a perfusing medium, using a suitable sensitive method of resolving and quantifying the compounds of interest (for example, HPLC). It is usually more convenient, however, to load tissues with the radioactively labeled transmitter or a precursor and then to measure the efflux of label by scintillation spectrometry.

Brain slices are popular for such studies because of the ease of preparation, as described above, although synaptosomes, which require much more time and equipment, have the advantage that release can be studied specifically from the presynaptic terminal. Various methods for preparing synaptosomes are available (Bradford, 1975; Morgan *et al.*, 1983; Dodd *et al.*, 1981).

Whether slices or synaptosomes are being used it is advisable, as for electrophysiological studies, to allow a period of at least 30 min for the tissue to recover from the trauma of execution. The radiolabel can then be added. Tritiated adenine or adenosine are popular in studies of purine release. The label used should be present at a concentration of about 0.1–1 μ*M*, sufficient to permit its selective uptake by any high-affinity processes, without causing saturation of those processes and consequently spilling over into low-affinity or nonspecific uptake areas that may cause difficulties of interpretation. Incubation with the radiolabel should for the same reasons be restricted to the shortest time consistent with the production of reasonable tissue levels and the subsequent release of measurable quantities of label. Although times of 1 min to 1 hr are used by different groups, a period of 10–20 min is widely employed.

After labeling, tissue may be transferred to a suitable superfusion chamber. For our own studies with brain slices, a continuous superfusion at 0.5 ml/min is used. As judged by the failure of uptake inhibitors to increase the resting efflux of label, this perfusion rate seems sufficient to wash out released material from the slices before it can be taken up again by the tissue. It is usual to subject the tissue to several complete changes of bathing fluid or to a period of 15–30 min of "washout" in order to remove nonspecifically bound or sequestered label.

Release of transmitter may be induced by electrical stimulation, high potassium solutions (10 to 60 m*M*), or veratridine (1–20 μ*M*). For electrical stimulation, it is usually necessary to employ a frequency of 5–20 Hz, using a current of about 10 mA, for several tens of seconds or even minutes in order to release sufficient material. It is therefore essential that nonpolarizable electrodes (platinum or chlorided silver) are used or that alternate stimulating pulses are reversed in polarity. This may involve a very expensive stimulator or the use of a very cheap inverting relay such as Type 349-434 produced by RS components (UK).

Whatever stimulus is chosen, it is essential to assess the validity of a system by confirming the calcium-dependence of release. This is most clearly achieved by perfusing with calcium-free solutions containing a depolarizing concentration of potassium ions and then providing a "calcium pulse" (2 m*M*) to evoke release (Haycock *et al.*, 1978).

Results from release studies can be highly variable, and a simple analysis of peak released radioactivity may yield an impossibly large variance. It is therefore customary to express release as a "fractional rate constant", i.e., as a fraction of the total tissue content at the start of perfusion. This is calculated by summing the release in all fractions over the course of the experiment with the counts present in the tissue at the end of the experiment. It may be considered wasteful and uneconomical, however, to collect and count *all* fractions (including washout), and, since the total efflux of label during perfusion is often only a few percent of the final tissue content, the latter is often used as the denominator for calculating the fractional release constant.

This may still leave much variability between experiments, and it is therefore becoming increasingly accepted practice to induce two peaks of release and to take the ratio of peak heights as the experimental result. This tends to be remarkably constant. The effects of release-modifying agents may then be tested on one (but only one) peak, as this should change the peak height ratio.

A. Results

Harms *et al.* (1978) were among the first to report an inhibitory action of adenosine on potassium-evoked release of labeled noradrenaline from rat cortex slices. In attempting to define the type of purine receptor involved in this action, we have tried various manipulations of experimental conditions including stimuli, calcium concentrations, and brain areas without succeeding in repeating the original observations of Harms *et al.* (1978).

In a study of tritiated D-aspartate release, however, we have found that adenosine at high concentrations (1 m*M*) does significantly inhibit evoked release. The use of analogs reveals that L-PIA causes inhibition at 10 μ*M*, but NECA does not, even at 100 μ*M*. While this potency series might suggest the involvement of an A_1 receptor, it should be emphasized that the effective concentrations of the compounds are several orders of magnitude greater than are effective in peripheral systems. It is interesting to note that Ebstein and Daly (1982), using a crude brain homogenate preparation, have also found that amine release can only be inhibited by high concentrations of purines and that D-PIA, which was not tested in our experiments, was equipotent with L-PIA. This similarity of potency is incompatible with an A_1 receptor.

Even when calcium uptake into synaptosomes is examined directly, the assignation of receptor type is made no easier. Thus, since L-PIA was only five times more active than D-PIA and 2-chloroadenosine was more potent than cyclohexyladenosine and L-PIA, properties consistent with a stimulation of adenylate cyclase (Bruns, 1980), the authors concluded that an A_2 receptor was involved in the inhibition of calcium uptake (Wu *et al.*, 1982). However, L-PIA was almost eight times more potent than NECA.

V. FUTURE PROBLEMS

In order to clarify the role of purines in the central nervous system, it will be necessary to examine their actions in systems other than the hippocampus, and there is, therefore, much scope for studying different areas of CNS both *in vivo* and *in vitro*.

There is in addition the extremely vexed question of the relationship between functional effects of purines (Stone, 1981, 1982a) and their modulation of the adenylate cyclase system. Thus, while the inhibitory effects of purines on spontaneous neuronal activity have been attributed to a presynaptic inhibitory action on the release of excitatory transmitters (Phillis *et al.*, 1979) it has become clear that there may be little relationship between inhibition of transmitter release and adenylate cyclase (Kuroda, 1978; Reddington and Schubert, 1979; Stone, 1981). Since the classifications of purine receptors by Van Calker *et al.* (1979) and Londos *et al.* (1980) were based on the modulation of cyclase, it is clearly an important point to establish whether these classifications are indeed applicable to studies of neuronal excitability. A similar problem has been raised in studies of purine receptors in peripheral tissues (Stone, 1983; Hughes and Stone, 1983; Baer *et al.*, 1983).

As presynaptic purine receptors appear to be classifiable as A_1 (Reddington *et al.*, 1982), whereas the receptors mediating neuronal depression and cyclase activation appear to be A_2 (Stone, 1982b; Phillis, 1982; Smellie *et al.*, 1979; Fredholm et al., 1982), one approach to this problem might be to examine the effects of purine analogs on postsynaptic neuronal excitability using intracellular methods (Segal, 1982; Siggins and Schubert, 1981).

It will be a special challenge to future investigators to correlate presynaptic and postsynaptic electrophysiological effects with the modulation of adenylate cyclase and with studies of receptor binding in the CNS, if such an ideal is attainable. It should be clear from much of the discussion in this chapter that many authors constrain their discussion to those aspects of their results that fit in with the concept of A_1 and A_2 purine receptors, though not many authors come to terms with the need to justify adequately the nonconsideration of their other results. The single most important question in purine research today, in my opinion, is whether the receptor classifications that have proved so popular in studies of cyclase activity are applicable to non-cyclase-modulated functional responses. I believe the evidence discussed above, and elsewhere, indicates that they are not.

REFERENCES

Baer, H. P., Muller, M. J., and Vriend, R. 1983. Adenosine receptors in smooth muscle. In: *Physiology and Pharmacology of Adenosine Derivatives*, pp. 77–84. Ed. by Daly, J. W., Kuroda, Y., Phillis, J. W., Shimizu, H., and Ui, M. Raven Press, New York.

Bloom, F. E. 1975. The role of cyclic nucleotides in central synaptic function. *Rev. Physiol. Biochem. Pharmacol., 74:*1–104.

Bradford, H. F. 1975. Isolated nerve terminals as an in vitro preparation for the study of dynamic aspects of transmitter metabolism and release. In: *Handbook of Psychopharmacology, Vol. 1*, pp. 191–252. Ed. by Iverson, L. L., Iversen, S. D., and Snyder, S. H. Plenum Press, New York.

Bradshaw, C. M., Szabadi, E., and Roberts, M. H. T. 1973. The reflection of ejecting and retaining currents in the time course of neuronal responses to microelectrophoretically applied drugs. *J. Pharm. Pharmac., 25:*513–520.

Bruns, R. F. 1980. Adenosine receptor activation in human fibroblasts: Nucleoside agonists and antagonists. *Can. J. Physiol. Pharmacol., 58:*673–691.

Burnstock, G. 1978. A basis for distinguishing two types of purinergic receptor. In: *Cell Membrane Receptors for Drugs and Hormones*, pp. 107–118. Ed. by Bolis, L., and Straub, R. W. Raven Press, New York.

De Groot, T. 1959. The rat forebrain in stereotaxic coordinates. *Trans. R. Neth. Acad. Sci., 52:*1–40.

Dodd, P. R., Hardy, J. A., Oakley, A. F., Edwardson, J. A., Perry, E. K., and Delannoy, J. P. 1981. A rapid method for preparing synaptosomes: Comparison with alternative procedures. *Brain Res., 226:*107–110.

Ebstein, R. P., and Daly, J. W. 1982. Release of norepinephrine and dopamine from brain vesicular preparations: Effects of adenosine analogues. *Cell. Mol. Neurobiol., 2:*193–204.

Frederickson, R. C., Jordan, L. M., and Phillis, J. W. 1971. The action of noradrenaline on central neurones: effect of pH. *Brain Res. 35:*556–560.

Fredholm, B. B., Jonson, B., Lindgren, E., and Lindström, K. 1982. Adenosine receptors mediating cyclic AMP production in the rat hippocampus. *J. Neurochem., 39:*165–175.

Harms, H. H., Wardeh, G., and Mulder, A. H. 1978. Adenosine modulates depolarisation induced release of (^{3}H)-noradrenaline from slices of rat brain neocortex. *Eur. J. Pharmacol., 49:*305–308.

Haycock, J. W., Levy, W. B., Denner, L. A., and Cotman, C. W., 1978. Effects of elevated (K^+)O on the release of neurotransmitters from cortical synaptosomes: efflux or secretion? *J. Neurochem., 30:*1113–1125.

Hughes, P. R., and Stone, T. W. 1983. Inhibition by purines of the ionotropic action of isoprenaline in rat atria. *Br. J. Pharmacol., 80:*149–153.

Kerkut, G. A., and Wheal, H. V. (eds.) 1981. *Electrophysiology of Isolated Mammalian CNS Preparations.* Academic Press, London.

König, J. F. R., and Klippel, R. A. 1963. *A Stereotaxic Atlas of the Rat Brain.* Williams and Wilkins, Baltimore.

Kuroda, Y. 1978. Physiological roles of adenosine derivatives which are released during neurotransmission in mammalian brain. *J. Physiol.* (*Paris*), *74:*463–470.

Londos, C., and Wolff, J. 1977. Two distinct adenosine sensitive sites on adenylate cyclase. *Proc. Natl. Acad. Sci. USA, 74:*5482–5486.

Londos, C., Cooper, D. M. F., and Wolff, J. 1980. Subclasses of external adenosine receptors. *Proc. Natl. Acad. Sci. USA, 77:*2551–2554.

McIlwain, H. 1975. *Practical Neurochemistry.* Churchill-Livingston, London.

Morgan, P. F., Lloyd, H. G. E., and Stone, T. W. 1983. Benzodiazepine inhibition of adenosine uptake is not prevented by benzodiazepine antagonists. *Eur. J. Pharmacol., 87:*121–126.

Paton, D. M. 1981. Structure activity relations for presynaptic inhibition of noradrenergic and cholinergic transmission by adenosine: evidence for action on A_1 receptors. *J. Autonom. Pharmacol., 1:*287–290.

Pellegrino, L. J., Pellegrino, A. S., and Cushman, A. J. 1979. *A Stereotaxic Atlas of the Rat Brain.* Plenum Press, New York.

Perkins, M. N., and Stone, T. W. 1980. Aminophylline and theophylline derivatives as antagonists of neuronal depression by adenosine: A microiontophoretic study. *Arch. Int. Pharmacodyn., 246:*205–214.

Perkins, M. N., Bowery, N. G., Hill, D. R., and Stone, T. W. 1981. Neuronal responses to ethylenediamine: preferential blockade by bicuculline. *Neurosci. Lett., 23:*325–328.

Phillis, J. W. 1982. Evidence for an A_2-like adenosine receptor on cerebral cortical neurones. *J. Pharm. Pharmacol., 34:*453–454.

Phillis, J. W., Edstrom, J. P., Kostopoulos, G. K., and Kirkpatrick, J. R. 1979. Effects of adenosine and adenine nucleotides on synaptic transmission in the cerebral cortex. *Can. J. Physiol. Pharmacol., 57:*1289–1312.

Reddington, M., and Schubert, P. 1979. Parallel investigations of the effects of adenosine on evoked potentials and cyclic AMP accumulation in hippocampus slices of the rat. *Neurosci. Lett., 14:*37–42.

Reddington, M., Lee, K. S., and Schubert, P. 1982. An A_1 adenosine receptor, characterised by (^{3}H)-cyclohexyladenosine binding, mediates the depression on evoked potentials in a rat hippocampal slice preparation. *Neurosci. Lett., 28:*275–280.

Segal, M. 1982. Intracellular analysis of a postsynaptic action of adenosine in the rat hippocampus. *Eur. J. Pharmacol., 79:*193–200.

Siggins, G. R., and Schubert, P. 1981. Adenosine depression of hippocampal neurons in vitro: An intracellular study of dose-dependent actions on synaptic and membrane potentials. *Neurosci. Lett., 23:*55–60.

Smellie, F. W., Daly, J. W., Dunwiddie, T. V., and Hoffer, B. J. 1979. The dextro and levorotatory isomers of N-phenylisopropyladenosine: Stereospecific effects on cyclic AMP formation and evoked synaptic responses in brain slices. *Life Sci., 25:*1739–1748.

Stone, T. W., 1972. Noradrenaline effects and pH. *J. Pharm. Pharmacol. 24:*422–423.

Stone, T. W. 1973. Cortical pyramidal tract interneurones and their sensitivity to L-glutamic acid. *J. Physiol., 233:*211–225.
Stone, T. W. 1981. Physiological roles for adenosine and ATP in the nervous system. *Neurosci., 6:*523–555.
Stone, T. W. 1982a. Purine receptors involved in the depression of neuronal firing in cerebral cortex. *Brain Res., 248:*367–370.
Stone, T. W. 1982b. Cell membrane receptors for purines. *Biosci. Rep., 2:*77–90.
Stone, T. W. 1983. Purine receptors in the rat anococcygeus muscle. *J. Physiol., 335:*591–608.
Stone, T. W. 1985. *Microiontophoresis and Pressure Ejection*, (IBRO Series Methods in Neurosciences). Wiley and Sons, Chichester.
Stone, T. W., and Perkins, M. N. 1981. Adenine dinucleotide effects on cortical neurones. *Brain Res., 229:*241–245.
Stone, T. W., and Taylor, D. A. 1977. Microiontophoretic studies of the effects of cyclic nucleotides on excitability of neurones in the rat cerebral cortex. *J. Physiol., 266:*523–543.
Stone, T. W., Taylor, D. A., and Bloom, F. E. 1975. Cyclic AMP and cyclic GMP may mediate opposite neuronal responses in the rat cerebral cortex. *Science, 187:*845–847.
Van Calker, D., Muller, M. and Hamprecht, B. 1979. Adenosine regulates via two different types of receptors, the accumulation of cyclic AMP in cultured brain cells. *J. Neurochem., 33:*999–1005.
Wu. P. H., Phillis, J. W., and Thierry, D. L. 1982. Adenosine receptor agonists inhibit potassium-evoked calcium uptake by rat brain cortical synaptosomes. *J. Neurochem., 39:*700–708.

Chapter **17**

Classification of Adenosine Receptors in Peripheral Tissues

David M. Paton

Department of Pharmacology and Clinical Pharmacology
University of Auckland
Auckland, New Zealand

I. INTRODUCTION

The numerous actions of adenosine on peripheral tissues have been extensively studied in the past 20 years. Most, if not all, of these actions apparently result from activation of discrete receptors by adenosine. The two main current classification systems for adenosine receptors are detailed and discussed elsewhere in this volume by Burnstock and Buckley (Chapter 11) and by Schwabe (Chapter 13) and have been reviewed by a number of authors including Londos *et al.* (1981), Stone (1982), and Daly *et al.* (1981). Consequently, they will not be further detailed in this review. The emphasis will be rather on a number of practical issues that arise in the classification of adenosine receptors in peripheral tissues and on a number of outstanding questions related to the activation of such receptors by adenosine.

II. USE OF ADENOSINE ANALOGS IN RECEPTOR CLASSIFICATION

The classification of adenosine receptors into P and R sites and the further subdivision of the R sites into R_i (A_1) and R_a (A_2) subtypes is dependent on determining the rank order of potency of adenosine analogs as agonists.

A. Selection of Adenosine Analogs for Study

In order to be able to classify adenosine receptors into P and R sites, information is required on the relative order of potency of adenosine analogs with modifications to the riboside at the 2′, 3′, and 5′ positions and to the adenine moiety at the 2 and 6 positions. For this purpose, the potencies of the following adenosine analogs should be obtained as a minimum, particularly if the tissue has not previously been studied:

Analogs with 2′ and/or 3′ substitutions (2′-deoxyadenosine or adenine arabinoside; 3′-deoxyadenosine or adenine xylofuranoside; 2′,3′-isopropylideneadenosine; 2′5′-dideoxyadenosine).

Analogs with 5′ substitutions [5′-*N*-ethylcarboxamidoadenosine (NECA) and/or 5′-*N*-cyclopropylcarboxamidoadenosine (NCPCA)].

Analogs with 2 substitutions (2-chloroadenosine).

Analogs with 6 substitutions [inosine; N^6-cyclohexyl-adenosine (CHA); N^6-(*R*)-and N^6-(*S*)-phenylisopropyladenosine (*R*- and *S*-PIA)].

For comparative classification purposes, it would be valuable if such studies could also include additional analogs, such as:

The L enantiomers of adenosine, NECA and 2-chloroadenosine (Cusack and Planker, 1979; Burnstock *et al.*, 1983).

Additional N^6 diastereomers, e.g., N^6-(*R*)- and N^6-(*S*)-phenethyladenosine and N^6-(*R*)- and N^6-(*S*)-1-phenyl-2-butyladenosine (Olsson, personal communication)

Additional N^6-substituted analogs, e.g., N^6-phenyladenosine, N^6-benzyladenosine, and N^6-phenethyladenosine (Bruns, 1980a; Paton and Webster, 1984).

B. Modification of Binding of Adenosine Analogs

As reviewed by Schwabe in this volume, the binding of radioligands, such as [^{3}H]-CHA and [^{3}H]R-PIA, to R_i (A_1) adenosine receptors is increased by pretreatment with adenosine deaminase and is reduced by GTP and by *N*-ethylmaleimide (NEM), whereas the binding of radioligands to R_a (A_2) adenosine receptors is not altered by these procedures. It would be informative to study the effects of these procedures on the potency of adenosine analogs at peripheral adenosine receptors, as this might provide additional insights into their classification and could be particularly helpful in those tissues in which the receptors appear to have both R_i (A_1) and R_a (A_2) characteristics, e.g., peripheral adrenergic and cholinergic nerves (Paton, 1981) and dog coronary artery (Kusachi *et al.*, 1983).

C. Inhibition of Sites of Loss for Adenosine

In any study of the rank order of potency of agonists, it is essential that potential sites of loss for the agonists are inhibited. In the case of adenosine and its analogs, these sites of loss are transport into cells and deamination by adenosine deaminase.

2-Deoxycoformycin is an irreversible inhibitor of adenosine deaminase and is a suitable agent to use in such studies (e.g., Muller and Paton, 1979).

A large number of drugs have been found to inhibit adenosine transport [see review by Paterson *et al.* (Chapter 9) in this volume]. In selecting an inhibitor of adenosine transport, consideration must be given to the selectivity and specificity of action of the compound. While dipyridamole has frequently been used for this purpose, it has been demonstrated to have additional actions that complicate the interpretation of results (e.g., Dowdle and Maske, 1980). We have found 2-amino-6-[(2-hydroxy-5-nitro)benzylthio]guanosine a useful agent to use in such studies (Muller and Paton, 1979).

D. Effect of Hypothermia on Responses to Adenosine

A reduction in the temperature of the bathing medium from 37°C to 30 or 27°C potentiated responses to adenosine and 2-chloroadenosine in rat paced left atria and transmurally stimulated rat vas deferens and guinea-pig ileum, but did not alter responses in guinea pig trachea (Broadley *et al.*, 1985). Thus, hypothermia caused supersensitivity of adenosine receptors considered to belong to the A_1 subtype, but not in trachea, where the receptors appear to belong to A_2 subtype. Whether hypothermia will affect all adenosine receptors similarly remains to be determined, but this may also represent a method for distinguishing between A_1 and A_2 receptors.

III. USE OF ADENOSINE NUCLEOTIDE ANALOGS IN RECEPTOR CLASSIFICATION

The classification of adenosine receptors into P_1 and P_2 purinoceptors depends, in part, on determining the rank order of potency of the 5′-adenine nucleotides as agonists.

A. Selection of Adenine Nucleotides For Study

Since the purinoceptor classification (Burnstock, 1978) depends in part on the relative order of potency as agonists of adenosine, AMP, ADP, and ATP, these must be included in any study of the type of purinoceptor present in a peripheral tissue.

Adenine nucleotide analogs that have also proved valuable in such studies include 2-chloro ATP and 2-methylthio ATP and their L enantiomers (Burnstock *et al.*, 1983). These workers demonstrated that 2-chloro ATP and 2-methylthio ATP were considerably more potent than ATP at P_2 receptors in guinea pig taenia, but were only approximately equipotent at P_2 receptors in guinea pig bladder and frog ventricle. In the taenia, there was a high degree of stereoselectivity, but a much lower degree of stereoselectivity in the guinea pig bladder and frog ventricle. Clearly these analogs deserve further study in other peripheral tissues.

Methylene-substituted adenine nucleotides, such as β,γ-methylene ATP, are frequently employed in such studies because of their reduced susceptibility to hydrolysis.

B. Determination of Whether Adenine Nucleotides Act Directly or Indirectly after Conversion to Adenosine

In many tissues, ectoenzymes such as 5′-nucleotidase rapidly hydrolyze the 5′-adenine nucleotides to adenosine. It thus needs to be determined in each tissue under study whether the adenine nucleotides act directly to produce their effects or indirectly following their conversion to adenosine, or by both mechanisms.

This situation may be considered conceptually as follows. Suppose there are two drugs, A and B, that produce qualitatively similar pharmacological actions. It is believed that A produces its actions, in whole or in part, only after its conversion to B, while B is considered to produce its actions through activation of specific receptors. The actions of B are terminated by inactivation. If this is indeed the case, then the following criteria should apply:

(a) Conversion of A to B should be demonstrable.

(b) Inhibition of the conversion of A to B should reduce or abolish the actions of A, while, conversely, increasing the conversion of A to B should accelerate or potentiate the actions of A.

(c) Drugs that act as receptor antagonists to B should also antagonize the actions of A.

(d) Increasing the inactivation of B should reduce the actions of both B and A, while, conversely, reducing the inactivation of B may prolong or potentiate the actions of both B and A.

As indicated earlier, it is known that ectoenzymes hydrolyze 5′-adenine nucleotides to adenosine, that adenosine produces its actions through activation of specific receptors, and that the actions of adenosine are terminated by its transport into cells and its deamination by adenosine deaminase. Accordingly, in examining the hypothesis that the actions of a given adenine nucleotide are dependent on its conversion to adenosine, the following tests may be applied.

1. Can Conversion to Adenosine be Demonstrated?

The metabolic fate of adenine nucleotides added to the bathing medium can be determined by subjecting aliquots of bathing medium to analysis of HPLC (see Chapter 2; Webster, this volume), or by using ^{3}H- or ^{14}C-labeled adenine nucleotides and subjecting aliquots of bathing medium to thin-layer chromatography followed by liquid scintillation spectrometry (e.g., Willemot and Paton, 1981).

Such studies provide definitive evidence for or against the hydrolysis of adenine nucleotides to adenosine and should thus be employed whenever possible. When conversion to adenosine is demonstrable, then clearly adenosine is contributing, at least in part, to the action of the nucleotide. However, as Bruns (1980b) has pointed out, the time taken for adenosine to appear in the bathing medium and/or the concentration of adenosine achieved in the bathing medium may not accurately reflect events in the region of the receptors, since the conversion of nucleotide to adenosine may occur in close proximity to the receptors.

We have used both these experimental approaches. In rat vas deferens, formation of adenosine from AMP, ADP, and ATP was readily demonstrable (Willemot and Paton, 1981), whereas no conversion to adenosine occurred from 2′-AMP, 3′-AMP, NADP, cyclic NADP, or 2′,3′-cyclic AMP (D. R. Webster and D. M. Paton, unpublished observations). In guinea pig ileum, formation of adenosine from 5′-AMP,2′-AMP, and NAD was readily demonstrable (D. R. Webster and D. M. Paton, unpublished observations).

2. *Does Inhibition of 5′-Nucleotidase Reduce or Abolish the Actions of the Adenine Nucleotides?*

α,β-Methylene ADP is a reasonably potent inhibitor of 5′-nucleotidase. In one study, 1 μ*M* produced about 85% inhibition and 100 μ*M* essentially abolished activity (Bruns, 1980b). In guinea pig atria, this inhibitor had no effect on responses to ATP, indicating that hydrolysis to AMP or adenosine is not a prerequisite for the action of ATP in this tissue (Collis and Pettinger, 1982).

However, α,β-methylene ADP has been reported to have additional effects. In guinea pig ileum, it caused a marked reduction in the twitch responses to transmural stimulation, the maximal reduction occuring at 1.6 μ*M* (Moody *et al.*, 1984). This action of α,β-methylene ADP was antagonized by theophylline, suggesting that it may have activated presynaptic adenosine receptors in this tissue or that, alternatively, there was a contaminant purine present.

It must be remembered that both ADP and ATP are themselves inhibitors of 5′-nucleotidase and this may also complicate the interpretation of such studies.

3. *Does Addition of 5′-Nucleotidase Accelerate or Potentiate the Actions of the Adenine Nucleotide?*

This approach has been used by Collis and Pettinger (1982) and Moody *et al.* (1984). In guinea pig atria, responses to ATP were not altered by 5′-nucleotidase (Collis and Pettinger, 1982).

4. *Do Receptor Antagonists for Adenosine Also Antagonize the Actions of the Adenine Nucleotide?*

The use of receptor antagonists is considered further in a later section in this review. In guinea pig atria, theophylline was a competitive antagonist for adenosine, ATP, and β,γ-methylene ATP. The pA_2 values for theophylline did not differ significantly, while Schild plot slopes were not significantly different from unity (Collis and Pettinger, 1982). This study illustrates the major problem with this criterion; namely, adenosine and the adenine nucleotide may both act directly at the same receptor and thus both will be antagonized by the same antagonist.

5. Does Increasing the Deamination of Adenosine Reduce the Actions of Both Adenosine and Adenine Nucleotide?

This criterion can be examined by determining the effect of addition of adenosine deaminase to the bathing medium. In rat vas deferens, addition of adenosine deaminase reduced responses to 5′-AMP, 5′-ADP, 5′-ATP, and NAD, but not those to 2′-AMP-3′-AMP, NADP, cyclic NADP, or 2′,3′-cyclic AMP (Willemot and Paton, 1981), in agreement with HPLC studies that have demonstrated the formation of adenosine from 5′-AMP, 5′-ADP, 5′-ATP and NAD, but not from the other nucleotides (D. R. Webster and D. M. Paton, unpublished observations). An experimental detail that we have observed is that the addition of adenosine deaminase greatly reduces the duration of responses to adenosine, 5′-AMP, 5′-ADP, and 5′-ATP in rat vas deferens, but has less effect on the immediate, initial response to these agents.

6. Does Reducing the Inactivation of Adenosine Prolong and/or Potentiate Not Only Responses to Adenosine but Also to the Adenine Nucleotides?

As discussed previously, the inactivation of adenosine results from transport into cells and deamination by adenosine deaminase. Before this criterion can be tested, one must first determine the effects on responses to adenosine of inhibiting its transport or deamination in the tissue under study. Agents that can be used for this purpose have already been discussed.

A number of studies have demonstrated that inhibitors of adenosine transport potentiate not only responses to adenosine but also those to adenine nucleotides (e.g., Willemot and Paton, 1981; Collis and Pettinger, 1982). Interpretation of such results has proved difficult. It is possible that inhibitors of adenosine transport may also inhibit the transport of adenine nucleotides (Collis and Pettinger, 1982), though it is generally held that nucleotides do not readily cross the plasma membrane. An alternative proposal is that inhibitors of adenosine transport may cause a conformational change to the receptors, thus potentiating responses to the nucleotides (Willemot and Paton, 1981). Clearly, however, this uncertainty over the mechanism(s) and specificity of action of adenosine transport inhibitors greatly reduces the value of this criterion.

In summary, therefore, results obtained to date have suggested that the most useful of these tests are the direct demonstration of the conversion of nucleotide to adenosine, and a careful, suitably controlled study of the effects of 5′-nucleotidase inhibitors and of added adenosine deaminase on responses to adenosine and adenine nucleotides.

C. Use of Methylene Isoteres of the Adenine Nucleotides

Methylene isosteres of the adenine nucleotides are more resistant to hydrolysis and have therefore been used extensively in studies designed to elucidate the mechanism of action of adenine nucleotides at receptors. In particular, α,β-methylene ADP, α,β-methylene ATP and β,γ-methylene ATP have been used (e.g., Maguire and Satchell, 1979; Brown and Burnstock, 1981; Taylor *et al.*, 1983; Moody *et al.*, 1984).

It must be realized, however, that results obtained using these methylene analogs require careful consideration and that adequate controls must be used in such studies. Their actions are not always qualitatively similar to those of the 5′-adenine nucleotides. For example, ATP produced relaxation of the guinea pig trachea and caused a rebound contraction due to prostaglandin production in guinea pig taenia coli, whereas α,β-methylene ATP and β,γ-methylene ATP failed to produce these effects (Brown and Burnstock, 1981). In rat vas deferens, β,γ-methylene ATP caused presynaptic inhibition of transmitter release apparently through activation of P_2 purinoceptors, whereas ATP activated P_1 purinoceptors in this tissue (Taylor *et al.*, 1983). In guinea-pig ileum, α,β-methylene ATP appeared to induce release of acetylcholine, while both this analog and β,γ-methylene ATP were degraded by this tissue (Moody and Burnstock, 1982).

If methylene isosteres of the adenine nucleotides are used to elucidate the mechanism of action of the 5′-adenine nucleotides, steps must be taken to determine whether:

(a) they act at the same site as the 5′-adenine nucleotides. Do they produce qualitatively similar responses and are their actions antagonized by the same drugs?

(b) they act directly or indirectly. Do they act, at least partially, following their hydrolysis to adenosine? It is frequently assumed in such studies that the methylene isosteres of ATP, for example, are not subject to hydrolysis. This should, however, be checked using a technique such as HPLC. Do they act, at least partially, by releasing transmitter stores or by increasing the synthesis of prostaglandins?

IV. USE OF ANTAGONISTS IN RECEPTOR CLASSIFICATION

The classification of any receptors is always very dependent on the availability of potent, specific, and selective antagonists, and the adenosine receptors are no exception. In examining the actions of presumed antagonists at adenosine receptors, the following general aspects of methodology are important to consider:

1. The solubility of the presumed antagonist. (Many of the methylxanthines have limited solubility in water, and agents that may increase their solubility, e.g., ethylenediamine, may have their own actions.)

2. The duration of exposure to the antagonist. (Preliminary studies should be performed to determine that the exposure time is sufficient for antagonism to be fully developed.)

3. Controls must be used to allow for any changes in tissue sensitivity with time.

4. Sites of loss for the agonist must be blocked. (In the case of adenosine, this will involve the use of inhibitors of adenosine deaminase and of adenosine

transport. Alternatively, an adenosine analog, such as 2-chloroadenosine or *R*-PIA, may be used, as these analogs are not subject to deamination or possibly transport.)

5. The specificity and selectivity of action of the antagonist will require careful study. (This will involve studies of the effects of the antagonist on the actions of agonists acting at other receptors; studies of pretreatment of tissues with antagonists at other receptors and with drugs inhibiting prostaglandin synthesis; the use of several different tissues and species, and so on.)

A comprehensive review of these methodological considerations may be found in Chapter 12 by Kenakin and Leighton (this volume) and in the review by Furchgott (1972).

A. Antagonists at P_1 Purinoceptors and at R Sites (the Methylxanthines)

The methylxanthine, theophylline, is a very important tool in the study of adenosine receptors, as it has been found to be an agonist at P_1 purinoceptors and at R sites of both subtypes (i.e., at R_i or A_1 and R_a or A_2 sites). However, theophylline is by no means an ideal antagonist, as it is not very potent (typical pA_2 values being in the region of 5.70) nor is it very soluble in water. In addition, it has other actions, e.g., inhibition of phosphodiesterase and changes in calcium transport.

Bruns *et al.* (1983) have employed a detailed structure–activity analysis of alkylxanthine derivatives at adenosine receptor binding sites in bovine brain membranes in order to design more potent antagonists. A 1-methyl substituent increased the affinity of xanthine about 40-fold, while an additional 3-methyl substituent (i.e., theophylline) caused a further doubling of affinity. 1,3-Dipropyl substitution enhanced potency about 20-fold compared to theophylline. An 8-phenyl substitution greatly increased affinity, 8-phenyltheophylline and 1,3-dipropyl-8-phenyltheophylline being 1000 and 10,000 times more potent than theophylline respectively. This increase in potency was further increased by certain para substitutions on the 8-phenyl ring (e.g., chloro), while a further substitution at the ortho position on the phenyl ring (e.g., amino) further increased potency. It was found that 1,3-dipropyl-8-(2-amino-4-chlorophenyl)xanthine was an extremely potent antagonist at A_1 (R_i) adenosine receptors in bovine brain having a K_i of 22 p*M*, thus being 70,000 times more potent than theophylline. It also behaved as a competitive antagonist. However, this agent is poorly soluble in water at neutral pH and has high nonspecific binding to tissue membranes and filters (Bruns *et al.*, 1983).

Further studies need to be performed with the newer, more potent xanthine antagonists such as 1,3-dipropyl-8-(2-amino-4-chlorophenyl)xanthine in order to determine how specific and selective they are and whether any of them are antagonists at only the A_1 (R_i) or A_2 (R_a) adenosine receptors subtypes. In rat vas deferens and guinea pig ileum, this new xanthine analog was over 10-fold more potent as an antagonist than theophylline against the presynaptic inhibitory actions of 2-chloroadenosine (D. M. Paton, unpublished observations).

B. Antagonists at P_2 Purinoceptors and at P Sites

There is a need for an antagonist at the intracellular P adenosine receptor on adenylate cyclase. Such an agent would help to clarify the role of this site.

The lack of potent, specific antagonists at P_2 purinoceptors has hindered attempts to determine whether they are a single homogenous group or whether they belong to additional subtypes. At present, there are several potential approaches that are being utilized in the study of P_2 purinoceptors. The use of the photoaffinity analog, amylazido aminopropronyl ATP ($ANAPP_3$) as a P_2-purinoceptor antagonist is detailed in Chapter 14 by Fedan *et al.* (this volume), while those of other antagonists are discussed in Chapter 11 by Burnstock and Buckley (this volume).

Burnstock and his colleagues have recently described the use of α,β-methylene ATP to desensensitize tissues to P_2-purinoceptor agonists (Kasakov and Burnstock, 1983; Meldrum and Burnstock, 1983).

V. CONCLUDING REMARKS

Much additional work is required before the classification of adenosine receptors in peripheral tissues can be considered to be firmly established. In addition to the questions already raised, the following topics also require attention:

1. What insights about the adenosine receptors in peripheral tissues can be obtained by the use of radioligands for the A_1 (R_i) and A_2 (R_a) subtypes. In this regard, the radioligand $[^{125}I]N^6$-*p*-hydroxyphenylisopropyladenosine would appear to have the greatest potential in view of its very high specific activity (Schwabe *et al.*, 1982).

2. What relationship is there, if any, between activation of adenosine receptors in peripheral tissues and changes in activity of adenylate cyclase in these tissues. This aspect has received relatively little attention to date. It is important to recall, however, that the classification of adenosine receptors into P and R sites or subtypes was based on the actions of adenosine on adenylate cyclase (Londos *et al.*, 1981) and has since been extrapolated to the pharmacological actions of adenosine on peripheral tissues. In a recent study, evidence was obtained that adenosine-induced relaxation of bovine coronary artery may involve cyclic AMP and activation of cyclic AMP-dependent protein kinase (Silver *et al.*, 1984).

ACKNOWLEDGMENT

Supported by a grant from the Medical Research Council of New Zealand.

REFERENCES

Broadley, K. J., Broome, S., and Paton, D. M., 1985. Hypothermia-induced supersensitivity to adenosine for responses mediated via A_1 receptors, but not A_2 receptors. *Br. J. Pharmacol.*, in press.

Brown, C. M., and Burnstock, G. 1981. The structural conformation of the polyphosphate chain of the ATP molecule is critical for its promotion of prostaglandin biosynthesis. *Eur. J. Pharmacol. 69*:81–86.

Bruns, R. F. 1980a. Adenosine receptor activation in human fibroblasts: nucleoside agonists and antagonists. *Can. J. Physiol. Pharmacol., 58*:673–691.

Bruns, R. F. 1980b. Adenosine receptor activation by adenosine nucleotides requires conversion of the nucleotides to adenosine. *Naunyn Schmiedebergs Arch. Pharmacol., 315*:5–13.

Bruns, R. F., Daly, J. W., and Snyder, S. H. 1983. Adenosine receptor binding: structure-activity analysis generates extremely potent xanthine antagonists. *Proc. Natl. Acad. Sci. USA, 80*:2077–2080.

Burnstock, G. 1978. A basis for distinguishing two types of purinergic receptors. In: *Cell Membrane Receptors for Drugs and Hormones: A Multidisciplinary Approach*, pp. 107–118. Ed. by Bolis, L., and Straub, R. W. Raven Press, New York.

Burnstock, G., Cusack, N. J., Hills, J. M., MacKenzie, I, and Meghji, P. 1983. Studies on the stereoselectivity of the P_2-purinoceptor. *Br. J. Pharmacol., 79*:907–913.

Collis, M. G., and Pettinger, S. J. 1983. Can ATP stimulate P_1-receptors in guinea-pig atrium without conversion to adenosine. *Eur. J. Pharmacol. 81*:521–529.

Cusack, N. J., and Planker, M. 1979. Relaxation of isolated taenia coli of guinea-pig by enantiomers of 2-azido analogues of adenosine and adenine nucleotides. *Br. J. Pharmacol., 67*:153–158.

Daly, J. W., Bruns, R. F., and Snyder, S. H. 1981. Adenosine receptors in the central nervous system: relationship to the central actions of methylxanthines. *Life Sci., 28*:2083–2097.

Dowdle, E. B., and Maske, R. 1980. The effects of dipyridamole on the guinea-pig ileal longitudinal muscle-myenteric plexus preparation. *Br. J. Pharmacol., 71*:235–244.

Furchgott, R. F. 1972. The classification of adrenoceptors (adrenergic receptors). An evaluation from the standpoint of receptor theory. In: *Handbook of Pharmacology*, *Catecholamines*, Volume 33, pp. 283–335. Ed. by Blashko H., and Muscholl, E. Springer, Berlin.

Kasakov, L., and Burnstock, G. 1983. The use of the slowly degradable analog, α,β-methyleneATP, to produce desensitisation of the P_2-purinoceptor effect on non-adrenergic, non-cholinergic responses of the guinea-pig urinary bladder. *Eur. J. Pharmacol., 86*:291–294.

Kusachi, S., Thompson, R. D., and Olsson, R. A. 1983. Ligand selectivity of dog coronary adenosine receptor resembles that of adenylate cyclase stimulatory (R_a) receptors. *J. Pharmacol. Exp. Ther., 227*:316–321.

Londos, C., Wolff, J., and Cooper, D. M. F. 1981. Adenosine as regulator of adenylate cyclase. In: *Purinergic Receptors, Receptors and Recognition*, Series B, Volume 12, pp. 289–323. Ed. by Burnstock, G. Chapman and Hall, London.

Maguire, M. H., and Satchell, D. G. 1979. The contribution of adenosine to the inhibitory actions of adenine nucleotides on the guinea-pig taenia coli: Studies with phosphate-modified adenine nucleotide analogs and dipyridamole. *J. Pharmacol. Exp. Ther., 211*:626–631.

Meldrum, L. A., and Burnstock, G. 1983. Evidence that ATP acts as a co-transmitter with noradrenaline in sympathetic nerves supplying the guinea pig vas deferens. *Eur. J. Pharmacol., 92*:161–163.

Moody, C. J., and Burnstock, G. 1982. Evidence for the presence of P_1-purinoceptors on cholinergic nerve terminals in the guinea-pig ileum. *Eur. J. Pharmacol., 77*:1–9.

Moody, C. J., Meghji, P., and Burnstock, G. 1984. Stimulation of P_1-purinoceptors by ATP depends partly on its conversion to AMP and adenosine and partly on direct action. *Eur. J. Pharmacol., 97*:55–65.

Muller, M. J., and Paton, D. M. 1979. Presynaptic inhibitory actions of 2-substituted adenosine derivatives on neurotransmission in rat vas deferens: effects of inhibitors of adenosine uptake and deamination. *Naunyn-Schmiedebergs. Arch. Pharmacol., 306*:23–28.

Paton, D. M. 1981. Structure–activity relations for presynaptic inhibition of noradrenergic and cholinergic transmission by adenosine: Evidence for action on A_1 receptors. *J. Auton. Pharmacol., 1*:287–290.

Paton, D. M., and Webster, D. R. 1984. On the classification of adenosine and purinergic receptors in rat atria and in peripheral adrenergic and cholinergic nerves. In: *Neuronal and Extraneuronal*

Events in Autonomic Pharmacology, pp. 193–204. Ed. by Fleming, W. W., Langer, S. Z., Graefe, K. H., and Weiner, N. Raven Press, New York.

Schwabe, U., Lenschow, V., Ukena, D., Ferry, D. R., and Glossman, H. 1982. [^{125}I]N^6-p-Hydroxyphenylisopropyl-adenosine, a new ligand for R_i adenosine receptors. *Naunyn-Schmiedebergs Arch. Pharmacol., 321:*84–87.

Silver, P. J., Walus, K., and DiSalvo, J. 1984. Adenosine mediated relaxation and activation of cyclic AMP-dependent protein kinase in coronary artery smooth muscle. *J. Pharmacol. Exp. Ther., 228:*342–347.

Stone, T. W. 1982. Cell-membrane receptors for purines. *Biosci. Rev., 2:*77–90.

Taylor, D. A., Wiese, S., Faison, E. P., and Yarbrough, G. G. 1983. Pharmacological characterization of purinergic receptors in the rat vas deferens. *J. Pharmacol. Exp. Ther., 224:*40–45.

Willemot, J., and Paton, D. M. 1981. Metabolism and presynaptic nucleotides in rat vas deferens. *Naunyn-Schmiedebergs Arch. Pharmacol., 317:*110–114.

V

Physiological Role of Adenosine

Chapter 18

Criteria for the Involvement of Adenosine in the Regulation of Blood Flow

Robert M. Berne

Department of Physiology
University of Virginia
School of Medicine
Charlottesville, Virginia

Any agent that is proposed as a mediator of the local regulation of blood flow must meet certain criteria, and it is the aim of this chapter to set forth these criteria and indicate to what extent adenosine fulfills them in different vascular beds. The major criteria are as follows:

1. The mediator must be a potent vasoactive substance (a vasodilator in the case of a metabolic mechanism) and its vasoactivity should be commensurate with its physiological concentration.
2. There must be an endogenous source of the mediator and it should be released under appropriate conditions (e.g., when parenchymal tissue oxygen supply is inadequate for tissue oxygen needs).
3. The agent should have access to the resistance vessels of the tissue.
4. The concentration of the mediator in the interstitial fluid must be sufficient to elicit vasodilation and the concentration should parallel the change in vascular resistance as well as the time course of tissue oxygen deficit (either increased oxygen demand or decreased oxygen supply).
5. The effects on vascular resistance of the endogenous mediator should be mimicked by equal concentrations of the agent when it is administered intraarterially or topically.
6. There should be a mechanism for removal of the substance (inactivation, uptake, washout) when the need for greater blood flow is removed.
7. Substances that potentiate or attenuate the effect of administered mediator should have the same effect on endogenous mediator.

8. The mechanism of action on vascular smooth muscle should be known.

Adenosine fulfills the first criterion since it dilates resistance vessels in the heart (Drury and Szent-Györgyi, 1929; Winbury *et al.*, 1953; Wolf and Berne, 1956), brain (Berne *et al.*, 1974), skeletal muscle (Bockman *et al.*, 1975, 1976; Dobson *et al.*, 1971; Proctor and Duling, 1982; Tominaga *et al.*, 1980), lung (Mentzer *et al.*, 1975), gastrointestinal tract (Granger *et al.*, 1978), and fat tissue (Sollevi and Fredholm, 1981). Furthermore, the magnitude of the vasodilation produced by adenosine is proportional to its concentration over physiological levels of the nucleoside (Schrader *et al.*, 1977; Wahl and Kuschinsky, 1976). A major problem with the dose–response curves for administered adenosine is that because of the large uptake by endothelial cells (Nees and Gerlach, 1983; Pearson *et al.*, 1983), it is not possible to determine the actual concentration of adenosine that reaches the target organ, the vascular smooth muscle. Nevertheless, there is a definite dose–response relationship even if the actual effective concentrations of adenosine are not known.

With respect to the second criterion, namely, an endogenous source of adenosine, it has been well documented that adenosine is formed in and released from hypoxic or ischemic myocardium (Olsson, 1970; Olsson *et al.*, 1978; Rubio *et al.*, 1969, 1974), brain (Berne *et al.*, 1974; Winn *et al.*, 1979, 1981), and skeletal muscle (Bockman *et al.*, 1975; Dobson *et al.*, 1971). It is also released from hypoxic cultured cardiac cells (Mustafa *et al.*, 1975). Furthermore, with enhanced oxygen consumption under free flow conditions, the concentration in and release from heart (Bacchus *et al.*, 1982; Knabb *et al.*, 1983; Miller *et al.*, 1979), brain (Berne *et al.*, 1974; Winn *et al.*, 1980), and skeletal muscle (Bockman *et al.*, 1975) increased significantly.

Since adenosine is formed from parenchymal AMP, which in turn arises from dephosphorylation of cellular ATP (Mustafa *et al.*, 1975), the nucleoside must reach the arterioles as it passes from the parenchymal tissue into the interstitial space where it comes in contact with the vascular smooth muscle. Hence, the third criterion is satisfied. Whether the adenosine is formed from AMP by 5′-nucleotidase within the parenchymal cells or at the cell membrane (Rubio *et al.*, 1973) or whether it arises from hydrolysis of *S*-adenosylhomocysteine (Schrader *et al.*, 1981) is not pertinent to the third criterion.

At the present time, it is not possible to obtain a reasonably accurate estimate of the interstitial fluid concentration of adenosine, although recent studies show promise for this determination (Hanley *et al.*, 1983). Consequently, an accurate correlation of interstitial fluid adenosine concentration with vascular resistance or with the time course of an oxygen deficit cannot yet be determined. In the case of the heart, a crude index of the interstitial adenosine concentration is obtainable. This is accomplished by injection of Krebs–Henseleit solution into the pericardial space of the dog heart, where it is left in contact with the epicardial surface of the heart for 4–5 min; it is then removed for analysis of its adenosine concentration (Miller *et al.*, 1979). Of course, equilibrium is not reached because of contact with only a small segment of the myocardial interstitial compartment and because of the brevity of this contact. Nevertheless, the direction and the magnitude of the changes of the adenosine concentration in the pericardial infusate parallels the changes in myocardial oxygen consumption and coronary blood flow under a wide variety of interventions in the anesthetized and unanesthetized dog (Bacchus *et al.*, 1982; Knabb *et al.*, 1983; Miller *et al.*, 1979; Watkinson *et al.*, 1979). In brief, the data are compatible with the fourth criterion but quantitative, and hence meaningful, support is lacking.

Intraarterial administration of adenosine produces a decrease in vascular resistance in all vascular beds except that of the kidney (Miller *et al.*, 1978). In the kidney, vasoconstriction is elicited by adenosine in the salt-depleted dog, and possibly acts via the renin–angiotensin system, (Osswald, 1983). On isolated vessels, including renal vessels, adenosine induces relaxation, and hence the direct action of adenosine on all vascular smooth muscle appears to be the same. Over a dose range of about 10^{-8} to 10^{-4} *M* exogenous adenosine exhibits a typical dose–response relationship (Schrader *et al.*, 1977; Wahl and Kuschinsky, 1976). As mentioned earlier, one cannot determine the concentration of exogenously administered adenosine in contact with the arteriolar vascular smooth muscle because of the avid uptake of the nucleoside by endothelial cells and by cellular elements of the blood. It is also impossible to determine the concentration of endogenous adenosine reaching the vascular smooth muscle, for the same reasons, as well as the possible release of adenosine from the endothelial cells. In heart, the concentrations of adenosine recovered in coronary venous blood probably represents a fraction of that present in the interstitial fluid. Attempts to estimate interstitial fluid levels of adenosine from measurements in cardiac lymph have not been successful, most likely due to the very slow lymph flow and the degradation by blood cells present in lymph. Despite the fact that interstitial fluid adenosine levels cannot be accurately quantified, the observations that vasodilation tends to parallel the increments in administered adenosine, as well as the release of endogenous adenosine at different levels of myocardial metabolic activity, strongly suggests that the vascular resistance changes in each case are caused by the same agent. Thus, the fifth criterion that the exogenous agent mimicks the endogenous agent is essentially met.

Adenosine is removed from its site of action by several mechanisms, thereby fulfilling the sixth criterion. Some is washed out by the perfusing blood and appears in the venous effluent as adenosine or its degradation products, inosine and hypoxanthine. The inosine and hypoxanthine are formed in the vascular cell walls and blood by adenosine deaminase and nucleoside phosphorylase, respectively (Rubio *et al.*, 1972), and do not exhibit significant vasoactivity. However, a large fraction of the adenosine is taken up by parenchymal tissue and is enzymatically phosphorylated to AMP by adenosine kinase and finally to ATP. In the case of the brain, released adenosine is essentially trapped in the cerebrospinal fluid because it crosses the blood–brain barrier very slowly (Berne *et al.*, 1974). Hence, there is almost complete recovery of endogenously released adenosine in the brain, whereas in other tissues, such as heart and skeletal muscle, some of the adenosine is carried away in one form or another by the blood.

With respect to potentiation and attenuation of exogenous and endogenous adenosine, there is controversy. General agreement exists that dipyridamole or lidoflazine, which block cellular uptake of adenosine and thereby protect against metabolism of the nucleoside, potentiate the vasodilation produced by administered adenosine. However, there are conflicting data about potentiation of blood flow under conditions when endogenous adenosine release is increased (e.g., reactive hyperemia). Some investigators have shown potentiation of reactive hyperemia (Bittar and Pauly, 1970; Juhran and Dietmann, 1970; Miura *et al.*, 1967), whereas others have not (Bittar and Pauly, 1971; Juhran *et al.*, 1971). The reason for these divergent results is not clear. A similar controversy exists concerning the attenuating effects of the methylxanthines, such as theophylline or aminophylline. These compounds presumably compete for the adenosine receptor and thereby reduce the response to a given dose of exogenous adenosine (Büngег *et al.*, 1975). However, results of theophylline or aminophylline on reactive hyperemia are not in agreement. Some investigators have observed attenuation of reactive hyperemia (Curnish *et al.*, 1972; Juhran *et al.*, 1971), whereas others have failed to observe any significant effect of theophylline or aminophylline on reactive hyperemia (Bittar and Pauly, 1971; Juhran and Dietman, 1970). In light of these discrepant results with potentiators and attenuators of adenosine in reactive hyperemia, no definitive conclusions can be drawn regarding the seventh criterion.

The mechanism whereby adenosine produces relaxation of vascular smooth muscle is not known, but there is suggestive evidence that the nucleoside interferes with calcium reaching the contractile machinery either by blocking cellular calcium uptake or its release from intracellular stores. In atrial and skeletal muscle, the contraction produced by caffeine (attributed to an increase in intracellular calcium) is attenuated by adenosine (Berne *et al.*, 1976; DeGubareff and Sleator, 1965). Furthermore, the slow inward calcium current (produced in guinea pig atria by blocking the fast sodium channels and stimulating electrically in the presence of norepinephrine) is abolished by the addition of 10^{-6} M adenosine to the bathing medium (Schrader *et al.*, 1975). One may question whether extrapolation of these results on cardiac and skeletal muscle to vascular smooth muscle is valid. However there is some evidence for a calcium-blocking effect on adenosine in vascular smooth muscle. The enhanced calcium uptake observed in vascular smooth muscle with partial depolarization with potassium is absent in the presence of $10^{-6}M$ adenosine (Fenton *et al.*, 1982). Hence, there is some support for the concept that adenosine induces relaxation of vascular smooth muscle by preventing access of calcium to the contractile apparatus. In contrast, there is no evidence that adenosine in physiological concentrations acts by increasing vascular smooth muscle cyclic AMP levels (Herlihy *et al.*, 1976), as could be inferred from studies by Triner *et al.* (1971). Finally, what links adenosine release to tissue metabolic activity is not known. There is suggestive evidence that 5′-nucleotidase activity is controlled in the intact tissue and that changes in phosphocreatine, magnesium, and AMP may be involved in the regulation of 5′-nucleotidase activity (Rubio *et al.*, 1979).

REFERENCES

Bacchus, A. N., Ely, S. W., Knabb, R. M., Rubio, R., and Berne, R. M. 1982. Adenosine and coronary blood flow in conscious dogs during normal physiological stimuli. *Am. J. Physiol.*, *243:*H628–H633.

Berne, R. M., Rubio, R., and Curnish, R. R. 1974. Release of adenosine from ischemic brain: effect on cerebral vascular resistance and incorporation into cerebral adenine nucleotides. *Circ. Res., 35:*262–271.

Berne, R. M., Herlihy, J. T., Schrader, J., and Rubio, R. 1976. Effect of adenosine on contraction of vascular smooth muscle. In: *Ionic Actions on Vascular Smooth Muscle*, pp. 137–140. Ed. by Betz, E. Springer-Verlag, Berlin.

Bittar, N., and Pauly, T. J. 1970. Potentiation by dipyridamole of myocardial reactive hyperemia in the dog. *Pharm. Res. Commun., 2:*231–242.

Bittar, N., and Pauly, T. J. 1971. Myocardial reactive hyperemia responses in the dog after aminophylline and lidoflazine. *Am. J. Physiol., 220:*812–815.

Bockman, E. L., Berne, R. M., and Rubio, R. 1975. Release of adenosine and lack of release of ATP from contracting skeletal muscle. *Pflügers Arch., 355:*229–241.

Bockman, E. L., Berne, R. M., and Rubio, R. 1976. Adenosine and active hyperemia in dog skeletal muscle. *Am. J. Physiol., 230:*1531–1537.

Bünger, R., Haddy, F. J., and Gerlach, E. 1975. Coronary responses to dilating substances and competitive inhibition by theophylline in the isolated perfused guinea pig heart. *Pflügers Arch., 358:*213–224.

Curnish, R. R., Berne, R. M., and Rubio, R. 1972. Effect of aminophylline on myocardial reactive hyperemia. *Proc. Soc. Exp. Biol. Med., 141:*593–598.

DeGubareff, T., and Sleator, W., Jr. 1965. Effects of caffeine on mammalian atrial muscle and its interaction with adenosine and calcium. *J. Pharmacol. Exp. Ther., 148:*202–214.

Dobson, J. G., Jr., Rubio, R., and Berne, R. M. 1971. Role of adenine nucleotides, adenosine, and inorganic phosphate in the regulation of skeletal muscle blood flow. *Circ. Res., 29:*375–384.

Drury, A. N., and Szent-Györgyi, A. 1929. The physiological activity of adenine compounds with special reference to their action upon the mammalian heart. *J. Physiol. London, 68:*213–237.

Fenton, R. A., Bruttig, S. P., Rubio, R., and Berne, R. M. 1982. Effect of adenosine on calcium uptake by intact and cultured vascular smooth muscle. *Am. J. Physiol., 242:*H797–H804.

Granger, D. N., Valleau, J. D., Parker, R. E., Lane, R. S., and Taylor, A. E. 1978. Effects of adenosine on intestinal hemodynamics, oxygen delivery, and capillary fluid exchange. *Am. J. Physiol., 235:*H707–H719.

Hanley, F., Messina, L. M., Baer, R. W., Uhlig, P. N., and Hoffman, J. I. E. 1983. Direct measurement of left ventricular interstitial adenosine. *Am. J. Physiol., 245:*H327–H335.

Herlihy, J. T., Bockman, E. L., Berne, R. M., and Rubio, R. 1976. Adenosine relaxation of isolated vascular smooth muscle. *Am. J. Physiol., 230:*1239–1243.

Juhran, W., and Dietmann, K. 1970. Zur Regelung der Coronardurchblutung im akuten Sauerstoffmangel. *Pflügers Arch., 315:*105–109.

Juhran, W., Voss, E. M., Dietmann, K., and Schaumann, W., 1971. Pharmacological effects on coronary reactive hyperemia in conscious dogs. *Naunyn Schmiedebergs Arch. Pharmacol., 269:*32–47.

Knabb, R. M., Ely, S. W., Bacchus, A. N., Rubio, R., and Berne, R. M. 1983. Consistent parallel relationships among myocardial oxygen consumption, coronary blood flow, and pericardial infusate adenosine concentration with various interventions and β-blockade in the dog. *Cir. Res., 53:*33–41.

Mentzer, R. M. Jr., Rubio, R., and Berne, R. M., 1975. Release of adenosine by hypoxic canine lung tissue and its possible role in pulmonary circulation. *Am. J. Physiol., 229:*1625–1631.

Miller, W. L., Thomas, R. A., Berne, R. M., and Rubio, R. 1978. Adenosine production in the ischemic kidney. *Circ. Res., 43:*390–397.

Miller, W. L., Belardinelli, L., Bacchus, N., Foley, D. H., Rubio, R., and Berne, R. M. 1979. Canine myocardial adenosine and lactate production, oxygen consumption and coronary blood flow during stellate ganglia stimulation. *Circ. Res., 45:*708–718.

Miura, M., Tominaga, S., and Hashimoto, K. 1967. Potentiation of reactive hyperemia in the coronary and femoral circulation by the selective use of 2,6-Bis (diethanolamine-4,8-dipiperidino-pyrimido [5,4]pyrimidine). *Arzneim. Forsch., 17:*976–979.

Mustafa, S. J., Berne, R. M., and Rubio, R. 1975. Adenosine metabolism in cultured chick embryo heart cells. *Am. J. Physiol., 228:*1474–1478.

Nees, S., and Gerlach, E. 1983. Adenine nucleotide and adenosine metabolism in cultured coronary endothelial cells: Formation and release of adenine compounds and possible functional implications. In: *Regulatory Function of Adenosine*, pp. 347–360. Ed. by Berne, R. M., Rall, T. W., and Rubio, R. Martinus Nijhoff, Boston.

Olsson, R. A. 1970. Changes in content of purine nucleoside in canine myocardium during coronary occlusion. *Circ. Res., 26:*301–306.

Olsson, R. A., Snow, J. A., and Gentry, M. K. 1978. Adenosine metabolism in canine myocardial reactive hyperemia. *Circ. Res., 42:*358–362.

Osswald, H. 1983. Adenosine and renal function. In: *Regulatory Function of Adenosine*, pp. 399–415. Ed. by Berne, R. M., Rall, T. W., and Rubio, R. Martinus Nijhoff, Boston.

Pearson, J. D., Hellewell, P. G., and Gordon, J. L. 1983. Adenosine uptake and adenine nucleotide metabolism by vascular endothelium. In: *Regulatory Function of Adenosine,* pp. 333–345. Ed. by Berne, R. M., Rall, T. W., and Rubio, R. Martinus Nijhoff, Boston.

Proctor, K. G., and Duling, B. R. 1982. Adenosine and free-flow functional hyperemia in striated muscle. *Am. J. Physiol., 242:*H688–H697.

Rubio, R., Berne, R. M., and Katori, M. 1969. Release of adenosine in reactive hyperemia of the dog heart. *Am. J. Physiol., 216:*56–62.

Rubio, R., Wiedmeier, V. T., and Berne, R. M. 1972. Nucleoside phosphorylase: localization and role in the myocardial distribution of purines. *Am. J. Physiol., 222:*550–555.

Rubio, R., Berne, R. M., and Dobson, J. G. Jr. 1973. Sites of adenosine production in cardiac and skeletal muscle. *Am. J. Physiol., 225:*938–953.

Rubio, R., Wiedmeier, V. T., and Berne, R. M. 1974. Relationship between coronary flow and adenosine production and release. *J. Mol. Cell. Cardiol., 6:*561–566.

Rubio, R., Belardinelli, L., Thompson, C. I., and Berne, R. M. 1979. Cardiac adenosine: electrophysiological effects, possible significance in cell function, and mechanisms controlling its release. In: *Physiological and Regulatory Functions of Adenosine and Adenine Nucleotides*, pp. 167–182. Ed. by Baer, H. P., and Drummond, G. I. Raven Press, New York.

Schrader, J., Rubio, R., and Berne, R. M. 1975. Inhibition of slow action potentials of guinea pig atrial muscle by adenosine: A possible effect on Ca^{2+} influx. *J. Mol. Cell. Cardiol., 7:*427–433.

Schrader, J., Haddy, F. J., and Gerlach, E. 1977. Release of adenosine, inosine and hypoxanthine from the isolated guinea pig heart during hypoxia, flow-autoregulation and reactive hyperemia. *Pflügers Arch., 369:*1–6.

Schrader, J., Schütz, W., and Bardenheuer, H. 1981. Role of S-adenosylhomocysteine hydrolase in adenosine metabolism in mammalian heart. *Biochem. J., 196:*65–70.

Sollevi, A., and Fredholm, B. B. 1981. Role of adenosine in adipose tissue circulation. *Acta Physiol. Scand., 112:*293–298.

Tominaga, S., Curnish, R. R., Belardinelli, L., Rubio, R., and Berne, R. M. 1980. Adenosine release during early and sustained exercise of canine skeletal muscle, *Am. J. Physiol., 238:*H156–H163.

Triner, L., Nahas, G. G., Vulliemoz, Y., Overweg, N. I. A., Verosky, M., Habif, D. V., and Ngai, S. H., 1971, Cyclic AMP and smooth muscle functions. *Ann. NY Acad. Sci., 185:*458–476.

Wahl, M., and Kuschinsky, W. 1976. The dilatory action of adenosine on pial arteries of cats and its inhibition by theophylline. *Pflügers Arch., 362:*55–59.

Watkinson, W. P., Foley, D. H., Rubio, R., and Berne, R. M. 1979. Myocardial adenosine formation with increased cardiac performance in the dog. *Am. J. Physiol., 236:*H13–H21.

Winbury, M. M., Papierski, D. H., Hemmer, M. L., and Hambourger, W. E. 1953. Coronary dilator action of the adenine-ATP series, *J. Pharmacol. Exp. Ther., 109:*255–260.

Winn, H. R., Rubio, R., and Berne, R. M. 1979. Brain adenosine production in the rat during 60 seconds of ischemia. *Circ. Res., 45:*486–492.

Winn, H. R., Welsh, J. E., Rubio, R., and Berne, R. M. 1980. Changes in brain adenosine during bicuculline-induced seizures in rats: effects of hypoxia and altered systemic blood pressure. *Circ. Res., 47:*568–577.

Winn, H. R., Rubio, R., and Berne, R. M. 1981. Brain adenosine concentration during hypoxia in rat. *Am. J. Physiol., 241:*H235–H242.

Wolf, M. M., and Berne, R. M. 1965. Coronary vasodilator properties of purine and pyrimidine derivatives. *Cir. Res., 4:*343–348.

Chapter **19**

Methods Used to Study the Involvement of Adenosine in the Regulation of Lipolysis

Bertil B. Fredholm

Department of Pharmacology
Karolinska Institute
Stockholm, Sweden

I. INTRODUCTION

The evidence that adenosine plays a role in the regulation of adipose tissue circulation and metabolism is impressive. Adipose tissue offers many special advantages when studying intraarterial adenosine effects. It is possible to study relevant phenomena in preparations ranging from cell free systems, via isolated purified cells and intact pieces of white adipose tissue *in vitro*, to intact tissue perfused *in situ*. Furthermore, the biochemical steps mediating receptor effects are particularly well delineated in this tissue. The present chapter will, however, neither describe the evidence that adenosine is physiologically important in adipose tissue nor review the evidence regarding the biochemical regulation of lipolysis, but will instead focus on the techniques that may be and have been used in studying the role of adenosine in the regulation of adipose tissue function.

II. ISOLATED FAT CELLS

A major advance in methodology was the introduction by Rodbell in 1964 of a method to isolate white fat cells. His method with minor modifications has since been used by most investigators in the field. Indeed, the ease and convenience of preparation of isolated fat cells have given this tissue the status of an established model system for a variety of biochemical and pharmacological applications.

A. Isolation of Fat Cells

The basis for Rodbell's (1964) procedure for isolating fat cells is digestion of the tissue with a crude collagenase preparation followed by flotation of the low-density cells in an albumin-containing medium. The procedure has been described in detail by Fain (1975) for white fat cells and by Nedergaard and Linberg (1982) for brown fat cells.

The source of the collagenase is critical. It must not be purified, since the procedure requires the presence of proteolytic enzymes. Instead crude preparations, such as the preparation from *Clostridium histolyticum* sold by Worthington, should be used. It is usually a good practice to test several batches of the enzyme and, when a satisfactory batch has been found, obtain a large quantity sufficient for a long period of use.

Bovine fraction V albumin is used both during the isolation and during incubation. Again, there may be considerable variations, and test runs are advisable. Of particular concern in the present context is the fact that many batches of bovine serum fraction V albumin contain very high adenosine deaminase activity. For economic reasons, albumin that is not defatted is often used in the isolation procedure even though defatted albumin is recommended for the actual incubations (Fain, 1975).

For the isolation procedure a Krebs–Ringer phosphate buffer is most convenient, but Rodbell (1964) originally suggested Krebs–Ringer Bicarbonate buffer. The buffer should be fortified with glucose (5–12 m*M*). If high concentrations of phosphate are disadvantageous for the intended experiment, HEPES (25 m*M*) buffers may be used.

White adipose tissue from an appropriate source is removed and kept in a salinic medium at 37°C and visible connective tissue removed. Rat epididymal (or parametrial) fat is the most common source. When young rats (less than 200 g) are used as donors, the cells obtained are remarkably stable and consistent in size and responsiveness. When fat from older rats or canine or human fat is used as the source, the cells are often much less stable and more variable. The difference is often already observed during the isolation procedure. When the cells are fragile, lipid droplets or even fat cakes appear at the top of the isolation vessel. It is often advisable, when this type of problem is encountered, to sacrifice completeness of digestion for brevity of exposure to the collagenase preparation. For example, we usually incubate adipose tissue from young rats for 30–45 min with collagenase, but subcutaneous canine adipose tissue for only 5 min. It was recently suggested by Londos that the addition of 0.2 μM adenosine to the buffer solution used in the preparation of fat cells markedly reduces the problem of cell lysis (personal communication).

The cut pieces of adipose tissue are placed in plastic or siliconized glass vessels containing 2 ml buffer with 4% albumin and 0.2–1.0 mg/ml collagenase. The tissue is incubated for the appropriate period of time in a shaking water bath

Table I. Inhibitory Effect of Adenosine on the Cyclic AMP Accumulation Induced by 3 μ*M* Noradrenaline (NA)

	NA-induced increase in cyclic AMP (pmoles/10^5 cells)		Percent inhibition by adenosine	
	pH 7.4	pH 7.0	pH 7.4	pH 7.0
Control	13.5 ± 0.7	5.5 ± 0.9		
Adenosine 0.1 μ*M*	10.2 ± 1.2	1.4 ± 0.4	24	75
Adenosine 1.0 μ*M*	5.5 ± 0.9	−0.2 ± 0.2	59	104

(approximately 100 cycles per minute). Very vigorous shaking can disrupt fragile fat cells.

After digestion the incubation mixture is filtered through nylon chiffon, silk cloth, or even pieces of nylon stocking. Mild pressure is often needed to speed up the filtration. The filtrate is diluted with albumin-containing medium without collagenase and briefly centrifuged at a low force (just sufficient to float the cells) in plastic centrifuge tubes. The medium underneath the floating cell layer is aspirated off, fresh buffer is added, and the cells are gently resuspended. This washing procedure is repeated twice (possibly more if insulin responses are studied). The cells are resuspended in an adequate amount of buffer and the cell density determined.

B. Incubation of Fat Cells

After counting, the cells are distributed in individual plastic flasks. The cell density should be between 20–250 × 10^3/ml. It was originally found by Schwabe and co-workers that the potency of adenosine as an antilipolytic agent was much higher in dilute than in dense cell suspensions (Schwabe *et al.*, 1973). The reason for this is at least twofold: (1) dense cell suspensions form much higher concentrations of adenosine, which provide a background against which the added adenosine has to compete; (2) the rate of inactivation via uptake and metabolism of added adenosine is faster in a dense than in a dilute cell suspension (cf. Fredholm, 1978a).

If Krebs–Ringer Bicarbonate is used as the buffer, it is essential that the atmosphere is well equilibrated with a suitable concentration of CO_2 in the gas phase, as otherwise the pH will rapidly change. It has been shown that lipolysis and cyclic AMP production are both very sensitive to pH changes (Fredholm and Hjemdahl, 1976). With other incubation buffers the composition of the gas medium is less critical, but, nonetheless, care must be taken that the pH does not change overly much during incubation. For example, using a phosphate buffer we found that the pH dropped as much as 0.5 pH units during 1-hr incubation (Fredholm and Hjemdahl, 1976). In this context it should be emphasized that even small changes in pH markedly affect the potency of adenosine (Hjemdahl and Fredholm, 1976a). This is demonstrated by the data presented in Table I.

After a brief period of equilibration, the lipolysis or cyclic AMP production is stimulated by a suitable agent. Noradrenaline is the physiologically most relevant agent and is very potent as a stimulator of lipolysis and cyclic AMP accumulation. EC_{50} for lipolysis is approximately 100 n*M* (Fredholm and Hjemdahl, 1976; Fredholm, 1978a,b) while the EC_{50} for cyclic AMP accumulation is approximately 1 μ*M* (Fredholm and Hjemdahl, 1976). The reason for this difference is that only small increases in cyclic AMP are sufficient to maximally activate lipolysis. For example, a doubling of cyclic AMP is associated with a 20-fold increase in lipolysis, even though the maximal increase in cyclic AMP may be more than 100-fold over control (Hjemdahl and Fredholm, 1976a). The potency of lipolytic agent is very strongly dependent upon the presence of endogenous inhibitory factor. It also has been described that there are seasonal differences (Londos, personal communication).

When the antilipolytic (and cyclic AMP inhibitory) effect of adenosine analogs is to be studied, it may be advantageous to add these drugs prior to the addition to the lipolytic agent. Similarly the effect of xanthine derivatives is larger if these drugs are added prior to the adenosine analog, the actions of which are to be antagonized. The timing should be rather exact to maximize reproducibility between experimental runs. The timing of stopping the incubation is similarly important, especially for cyclic AMP, as these incubations are commonly briefer than those for the estimation of lipolysis.

C. Measurement of Lipolysis and Cyclic AMP

Lipolysis is the process whereby stored triglycerides are hydrolyzed to form nonesterified fatty acids and glycerol; three moles of fatty acids being formed per mole of glycerol. The process is catalyzed by a series of enzymes, the rate-limiting one being the first in the sequence, triglyceride lipase (Steinberg *et al.*, 1975). This enzyme is regulated by phosphorylation–dephosphorylation reactions catalyzed by cyclic AMP-dependent protein kinase and a relatively specific protein phosphatase (Strålfors and Belfrage, 1984). The degree of activation of the protein kinase is a function of the cellular cyclic AMP content.

Lipolysis may be assessed by determining the release of either glycerol or FFA. The former is generally to be preferred since glycerol is, in the majority of species, reutilized to a very minor extent by adipose tissue and hence gives a good measure of the hydrolytic process. FFA, by contrast, may be formed not only by complete hydrolysis of triglycerides but also by a partial hydrolysis to di- and monoglycerides. This can be a problem for example when the rate of lipolysis is very strongly stimulated (e.g., Fredholm *et al.*, 1973). Another complicating factor is that FFA are reutilized by the fat cells. They are used as substrates for oxidation and more importantly they are re-esterified with glycerol-3-phosphate formed via a branch in the Embden–Meyerhof pathway (see Fredholm, 1970). When FFA are used to assess the rate of lipolysis, the rate may be either overestimated (partial hydrolysis or triglycerides, for example, after stimulation with high doses of theophylline; Fredholm *et al.*, 1973) or underestimated (re-esterification of FFA stimulated, e.g., by insulin, prostaglandins, glucose, and pyruvate; Fredholm, 1970, 1971).

Several methods to measure glycerol have been published. My own experience is limited to the method described by Laurell and Tibbling (1966), which involves the fluorimetric measurement of NADH formed by glycerol-3-phosphate dehydrogenase acting on glycerol-3-phosphate formed from ATP and the glycerol in the sample by the action of glycerol kinase. In its original version, the samples are deproteinized with $ZnSO_4$ and $Ba(OH)_2$ leading to a 10-fold dilution of the samples. This is possible in some applications, such as the perifusion model described below, when the absolute level of glycerol is low. Glycerol release is difficult to determine accurately after short periods of incubation and 1 hr is the most commonly used time interval.

Recently, a method to measure continuously the release of fatty acids was described (Nilsson and Belfrage, 1981). When fatty acids are released into the medium at pH 7.4, there is an essentially stoichiometric production of protons that may be determined by continuous titration with NaOH using a pH-stat titration apparatus. The described modification allows the continuous determination of lipolytic rate, which, of course, makes it possible to do kinetic experiments and also allows measurements of lipolysis at much shorter time intervals than is practicable with the glycerol methods.

Cyclic AMP may be measured in samples of the incubated fat cells at the same time intervals as glycerol is determined. However, the time course for cyclic AMP accumulation is quite different, a peak of cyclic AMP usually being observed within a few minutes after incubation with the lipolytic drugs. Since small cyclic AMP changes are produced with physiologically relevant concentrations of lipolytic drugs, it is usually preferable to measure cyclic AMP at shorter time intervals than are used in the assay for lipolysis, since the changes in cyclic AMP content may otherwise be below the detection limit.

An easy and valid method is to deproteinize aliquots of the incubates with perchloric acid, neutralize with KOH and Tris, and determine cyclic AMP content by one of the common competitive binding methods, e.g., that described by Brown *et al.* (1972).

Another method that can be used to study qualitative aspects is to prelabel the fat cell ATP stores with [^{3}H]adenine (or [^{3}H]adenosine) for 15 min (Schönhöfer and Skidmore, 1971). After incubation with the lipolytic drug to be studied, labeled cyclic AMP is separated from other labeled compounds by chromatographic methods and by $ZnSO_4/Ba(OH)_2$ precipitation (Fredholm and Hjemdahl, 1976; Fredholm *et al.*, 1982). Provided that cyclic AMP breakdown is completely abolished, this method may be used to obtain a semiquantitative estimate of adenylate cyclase activity in intact cells.

A methodology to determine the degree of phosphorylation of the hormone-sensitive triglyceride lipase in intact adipocytes in parallel with measurements of lipolysis has also been described (Nilsson, 1981). The method involves incubation of fat cells with radiolabeled orthophosphate to label the adipocyte ATP stores. At fixed intervals, the reaction is terminated and the radioactivity comigrating with hormone sensitive lipase on an SDS–PAGE is determined. The method has

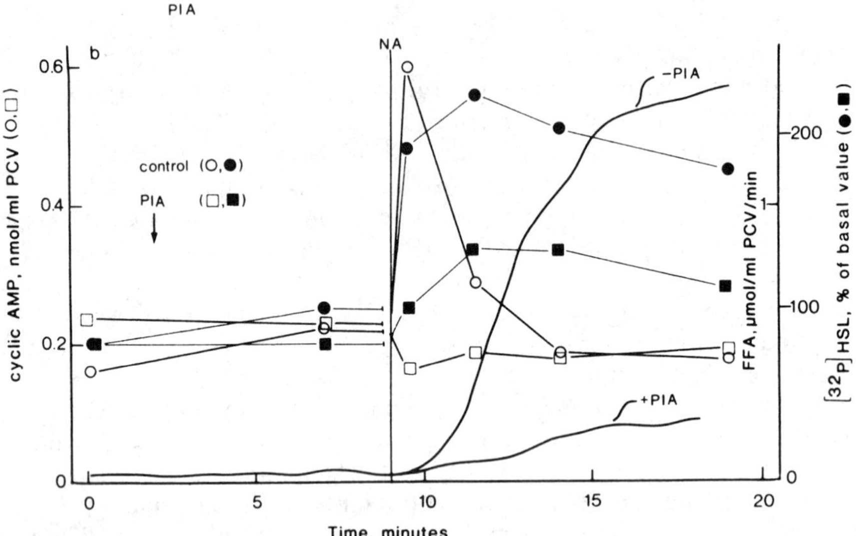

Figure 1. Effect of phenylisopropyladenosine (PIA, 100 n*M*) on basal and nordrenaline (NA; 0.5 μ*M*)-induced level of cyclic AMP, phosphorylation of hormone-sensitive lipase (HSL), and release of free fatty acids (FFA). Unpublished results from Nilsson and Belfrage, by permission.

been used to determine the relationship between the lipolytic response to adenosine deaminase and the degree of phosphorylation of hormone sensitive lipase (Figure 1).

D. Measurement of Adenosine Levels and Adenosine Metabolism

1. Uptake

Several techniques have been used to determine the uptake of nucleosides by fat cells: centrifugation followed by aspiration of medium (Ebert and Schwabe, 1973); filtration through glass fiber filters (Fain *et al.*, 1978); or separation of fat cells from medium by centrifugation through oil of silicon oil (Rosenblit and Levy, 1980; Fredholm, unpublished). The basis for the latter method has been described by Gammeltoft *et al.* (1972). Even with these techniques it is apparent that not only uptake but also phosphorylation is measured. Thus, after 20 sec, 5 times more radioactivity is already present as nucleotides than is present as free adenosine (Fain *et al.*, 1978). Rosenblit and Levy (1980) reported that the initial rate of accumulation of labeled adenosine (1 min) followed Michaelis–Menten kinetics, but others have failed to provide firm evidence for saturability (Fain *et al.*, 1978). The initial rate of nucleotide accumulation is a saturable process with an apparent K_m of 1–5 μ*M* (Fredholm and Hjemdahl, 1979). It is interesting that in fat cells the rate of phosphorylation of adenine is higher than that seen with adenosine. Hypoxanthine is apparently also rapidly phosphorylated in fat cells. This fact could possibly explain the curious finding that under some circumstances the rate of incorporation of label into nucleotides from [^{3}H]adenosine is blocked by in-

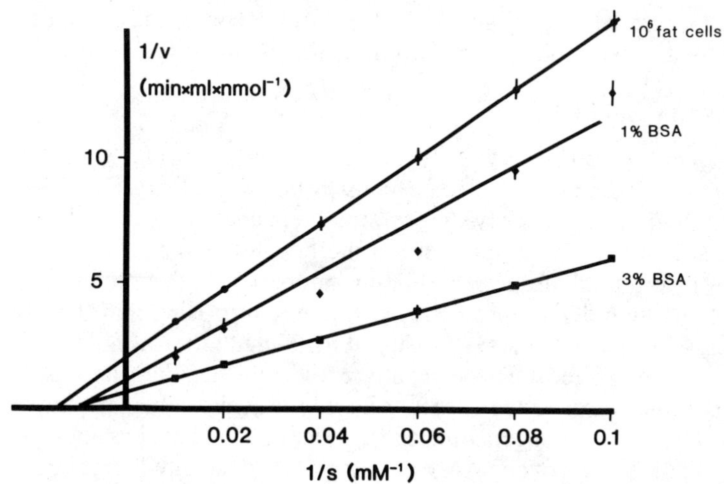

Figure 2. Adenosine deaminase activity in isolated rat fat cells and in a preparation of bovine serum albumin (BSA). The 286,000 cells were washed in a albumin-free medium before homogenization in 0.5 ml assay medium. BSA was dissolved directly in the assay medium. Mean ± S.D. of triplicate determinations.

hibitors of adenosine metabolism to inosine and hypoxanthine (Fredholm, unpublished). Much more work on the mechanism of uptake and further metabolism of adenosine is necessary in the fat cell system. The methods described in earlier chapters of this volume should be employed. Furthermore, account should be taken of the fact that there are saturable binding sites for adenosine intracellularly (e.g., SAH hydrolase).

2. *Adenosine Deamination*

Deamination of adenosine to inosine leads to loss of biological activity. Whereas the bulk of the adenosine kinase activity in adipose tissue is present in fat cells, the adenosine deaminase activity is mainly present in other cell types (Green and Newsholme, 1981; Sollevi and Fredholm, 1981b). Moreover, as already mentioned, considerable deaminase activity may be provided by fraction V albumin preparations. This is illustrated in Figure 2. This may complicate the interpretation of some results regarding the metabolic fate of adenosine in adipose tissue.

3. *Adenosine Release*

The release of endogenous adenosine from adipocytes has, to my knowledge, not been studied directly. On the other hand, there have been some studies of the release of labeled adenosine after prelabeling of the adenine nucleotide stores essentially as described above (Fredholm and Hjemdahl, 1979; Fain, 1979). However, the results obtained have been mainly qualitative and the results obtained, e.g., that noradrenaline can increase release of adenosine, have not been followed up with quantitative study of the mechanisms involved.

4. *Adenosine Levels*

In their pioneering study, Schwabe and co-workers (1973) reported that the medium during incubation with fat cells contained adenosine. Since that time several methods to accurately determine adenosine levels have been published, mostly based on HPLC. Using such a method we find that the adenosine concentration in the medium after a 30-min incubation with fat cells is 42 ± 10 n*M*. In view of the high deaminase activity, it is not surprising that the inosine levels are higher. The net increase in inosine during incubation was increased by noradrenaline (unpublished). These results could indicate that the concentration of adenosine in the water space surrounding the fat cells is higher than 50 n*M*. This would explain the data suggesting that endogenous adenosine does play a role in regulating lipolysis and cyclic AMP accumulation in isolated rat fat cells (Schwabe *et al.*, 1973).

E. Perifusion of Fat Cells

A method has been described whereby white fat cells may be perifused (Allen *et al.*, 1975). This method offers some advantages over conventional incubation techniques. Thus, rapid changes in lipolytic rate may be followed with this technique and the problem of interfering products (such as endogenous adenosine) accumulating in the medium is circumvented.

Perifused fat cells have been used to study the release and actions of adenosine (Turpin *et al.*, 1977; Solomon *et al.*, 1980; Hjemdahl and Sollevi, 1978; Fredholm and Hjemdahl, 1979). Using this technique, Turpin and co-workers (1977) could confirm the finding of Schwabe and others (1973) that medium used for incubation of fat cells contains an antilipolytic factor. This factor is removed by the addition of adenosine deaminase. Turpin and co-workers (1977) found that adenosine deaminase per se caused a substantial stimulation of lipolysis, but this could not be confirmed by Hjemdahl and Sollevi (1978). There are also other discrepancies in the literature. Thus, Turpin and co-workers (1977) found that 0.1 μM adenosine completely abolished the lipolytic response to 0.3 μM noradrenaline, whereas Hjemdahl and Sollevi (1978) reported only a 30% inhibition by a ten times higher concentration of adenosine. Further studies are necessary to explain the reported difference in adenosine potency, which amounts to two orders of magnitude, and in sensitivity to adenosine deaminase. It should be pointed out that the basal concentration of adenosine is between 0.1 and 1 μM in most tissues and body fluids (see below). If fat cells are indeed as sensitive to the effects of adenosine as the results of Turpin *et al.* (1977) suggest, then an essentially complete inhibition of lipolysis under physiological conditions can be expected.

III. CELL-FREE SYSTEMS

Many of the biochemical events underlying the actions of adenosine in adipose tissue have also been studied in cell-free systems. Even though pertinent studies have been performed on cyclic nucleotide phosphodiesterases, protein kinases, and the lipases, I will forego these and focus on the studies of binding of adenosine analogs and of adenylate cyclase regulation.

Both these types of study require the use of a purified preparation of cell membranes from fat cells. A method to prepare such membranes has been described by Jarett (1974). Briefly, fat cells are prepared as described above and extensively washed in 0.25 *M* sucrose containing 10 m*M* tris-C1 (pH 7.4) and 1 m*M* EDTA. They are homogenized in a glass–teflon homogenizer in the same medium. After centrifugation at 1000*g* for 10 min the supernatant is centrifuged at 17,000*g* for 20 min and the pellet resuspended and placed on a discontinuous Ficoll gradient. The resulting membrane fraction has been characterized biochemically and morphologically. This method or a variation of it has been used in most studies on adipocyte cell membranes.

A. Studies of Adenosine Analog Binding

The general methodology involved in the study of adenosine receptors has been described in detail in earlier sections of this volume. The major study in relation to fat cells is the paper by Trost and Schwabe (1981), who studied the binding of ^{3}H-phenyliso-propyladenosine (PIA) to fat cell membranes, and reported that K_D was 2–6 n*M*, using several independent means of determination. The (+)-isomer was some 10 times less potent than the (−)-isomer. Using a modification of the assay, the authors found adenosine itself to be about 8 times less potent than (−)-PIA. However, using this modification, the potency of the ligand itself was reduced at least 10-fold, and the only safe conclusion is that the K_D for adenosine is somewhere between 20 and 1000 n*M*.

B. Adenylate Cyclase

An inhibitory effect of adenosine and some adenosine analogues on adenylate cyclase was observed by Fain *et al.* (1972). The most potent compound was 2′,5′-dideoxyadenosine, whereas PIA was virtually ineffective. The reverse order or potency was found when lipolysis was studied.

Trost and Stock (1977) later observed that adenosine was much more potent then 2′,5′-dideoxyadenosine as an inhibitor of cyclic AMP accumulation in isolated rat fat cells, but less potent as an inhibitor of adenylate cyclase activity. These apparent discrepancies were largely resolved by the studies of Londos and coworkers (see Londos *et al.*, 1979). As described elsewhere in this volume, these authors found that adenosine derivatives could inhibit adenylate cyclase activity both by interacting with a so-called P site, presumably localized on the internal aspect of the cell membrane, and by interacting with a so-called R site on the external surface of the membrane. In the studies of Fain *et al.* (1972) the latter site might have remained undetectable because adenosine, formed from the substrate ATP, was already exerting an almost maximal effect. As discussed by Londos *et al.* (1979), the assay conditions are critical. In order to detect the full potency of R-site agonists; deoxy ATP should be substrate, adenosine deaminase be included in the assay, and xanthine phosphodiesterase inhibitors be omitted.

The effect of adenosine acting on R sites is dependent on the presence of GTP and it is amplified by sodium ions (Aktories *et al.*, 1981a), even though sodium ions may not be of importance in intact fat cells. Further studies from this group (Aktories *et al.*, 1981b) demonstrated that phenylisopropyladenosine enhanced the rate of GTP hydrolysis. This could be a primary site of action or it could be a reflection of an enhanced rate of dissociation of quanine nucleotides from the N-protein.

Since fat cells are pure, the use of fat cell membranes to elucidate the detailed mechanisms underlying the coupling of adenosine R-type receptors to inhibition of adenylate cyclase in a single cell type may be performed. It is not easy to study binding and adenylate cyclase inhibition in parallel in most other preparations. Fat cell membranes will therefore probably be used in studies of general significance to elucidate the mechanisms underlying R_i-receptor activation. It may even be found that the inhibition of adenylate cyclase is not the sole mechanism of action of adenosine in adipocytes.

IV. *IN SITU* PERFUSED ADIPOSE TISSUE

A. Preparation

In 1965, Orö *et al.* described a method to study blood flow and lipolysis in the intact canine subcutaneous adipose tissue. A full description of the method was later published (Rosell, 1966). The method depends on the fact that most mammals have, in the inguinal region, a well-circumscribed pad of subcutaneous adipose tissue on either side of the abdominal midline. This fat pad may be completely isolated from all surrounding tissues including the underlying muscle and the overlying mammary tissue and skin. The tissue is supplied by one artery and drained by one vein. There is also a mixed nerve containing intraarterial sympathetic fibers that runs along the artery and vein. The nerve may be cut at the level of the external hiatus of the inguinal canal, placed on bipolar stimulating electrodes, and electrically activated. Similarly the arterial and venous blood lines can be cannulated to allow infusions, to determine various circulatory parameters, and, finally, to allow sampling of arterial and venous blood for determination of metabolic parameters.

B. Blood Flow

Contrary to a commonly held opinion, the resting blood flow in subcutaneous adipose tissue is rather high (between 2 and 10 ml/min per 100 g tissue; Fredholm, 1970). There is evidence that adenosine plays a role in regulating adipose tissue blood flow already under basal conditions (Sollevi and Fredholm, 1981a), while its role in determining other vascular functions is less clear.

In the subcutaneous adipose tissue, it is possible to study simultaneously not only the arteriolar resistance section, which determines blood flow, but also the

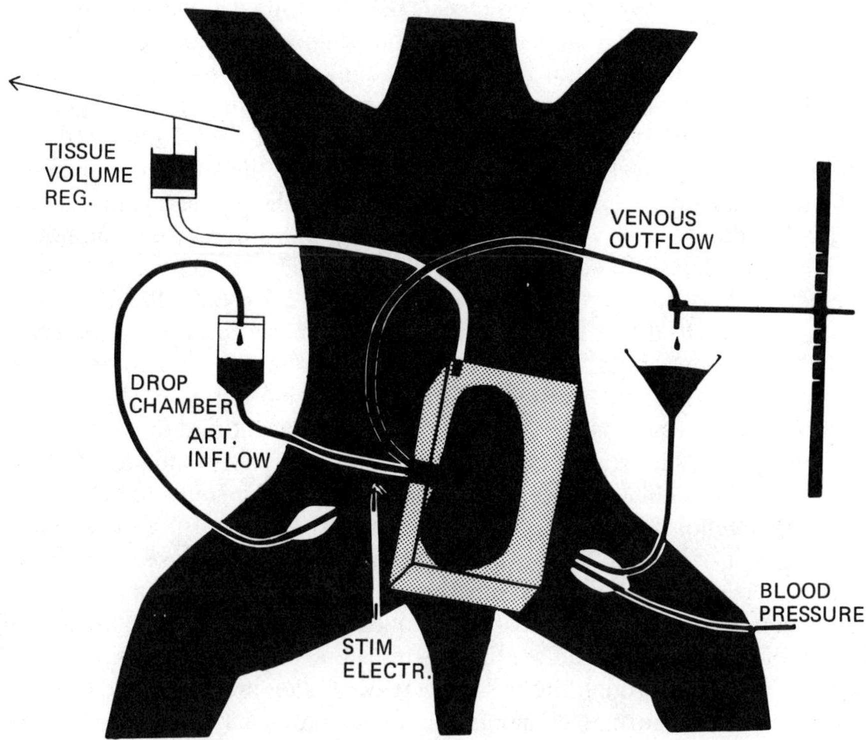

Figure 3. Schematic representation of the canine subcutaneous adipose tissue preparation set up for the study of series-coupled vascular sections. For details see text and Fredholm *et al.* (1970).

exchange section, which is responsible for the capillary exchange, and the venous section, responsible for the vascular capacitance (Öberg and Rosell, 1967). The preparation used is schematically represented in Figure 3. The tissue is enclosed in a water-filled plethysmograph, connected to a volume recorder. The volume changes are an adequate measure of the changes in the venous capacitance section of the tissue. The venous outflow may be adjusted to different heights above the preparation. The bulk of the increase in pressure is transmitted to the capillary exchange section, which thus experiences an increased hydrostatic pressure head. This leads to an outward filtration of fluid, which can be observed as a continuous increase in tissue volume. Based on the increase in venous outflow pressure and the observed volume increase, the so-called capillary filtration coefficient can be determined. This parameter is a measure of the dimensions of the exchange section (or more strictly the dimensions of the pore systems capable of filtering water). In addition several techniques to study the diffusion of water- and lipid-soluble drugs in adipose tissue have been established (see Linde, 1976).

The resistance section of adipose tissue may be studied either by determining the changes in blood flow at an essentially constant arterial blood pressure (e.g., Sollevi and Fredholm, 1981a) or by studying changes in perfusion pressure when the blood flow through the tissue is kept constant by some kind of perfusion apparatus (cf. Rosell, 1966; Fredholm, 1970; Sollevi and Fredholm, 1981a). The former method is obviously the more physiological, but the latter has some other advantages. Thus, adenosine, as well as lipolytic catecholamines, is rapidly eliminated by the adipose tissue. Therefore, the response *in situ* may depend not only on the concentration of the drug in the arterial inlet but also on the total amount of drug administered to the tissue (cf. Hjemdahl and Fredholm, 1976b). Furthermore it can be quite difficult to adjust the rate of intraarterial drug delivery to match the changes in blood flow exactly when, for example, a potent vasodilator such as adenosine is given. Assume that the resting blood flow is 2 ml/min in a given preparation of adipose tissue. Adenosine is then infused at the rate of 20 nmoles/min, giving an arterial concentration of adenosine (nominal) of 10 μM, which is clearly vasodilatory, increasing the blood flow by some 200%. The concentration of adenosine is then reduced, blood flow falls, causing the adenosine concentration to rise and flow to increase, and so on. The dose adjustment is particularly hazardous when the sympathetic vasoconstrictor fibers are activated during the administration of adenosine. On one hand, the nominal adenosine concentration increases due to the continuous infusion, while on the other hand, the transit time of blood through the tissue decreases; allowing more time of contact of adenosine with the formed elements and the degrading enzymes. The net result is very difficult to predict. The above discussion has, I hope, made it clear that constant flow and constant pressure arrangements should preferrably both be used to allow firm conclusions to be drawn.

Instead of adding exogenous adenosine, it is possible to raise the endogenous adenosine content by, for example, giving an adenosine uptake inhibitor or an inhibitor of adenosine deaminase, or both. Provided that a methodology to determine the resulting changes in adenosine levels is used, this method can also be used to generate dose–response curves (cf. Fredholm and Sollevi, 1981; Sollevi and Fredholm, 1981a).

Finally, it can be mentioned in this context that adipose tissue is a convenient source not only of fat cells but also of small vessels. Such vessel preparations may be used to advantage to determine the mechanism of action of adenosine analogues in the vasculature.

C. Lipolysis

The rate of lipolysis *in vivo* is assessed by determining the rate of glycerol release from adipose tissue. To this end, arterial blood and blood leaving the adipose tissue is sampled and the veno-arterial concentration difference in plasma is determined. This value is multipled by the rate of plasma flow (blood flow × hematocrit). The basal rate of lipolysis is usually about 1 nmole/min per g tissue, but increases markedly after a period of starvation (Fredholm *et al*., 1973).

Table II. Release of Glycerol and of Noradrenaline Induced by Sympathetic Nerve Stimulation (2, 4, and 8 Hz) for 2 min[a,b]

	2 Hz	4 Hz	8 Hz
Glycerol outflow (μmoles/100 g)	8.7 ± 1.3 (5)	18.1 + 1.2 (5)	28.9 ± 1 (5)
Noradrenaline outflow (pmoles/100 g)	30.7 ± 4.2 (5)	70.5 ± 14.2 (5)	157.6 ± 21.6 (5)

[a] Adipose tissue weight 18 to 54 g (mean 34 g).
[b] Number of observations given in parentheses.

There is good evidence that the physiologically relevant stimulus to enhance lipolysis is sympathetic nerve activity (cf. Fredholm, 1970, 1984). The magnitude of the lipolytic response to sympathetic nerve stimulation is a function of the stimulation frequency (Sollevi *et al.*, 1981; Table II), and the time of stimulation (Fredholm, 1970; Table III). On the other hand, the lipolytic response is virtually identical in free flow and constant flow perfused adipose tissue (Table III). The size of the adipose tissue is a factor in determining the magnitude of the lipolytic response. Thus, adipose tissue from obese individuals appears to release less glycerol per unit fat weight than does adipose tissue from lean individuals.

When lipolysis is measured *in vivo*, it is even more important to use glycerol release as the index than it is *in vitro* (see above). The reason is that re-esterification may be so promiment that all the fatty acids liberated are re-esterified by the adipose tissue before any mobilization takes place (e.g., Fredholm and Rosell, 1970). The factors determining the magnitude of this re-esterification are the availability of α-glycerolphosphate and the concentration of fatty acids. The availability of α-glycerolphosphate is enhanced by increasing glucose uptake and by increasing the cytoplasmic NADH/NAD ratio. The availability of nonesterified fatty acids is increased by enhancing the rate of lipolysis and also by decreasing

Table III. Glycerol Release following Stimulation of the Sympathetic Nerve Supply by 4 Hz for Different Periods of Time (5, 10, and 20 min)[a,b]

	μmoles/100 g		
	5 min	10 min	20 min
Constant outflow	14 ± 6 (18)	23 + 10 (19)	
Free flow	11 ± 3 (5)	25 ± 9 (7)	44 ± 15 (6)

[a] Adipose tissue weight 20–110 g (mean 51 g).
[b] Number of observations given in parentheses.

the rate of transport of the fatty acids away from the tissue, by, e.g., decreasing the blood flow (Belfrage *et al.*, 1979). Thus, the proportions of the two products of lipolysis, glycerol and FFA, may be altered by changes in blood flow.

Not only re-esterification but also lipolysis may be altered by decreases in blood flow. Thus, during sympathetic nerve stimulation, there is a decrease in blood flow and in the number of capillaries, while glycerol outflow increases only slowly, with the bulk of the release occurring after the period of stimulation (cf. Fredholm, 1970). This pattern of glycerol efflux from adipose tissue is altered if α-adrenoceptors are blocked (Fredholm and Rosell, 1968). Furthermore, the total release of lipolytic products is much higher after α-adrenoceptor blockade. The following factors contribute to this effect:

1. During severe vasoconstriction products formed of lipolysis are trapped within the tissue and are released only after cessation of stimulation.
2. During severe vasoconstriction, the activation of lipolysis per se is delayed, possibly because the neurotransmitter itself is trapped and reaches the fat cells that are not directly innervated, with a more delayed time course.
3. Blockade of presynaptic α-adrenoceptors causes more NA to be released and hence lipolysis to increase.
4. Simultaneous activation of α- and β-adrenoceptors stimulates the formation of adenosine, which inhibits lipolysis and decreases the release of NA (Hedqvist and Fredholm, 1976). The last-mentioned aspect will be discussed further below.

In order to study the role of adenosine in intact adipose tissue, several approaches can be used. For example, the dose–response curve for exogenous adenosine may be compared with the levels of adenosine actually found in the tissue. The levels of endogenous adenosine can be altered by drugs that influence its inactivation, while the effects of adenosine antagonists, e.g., xanthine derivatives, may be studied. All these approaches have been used.

When the antilipolytic effect of exogenous adenosine is to be studied in blood perfused adipose tissue, there are problems because of the rapid rate of degradation of adenosine. Thus, when adenosine is infused intraarterially and blood samples are taken on the venous side, after a transit of 40 sec, only 5% of the added adenosine is recovered intact. A transit period of 20 sec resulted in recovery of about 40% of the added adenosine (Fredholm and Sollevi, 1981). It has been shown by tracer techniques that the transit time through adipose tissue is between 10 and 20 sec (Linde *et al.*, 1974). Thus, during a normal transit through adipose tissue, the blood cells eliminate about half of the added adenosine. In addition there is elimination of adenosine by the adipose tissue. During intraarterial infusion of adenosine (3–40 nmoles/min), 11% was recovered on the venous side as adenosine and an additional 10% as inosine (Fredholm and Sollevi, 1981).The recovery of adenosine is much enhanced by inhibiting adenosine deaminase with EHNA (2–5 μM) and even further by also adding dipyridamole (2 μM). This combination reduces the elimination of adenosine by elements formed in blood

Table IV. Relationship between Arterial and Venous Adenosine Concentration and the Inhibition of Lipolysis Induced by Sympathetic Nerve Stimulation

Intraarterial infusion	Adenosine concentration (μM)		Lipolysis (% of control)
	Arterial	Venous	
NaCl	0.24 ± 0.03	0.31 ± 0.04	100
Adenosine	3.2	0.33	100
EHNA	0.30 ± 0.09	0.40 ± 0.09	104
EHNA + dipyridamole	0.27 ± 0.03	0.7 ± 0.1	60
		$p < 0.01$	$p < 0.05$
	2-Chloroadenosine (μM)		
	Arterial	Venous	
2-chloroadenosine	2.0	1.8	5

to nearly zero and the elimination of adenosine by adipose tissue to about 30% (Fredholm and Sollevi, 1981).

Thus, when the dose–response curve for adenosine as an antilipolytic drug *in vivo* is to be determined, it is not sufficient merely to plot administered dose versus lipolysis, since this will markedly underestimate the potency of adenosine, but the actual concentrations of adenosine have to be measured. When this is done, it is found that the IC_{50} of adenosine against nerve-stimualtion-induced lipolysis is close to 1 μM (Sollevi and Fredholm, 1981b). The results presented in Table IV show the lack of correlation between the arterial adenosine concentration and lipolysis but show a relationship between venous adenosine concentration and antilipolytic effect.

The methylxanthines (theophylline, caffeine, and 8-phenyl-theophylline) may also be used to assess the role of adenosine in the regulation of lipolysis. Adenosine may be given by intraarterial infusion or given systemically (10 mg/kg b.w.). The arterial plasma concentrations of theophylline must be kept below 100 μM. When this is done, theophylline has no lipolytic effect per se nor does it potentiate lipolysis induced by a brief (2 min) nerve stimulation, but it does enhance lipolysis induced by prolonged nerve stimulation (Sollevi *et al.*, 1981). The reason for this is that only during a prolonged nerve stimulation is the adenosine level enhanced (see below). Similarly, these doses of theophylline can antagonize the antilipolytic effect of dipyridamole. Hence, in this low-concentration range, theophylline is lipolytic when the influence of endogenous adenosine is raised, but not otherwise. 8-Phenyl-theophylline is a more selective adenosine receptor antagonist and may offer advantages as a tool. However, this has not been tested and the extreme lipophilicity of the drug may present complications. Conversely, enprofylline, a xanthine derivative with a lower potency as an adenosine antagonist in adipose tissue (Fredholm and Lindgren, 1983), may be a useful tool by mimicking aspects of theophylline effects that are unrelated to adenosine antagonism. It is interesting

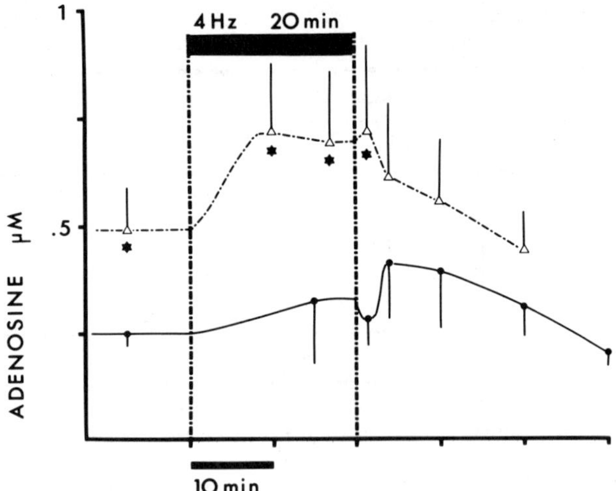

Figure 4. The effect of sympathetic nerve stimulation (4 Hz, 20 min) on venous adenosine concentration and on the fractional release of labelled purines in the absence (●) and presence (△) of dipyridamole (0.5–1 mg/kg i.v.). From Sollevi and Fredholm (1981b), by permission. The stars indicate statistical difference ($p < 0.05$) versus control.

in this context that enprofylline does not raise plasma FFA levels in man, which theophylline does (Persson, personal communication).

D. Adenosine Release and Levels of Adenosine

In order to determine the physiological role of adenosine in adipose tissue, a detailed knowledge of the conditions under which adenosine formation and/or adenosine levels are increased is of utmost importance. There are two main methods to study adenosine release: (1) release of radioactive purines from prelabeled tissue (Fredholm, 1976) or (2) release of endogenous adenosine by determining veno-arterial concentration differences (Fredholm and Sollevi, 1981). Each method has its advantages and disadvantages. The former method in principle measures unidirectional flux of purines, whereas the latter method determines the net effect of release, uptake, and metabolism. On the other hand, the prelabel method may at best be semiquantitative since one cannot be certain that labeling is uniform. A combination of the two methods may therefore yield the most relevant results.

As shown in Figure 4 the two methods may give not only quantitatively, but also qualitatively, different results. Thus, dipyridamole significantly increased basal adenosine levels but decreased the basal fractional release of [^{3}H]purines. This is largely due to the fact that dipyridamole decreases the deamination of adenosine to inosine (the radioactive method determines not only [^{3}H]adenosine release but also the outflow of the metabolites (cf. Fredholm and Sollevi, 1981). Moreover, dipyridamole enhanced the release of adenosine induced by nerve stimulation, whereas the release of [^{3}H]purines was reduced. The explanation for this surprising finding is probably that dipyridamole antagonizes not only carrier-

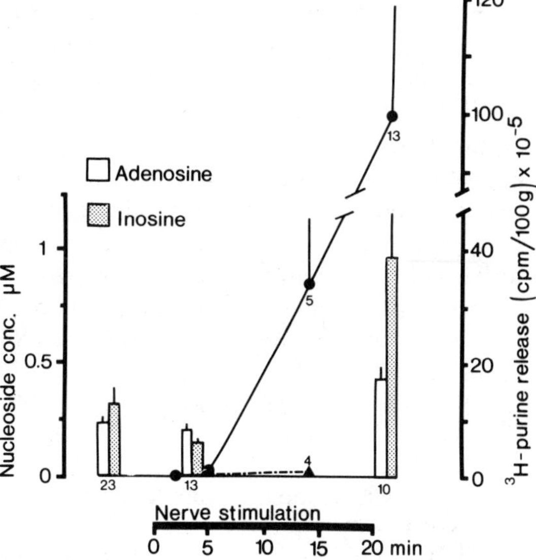

Figure 5. Outflow of purines from subcutaneous adipose tissue induced by sympathetic nerve stimulation (4 Hz, 12V for 2, 5, 15, and 20 min). The bars indicate the venous plasma concentrations of adenosine (open bars) and its primary metabolite inosine (closed bars). The solid lines show the net outflow of [^{3}H]-purines from prelabeled adipose tissue and the broken line the release after α-adrenoceptor blockade. Mean ± S.E.M. The number of observations is given in the figure. From Sollevi and Fredholm (1983), by permission.

mediated influx but also efflux of purines. Finally, the time course of release of endogenous adenosine and radioactive purines was quite different. Again the explanation appears to be that the radioactive purines are composed mainly of adenosine metabolites (Fredholm and Sollevi, 1981).

The findings, however, clearly show that sympathetic nerve stimulation is able to increase adenosine release from adipose tissue. This release has been shown to be entirely dependent on the stimulation of α-adrenoceptors (Fredholm, 1976; Fredholm and Sollevi, 1981). The reason for this is probably that the most important stimulus for adenosine release is tissue hypoxia induced by a decreased blood flow and a decreased number of open capillaries. In particular, the finding that α-adrenoceptor blockade inhibits adenosine release shows that the bulk of the purines do not originate from ATP released from sympathetic nerves as a cotransmitter with noradrenaline. However, β-adrenoceptor stimulation is also of importance (Sollevi and Fredholm, 1983), in agreement with previous findings that the decrease of tissue P_{O_2} is a consequence of a simultaneous reduction in oxygen delivery and stimulation of oxygen consumption (Fredholm *et al.*, 1976).

Further evidence for the view that increased purine release is a secondary consequence of the nerve stimulation is provided by the time course of purine release (Figure 5). Thus, brief nerve stimulation (5 min or less) has little effect, but prolonged nerve stimulation is a powerful stimulus. This finding provides the explanation for our finding that adenosine is a physiologically important regulator of lipolysis induced by prolonged, but not by short periods of nerve stimulation.

V. CONCLUSIONS

This brief overview has demonstrated that a variety of methods to study the role of adenosine in the regulation of lipolysis have been established. The methodology ranges from purely biochemical methods in cell-free systems to techniques to assess the physiology of adenosine.

It has been shown that adenosine binds to structures with properties similar to A_1-(R_i)-adenosine receptors and that it inhibits adenylate cyclase, cyclic AMP accumulation, and the phosphorylation of hormone-sensitive lipase. Adenosine is continuously formed by fat cells and is taken up by these cells and phosphorylated to adenine nucleotides. These processes occur also under *in vivo* conditions, and in unstimulated adipose tissue the concentration of adenosine is close to 0.25 μM. Activation of the sympathetic nerve supply to the tissue increases the adenosine formation and the levels increase. When this occurs, lipolysis is inhibited. Thus, adenosine appears to be a physiologically important modulator of lipolysis.

However, several important questions are still open. Some of these are listed below:

1. How is occupancy of adenosine receptors linked to inhibition of adenylate cyclase?
2. Is inhibition of cyclic AMP formation the only mechanism of action of adenosine in adipose tissue?
3. Is adenosine formed only by direct dephosphorylation of AMP, and, if so, where does it occur?
4. Can one and the same cell both release and take up adenosine? Are the two processes linked?
5. Is adenosine metabolized to SAH to any significant extent in adipose tissue? If so, what are the consequences of this?
6. Is the rate of adenosine formation or metabolism altered by hormonal and nutritional states?
7. Is the adenosine receptor number subject to physiological or pharmacological regulation?
8. What is the role of adenosine in the regulation of fat metabolism in man?

All these questions are amenable to experimental study using slight modifications of presently established methodology. The answers will be not only of importance for our understanding of adipose tissue physiology but also of more general significance for our understanding of the role of adenosine in physiological regulation. Adipose tissue will continue to provide a convenient preparation for important studies in the adenosine field.

ACKNOWLEDGMENTS

Many of the studies briefly reviewed here were carried out in collaboration with Drs. Per Hedqvist, Paul Hjemdahl, Sune Rosell, and Alf Sollevi. The studies were supported primarily by the Swedish Medical Research Council (Prof. no. 2553), by Magnus Bergvalls Foundation, and by Karolinska Institutet.

REFERENCES

Aktories, K., Schultz, G., and Jakobs, K. H. 1981. Na^+ amplifies adenosine receptor-mediated inhibition of adipocyte adenylate cyclase. *Eur. J. Pharmacol., 71*:157–160.

Aktories, K., Schultz, G., and Jakobs, K. H. 1981b. Adenosine receptor-mediated stimulation of GTP hydrolysis in adipocyte membranes. *Life Sci., 30*:269–275.

Allen, D. O., Largis, E. E., Katocs, A. S., Jr., and Ashmore, J. 1975. Perifused fat cells. *Methods Enzymol. 35*:607–612.

Belfrage, E., Hjemdahl, P., and Fredholm, B. B. 1979. Metabolic effects of blood flow restriction in adipose tissue. *Acta Physiol. Scand., 105*:222–227.

Brown, B. L., Eakins, R. P., and Albano, J. D. M. 1972. Saturation assay for cyclic AMP using endogenous binding protein, *Adv. Cyclic Nucleotide Res., 2*:25–40.

Ebert, R., and Schwabe, U. 1973. Studies on the antilipolytic effect of adenosine and related compounds in isolated fat cells. *Naunyn Schmiedebergs Arch. Pharmacol., 278*:247–259.

Fain, J. N. 1975. Isolation of free brown and white fat cells. *Methods Enzymol. 35*:555–561.

Fain, J. N. 1979. Effect of lipolytic agents on adenosine and AMP formation by fat cells. *Biochim. Biophys. Acta, 573*:510–520.

Fain, J. N., Pointer, R. H., and Ward, W. F. 1972. Effects of adenosine nucleosides on adenylate cyclase, phosphodiesterase, cyclic adenosine monophosphate accumulation, and lipolysis in fat cells. *J. Biol. Chem., 247*:6866–6872.

Fain, J. N., Shepherd, R. E., Malbon, C. C., and Moreno, F. J. 1978. Hormonal regulation of triglyceride breakdown in adipocytes. In: *Disturbance in Lipid and Lipoprotein Metabolism*, American Physiological Society pp. 213–228. Ed. by Dietschy, J. M., Gotto, A. M., and Ontko, J. A. Williams & Wilkins, Baltimore.

Fredholm, B. B. 1970. Studies on the sympathetic regulation of circulation and metabolism in isolated canine subcutaneous adipose tissue, *Acta Physiol. Scand.* (*Suppl.*), *354*:1–47.

Fredholm, B. B. 1971. The effect of lactate in canine subcutaneous adipose tissue in situ. *Acta Physiol. Scand., 81*:110–123.

Fredholm, B. B. 1976. Release of adenosine-like material from isolated perfused dog adipose tissue following sympathetic nerve stimulation and its inhibition by adrenergic α-receptor blockade. *Acta Physiol. Scand., 96*:422–430.

Fredholm, B. B. 1978a. Local regulation of lipolysis by fatty acids, prostaglandins and adenosine. *Med. Biol., 56*:249–261.

Fredholm, B. B. 1978b. Effect of adenosine, adenosine analogues and drugs inhibiting adenosine inactivation on lipolysis in rat fat cells. *Acta Physiol. Scand., 102*:191–198.

Fredholm, B. B. 1984. Nervous control of circulation and metabolism in white adipose tissue. In: *New Perspective in Adipose Tissue Structure, Function and Development,* pp. 45–64. Ed. by Van, R. L. R., and Cryer, A. Butterworths, London.

Fredholm, B. B., and Hjemdahl, P. 1976. Inhibition by acidosis of adenosine 3′,5′-cyclic monophosphate accumulation and lipolysis in isolated rat fat cells. *Acta Physiol. Scand., 96*:160–169.

Fredholm, B. B., and Hjemdahl, P. 1979. Uptake and release of adenosine in isolated rat fat cells. *Acta Physiol. Scand., 105*:257–267.

Fredholm, B. B., and Lindgren, E. 1983. The effect of alkylxanthines and other phosphodiesterase inhibitors on adenosine-receptor mediated decrease in lipolysis and cyclic AMP accumulation in rat fat cells. *Acta Pharmacol. Toxicol., 54*:64–71.

Fredholm, B. B., and Rosell, S. 1968. Effect of adrenergic blocking agents on lipid mobilization from canine subcutaneous adipose tissue after sympathetic nerve stimulation. *J. Pharmacol. Exp. Ther., 159*:1–7.

Fredholm, B. B., and Rosell, S. 1970. Effects of prostaglandin E_1 in canine subcutaneous adipose tissue in situ. *Acta Physiol. Scand., 80*:450–458.

Fredholm, B. B., and Sollevi, A. 1981. The release of adenosine and inosine from canine subcutaneous adipose tissue by nerve stimulation and noradrenaline. *J. Physiol., 313*:351–367.

Fredholm, B. B., Jonzon, B., Lindgren, E., and Lindström, K. 1982. Adenosine receptors mediating cyclic AMP production in the rat hippocampus. *J. Neurochem., 39*:165–175.

Fredholm, B. B., Linde, B., and Persson, B. 1973. Effects of fasting on adipose tissue perfused in situ in young dogs. *Scand. J. Clin. Lab. Invest., 31:*79–86.

Fredholm, B. B., Linde, B., Prewitt, R., Jr., and Johnson, P. C. 1976. Oxygen uptake and tissue oxygen tension in canine subcutaneous adipose tissue during adrenergic stimulation. *Acta Physiol. Scand., 97:*48–59.

Fredholm, B. B., Oberg, B., and Rosell, S. 1970. Effect of vasoactive drugs on circulation in canine subcutaneous adipose tissue. *Acta Physiol. Scand., 79:*564–574.

Gammeltoft, S., Glieman, J., Vinter, J., and Osterlind, K. 1972. A technique for rapid separation of isolated fat cells from their incubation medium. *Acta Physiol. Scand., 84:*16–32.

Green, A., and Newsholme, E. A. 1981. Distribution of adenosine metabolizing enzymes between adipocyte and stroma-vascular cells of adipose tissue. *Biochim. Biophys. Acta, 676:*122–124.

Hedqvist, P., and Fredholm, B. B. 1976. Effects of adenosine on adrenergic neurotransmission: prejunctional inhibition and postjunctional enhancement. *Naunyn Schmiedebergs Arch. Pharmacol., 293:*217–223.

Hjemdahl, P., and Fredholm, B. B. 1976a. Cyclic AMP-dependent and independent inhibition of lipolysis by adenosine and decreased pH. *Acta Physiol. Scand., 96:*170–179.

Hjemdahl, P., and Fredholm, B. B. 1976b. Influence of adipose tissue blood flow on the lipolytic response to circulating noradrenaline of normal and reduced pH. *Acta Physiol. Scand., 98:*74–79.

Hjemdahl, P., and Sollevi, A. 1978. Antilipolytic effect of adenosine in isolated perfused fat cells. *Acta Physiol. Scand., 103:*270–274.

Jarett, L. 1974. Subcellular fractionation of adipocytes. In: *Methods in Enzymology*, Volume 31, pp. 60–71. Ed. by Fleischer, S., and Parker, L., Academic Press, New York.

Laurell, S., and Tibbling, G. 1966. An enzymatic fluorimetric micromethod for the determination of glycerol. *Clin. Chim. Acta, 13:*317–322.

Linde, B. 1976. Studies on the vascular exchange function in canine subcutaneous adipose tissue. *Acta Physiol. Scand.* (*Suppl.*), 433:1–43.

Linde, B., Chisholm, G., and Rosell, S. 1974. The influence of sympathetic activity and histamine on the blood-tissue exchange of solutes in canine adipose tissue. *Acta Physiol. Scand., 92:*154–155.

Londos, C., Wolff, J., and Cooper, D. M. F. 1979. Action of adenosine on adenylate cyclase. In: *Physiological and Regulatory Functions of Adenosine and Adenine Nucleotides*, pp. 271–281 Ed. by Baer H. P., and Drummond, G. I. Raven Press, New York,

Nedergaard, J., and Lindberg, O. 1982. The brown fat cell. *Int. Rev. Cytol.,* 187–286.

Nilsson, N. O. 1981. Studies on the short term regulation of lipolysis in rat fat cells with special regard to the anti-lipolytic effect of insulin. *Doctoral Thesis for the Department of Biochemistry*, Lund, pp. 1–43.

Nilsson, N. O., and Belfrage, P. 1981. Continuous measurement of free fatty acid release from intact adipocytes by pH-stat titration. *Methods Enzymol. 72:*319–325.

Öberg, B., and Rosell, S. 1967. Sympathetic control of consecutive vascular sections in canine subcutaneous adipose tissue. *Acta Physiol. Scand., 71:*47–56.

Orö, L., Rosell, S., and Wallenberg, L. 1965. Circulatory and metabolic processes in adipose tissue in vivo. *Nature, 205:*178–179.

Rodbell, M. 1964. Metabolism of isolated fat cells. I. Effects of hormones on glucose metabolism and lipolysis. *J. Biol. Chem., 239:*375–380.

Rosell, S. 1966. Release of free fatty acids from subcutaneous adipose tissue in dogs following sympathetic nerve stimulation. *Acta Physiol. Scand., 67:*343–351.

Rosenblit, P. D., and Levy, D. 1980. Photoaffinity labelling of the adenosine transport system in adipocyte plasma membranes. *Arch. Biochem. Biophys., 204:*331–339.

Schönhöfer, P. S., and Skidmore, I. F. 1971. Studies on the conditions for cyclic AMP formation in homogenized and intact fat cells by use of ^{3}H-ATP and ^{3}H-adenine. *Pharmacology, 6:*109–125.

Schwabe, U., Ebert, R., and Erbler, H. C. 1973. Adenosine release from isolated fat cells and its significance for the effects of hormones on cyclic 3′,5′-AMP levels and lipolysis. *Naunyn Schmiedebergs Arch. Pharmacol., 275:*133–148.

Sollevi, A., and Fredholm, B. B. 1981a. Role of adenosine in adipose tissue circulation. *Acta Physiol. Scand., 112:*293–298.

Sollevi, A., and Fredholm, B. B. 1981b. The antilipolytic effect of endogenous and exogenous adenosine in canine adipose tissue in situ. *Acta Physiol. Scand., 113*:53–60.

Sollevi, A., and Fredholm, B. B. 1983. Influence of adenosine on the vascular responses to sympathetic nerve stimulation in the canine subcutaneous adipose tissue. *Acta Physiol. Scand., 119*:15–24.

Sollevi, A., Hjemdahl, P., and Fredholm, B. B. 1981. Endogenous adenosine inhibits lipolysis induced by nerve stimulation without inhibiting noradrenaline release in canine subcutaneous adipose tissue in vivo, *Naunyn Schmiedebergs Arch. Pharmacol., 316*:112–119.

Solomon, S. S., Turpin, B. P., and Duckworth, W. C. 1980. Comparative studies of the antilipolytic effect of insulin and adenosine in the perifused isolated cell. *Horm. Metab. Res., 12*:601–604.

Steinberg, D., Mayer, S. E., Khoo, J. C., Miller, E. A., Miller, R. E., Fredholm, B. B., and Eichner, R. 1975. Hormonal regulation of lipase, phosphorylase and glycogen synthase in adipose tissue. *Adv. Cyclic Nucleotide Res., 5*:549–568.

Strålfors, P., and Belfrage, P. 1984. Reversible phosphorylation of hormone-sensitive lipase/cholesterol ester hydrolase in the hormonal control of adipose tissue lipolysis and of adrenal stereoidogenesis. In: *Molecular Aspects of Cellular Regulation. Recently Discovered Systems of Enzyme Regulation by Reversible Phosphorylation—Further Advances*, pp. 27–62. Ed. by Cohen, P., Elseiver, Amsterdam. In press.

Trost, T., and Schwabe, U. 1981. Adenosine receptors in fat cells. Identification by (-)-N^6-[^{3}H]-phenylisopropyladenosine binding. *Mol. Pharmacol., 19*:228–235.

Trost, T., and Stock, K. 1977. Effects of adenosine derivatives on cAMP accumulation and lipolysis in rat adipocytes and on adenylate cyclase in adipocyte plasma membranes. *Naunyn Schmiedeberg's Arch. Pharmacol., 299*:33–40.

Turpin, B. P., Duckworth, W. C., and Solomon, S. S. 1977. Perifusion of isolated rat adipose cells. Modulation of lipolysis by adenosine. *J. Clin. Invest., 60*:442–448.

Chapter **20**

Criteria for the Involvement of Adenosine and Adenine Nucleotides in Nonadrenergic, Noncholinergic Transmission

Lowie P. Jager* and Adriaan den Hertog†

Department of Pharmacology
Central Veterinary Institute, Lelystad* and Department of Pharmacology
State University, Groningen†
The Netherlands

I. INTRODUCTION

In his synthetic overview of the physiology of synaptic transmission, Eccles (1964) summarized the criteria put forward up to then. Since that time, knowledge of neurohumoral transmission has vastly increased, but Eccles's criteria still provide a good starting point for an appraisal of data and methods used in research concerning the involvement of "purines" in neurotransmission. However, there is a need to incorporate into these five criteria the significant new concepts concerning neurohumoral transmission that have emerged during the past two decades. Among these are:

- Feedback regulation to the presynaptic terminal by the released neurotransmitter or by substances released simultaneously.
- Histochemical identification of nerves based on the neurotransmitter released.
- Release of more than one functional neurotransmitter from one nerve terminal.

Furthermore, we have to take into account that most of the data concerning nonadrenergic, noncholinergic (NANC) nerves indicates that they innervate visceral organs, that the excitation in NANC nerves induces release of neurotransmitter "*en passage*" from nerve varicosities and that the distance between presynaptic terminal and effector organ (mostly smooth muscle cell) is considerably larger than in synapses in the central nervous system or in the endplate in skeletal muscle. In some preparations, interstitial cells of Cajal may also mediate, coordinate, or modulate the transmission between smooth muscle cell and nerve varicosity.

In a commentary, Orrego (1979) updated the criteria for application in studies with preparations of central nervous tissue. Although the proposed division of the criteria into a set of primary and secondary ones seems not wholly appropriate for the present discussion, they reflect a differential assessment of experimental observations that might not be tissue specific. Our adherence to Eccles's criteria is mostly due to the fact that he used the same order as the sequence in the physiological phenomenon studied: presynaptic presence, release, postsynaptic action, inactivation, and pharmacological interference. In the present discussion, we start each section by quoting the relevant criterion, discuss its discriminating power in general, and subsequently consider the physiological and pharmacological data available concerning the NANC nerves and the purinergic nerve hypothesis.

NANC nerves or responses supposedly mediated via intramural NANC nerves are reported from almost all visceral organs of entodermal origin. However, most reports deal with gastrointestinal preparations, among which the guinea pig taenia caecum figures as the "top hit," and far less detailed information is available concerning other organ systems, such as the respiratory tract, esophagus and the urogenital tract. We have therefore chosen to discuss the criteria in relation to the purinergic nerve hypothesis firstly with taenia caecum data and to deal more superficially with information from other preparations. Throughout this chapter, background information as summarized in earlier reviews (Burnstock, 1969, 1972, 1979 and 1981) is assumed and is not specifically mentioned as reference.

As part of the preparation for this discussion, a literature search was carried out. The search strategies are given at the end of this chapter. They are certainly not sophisticated and were developed on the spot, while reacting to the "number of hits" indicated. Subsequent searchers might benefit from our surprises.

II. FIRST CRITERION

The putative neurohumoral transmitter substance must exist in sufficient quantities in the presynaptic terminals, which must also contain a synthesizing enzyme system.

The question arises whether this is a useful criterion in testing the "purinergic nerve" hypothesis. In view of the central role of ATP in energy transport in living cells and regulatory functions of adenosine and adenine nucleotides in many pro-

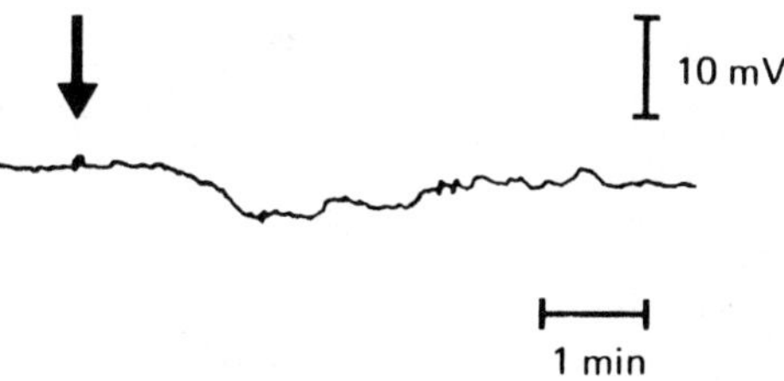

Figure 1. Single sucrose-gap recording from the opossum esophageal circular smooth muscle; upstream in the superfusion medium another preparation was stimulated supramaximally for 5 sec (arrow). Note the hyperpolarizing response due to the elicited release of an active principle from the upstream preparation, presumably the NANC mediator. Courtesy of J. Jury.

cesses, it is unimaginable that there could be nerve varicosities that do not contain "purines" and their synthesizing enzyme system. Due to this lack of possible falsification of the hypothesis, this criterion is at least qualitatively useless. It might, however, be possible to use this criterion on a quantitative basis, if NANC nerves contained significantly more "purines" than other nerves. A quantitive study of the "purine" content of nerve varicosities that might be feasible with fluorizing probes or autoradiographical methods has not yet been reported for autonomic nerves (see Bloom *et al.*, 1972).

An alternative approach to identify NANC nerve varicosities by anatomical characteristics (large opaque vesicles; Robinson *et al.*, 1971) generated a still ongoing debate (Daniel *et al.*, 1977; Gibbins, 1982). This discussion centers on the question whether all NANC nerve-mediated responses are attributable to only one type of NANC neuron. The different opinions might reflect differences between the preparations studied. An intriguing sequel to the Robinson *et al.* (1971) paper is the conclusion by Downes and Taylor (1983) that in toad lungs the NANC-relaxation is not mediated by purinergic nerves.

III. SECOND CRITERION

Stimulation of the presynaptic nerves must release the substance in adequate quantities from the presynaptic terminals.

Although this criterion is usually referred to as the "release" criterion, and interpreted as only demanding evidence that the putative neurotransmitter should be released—the classical Lowei experiment (1921) (Figure 1)—there are at least three different questions hidden in this criterion: (1) are "purines" released after field stimulation, (2) are these "purines" released from NANC nerve, and (3) are they released in sufficient quantities to account for both the transmitter and the modulating cotransmitter functions? In the phrasing of these questions, we have taken into account that the adenine nucleotides are rapidly degraded, with adenosine as a relatively stable product.

With regard to the first question there is now ample evidence that indeed "purines" are released after field stimulation (Burnstock *et al.*, 1978; Huizinga, 1981) (Figure 2).

Concerning the source of the released "purines" the answer is less certain. The release of neurotransmitter from nerve varicosities can be inhibited by substances such as TTX, which block the propagation of nerve action potentials or

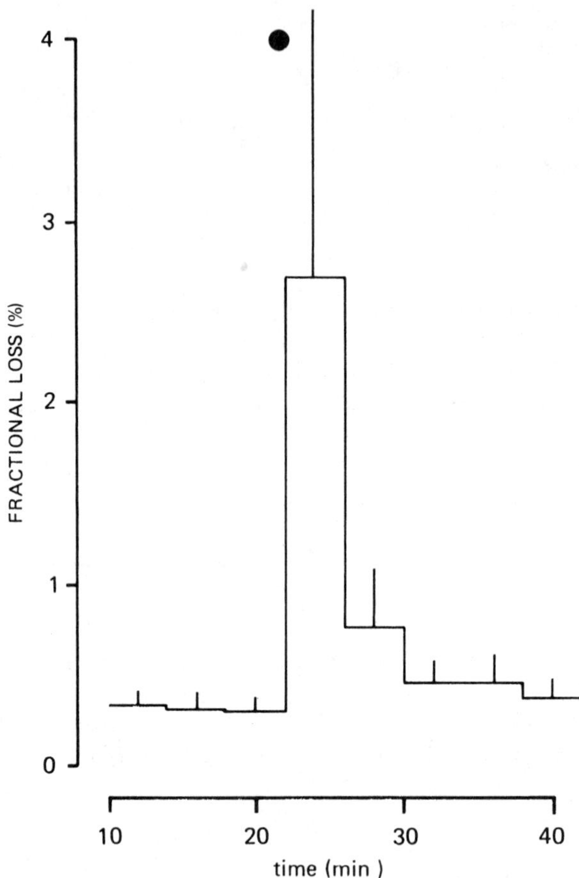

Figure 2. The increase in [^{3}H]-purine loss from taenia caeci (37°C) induced by field stimulation (dot: 20 pps for 4 sec). Bars: the S.E.M. for four different preparations. Courtesy of J. D. Huizinga.

by scorpion venom, which depletes the neurotransmitter stores in nerve varicosities (Kao, 1966; Blaustein and Goldring, 1975). The subsequent disappearance of the smooth muscle cell response indicates both the effectiveness of the interference with transmitter release (Bülbring and Tomita, 1967) and the presence of a possible source of "purines" that is indirectly TTX sensitive. Also the masked release from adrenergic and cholinergic nerves (when smooth muscle responses are suppressed by the presence of postsynaptic receptor antagonists) of "purines" as modulatory cotransmitters is also sensitive to these toxins. Thus, the TTX-sensitive fraction of the "purines" released might still originate from the smooth muscle or from other than NANC nerve endings.

The third question is not yet answerable. We can however envisage an experiment where the adrenergic and cholinergic nerves are selectively made nonfunctional (e.g., with reserpine and hemicholinium) and where the TTX-sensitive release of "purines" is not or only partly affected by a selective postsynaptic inhibitor, which blocks the smooth muscle response to field stimulation.

IV. THIRD CRITERION

The action of the substance on the postsynaptic cell must be identical with that of the synaptic action, particularly when applied by micro-electrophoretic techniques.

Compared with the now twenty-five-year-old experiment of Krnjević and Miledi, which Eccles used as an illustration of this criterion, most reports concerning the purinergic hypothesis are a far cry from applying this "identity of action" criterion (Orrego, 1979) as it was intended.

There are reports concerning the electrophoretic application of purines to excitable tissues (see Phillis *et al.*, 1979) however, with regard to the NANC nerves the putative transmitters are at best added to the superfusion medium but are generally added to the organ bath, where they are subjected not only to "spontaneous" degradation but also to extracellular degradation and uptake by the tissue (McKenzie *et al.*, 1977; Huizinga *et al.*, 1981) and to electrochemical degradation if field stimulation is applied (Nakatsu and Bartlett, 1979). Needless to say, the value as an argument for or against the purinergic hypothesis of conclusions drawn from mechanical responses measured in organ bath experiments is questionable. The most convincing way to deal with this criterion would be experiments in which both binding and activation of the postsynaptic receptors by the contenders could be studied. As this type of experiment is only described in science fiction, we will have to do the next best thing.

Although all known neurotransmitters exhibit binding to postsynaptic receptors, the reverse is not true, as illustrated by competitive antagonists. Thus, binding studies yield less than half of the information sought and should be regarded with caution if they are not accompanied with substantial information concerning the activation of the receptor involved. A comparable conclusion is reached by Orrego with respect to binding studies in nervous tissue, where this type of study is far more *en vogue* than in visceral organs. Far more definitive are experiments which measure a result of receptor activation, as activation implies binding to the receptor. From receptor activation to contractile response of the muscle reflects a descending order of conclusiveness from observations made of intermediate steps. With each next step in the reaction sequence, other factors can cloud the answer sought.

A way to tackle this criterion is to solve the physiology of the NANC nerve mediated response—mechanisms of action of the endogenously released neurotransmitter—and compare it with the pharmacology of the putative transmitter—mechanism of action of the exogenously applied contender. In order to have maximal conclusiveness the first question thus becomes, "Which membrane responses mediated via NANC nerves are known and is there knowledge about the membrane response of the same preparation evoked by "purines"? Up to now all NANC nerve-mediated responses have been thought to result from modifications to ion channels and not primarily via enzymatic functions without changes of the membrane potential. Data concerning mechanical responses (relaxation, contraction, rebound, and inhibition) have to be judged as preliminary evidence, awaiting further confirmation.

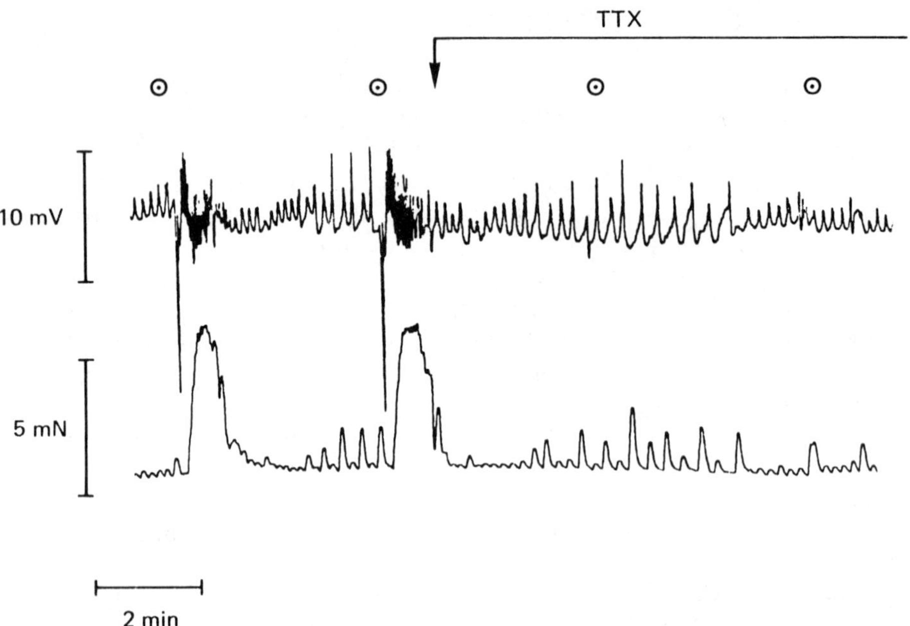

Figure 3. Sucrose-gap recording of the membrane (upper trace) and the mechanical responses of the guinea pig taenia caecum to field stimulation (⊙: 20 pps for 0.5 sec) in the presence of agents, which inhibit responses mediated by cholinergic and adrenergic nerves, before and during superfusion with TTX (3×10^{-6} *M*) at 22°C. Courtesy of A. J. J. Maas.

In retrospect, the first reports concerning responses mediated via NANC nerves originate from the end of the last century (e.g., Langley, 1898). Research concerning this response gained momentum when it was found that transmembrane potentials could also be measured in smooth muscle cells with microelectrodes (Bülbring, 1954) and that changes in membrane potential could be measured with the sucrose gap technique (Burnstock and Straub, 1958; Berger, 1963) simultaneously with changes in membrane resistance and in contractility. The new experimental techniques were first used with the guinea pig taenia caecum and most of our knowledge concerning the mechanisms underlying the NANC nerve-mediated responses applies to this preparation. With regard to other preparations supposedly having NANC nerves, the electrophysiological information is rather scanty. Therefore we have chosen to employ the guinea pig taenia caecum as a model in this discussion.

Field stimulation of the guinea pig taenia caecum induces a transient hyperpolarization of the smooth muscle cell membrane (IJP), followed by a 'rebound' or "off" depolarization accompanied by an increased spike activity (Figure 3). Depending on the tone of the preparation the mechanical response is characterized by a relaxation with a "rebound" contraction or by a "rebound" contraction only (Bennett *et al.*, 1963; 1966a,b). The response was inhibited by agents like TTX, which prevent the development of action potentials carried by sodium ions, as in

EQUILIBRIUM POTENTIAL (mV)	INTRACELLULAR CONCENTRATIONS (mM)	EXTRACELLULAR CONCENTRATIONS (mM)
+ 52 ———	Na^+: 29	Na^+: 150
0 ———		
–24 ———	Cl^-: 55	Cl^-: 143
RP – – – – –		
–89 ———	K^+: 164	K^+: 4.8

Figure 4. Generalized values for electrochemical gradients across the smooth muscle cell membrane from the mammalian intestinal tract at 37°C. RP: resting membrane potential.

nerve fibers, suggesting that a nervous structure is involved in the generation of the response (Bülbring and Tomita, 1967).

A first estimate of the process underlying the postsynaptic effects can be based on the determination of the membrane conductance during the IJP. The overall conductance (reciprocal resistance) of the smooth muscle cell membrane is a composite from the membrane permeabilities toward ions and molecules present in the system. Electrotonic potentials generated by application of constant current pulses through the membrane can be used to monitor changes in the membrane conductance. It was shown that the electronic potentials decrease during the IJP (Tomita, 1972; Den Hertog and Jager, 1975). Due to its transient nature, the duration of the IJP relative to the rise time of electronic potentials is too short, so that accurate data with respect to the change in electronic potentials cannot be obtiained. An overall change of about 50% was found, suggesting an increased membrane permeability during the response.

The next question that arises is for which ions, present in the system, is the permeability changed during the IJP. This can be studied by changing the concentration gradients of the respective ions which power movement of ions through the cell membrane (Figure 4). It has to be kept in mind, however, that not only smooth muscle cells, but also nervous structures, are influenced by changes in ion gradients. Experiments in which the IJP was evoked in the presence of reduced gradients of sodium or chloride ions, by lowering the extracellular ion concentration, showed that these ions did not contribute to the development of the hyperpolarization of the smooth muscle cell membrane (Jager, 1974; Maas, 1981). The IJP appeared to be dependent on the extracellular calcium concentration. However, transmitter release from nerve endings is assumed to be dependent on the presence of this cation in the extracellular medium. Thus, a specific postsynaptic effect due to changes in the calcium ion concentrations cannot be expected (Maas, 1980). Increasing the extracellular potassium concentration in order to decrease the potassium gradient, however, caused reduced amplitudes of the IJP (Bennett *et al.*, 1963; Tomita, 1972; Den Hertog and Jager, 1975). Furthermore, the amplitude of the IJP decreased with increasing membrane potential and a reversal potential was observed. This reversal potential of the IJP varied with the extracellular potassium concentration in a manner predicted by the Goldman equation for a selective increase in the membrane permeability for potassium (Jager, 1979).

These results imply that the substance released upon transmural stimulation from intramural nerves causes an increase in the potassium permeability of the smooth muscle cells. In view of the direction of the potassium gradient this should be accompanied by an increased efflux of potassium ions from the smooth muscle cells. Thus, direct evidence can be obtained by labeling the intracellular medium with a potassium isotope and detecting the amount of isotope leaving the tissue in the absence and in the presence of evoked IJPs. Such an experiment showed that the potassium efflux from the tissue was markedly enhanced during field stimulation (Den Hertog and Jager, 1975). Hence, electrical stimulation of non-adrenergic, noncholinergic inhibitory nerves caused the opening of receptor-operated potassium channels, followed by an enhanced potassium efflux and hyperpolarization of the smooth muscle cells of the guinea pig taenia caecum.

Another approach to studying the ionic currents underlying junction potentials is to determine the changes in currents across the cell membrane during the transient response, keeping the membrane potential constant. However, voltage clamp experiments on smooth muscle cells preparations have not yet reached the stage of accepted investigational tools. The technical difficulties and interpretative ambuigities of voltage clamp methods, as well as those of the sucrose gap method, are extensively reviewed by Coburn *et al.* (1975), Bolton (1979), and Bolton *et al.*, (1981).

Although the IJP is the first manifestation of the postsynaptic action of the NANC transmitter, the "rebound" or "off" response following it has to be taken into account. Strictly taken the adjectives "rebound" and "off" are not synonymous, although they are used here as such. "Off" response refers to the observation that the response (i.e., depolarization, enhancement of spike activity, and contraction of the smooth muscle) occurs after the cessation of (prolonged) stimulation, whereas "rebound" implies that this is due to characteristics of the smooth muscle cell membrane acting in the wake of the junction potential. Similar effects were observed on the "off" response as on the IJP by blocking the activity of NANC nerves or by changing the ion concentration gradients, as long as direct stimulation of the muscle cells had been avoided. Thus, the rebound depolarization is not carried by sodium or chloride ions but might be due to calcium ions entering the smooth muscle cells. It was reported that IJP could be evoked in the presence of low calcium concentrations in the superfusion medium, although the amplitude was somewhat reduced, but the rebound depolarization could not be detected (Maas and Den Hertog, 1980).

The release of endogenous NANC transmitter by field stimulation is rather narrowly distributed in time and space and is thus hardly mimicked by the more diffuse application of putative transmitters by superfusion with regard to the time course of the response of the smooth muscle. An alternative comparison might be obtained by releasing endogenous NANC transmitter via chemical stimulation of nerve varicosities. In this respect scorpion venom and especially 4-aminopyridine seem to be promising tools. Both these agents prolong the duration of the nerve action potential but via different mechanisms: preventing the closure of

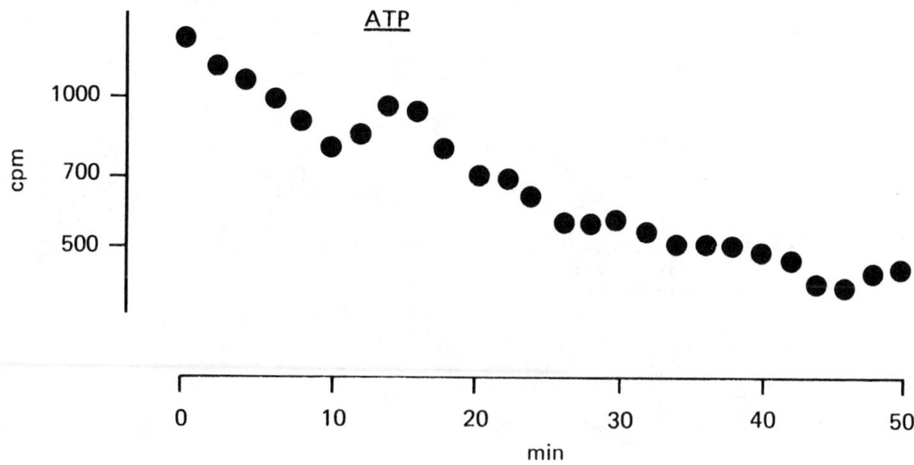

Figure 5. The increase in ^{42}K loss from taenia caecum (22°C) induced by ATP (4×10^{-4} *M*). Courtesy of J. D. Huizinga.

sodium channels opened during the upstroke of the action potential and inhibiting the potassium channels involved in the repolarization, respectively.

Application of adenosine and adenine nucleotides induces a hyperpolarization and increases the conductance of the smooth muscle cell membrane: adenine and related nucleotides were hardly effective in this respect, but the phosphorylated nucleotides, especially ATP, were effective. The different orders of potency of the "purines" have led to the development of the concept of different receptors for these compounds, namely P_1 receptors (adenosine more potent than ATP) and P_2 receptors (ATP more potent than adenosine) (Maguire and Satchell, 1981). P_1 receptors are supposedly involved in metabolic feedback functions of adenosine (e.g., release of neurotransmitter, regulation of vasotonus) and are located both pre- and postsynaptic. To date P_2 receptors have been found to be localized only postsynaptically and the responses mediated via these receptors are comparable to those evoked by stimulation of NANC nerves. Maas *et al.* (1980) reported an increased efflux of potassium ions from the guinea pig taenia caecum following application of ATP (Figure 5), but not with adenosine (unpublished observations).

The postsynaptic localized P_1 and P_2 receptors appear to activate different processes in the smooth muscle cell, as can be concluded from the following observations.

1. In calcium-free medium, ATP induces a transient hyperpolarization that cannot be repeated by a second application (Den Hertog, 1982). However, the response evoked by adenosine is sustained and can be repeated (Ferrero and Frischknecht, 1983). Thus, the P_2 receptor-mediated response involves the dislodging of calcium from a limited, membrane-bound compartment, a mechanism presumably not activated by adenosine. Apparently, two subsequent steps are involved in the ATP response, namely; calcium mobilization and opening of potassium channels.

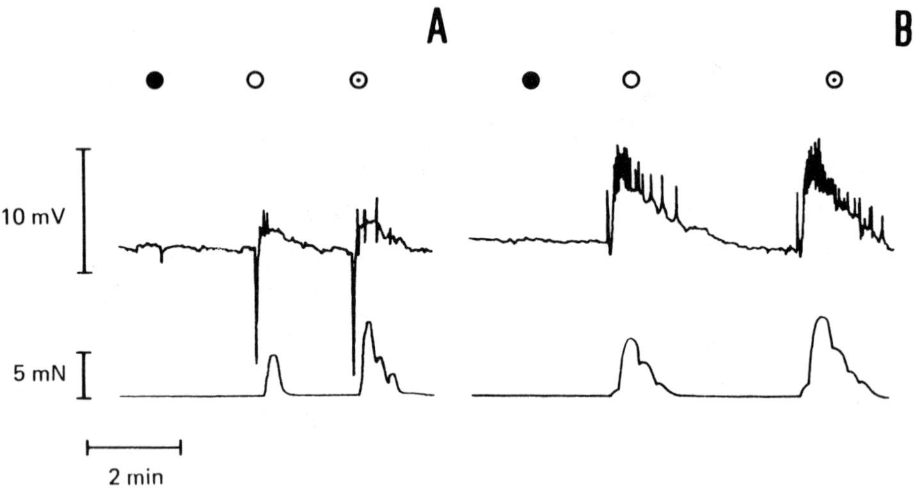

Figure 6. Sucrose-gap recording of the membrane (upper trace) and mechanical response of the taenia caecum (22°C) to field stimulation (20 pps for 0.5 sec) at increasing pulse intensities (●, ○, ⊙). A: control responses; B: same stimulations in the presence of apamin (10^{-7} *M* for 20 min). With permission from Maas, 1981.

2. The opening of these potassium channels can be prevented by apamin, which thus inhibits the hyperpolarization induced by ATP and unmasks a calcium dependent depolarization, reflecting the calcium mobilization of an earlier step. Comparable changes were observed in the response following NANC nerve stimulation (Maas, 1981) (Figure 6). The response evoked by adenosine was not affected by apamin. The calcium mobilization observed with the IJP can be regarded as a calcium influx which might at least in part be responsible for the 'off' response. A complementary and complicating possibility is the postulated existence of a second, excitatory NANC cotransmitter.

Comparison of the characteristics of the responses evoked by ATP or by NANC nerve stimulation imply that both the P_2 receptor operated by ATP and the receptor operated by the NANC neurotransmitter control the same set of calcium-dependent potassium channels within the smooth muscle cell membrane. To put this conclusion into perspective it should be noticed that the α-adrenoceptor also controls these channels (Den Hertog, 1981).

With respect to other smooth muscle preparations the above given picture becomes clouded by incomplete and/or conflicting evidence. The circular smooth muscle of the body of the opossum esophagus seems to be innervated by NANC nerves only and the characteristics of the IJP evoked by field stimulation are comparable to those observed in the taenia caecum (Daniel *et al.*, 1983). The potassium channels involved in the IJP are not, however, blocked by apamin, or by any other of the known potassium channel blockers (Jager *et al.*, 1984). Furthermore, none of the "purines" induced responses comparable to that following

NANC nerve stimulation and are thus ruled out as possible candidates for the role of NANC transmitter (Daniel *et al.*, 1983).

With regard to the off-response the differences between opossum and guinea pig are more pronounced than with the IJP. The off-response in the opossum esophagus is chloride dependent (Daniel *et al.*, 1984). With regard to the postulated excitatory cotransmitter, vasoactive intestinal polypeptide (VIP) is a possible candidate. Another complication is that a NANC transmitter might influence smooth muscle cells not only directly, but also indirectly, via the interstitial cells of Cajal (Stach, 1972; Thuneberg, 1982; Daniel and Posey-Daniel, 1984).

The electrophysiological studies of other preparations with NANC nerve-mediated inhibitory responses can be divided speculatively into three groups, although the currently available data are generally too preliminary to make a clear classification.

1. The electrophysiological data imply a postsynaptic mechanism identical to that found in the guinea pig taenia coli, namely NANC-transmitter-operated potassium channels that can be blocked by apamin. The response elicited by application of "purines" mimick that of the NANC-nerve-mediated IJP and seems to be mediated via postsynaptic P_2 receptors. The preparations within this group are all derived from the guinea pig: circular muscle strips from the fundus (Huizinga and Den Hertog, 1980), internal anal sphincter (Lim and Muir, 1984), and the ileocecal sphincter (Kubota, 1982).
2. The electrophysiological data indicate a postsynaptic action of the NANC nerve transmitter on potassium channels that are insensitive to apamin. The IJP in these preparations is not mimicked by "purines." Within this group, preparations are derived from more than one species. Besides the opossum preparation mentioned, the bovine receptor penis (Lim and Muir, 1984), the anococcygeus muscle of rat (Creed *et al.*, 1975) and rabbit (Creed and Gillespie, 1977), and the longitudinal cardiac muscle of porcine stomach (Ohga and Taneike, 1977) all seem to possess NANC nerves that are seemingly nonpurinergic.
3. The postsynaptic action of the NANC nerve transmitter induces a muscle relaxation apparently without a change in membrane potential. This response can be mimicked by ATP as observed in cat trachea (Ito and Takeda, 1982).

From the speculations summarized above, the conclusion should be drawn that the inhibitory responses mediated by NANC nerves in organs of entodermal origin by no means constitue a coherent group. Whether the responding smooth muscles have different characteristics or that the term NANC neurotransmitter signifies several different, so far unidentified substances, is as yet an unsettled question. It would be a tremendous improvement in our understanding of these nerves if electrophysiological data were available for all smooth muscles with mechanical responses attributed to NANC nerves.

V. FOURTH CRITERION

There should be an inactivating enzyme system in the region of the synaptic cleft.

This is another criterion that, due to the fact that adenosine and adenine nucleotides are involved in other processes in living cells, can hardly be used to test the "purinergic" nerve hypothesis. The inactivation system for the released NANC transmitter according to the purinergic nerve hypothesis was readily composed from known enzyme systems (Burnstock, 1972). The energy-rich phosphorylated purines are rapidly hydrolyzed extracellularly into adenosine, which is actively taken up by cells (Pearson *et al.*, 1978) or deaminated into inosine, which is devoid of NANC-transmitter-like activities.

Early attempts to test this part of the purinergic nerve hypothesis by interference with the inactivation system in guinea pig taenia caecum were inconclusive. Inhibition of the uptake of adenosine by dipyridamole enhanced the relaxation induced by both exogenously applied ATP and stimulation of the NANC nerves (Satchell *et al.*, 1972), but the hyperpolarization of the smooth muscle cells preceeding the mechanical response was unchanged (Jager, 1976). The potentiation of the relaxant response by dipyridamole might be due to an adenosine-independent action (Klabunde, 1983). The usefulness of adenosine-uptake inhibitors is seriously limited by the variety of adenosine sources present in most preparations. How can one discriminate between adenosine released from nerves as a "modulatory cotransmitter" and adenosine generated as an intermediate during inactivation of the NANC transmitter?

During the past decade this criterion has been used with a peculiar one-sidedness. The system via which the endogenously released NANC transmitter is inactivated is taken for granted. Only for the putative neurotransmitter has the presence of an efficient inactivating system been investigated. Evidence for the existence of an inactivating enzyme system with respect to ATP was obtained by comparing the action of slowly degradable analogs (Maguire and Satchell, 1979) in guinea pig taenia caecum. Comparable enzyme systems seem to be present in other smooth muscle preparations with NANC nerves (Kasakov and Burnstock, 1982; Meldrum and Burnstock, 1983). It is notable that most research is centered on adenosine (using nondegradable phosphorylated analogs, uptake inhibitors, deaminaze inhibitors) and that the results concerning the "purinergic nerve transmitter inactivation system" are significant for our understanding of the modulatory functions of adenosine.

VI. FIFTH CRITERION

When the action of drugs is tested by microelectrophoretic injection, the pharmacology of the synaptic transmission and of the postsynaptic transmission and of the postsynaptic action of the substance must be similar.

This criterion implies the detailed knowledge of the physiology of synaptic transmission, as given in the four preceding criteria and the pharmacological manipulation of the processes involved. With regard to the first criteria "presence in presynaptic terminal" and "release nervous stimulation," some agents, such as TTX and scorpion venom, have been already mentioned as "physiological tools." A more specific interference with the purines in nerve endings is barred by the pivotal role they play in virtually all functions of living cells. Hence, attempts to introduce adenosine analogs that might generate intracellularly "false transmitters" have not been reported. The involvement of adenosine or P_1 receptors in the regulation of transmitter release from adrenergic, cholinergic, and NANC nerves (Su, 1983; Ginsborg and Hirst, 1972; Daniel *et al.*, 1983) has already been mentioned. Pharmacological interference with this feedback mechanism will probably not yield data pertinent to the central question: are "purines" acting as transmitters of information to postsynaptic sites?

Pharmacological interference with postsynaptic receptors will be discussed in two parts, namely agonists that activate the receptors and antagonists that prevent this activation.

As pointed out in the discussion regarding the "identity of action" criterion, ATP is the most obvious candidate of the "purines" to fulfill the role of NANC transmitter in guinea pig taenia caecum. The concentrations of ATP (10^4–10^3 M) which have to be used to generate responses of a size comparable with the IJP are still a matter of debate (Tomita and Watanabe, 1973; Jager and Schevers, 1980). Desensitization experiments with ATP have been reported from several preparations (e.g. Weston 1973a,b; Ohga and Taneike, 1977; Baer and Frew, 1979), but not from guinea pig taenia caecum. All these observations were based on mechanical responses and were hampered by the metabolic degradation of ATP (Frew and Lundy, 1982). A more promising approach might be the use of a metabolicaly stable ATP analog, such as αβ-methylene ATP, as used in the vas deferens (Meldrum and Burnstock, 1983) and bladder (Kasakov and Burnstock 1982), where both the NANC neurotransmitter and ATP cause contractions. The question remains whether the hyperpolarizing membrane response to ATP in other preparations as well as the IJP can be suppressed by desensitization of P_2 receptors.

A variety of drugs have been put forward as selective antagonists for the P_2 receptor but were subsequently found to be functional antagonists, acting at steps following receptor activation, e.g., apamin. Recently, two compounds have been reported to meet the requirements of selective receptor antagonists, namely arylazido-aminopropionyl ATP (Fedan *et al.*, 1982) and oxyhaemoglobin (Bowman *et al.*, 1982). The photoaffinity antagonist arylazido-aminopropionyl ATP seems to complement the photoaffinity agonists (2-azido analog of the purines; Cusack and Planker, 1979), but both these groups of substances have been studied in different organs and so far only mechanical responses have been used as a measure of drug action. With regard to oxyhaemoglobin, electrophysiological studies are beginning to appear (Lim and Muir, 1984) in a follow-up to the mechanical studies (Bowman and Gillespie, 1982). In so far as conclusions are permissible at this point in time, it seems that in those preparations in which the IJP cannot be inhibited by the potassium-channel blocker apamin (see criterion 3), oxyhaemoglobin is an effective antagonist, whereas it seems not to antagonize NANC nerve-mediated relaxations in preparations like the guinea pig taenia coli. No evidence has been presented so far to determine the nature of this antagonism: a physiological antagonist like apamin or a competitive antagonist at the postsynaptic NANC nerve receptor.

The lack of a powerful tool as a competitive, selective antagonist is probably the reason why so much effort has been directed to pharmacological manipulation of the inactivation of the NANC transmitter. The rationale for the use of drugs such as dipyridamole and hexobendine (Satchell *et al.*, 1972) is twofold; by way of product inhibition in the degradation processes, a measurable increase in NANC transmitter or exogenously applied ATP at the receptor site might be achieved, and a selective interference with the uptake mechanism of adenosine might produce evidence that NANC transmitter is a "purine." The potentiation of the mechanical responses mediated by the NANC transmitter and ATP was subsequently found not to be present at the level of membrane responses and might be due to a nonspecific inhibitory action of dipyridamole on the smooth muscle (Jager, 1976). The involvement of adenosine in the feedback regulation of transmitter release seriously complicates the interpretation of these experiments. Discrimination between adenosine released as a modulating cotransmitter and adenosine originating from NANC transmitter metabolism is not feasible.

In overview, the pharmacology of NANC synaptic transmission is rather limited. Paramount is the lack of an established competitive and selective receptor antagonist. While the reports concerning antagonists of NANC nerve-mediated contractions are promising, they need further corroboration with electrophysiological measurements. It is possible that the competition reported so far does not apply to inhibitory responses. Assuming one type of postsynaptic NANC receptor, interference with drugs should lead to qualitative similar changes in NANC-nerve mediated responses, irrespective of the transduction mechanism (relaxation or contraction) following receptor activation.

VII. CONCLUSIONS

At the end of this rather limited exercise using Eccles's yardsticks in the domain of the purinergic nerve hypothesis, comments can be made regarding both the measures and their subject.

Within the set of criteria formulated by Eccles, that of identical actions of endogenous and putative transmitters and that of pharmacological identity seem to be the cornerstones for an evaluation. Gaddum refered to pharmacology as a jack of all trades, and along the same lines Werman (1966) rearranged pharmacology into the seven criteria linked to the physiology of synaptic transmission that he discerned. In this chapter we have followed the same line, but, although Werman formulated an eighth criterion concerning postsynaptic pharmacology and subsequently included that in the identity of action criterion, we chose to narrow further the definition of a separate pharmacology criterion. Postsynaptic pharmacology beyond the receptor produces insight into the mode of action of the neurotransmitter and the physiology of the effector organ and should thus be included in the identical actions criterion. Interactions, especially competitive, at the postsynaptic receptor between endogenous neurotransmitter, putative agonists, and antagonists provide a separate and indispensable measure for the evaluation of any -ergic nerve hypothesis.

Concerning the purinergic nerve hypothesis, one of its most enticing elements is at least questionable. Described in sweeping vistas (e.g., Burnstock, 1972) is the suggestion that the "purinergic" nerves are evolutionary old nerves and that throughout the vertebrate realm they are essential similar. The possibility that NANC nerves are old cannot be discarded, but essentially similarity does not imply the same neurotransmitter. In some preparations, all available data are explainable if the NANC nerves are purinergic nerves, e.g., guinea pig taenia caecum. In other preparations, the available data exclude the possibility that the NANC nerves are purinergic nerves, e.g., opossum esophageal circular muscle.

In this chapter, preparations in which NANC nerves mediate excitatory responses in smooth muscle have hardly been mentioned in order to keep the subject manageable. The sparsely available information seems to indicate, however, that some excitatory NANC nerves might also be "purinergic", e.g., detrusor muscle from guinea pig urinary bladder (Sjögren and Andersson, 1979a,b; Muir and Smart, 1983).

In view of the criteria set, unambiguous proof for the purinergic hypothesis is lacking, whereas serious arguments against can be raised. Nevertheless, it is tempting to speculate that the intramural NANC nerves are evolutionary old nerves, which along some developmental lines obtained phosphorylated purines (ATP) as neurotransmitter, while some lines only have them as cotransmitter (Fedan *et al.*, 1981) and other lines developed other substances, such as vasoactive intestinal polypeptide (VIP), as transmitter. As far as our current knowledge is concerned, the only common traits of all NANC nerves reported is that they are intramural and that the nonphosphorylated "purines" (adenosine) are cotransmitters acting presynaptically as release modulators.

As long as so many facets of NANC nervous control of smooth muscle function have not been studied, the current state of affairs renders it counterproductive to hypothesize that all NANC nerves are "purinergic" or "peptidergic" (Hakanson *et al.*, 1981) or anything else. There are always preparations to be found in which a NANC-nerve-mediated response can be measured in such a way that it seems to favor a petyergic nerve hypothesis. Detailed and verified information is available from only one preparation; the taenia, and that has yielded inconclusive evidence concerning the purinergic hypothesis for these NANC nerves. An assessment of the purinergic hypothesis will be possible when comparable amounts of information are available from other preparations and from other species and other classes in the chordate phylum and when a proven competitive P_2-purinoceptor antagonist can be employed. Till then, the purinergic nerve hypothesis will continue to function as a challenging starting point to enlarge the physiology of the intramural, nonadrenergic, noncholinergic neural control of smooth muscles.

Table I. List of Descriptors and Conditions Used in the Literature Search[a]

Masterset I:	Smooth (w) muscle? *or* taenia (w) coil *or* caecum *or* caeci *or* vas (w) deferens *or* trachealis *or* detrusor *or* anococcygeus *or* retractor *or* intestinal (w) muscle?
Subset I:	Masterset I *and* nerve?
Workset I:	Subset I *and* membrane?
Workset I A:	Masterset I *and* membrane?
Workset II:	Masterset I *and* dipyridamole?
Workset III:	Subset I *and* (methylxanthine? *or* aminophyllin? *or* theophyllin? or caffein?)
Workset IV:	Subset I *and* quini?
Workset V:	Subset I *and* [apamin? *or* bee (w) venom]
Workset VI:	Subset I *and* (imidazolin? *or* phentolamin?)
Workset VII:	Subset I *and* pyridylisatogen
Workset VIII:	Subset I *and* (temperature? *or* tetrodotoxin? *or* ttx? *or* scorpion (w) venom *or* calcium)
Workset IX:	Workset VIII *and* (purinerg? *or* nanc? *or* nai?)
Masterset II:	Nerv?/DE, TI *and* (terminal?/DE, TI *or* releas?/DE, TI *or* varicosit?/DE, TI *or* synap?/DE, TI)
Workset X:	Masterset II *and* (ATP/DE, TI *or* purine?/DE, TI *or* adenosin?/DE, TI *or* ADP/DE, TI *or* AMP/DE, TI *or* adenin?/DE, TI)
Workset XI:	Workset X *not* [brain? *or* central (w) nerv?]

[a] Dialogue files 152, 153, and 154 (Medline U.S. Nat. Libr. Med. 1966–72, 1972–79, and 1979-present, respectively) and 77 (Conference Papers).

VIII. LITERATURE SEARCH

Initially we tried to compile a set of references that among many others would contain all papers published that might be of pertinence for this study. To our knowledge the "purinergic" nerve hypothesis is only implied in visceral organs and thus the entry "smooth muscle" should generate our base. Surprisingly, we found that it did not contain some papers that we were certain ought to be included. Subsequently we found that naming individual smooth muscles increased our master set. In hindsight we could have included smooth muscles other than those mentioned, such as the nictitating membrane.

To generate a set of the most pertinent or least ambiguous papers concerning the postsynaptic actions of endogenous released neurotransmitters we employed the descriptors: nerve and membrane. Because the NANC-nerve-mediated response is known under different full names and abbrevations, Table I shows the sets of literature data that were used and how they were generated.

A separate set of literature references was made in order to gain insight about the literature concerning the reported involvement of "purines" in neurohumoral transmission. As this proved to be an unmanegeable amount of data, which included references concerning the involvement of "purines" in metabolic processes, the selection was restricted to the title (TI) and descriptors (DE) mentioned in the files, thus excluding abstracts.

The main problem encountered during our search was traceble to the fact that the "purinergic" nerves are still largely defined by what they are not, e.g., nonadrenergic, noncholinergic, or do not have, e.g., large granular vesicles. Thus

Table II. Yield of the Literature Search with the Descriptors and Conditions Given in Table I

	File 154		File 153		File 152		File 77	
	Hits (n)	Precision (%)	Hits (n)	Precision (%)	Hits (n)	Precision (%)	Hits (n)	Precision (%)
I	106	22	98	12	28	25	0	—
IA	—		—		—		60	9
II	21	24	33	43	1	0	—	
III	15	60	10	30	42	17	—	
IV	6	100	2	100	0	—	—	
V	10	100	1	100	0	—	—	
VI	54	22	77	16	13	23	—	
VII	2	100	—		—		—	
VIII	102	—	76	—	19	16	—	
IX	4	100	3	100	0	—		
X	129	28	234	—	74	14	—	
XI	—		132	28	—		—	

the work sets generated still contained quite a lot of "garbage" that had to be weeded out by hand on the prints (Table II). Because there is still considerable debate as to whether "purinergic" nerves have a characteristic nerve profile in electronmicroscopic view and what that might be, we have refrained from a search in that area. With "key articles" this search might have been fruitful in the (more expensive) SCI search files.

ACKNOWLEDGMENTS

The assistance of Drs. P. W. van Olm and P. Tieleman (University of Amsterdam) in the literature search is gratefully acknowledged. We wish to thank Mrs. M. Schipper and Mrs. J. L. v.d. Valk for their assistance in the preparation of the manuscript and Mr. J. Pleiter and Mr. F. Propsma for the illustrations.

REFERENCES

Baer, H. P., and Frew, R. 1979. Relaxation of guinea-pig fundic strip by adenosine, adenosine, adenosine triphosphate and electrical stimulation: Lack of antagonism by theophylline or ATP treatment. *Br. J. Pharmacol., 67*:293–299.

Bennett, M. R., Burnstock, G., and Holman, M. E. 1963. The effect of potassium and chloride ions on the inhibitory potential recorded in the guinea-pig tanea coli. *J. Physiol., 164*:33p–34p.

Bennett, M. R., Burnstock, G., and Holman, M. E. 1966a. Transmission from perivascular inhibitory nerves to the smooth muscle of the guinea-pig taenia coli. *J. Physiol., 182*:527–540.

Bennett, M. R., Burnstock, G., and Holman, M. E. 1966b. Transmission from intramural inhibitory nerves to the smooth muscle of the guinea-pig taenia coli. *J. Physiol., 182*:541–558.

Berger, W. 1963. Die Doppelsaccharosetrennwandtechnik; Eine Methode zur Untersuchung des Membranpotentials und der Membraneigenschaften glatter Muskelzellen. *Pflügers Arch., 277*:570–576.

Blaustein, M. P., and Goldring, J. M. 1975. Effects of potassium veratridine and Scorpion Venom on calcium accumulation and transmitter release by nerve terminals in vitro. *J. Physiol., 247:*617–655.

Bloom, F. E., Hoffer, B. J., Battenberg, E. R., Siggins, G. R., Steiner, A. L., Parker, C. W., and Wedner, H. J. 1972. Adenosine 3′,5′-monophosphate is localized in cerebellar neurons: Immunofluorescence evidence. *Science, 177:*436–438.

Bolton, T. B. 1979. Mechanisms of action of transmitters and other substances on smooth muscle. *Physiol. Rev., 59:*606–718.

Bolton, T. B., Tomita, T., and Vassort, G. 1981. Voltage clamp and the measurement of ionic conductances in smooth muscle. In: *Smooth Muscle,* pp. 47–63. Ed. by Bülbring, E., Brading, A. F., Jones, A. W., and Tomita, T. Edward Arnold, London.

Bowman, A., and Gillespie, J. S. 1982. Block of some non-adrenergic inhibitory responses of smooth muscle by a substance from haemolysed erythrocytes. *J. Physiol., 328:*12–25.

Bowman, A., Gillespie, J. S., and Pollock, D. 1982. Oxyhaemoglobin blocks nonadrenergic non-cholinergic inhibition in the bovine retractor penis muscle. *Eur. J. Pharmacol., 85:*221–224.

Bülbring, E. 1954. Membrane potentials of smooth muscle fibres of the taenia coli of the guinea-pig. *J. Physiol., 125:*302–315.

Bülbring, E., and Tomita, T. 1967. Properties of the inhibitory potential of smooth muscle as observed in the response to field stimulation of the guinea-pig taenia coli. *J. Physiol., 189:*299–315.

Burnstock, G. 1969. Evolution of the autonomic innervation of visceral and cardiovascular systems in vertebrates. *Pharmacol. Rev., 21:*247–324.

Burnstock, G. 1972. Purinergic nerves. *Pharmacol. Rev., 24:*509–581.

Burnstock, G. 1979. Past and current evidence for the purinergic nerve hypothesis, in: *Physiological and Regulatory Functions of Adenosine and Adenine Nucleotides,* pp. 3–32. Ed. by Baer, H. P., and Drummond, G. J. Raven Press, New York.

Burnstock, G. 1981. An introduction to purinergic receptors. In: *Purinergic Receptors*, pp. 1–45. Ed. by Burnstock, G. Chapman and Hall, London.

Burnstock, G., and Straub, R. W. 1958. A method for studying the effects of ions and drugs on the resting and action potentials in smooth muscle with external electrodes. *J. Physiol., 140:*156–167.

Burnstock, G., Cocks, T., Kasakov, L., and Wong, H. K. 1978. Direct evidence for ATP release from non-adrenergic, non-cholinergic ('purinergic') nerves in the guinea-pig taenia coli and bladder. *Eur. J. Pharmacol., 49:*145–149.

Coburn, R. F., Ohba, M., and Tomita, T. 1975. Recording of intracellular electrical activity with the sucrose-gap method. In: *Methods in Pharmacology*, volume 3, pp. 231–245. Ed. By Daniel, E. E., and Paton, D. M. Plenum Press, New York.

Creed, K. E., and Gillespie, J. S. 1977. Some electrical properties of the rabbit anococcygeus muscle and a comparison of the effects of inhibitory nerve stimulation in the rat and rabbit. *J. Physiol., 273:*137–153.

Creed, K. E., Gillespie, J. S., and Muir, T. C. 1975. The electrical basis of excitation and inhibition in the rat anococcygeus muscle. *J. Physiol., 245:*33–47.

Cusack, N. J., and Planker, M. 1979. Relaxation of isolated taenia coli of guinea-pig by enantiomers of 2-azido analogues of adenosine and adenine nucleotides. *Br. J. Pharmacol., 67:*153–158.

Daniel, E. E., and Posey-Daniel, V. 1984. The structural comparison of esophageal lower sphincter (LES) and body circular muscle (BCM) from opossum. Role of interstitial cells of Cajal. *Am. J. Physiol., 246:*G305–G315.

Daniel, E. E., Taylor, G. S., Daniel, V. P., and Holman, M. E. 1977. Can non-adrenergic inhibitory varicosities be identified structurally? *Can. J. Physiol. Pharmacol., 55:*243–250.

Daniel, E. E., Helmy-Elkholy, A., Jager, L. P., and Kannan, M. S. 1983. Neither a purine nor VIP is the mediator of inhibitory nerves of opossum oesophageal smooth muscle. *J. Physiol., 336:*243–260.

Daniel, E. E., Jager, L. P., Jury, J., Helmy-Elkholy, A., Kannan, M. S., Posey-Daniel, V. 1984. The mediators and mechanisms causing the non-adrenergic, non-cholinergic nerve responses in opossum esophagus. Role of interstitial cells of Cajal. *Biomed. Res.,* in press.

Den Hertog, A. 1981. Calcium and the α-action of catecholamines on guinea-pig taenia caeci. *J. Physiol., 316:*109–125.

Den Hertog, A. 1982. Calcium and the action of adrenaline, adenosine triphosphate and carbachol on guinea-pig taenia caeci. *J. Physiol., 423:*423–439.

Den Hertog, A., and Jager, L. P. 1975. Ion fluxes during the inhibitory junction potential in the guinea-pig taenia coli. *J. Physiol., 250:*681–691.

Downes, H., and Taylor, S. M. 1983. Distinctive pharmacological profile of a nonadrenergic inhibitory system in bullfrog lung. *Br. J. Pharmacol., 78:*339–351.

Eccles, J. C. 1964. *The Physiology of Synapses.* Springer Verlag, Berlin.

Fedan, J. S., Hogaboom, G. K., O'Donnell, J. P., Colby, J., and Westfall, D. P. 1981. Contribution by purines to the neurogenic response of the vas deferens of the guinea pig. *Europ. J. Pharmacol., 69:*41–53.

Fedan, J. S., Hogaboom, G. K., Westfall, D. P., and O'Donnell, J. P. 1982. Comparison of the effects of arylazido aminopropionyl ATP ($ANAPP_3$), an ATP antagonist, on responses of the smooth muscle of the guinea-pig vas deferens to ATP and related nucleotides. *Eur. J. Pharmacol., 85:*277–290.

Ferrero, J. D., and Frischknecht, R. 1983. Different effector mechanisms for ATP and adenosine hyperpolarization in guinea-pig taenia coli. *Eur. J. Pharmacol., 87:*151–154.

Frew, R., and Lundy, P. M. 1982. Evidence against ATP being the nonadrenergic, noncholinergic inhibitory transmitter in guinea pig stomach. *Eur. J. Pharmacol., 81:*333–336.

Gibbins, I. L. 1982. Lack of correlation between ultrastructural and pharmacological types of non-adrenergic autonomic nerves. *Cell Tissue Res., 221:*551–581.

Ginsborg, B. L., and Hirst, G. D. S. 1972. The effect of adenosine on the release of the transmitter from the phrenic nerve of the rat. *J. Physiol., 224:*629–645.

Hakanson, R., Leander, S., Sundler, F., and Uddman, R. 1981. P-type nerves: purinergic or peptidergic? In: *Cellular Basis of Chemical Messengers in the Digestive System*, pp. 169–200. (UCLA Forum Med. Sc., *23*), Academic Press, London.

Huizinga, J. D. 1981. *Intestinal motility; regulatory function of adenosine and adenosine triphosphate.* Thesis, State University, Groningen, the Netherlands.

Huizinga, J. D., and Den Hertog, A. 1980. Inhibition of fundic strips from guinea-pig stomach: the effect of theophylline on responses to adenosine, ATP and intramural nerve stimulation. *Eur. J. Pharmacol., 63:*259–265.

Huizinga, J. D., Pielkenrood, J. M., and Den Hertog, A. 1981. Dual action of high energy adenine nucleotides in comparison with responses evoked by other adenine derivatives and intramural nerve stimulation on smooth muscle. *Eur. J. Pharmacol., 74:*175–180.

Ito, Y., and Takeda, K. 1982. Non-adrenergic inhibitory nerves and putative transmitters in the smooth muscle of cat trachea. *J. Physiol., 330:*497–511.

Jager, L. P. 1974. The effect of catecholamines and ATP on the smooth muscle cell membrane of the guinea-pig taenia coli. *Eur. J. Pharmacol., 25:*372–382.

Jager, L. P. 1976. Effects of dipyridamole on the smooth muscle cells of the guinea-pig's taenia coli. *Arch. Int. Pharmacodyn. Therap., 221:*40–53.

Jager, L. P. 1979. Effects of purinergic compounds on excitable membranes. in: *Physiological and Regulatory Functions of Adenosine and Adenine Nucleotides*, pp. 369–376. Ed. by Baer, H. P., and Drummond, G. I. Raven Press, New York.

Jager, L. P., and Schevers, J. A. M. 1980. A comparison of effects evoked in guinea-pig taenia caecum by purine nucleotides and by "purinergic" nerve stimulation. *J. Physiol., 299:*75–83.

Jager, L. P., Jury, J., and Daniel, E. E. 1984. Electrophysiological and pharmacological characterization of the NANC-nerve mediated inhibition of the circular muscle layer of the opossum esophagus. In: *Gastrointestinal motility*, pp. 9–16. Ed. by Roman, Cl. MTP, Lancaster.

Kao, C. Y. 1966. Tetrodotoxin, saxitoxin and their significance in the study of excitation phenomena. *Pharmacol. Rev., 18:*997–1049.

Kasakov, L., and Burnstock, G. 1982. The use of the slowly degradable analog, α-β methylene ATP, to produce desensitisation of the P_2-purinoceptor: Effect on non-adrenergic, non-cholinergic responses of the guinea-pig urinary bladder. *Eur. J. Pharmacol., 86:*291–295.

Klabunde, R. E. 1983. Effects of dipyridamole on postischemic vasodilation and extracellular adenosine. *Am. J. Physiol., 244:*H273–H280.

Kubota, M. 1982. Electrical and mechanical properties and neuro-effector transmission in the smooth muscle layer of the guinea-pig ileocecal junction. *Pflügers Arch., 394:*355–361.

Langley, J. N. 1898. On inhibitory fibres in the vagus for the end of the oesophagus and the stomach. *J. Physiol., 23:*407–414.

Lim, S. P., and Muir, T. C. 1984. The electrical basis for the inhibitory response of the guinea pig internal anal sphincter to nerve stimulation and drugs. In: *Gastrointestinal Motility*, pp. 413–420. Ed. by Roman, Cl. MTP Lancaster.

Loewi, O. 1921. Über humorale Übertragbarkeit der Herznervenwirkung, I, Mitteilung. *Pfügers Arch., 189:*239–242.

Maas, A. J. J. 1980. *Inhibition and post inhibitory excitation in guinea-pig taenia caeci.* Thesis, State University, Groningen, the Netherlands.

Maas, A. J. J. 1981. The effect of apamin in responses evoked by field stimulation in guinea-pig taenia caeci. *Eur. J. Pharmacol., 73:*1–19.

Maas, A. J. J., and Den Hertog, A. 1980. The effect of the phenyl phosphonate N-0164 on prostaglandin action and on post inhibitory excitation in the taenia of guinea-pig caecum. *Eur. J. Pharmacol., 62:*157–166.

Maas, A. J. J., Den Hertog, A., Ras, R., and Van der Akker, J. 1980. The action of apamin on guinea-pig taenia caeci. *Eur. J. Pharmacol., 67:*265–274.

Maguire, M. H., and Satchell, D. G. 1979. The contribution of adenosine to the inhibitory actions of adenine nucleotides on the guinea-pig taenia coli: Studies with phosphate-modified adenine nucleotide analogs and dipyridamole. *J. Pharmacol. Exp. Therap, 211:*626–631.

Maguire, M. H., and Satchell, D. G. 1981. Purinergic receptors in visceral smooth muscle. In: *Purinergic Receptors,* pp. 47–92 Ed. by Burnstock, G. Chapman and Hall, London.

McKenzie, S. G., Frew, R., and Bär, H. P. 1977. Effects of adenosine and related compounds on adenylate cyclase and cyclic AMP levels in smooth muscle. *Eur. J. Pharmacol., 41:*193–203.

Meldrum, L. A., and Burnstock, G. 1983. Evidence that ATP acts as a cotransmitter with nonadrenaline in sympathetic nerve supplying the guinea-pig vas deferens. *Eur. J. Pharmacol., 92:*161–165.

Muir, T. C., and Smart, N. G. 1983. The effect of clonidine on the response to stimulation of non-adrenergic non-cholinergic nerves in the guinea-pig urinary bladder in-vitro. *J. Pharm. Pharmacol., 35:*234–237.

Nakatsu, K., and Bartlett, V. 1979. Multiple adenine derivative receptors in rat ileum and electrical degradation of purine drugs. In: *Physiological and Regulatory Functions of Adenosine and Adenine Nucleotides*, pp. 79–84. Ed. by Baer, H. P., and Drummond, G. I. Raven Press, New York.

Ohga, A., and Taneike, T. 1977. Dissimilarity between the responses to adenosine triphosphate or its related compounds and non-adrenergic inhibitory nerve stimulation in the longitudinal smooth muscle of pig stomach. *Br. J. Pharmacol., 60:*221–231.

Orrego, F. 1979. Criteria for the identification of central neurotransmitters, and their application to studies with some nerve tissue preparations *in vitro. Neuroscience, 4:*1037–1057.

Pearson, J. D., Carleton, J. S., Hutchings, A., and Gordon, J. L. 1978. Uptake and metabolism of adenosine by pig aortic endothelial and smooth muscle cells in culture. *Biochem. J., 170:*265–271.

Phillis, J. W., Edstrom, J. P., Kostopoulos, G. K., and Kirkpatrick, J. R. 1979. Effects of adenosine and adenine nucleotides on synaptic transmission in the cerebral cortex. *Can. J. Physiol. Pharmacol., 57:*1289–1312.

Robinson, P. M., McLean, J. R., and Burnstock, G. 1971. Ultrastructural identification of non-adrenergic inhibitory nerve fibres. *J. Pharmacol. Exp. Therap., 179:*149–160.

Satchell, D. G., Lynch, A., Bourke, P. M., and Burnstock, G. 1972. Potentiation of the effects of exogenously applied ATP and purinergic nerve stimulation on the guinea-pig taenia coli by dipyridamole and hexobendine. *Eur. J. Pharmacol., 19:*343–350.

Sjögren, C., and Andersson, K. E. 1979a. Inhibition of ATP-induced contraction in the guinea-pig urinary bladder *in vitro* and *in vivo. Acta Pharmacol. Toxicol., 44:*221–227.

Sjögren, C., and Andersson, K. E. 1979b. Effects of cholinoceptor blocking drugs, adrenoceptor stimulants, and calcium antagonists on the transmurally stimulated guinea-pig urinary bladder *in vitro* and *in vivo. Acta Pharmacol. Toxicol., 44:*228–234.

Stach, W., 1972, Der Plexus entericus extremus des Dickdarmes und seine Beziehungen zu den interstitiellen Zellen (Cajal). *Z. Mikrosk. Anatl. Forsch., 82:*245–272.

Su, C. 1983. Purinergic neurotransmission and neuromodulation. *Ann. Rev. Pharmacol. Toxicol., 23:*397–411.

Thuneberg, L. 1982. Interstitial cells of Cajal: Intestinal pacemaker cells? *Adv. Anat. Embryol. Cell Biol., 71:*1–130.

Tomita, T. 1972. Conductance change during the inhibition potential in the guinea-pig taenia coli. *J. Physiol., 225:*693–703.

Tomita, T., and Watanabe, H. 1973. A comparison of the effects of adenosine triphosphate with noradrenaline and with the inhibitory potential of the guinea-pig taenia coli. *J. Physiol., 231:*167–177.

Werman, R. 1966. Criteria for identification of a central nervous system transmitter. *Comp. Biochem. Physiol., 18:*745–766.

Weston, A. H. 1973a. The effect of desensitization to adenosine triphosphate on the peristaltic reflex in guinea-pig ileum. *Br. J. Pharmacol., 47:*606–608.

Weston, A. H. 1973b. Nerve-mediated inhibition of mechanical activity in rabbit duodenum and the effects of desensitization to adenosine and several of its derivatives. *Br. J. Pharmacol., 48:*302–308.

Index